Introduction to Auditory Rehabilitation

A Contemporary Issues Approach

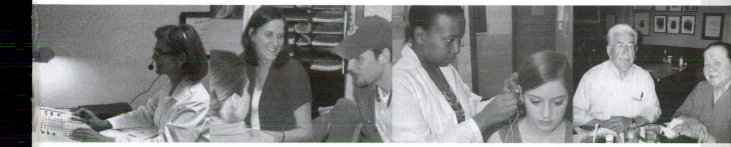

Carole E. Johnson
Auburn University

D0166083

Boston Columbus Indianapolis New York San Francisco Upper Saddle River
Amsterdam Cape Town Dubai London Madrid Milan Munich Paris Montreal Toronto
Delhi Mexico City São Paulo Sydney Hong Kong Seoul Singapore Taipei Tokyo

Vice President and Editorial Director: Jeffery W. Johnston
Executive Editor and Publisher: Stephen D. Dragin
Editorial Assistant: Jamie Bushell
Vice President, Director of Marketing: Margaret Waples
Marketing Manager: Weslie Sellinger
Senior Managing Editor: Pamela D. Bennett
Senior Project Manager: Linda Hillis Bayma
Senior Operations Supervisor: Matthew Ottenweller
Senior Art Director: Diane C. Lorenzo

Cover Designer: Diane C. Lorenzo
Cover Image: Shutterstock
Media Project Manager: Rebecca Norsic
Full-Service Project Management: Mary Tindle, S4Carlisle Publishing Services
Composition: S4Carlisle Publishing Services
Printer/Binder: R.R. Donnelley & Sons Company
Cover Printer: R.R. Donnelley & Sons Company
Text Font: Times LT Std

Additional Photo Credits: Bettie Borton, pp. i (left), 1, 432; Carole Johnson, pp. i (2nd from left & right), 27, 86, 107, 160, 229, 245, 394, 444, 473, 478; Picture provided courtesy of Cochlear™ Americas, © 2005, Cochlear Americas, pp. 52, 264, 307; Amy Bradley, pp. i (2nd from right), 153, 158, 159 (top), 161, 162 (bottom), 163 (bottom), 164 (top), 174, 176 (both), 177, 204, 205 (both), 230, 236 (both), 237 (all), 239 (both), 240 (both), 241, 248, 333, 395 (both), 467 (all), 471; Ronnie Ranew, p. 364. All other photos are credited on the text pages on which they appear.

Library of Congress Cataloging-in-Publication Data
Johnson, Carole E.
  Introduction to auditory rehabilitation : a contemporary issues approach / Carole E. Johnson, Auburn University.
    p. ; cm.
  Includes bibliographical references.
  ISBN-13: 978-0-205-42417-7
  ISBN-10: 0-205-42417-1
  1. Hearing impaired—Rehabilitation.   I. Title.
  [DNLM: 1. Rehabilitation of Hearing Impaired. WV 270]
  RF297.J64 2012
  362.4'20832—dc22

                                                             2010048785

10 9 8 7 6 5 4 3 2 1

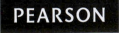

ISBN-13: 978-0-205-42417-7
ISBN-10:   0-205-42417-1

To my parents, Irma and Arthur Johnson;
my best friend, Ronnie Ranew;
my colleague and mentor, Dr. Jeffrey L. Danhauer;
and all of my students at Auburn University.

Preface

In writing an *Introduction to Auditory Rehabilitation: A Contemporary Issues Approach,* the following questions were considered: What do students need to know in preparation for serving patients with hearing impairment and their families? How have changes in healthcare, professional issues in audiology, and speech-language pathology, demographic trends in patient populations, and advancements in technology impacted how auditory rehabilitation is defined and practiced? What are the best ways to engage students in the learning process? The major aim of this textbook is to provide a requisite foundation for auditory rehabilitation service provision to diverse patient populations across the life span and in the real world. Critical knowledge and skills are presented within the context of contemporary issues integrating patient, professional, and treatment perspectives. *Zeitgeist* is a German term meaning the "sign of the times"—the accessibility to hearing healthcare is certainly an example of what is happening in the real world.

Organization of This Text

The first section of the textbook provides an introduction to auditory rehabilitation, psychosocial aspects of hearing impairment and counseling, and in-depth discussion of multicultural and professional issues. A full chapter is devoted to evidence-based practice and provides knowledge and tools for its use in clinical decision-making. The second section focuses on technology with informative chapters on hearing aids, hearing assistive technology, and cochlear implants. The final section focuses on the effects of and treatments for hearing impairment across the life span using a process-driven approach. Separate chapters cover infants/toddlers, school-aged children, young to middle-aged adults, and the elderly, and follow patients and their family members through identification, diagnosis, and management of hearing loss. These chapters highlight the complementary, interrelated, and overlapping roles of audiologists and speech-language pathologists across service-delivery sites using patient- and family-centered philosophies.

While a "rubber hits the road approach" engages and immerses students in the real world of clinical practice and decision-making, a variety of pedagogical feature—learning objectives, casebook reflections, and learning activities—help readers to process, apply, and internalize the central issues, tools, and contemporary philosophies in the field. For example, a feature called "What Does the Evidence Show?" in many chapters serves to infuse evidence-based practice within the context of patient management. I hope readers will learn from and enjoy *Introduction to Auditory Rehabilitation: A Contemporary Issues Approach.*

New! CourseSmart eTextbook Available

CourseSmart is an exciting new choice for students looking to save money. As an alternative to purchasing the printed textbook, students can purchase an electronic version of the same content. With a CourseSmart eTextbook, students can search the text, make notes online, print out reading assignments that incorporate lecture notes, and bookmark important passages for later review. For more information, or to purchase access to the CourseSmart eTextbook, visit www.coursesmart.com.

Supplementary Materials: A Wealth of Resources for Students and Professors

The text is designed to support learning and facilitate better understanding of chapter concepts through the features discussed earlier. In addition, both students and professors can benefit from a wealth of supplementary materials.

Companion Website

Located at www.pearsonhighered.com/johnson, the Companion Website for this text includes informative resources such as chapter overviews, reflection questions, suggested reading, updated clinical cases, and self-assessment study guide material.

Instructor's Resource Manual and Test Bank

Instructors will find many resources to support their course within the text itself. Each text chapter contains learning objectives, key terms, chapter summaries, cases for discussion and reflection, and end-of-chapter learning activities. To help prepare coursework, an online Instructor's Resource Manual and Test Bank is available. Please contact your Pearson representative for information or go to www.pearsonhighered.com and then click on "Educators" to download and print resource files.

Acknowledgments

I would like to acknowledge the following individuals who reviewed the manuscript and provided helpful comments and suggestions: Amy Engler Booth, University of Maine; Debra Busacco; Gail D. Chermak, Washington State University; Holly Kaplan; Jean E. Lundy, Metropolitan State College of Denver; Douglas Martin, University of Cincinnati; James McCartney, California State University, Sacramento; June McCullough, San Jose State University; Lisa Lucks Mendel, University of Memphis; Joseph Montano, Long Island University; Barbara J. Parker, Southwest Speech & Hearing Center, DeSoto, Texas; Sheila Pratt, University of Pittsburgh; Harry Rizer, New Jersey's William Paterson University; Deborah von Hapsburg, University of Tennessee, Knoxville; Barbara Weinstein, Lehman College; and Thomas R. Zalewski, Bloomsburg University. I would also like to acknowledge my graduate student assistants: Amber Reith Rolfes, Lindsey Koch, Charles Cresawn, and Sarah Beam.

Carole E. Johnson
Auburn University

Contents

CHAPTER *2*

Psychosocial Aspects of Hearing Impairment
and Counseling   27

CHAPTER *3*

Multicultural Issues in Auditory Rehabilitation   52

CHAPTER *4*

Professional Issues in Auditory Rehabilitation   86

CHAPTER *5*

Evidence-Based Practice in Auditory Rehabilitation   107

Section II   Sensory Aids for Auditory Rehabilitation

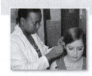

CHAPTER 6

An Introduction to Amplification   153

CHAPTER *7*

Introduction to Hearing Assistive Technology   229

CHAPTER *8*

An Introduction to Cochlear Implants   264

Section III   Auditory Rehabilitation Across the Lifespan

CHAPTER *9*

Auditory Habilitation for Young Children and Their Families   307

CHAPTER *10*

Auditory Habilitation for School-Aged Children   364

CHAPTER *11*

Auditory Rehabilitation for Young to Middle-Aged Adults   432

CHAPTER *12*

Auditory Rehabilitation for Elderly Adults   478

CHAPTER *one*

Introduction to Auditory Rehabilitation

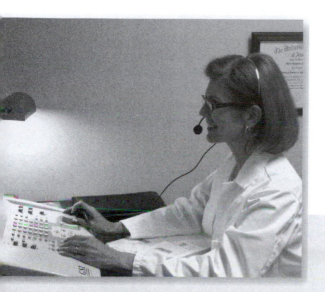

LEARNING *objectives*

After reading this chapter, you should be able to:

1. Define *prevalence* and *incidence* as they pertain to hearing loss.

2. Define *audiologic rehabilitation, aural rehabilitation, auditory rehabilitation,* and *auditory habilitation.*

3. Interrelate the roles of various professionals involved in auditory rehabilitation across service delivery sites.

4. Interpret audiograms.

5. Describe the effects of hearing loss.

6. Explain a model for auditory rehabilitation.

7. Acknowledge other areas of auditory rehabilitation.

W hat does it mean to have a hearing loss or know someone with a hearing loss? Most people rarely think about hearing loss unless it happens to them, or an acquaintance, friend, or family member. Let's see how hearing loss is soon to become a major issue for the Smiths and the Washingtons.

Casebook Reflection

Charles's Story

Charles Smith and his wife, Irene, were waiting to be seated at their favorite restaurant. Charles, 70, was professor emeritus in the biology department at the local university. He maintained an office in the department and enjoyed going into work three mornings a week. He looked forward to teaching one class a year and felt the students "kept him young." The Smiths were parents of two children with families of their own. Irene was very active in the community and enjoyed babysitting her grandchildren. Eating out on Friday night was a ritual for this busy couple.

"Dear, I'm going to the restroom," Irene said. "I think I've got time before we're seated."

Charles was busy looking at the basketball game on the bar TV visible to those seated in the waiting area.

"Dear, I'm going to the restroom," Irene said, tapping Charles on the hand.

"OK, OK . . . ," Charles said, not looking up at his wife.

"Smith, party of two, Smith," the hostess said. "Smith, party of two, Smith."

Irene heard the announcement in the restroom while she was combing her hair. She immediately rushed out and went to the hostess station.

"Yes, yes . . . that's us," Irene said to the hostess.

"Charles, CHARLES. . . . Come on!" Irene said.

"OK . . . ," Charles said with his finger up. "Wait just a second until the boy makes the free throw."

"Charles, now!" Irene said in a loud voice, "Charles!"

Irene was embarrassed when she saw that everyone in the waiting area was looking at her. She had been frustrated with her husband over the past several months. She felt he was ignoring her and what was going on around him.

"How is this table?" the hostess asked.

"Fine," Irene said. "Charles, does this suit you?"

Charles, not hearing what was said, just nodded as he sat down.

"Here are your menus. I hope you enjoy your meal, and your server will be with you shortly."

"Didn't you hear our name being called out there? Didn't you hear me?" Irene asked.

"I guess not. I was so wrapped up in watching the game."

At that moment, a young woman walked up to their table. "Hi, my name is Stacy and I'll be taking care of you tonight. Have you decided what you want to drink?"

"I'll have some iced tea," Irene said.

"I'll have the same," Charles said.

"Very well, I'll go get your drinks for you right now," Stacy said.

"Oh Lacy, could you tell me what the special is tonight?" Charles asked.

"Dear, her name is Stacy," Irene corrected.

"Stacy . . . sorry," Charles apologized.

"No problem. . . . Our special is prime rib, baked potato, and asparagus," Stacy explained. "I'll go get those drinks now."

"It is a problem! I think there is something wrong with your hearing!" Irene said.

"I don't think so. Everyone just mumbles. . . ."

Joshua's Story

Debbie, 32, and Leon Washington, 35, were on their way from the hospital with their newborn baby, Joshua, a healthy, full-term baby who weighed in at 7 pounds, 2 ounces. They had only a 10-minute drive from the hospital to their home, which was full of family members anxiously awaiting their arrival.

"Look, Leon, he's fast asleep!" remarked Debbie from the backseat while looking over at her baby.

"Yeah, I can't wait to get to bed. I'm bushed!" Leon said, looking back at her through the rearview mirror. "How do you feel, dear?"

"I'm exhausted too, but very excited!" Debbie answered. "Look! My parents and my sister are here!"

"I hope they don't stay too long," Leon groaned as he pulled into the driveway.

"They're here!" Sue Jefferson, Debbie's mother, said, looking through the living room window.

"Henry? Henry! Let's go help our daughter into the house!" Sue requested.

"Alright, alright . . . ," said Henry, slowly getting up out of the easy chair and out the front door.

"I bet you're glad to be home!" remarked Sue to the young couple.

"Oh yes! Joshua, Grandma and Grandpa Jefferson are here!" Debbie said, gently lifting Joshua out of the car seat.

"Yes, Grandma is here," Sue said, lifting Joshua into her arms. "I believe he's grown in just two days!"

"We won't stay long, honey," Henry said, carrying Debbie's bags. "Joshua's room is all ready to go!"

"The refrigerator is full of food," Sue added as everyone went up the front steps inside.

"Thanks, Mom," Debbie said as she and Sue walked into Joshua's room. "Mom, I'm a little concerned because a nurse notified me that Joshua did not pass his hearing screening test. We have an appointment with a doctor to have his hearing tested. I'm worried because my personal trainer at the gym has a little girl with a hearing loss who has speech problems and goes to a special school."

"Oh, Joshua is probably just stubborn like his grandfather. He probably hears only what he wants to!" Sue said with a concerned look on her face.

Hearing loss is more common than people may think. **Prevalence** is the number of individuals per segment of the population that have a particular condition. It has been estimated that 32 million individuals in the United States have hearing loss or about 10% of the population (Kochkin, 2010). Prevalence of hearing loss is greater or about 30% for those individuals over 60 years of age (Kochkin, 2004). The **incidence**, or the number of persons diagnosed with hearing loss per a given time period, is more elusive because so many individuals failed to get tested. Because the majority of states have mandated universal newborns hearing screening, it has been estimated that the incidence of hearing loss among newborns is 12,000 per year (Joint Committee on Infant Hearing, 2007).

Hearing loss in a newborn or an elderly person affects the person with the impairment as well as the individual's significant others. For example, Charles knew something was wrong but didn't want to admit it. He felt anxious and frustrated about not being able to hear at restaurants and having to turn the television up louder to be able to understand what was being said. Charles and Irene have had issues over his difficulty hearing for several years. Their grown children have become increasingly concerned about their dad: "What's wrong with Dad? Is he in the early stages of dementia? Why does he ignore questions or provide 'off-the-wall' answers?" Similarly, Debbie and Sue were already worried about Joshua: "What if he has a significant hearing loss? What will we do? Will Joshua be able to talk? Will he be able to go to school? Will he have to wear hearing aids?"

We will follow the Smiths and the Washingtons on their journeys with hearing loss. We will also begin our journey learning about auditory rehabilitation and the roles of communication sciences and disorders professionals in serving patients with hearing losses and their families. We will begin by reviewing the definitions and changes in auditory terminology.

DEFINING AUDITORY REHABILITATION

The text's title, *Introduction to Auditory Rehabilitation: A Contemporary Issues Approach*, is appropriate because even when defining auditory rehabilitation, we must acknowledge how terminology has changed to reflect advancements in technology and expansions of the scope of practice for audiologists and speech-language pathologists. A **scope of practice** is an official document of a professional organization that specifies appropriate areas of practices for its members. These documents for the professions are discussed in more detail later on in this chapter and in Chapter 4 on professional issues. Figure 1.1 displays examples of some of the roles of audiologists and speech-language pathologists in providing auditory rehabilitative services. Some auditory rehabilitative services may be provided by audiologists, some by

Audiologist	Speech-Language Pathologist
• Fitting and dispensing hearing aids • Mapping cochlear implant speech processor • Evaluating and dispensing hearing assistive technology • Treatment of balance disorders	• Evaluating receptive and expressive skills • Comprehension of language: oral, signed, or written models • Treatment of speech and voice disorders

Both

Speechreading training
Development of communication strategies

figure *1.1*

Examples of services provided primarily by audiologists, speech-language pathologists, or both.

speech-language pathologists, and some by both. For example, audiologists, not speech-language pathologists, select, evaluate, and fit hearing aids, sensory aids, and hearing assistive technology. On the other hand, speech-language pathologists, not audiologists, typically provide speech and language therapy and auditory training to children with hearing impairment. In this way, the roles of audiologists and speech-language pathologists are complementary, meaning that auditory rehabilitative efforts of both professions combine well to ameliorate the effects of hearing impairment on patients' lives. Their services are also interrelated, meaning that both professions may deal with speech perception, for example, but approach it from different perspectives. Audiologists are concerned with what phonemes patients can and cannot perceive with their hearing aids, whereas speech-language pathologists are concerned with how errors in speech perception affect those in speech production. However, audiologists and speech-language pathologists can both provide training in speechreading and communication strategies.

Over 25 years ago, the Committee of the American Speech-Language-Hearing Association defined the term *aural rehabilitation* and its related areas (see Figure 1.2). This definition focused on the services received by individuals with hearing loss, but not on the relevance of those services to the specific patient (ASHA, 2001). In 2001, the Working Group on Audiologic Rehabilitation of the American Speech-Language-Hearing Association (ASHA) updated terminology to include two terms, **audiologic rehabilitation** and **aural rehabilitation**, which are defined as "an ecological, interactive process that facilitates one's ability to minimize or prevent the limitations and restrictions that auditory dysfunctions can impose on well-being and communication, including interpersonal, psychosocial, educational, and vocational functioning." Audiologic rehabilitation has referred to services audiologists provide; aural rehabilitation has been often associated with services provided by audiologists and speech-language pathologists. Use of different terms for the two different professions has had some impact on whether audiologists have been paid for services rendered. Customarily, audiologists and speech-language pathologists use a coding system to indicate services rendered so that they may be reimbursed by **third-party payers**. Third-party payers are entities (e.g., insurance company) other than the healthcare provider (audiologist or speech-language pathologist) or patient who reimburses for procedures performed, diagnoses made, and certain devices, supplies, and/or other equipment for clients (ASHA, 1996). So, some claims submitted by audiologists using codes with the term "aural rehabilitation" typically submitted by speech-language pathologists were denied (White, 2006, 2009). Recognizing this, the ASHA Health Care Economics Committee recommended and had the term "aural rehabilitation" replaced with the more professionally neutral term of **auditory rehabilitation** for use in coding (White, 2006, 2009). Therefore, we will replace the terms "audiologic rehabilitation/aural rehabilitation" used in the above definition with "auditory rehabilitation" to represent current thinking and the collaborative nature among professionals in this area of practice. In addition, it should be noted that **auditory habilitation** refers to serving patients under 18 years of age with hearing loss and their families. Third-party payment is one professional issue discussed in more detail in Chapter 4.

Besides this change in terminology for the above definition, it is important to note that an ecological approach to rehabilitation centers on the whole person, facilitating functioning and interaction within patient-specific contexts (ASHA, 2001). In other words, rehabilitation for Charles should be more than just a listing of services (e.g., evaluation, fitting, and monitoring of hearing aids, counseling). It should focus on improving communication with his wife and their children and families. Similarly, initially, therapeutic efforts for Joshua should focus on communication within the context of family life in the home environment.

Aural rehabilitation refers to services and procedures for facilitating adequate receptive and expressive communication in individuals with hearing impairment. These services and procedures are intended for those persons who demonstrate a loss of hearing sensitivity or function in communication situations as if they possess a loss of hearing sensitivity. The services and procedures include, but are not limited to:

I. Identification and Evaluation of Sensory Capabilities
    A. Identification and evaluation of the extent of the impairment, including assessment, periodic monitoring and re-evaluation of auditory abilities.
    B. Monitoring of other sensory capabilities (e.g., visual and tactile-kinesthetic) as they relate to receptive and expressive communication.
    C. Evaluation, fitting, and monitoring of auditory aids and monitoring of other sensory aids (e.g., visual and vibro-tactile) used by the auditorily handicapped person in various communication environments (e.g., home, work, and school). Such auditory and sensory aids are taken to include all amplification systems (group and individual), as well as such supplementary devices as telephone amplifiers, alarm systems, and so on.
    D. Evaluation and monitoring of the acoustic characteristics of the communication environments confronted by the hearing-impaired person.

II. Interpretation of Results, Counseling, and Referral
    A. Interpretation of audiologic findings to the client, his/her family, employer, teachers, and significant others involved in communication with the hearing-impaired person.
    B. Guidance and counseling for the client, his/her family, employer, caregiver, teachers, and significant others concerning the educational, psychosocial, and communication effects of hearing impairment.
    C. Guidance and counseling for the parent/caregiver regarding: educational options available; selection of educational programs; and facilitation of communication and cognitive development.
    D. Individual and/or family counseling regarding: acceptance and understanding of the hearing impairment; functioning within difficult listening situations; facilitation of effective strategies and attitudes toward communication; modification of communication behavior in keeping with those strategies and attitudes; and promotion of independent management of communication-related problems.
    E. Referral for additional services (e.g., medical, psychological, social, and educational) as appropriate.

III. Intervention for Communication Difficulties
    A. Development and provision of an intervention program to facilitate expressive and receptive communication.
    B. Provision of hearing and speech conservation programming.
    C. Service as a liaison between the client, family, and other agencies concerned with the management of communication disorders related to hearing impairment.

IV. Reevaluation of the Client's Status

V. Evaluation and Modification of the Intervention Program

figure *1.2*

Definition of aural rehabilitation and its services and procedures.

Source: Reprinted with permission from *Definition of and Competencies for Aural Rehabilitation* [Relevant paper]. Available from www.asha.org/policy. Copyright 1984 by American Speech-Language-Hearing Association. All rights reserved.

Audiologists and speech-language pathologists must take a patient-centered approach to rehabilitation, tailoring therapy to meet specific needs of patients and families. The effects of hearing impairment are pervasive, impacting not only communication, but interpersonal, psychosocial, educational, and vocational functioning, necessitating interaction between and among other professionals in meeting patients' needs. Further, within the previously stated definition the term "auditory dysfunction" also includes (central) auditory processing disorders, tinnitus, and hyperacusis, which are discussed later on in the chapter.

PROVIDERS OF AUDITORY REHABILITATION ACROSS SERVICE DELIVERY SITES

Audiologists and speech-language pathologists certified by the American Speech-Language-Hearing Association collaborate to provide auditory rehabilitative services. Audiologists may also be certified by the American Board of Audiology (ABA); some professionals may not be certified at all and opt for state licensure. The roles of audiologists and speech-language pathologists in providing auditory rehabilitative services are *complementary*, *interrelated*, and *overlapping*, requiring a breadth of knowledge and skills to meet the communication needs of patients with hearing impairment and their families (ASHA, 2001).

Other professionals assist in the delivery of auditory rehabilitative services depending on the **service delivery site**, a place where services are provided that depend on the age or other characteristics of the patient. For example, educational audiologists provide auditory (re)habilitation services to children in public schools. Furthermore, other professionals may play a role in the delivery of those services, such as early childhood special educators, hearing aid dispensers, interpreters, public school nurses, physicians, psychologists, teachers, and so on. Teachers of children who are deaf or hard of hearing may play an important role by either providing direct auditory rehabilitative services or critical information regarding a child's educational needs in a consultative role. An adult who has served his or her country in the armed forces may receive auditory rehabilitative services at a Department of Veterans Affairs Medical Center, or an elderly person with medical needs may receive those services within a skilled nursing facility. Table 1.1 shows which patient groups are served by various service delivery sites depending on the purpose of the site.

Auditory (re)habilitative services are often provided within a context of a team approach, with audiologists leading the way on issues of hearing healthcare. A **team approach** in auditory rehabilitation involves a group of healthcare professionals collaborating to lessen the effects of hearing impairment on patients and their families. Using the previous example, educational audiologists may lead the children's individualized education plan team in understanding the importance of using hearing assistive technology within the classroom. Similarly, audiologists lead hearing conservation teams (e.g., engineers, industrial hygiene technicians, managers, nurses, physicians, and so on) in industry to protect the hearing of workers exposed to excessive noise levels in the workplace. Another example of teamwork is a cochlear implant team in which audiologists, otologists, psychologists, social workers, speech-language pathologists, and so on work together in assisting a child with hearing loss and his or her family through the process of receiving a cochlear prosthesis.

table *1.1* Professionals, Service Delivery Sites, and Patient Groups Involved in the Provision of Auditory Rehabilitation Services

Patient Groups	Infants and Toddlers (0 to 2 Years)	Preschool Children (3 to 5 Years)	School-Age Children (6 to 18 Years)	Adults (19 to 64 Years)	The Elderly (65 Years and Over)
Professionals					
Audiologists	X	X	X	X	X
Early Childhood Special Educators	X	X			
Early Interventionists	X				
Geriatric Care Specialists					X
Hearing Aid Dispensers	X	X	X	X	X
Interpreters		X	X	X	X
Nurses	X	X	X	X	X
Nurse's Aides	X	X	X	X	X
Otologists	X	X	X	X	X
Otorhinolaryngologists	X	X	X	X	X
Pediatricians	X	X	X		
Psychologists	X	X	X	X	X
Primary Care Physicians	X	X	X	X	X
Public School Teachers		X	X	X	
Teachers of the Deaf	X	X	X		
Social Workers	X	X	X	X	X
Speech-Language Pathologists	X	X	X	X	X
Vocational Rehabilitation Counselors				X	
Service Delivery Sites					X
Assistive Living Facilities					X
Child's Medical Homes	X	X	X		
Daycare Centers	X	X	X		X
Doctors' Offices	X	X	X	X	X
Early Intervention Centers	X				
Hospitals	X	X	X	X	X
Long-Term Residential Care Facilities					X
Patients' Homes	X	X	X	X	X
Preschools		X			
Private Clinical Practices	X	X	X	X	X
Public Schools		X	X		
Speech and Hearing Centers	X	X	X	X	X
Senior Centers					X
State Departments of Health	X	X	X	X	X
Universities	X	X	X	X	X

THE AUDIOGRAM: BASIC CONCEPTS

Many readers of this textbook will have some background information on audiologic evaluations from an introductory audiology course. However, a review of some basic concepts is needed before we further discuss auditory rehabilitation. Audiologists have a wide variety of instruments with which to assess patients' auditory functions. Audiologic assessment can involve nonbehavioral or behavioral testing. **Nonbehavioral tests** are those that measure physiological responses to sound; **behavioral tests** assess patients' conscious responses to auditory stimuli. The major advantage of nonbehavioral testing is objectivity, but it does not provide information about how patients consciously respond to auditory stimuli.

Audiologists measure hearing sensitivity, or the softest sounds patients can hear, with an **audiometer**. These instruments range in their sophistication from portable units used for screening to elaborate computerized systems for diagnosis of hearing loss. Audiologic assessments that use an audiometer involve behavioral testing, although audiologists frequently confirm behavioral assessments with nonbehavioral results, which is known as the **cross-check principle** (Jerger & Hayes, 1976). **Screening** is a short testing process that serves to distinguish persons who may have a condition, such as a hearing loss, that needs further evaluation from those who do not. Patients who test positive (fail the screening) often undergo a complete **diagnostic evaluation** that involves a recognized "gold standard" test to confirm the type, degree, and configuration of a hearing loss. The audiometer allows audiologists to present **pure-tone stimuli** of varying frequencies and hearing levels to patients who are seated in a sound-treated booth wearing earphones. Alternatively patients are also tested when sounds are transmitted via loudspeakers (i.e., via air conduction) and/or through a bone oscillator (i.e., bone conduction) that is placed on the mastoid bone behind the ear or on the forehead. **Air-conduction stimuli** travel through the air to the outer ear, middle ear, and inner ear. **Bone-conduction stimuli** bypass the outer and middle ears (i.e., conductive mechanism) to stimulate directly the inner ear (i.e., sensorineural mechanism) through vibration of the bones of the skull.

Pure-tone threshold is defined as the softest pure tone that a patient can detect 50% of the time. Pure-tone thresholds are measured at various frequencies measured in hertz (Hz) that indicate the various pitches that we can hear. Customarily, the octave frequencies of 250 through 8000 Hz are assessed for air conduction and 250 through 4000 Hz for bone conduction. Patients' thresholds are recorded on an **audiogram**, a graph used to document the results of an audiologic evaluation. Figure 1.3 shows a typical audiogram with two axes. The horizontal axis represents frequency, and the vertical axis is for hearing level (HL) measured in decibels (dB). Patients' thresholds are plotted using special symbols according to the legend on the audiogram. For example, for a patient who indicates hearing a 1000 Hz tone at 10 dB HL 50% of the time via air conduction in the right ear, the audiologist marks a circle at the appropriate coordinate. Similarly, the air-conduction symbol for the left ear is a "X." Many other symbols are used and are found on the legend, and they vary based on the ear, transducer, and whether a procedure called **masking** was used. Masking is a procedure used by audiologists to ensure that the non-test ear does not participate; otherwise it interferes with audiometric testing. For example, a blue ">" is used to denote an unmasked bone-conduction threshold obtained in the left ear. Masking procedures are beyond the scope of this textbook; see Stach (2010) or Martin and Clark (2008) for further explanation. The audiologist compares the relationship between the air- and bone-conduction symbols to determine the degree, type, and configuration of hearing loss.

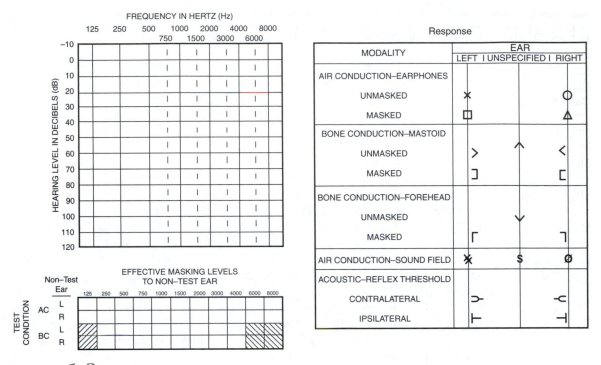

figure *1.3*

An audiogram.

Most patients can press a button or raise their hands to indicate when they hear a tone. Patients' thresholds are obtained for both ears via air- and bone-conduction audiometry to obtain their pure-tone thresholds. However, special testing paradigms are used for evaluating the hearing sensitivity of young children. **Visual reinforcement audiometry** (VRA), a testing paradigm for children 6 months to 2 years, uses animated toys hidden behind smoked Plexiglas on top of the loudspeakers. Children are conditioned to turn their heads in response to hearing a stimulus delivered via loudspeakers or through earphones. The child sits on his or her parent's lap with loudspeakers positioned at 90 and 270 degrees to the right and left, respectively. An assistant positioned directly in front of the child (at a zero-degree azimuth) keeps the child's attention focused toward midline between stimulus-presentation trials. Reinforcement techniques are used to bring the child under stimulus control such that a head-turn response to auditory stimuli results in animation of the toys. With VRA, the child is rewarded for a head-turn response, regardless of whether the child localizes to the correct side or loudspeaker. **Conditioned oriented response audiometry** (COR) is similar to VRA, but requires localization to the correct side or loudspeaker for reinforcement. It is also appropriate for children 6 months to 2 years of age. **Play audiometry** is a testing paradigm for children ages 2 to 5 years who are conditioned to complete a repetitive, motoric task (e.g., dropping blocks in a bucket, putting pegs in a board) to indicate detection of an auditory stimulus.

table *1.2* Classification Scheme for Degree of Hearing Loss, Range of Decibel Values in Hearing Level (dB HL), and Ability to Understand Speech

Classification for Degree of Hearing Loss	Range in dB HL	Ability to Understand Speech
Normal	–10 to 15	Has no difficulty understanding faint or distant speech
Minimal	16 to 25	May have difficulty hearing faint or distant speech
Mild	26 to 40	Can "hear" speech, but misses pieces of words, causing misunderstanding
Moderate	41 to 55	May understand familiar conversational speech at a distance of 3 to 5 feet
Moderately Severe	56 to 70	May understand only loud speech
Severe	71 to 90	May hear a loud shout 1 foot from the ear
Profound	91 and greater	Not able to use hearing for communication

Source: Information from *Hearing Loss Counseling Sheets*, by K. Anderson and N. Matkin, 1998, Tampa, FL: Educational Audiology Association.

Degree of Hearing Loss

A complete audiometric evaluation results in an audiogram with air- and bone-conduction thresholds recorded for both ears. **Degree of hearing loss** describes the severity of hearing impairment based on predefined categories that may vary slightly among instructors, clinical supervisors, and textbooks.

Table 1.2 shows a classification scheme for degree of hearing loss based on hearing level measured in decibels (dB HL) with a corresponding description of ability to understand speech. As a reference, a whisper at 1 meter away is about 25 dB HL, conversational speech about 45 dB HL, and a loud shout about 65 dB HL. Furthermore, it is important to remember that audiometric thresholds represent the hearing level that pure-tone stimuli are detected about 50% of the time. In other words, they do not represent hearing levels consistently heard by patients. Patients' pure-tone thresholds that fall between plus and minus 10 to 15 dB HL have normal hearing sensitivity and can understand faint and/or distant speech, although some consider the normal hearing range to extend to 20 dB HL. With minimal hearing loss, patients may have difficulty understanding soft or distant speech. Alternatively, those with severe hearing losses can just barely hear loud speech at 1 foot from the ear.

Type of Hearing Loss

Pure-tone audiometry assists in determining the type of hearing loss. As stated earlier, the conductive mechanism consists of the outer and middle ears. The outer ear consists of the pinna and ear canal, a conduit that collects sound and funnels acoustic energy toward the tympanic membrane, respectively. The middle ear consists of the tympanic membrane, the ossicles, middle ear space, tendons, ligaments, and so on. Sound energy sets the tympanic membrane into vibration, which is the beginning of the middle ear's complex transformation function. The vibrational process ends with the stapes footplate moving in and out of the oval window, converting mechanical-vibrational energy into hydrodynamic wave forces in the inner ear.

The inner ear consists of three main parts: (1) the cochlea, (2) the vestibule, and (3) the semicircular canals. The vestibule and the semicircular canals contain the end organs for balance. The cochlea, the end organ of hearing, contains sensory hair cells. Through an equally complex process, the hair cells within the cochlea are stimulated by the inner ear waves that are part of the transduction process converting hydrodynamic waves into neural impulses. The nerve impulses, or action potentials, are sent from the peripheral auditory system via cranial nerve VIII, or the statoacoustic nerve, which is the starting point for the journey to the central auditory mechanism. A complete discussion of these processes is beyond the scope of this textbook; see Bellis (2003) for further explanation.

Air-conduction stimuli must travel through the conductive mechanism (i.e., outer and middle ear) and on through to the inner ear, and so on. Any pathology in either the conductive or sensorineural mechanisms may result in loss of hearing sensitivity measured by air-conduction audiometry. However, bone-conduction stimuli (generated by a bone oscillator) transmit energy directly to the inner ear when placed on the mastoid or any other bone of the skull, bypassing the conductive mechanism. Bone-conduction thresholds are a direct measure of the status of the sensorineural mechanism. Further distinction is now made between **sensory losses** and **neural losses**. Sensory losses are those in which there is a destruction of the sensory hair cells within the cochlea. Neural hearing losses occur due to difficulties that cranial nerve VIII (i.e., statoacoustic nerve) has in transmitting electrical impulses from the peripheral to the central auditory nervous system. These two types of hearing loss will be discussed further in Chapter 9.

A **conductive hearing loss** is a loss of hearing sensitivity due to a problem in the outer or middle ear that impedes transmission of sound energy into the inner ear. Possible problems in the outer ear include impacted ear wax (i.e., cerumen), growths, or infections that may obstruct the ear canal. Middle-ear pathologies include such conditions as a perforation in the tympanic membrane, a presence of fluid, otitis media, a cholesteatoma, and so on. Recall that conductive hearing losses are those in which all of the bone-conduction thresholds are within normal hearing limits, but some or all of the air-conduction thresholds are not resulting in air-bone gaps. **Air-bone gaps** are a difference of more than 10 dB between bone- and air-conduction thresholds at the same frequency and in the same ear. The air-bone gaps are the result of lower thresholds obtained when using a bone oscillator to assess the sensorineural mechanism directly, bypassing the conductive mechanism. Figure 1.4 shows an audiogram of a bilateral, conductive hearing loss.

Sensorineural hearing losses result from a problem in the inner ear, usually the result of hair cell damage from excessive noise exposure, ototoxic drugs, aging, and so on, but may also involve the auditory nerve. Most sensorineural hearing losses are not

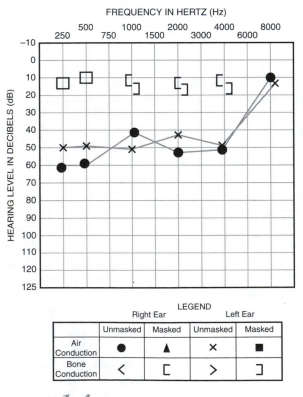

figure *1.4*

Audiogram of a moderate conductive hearing loss in the left ear and a moderately severe conductive hearing loss in the right ear.

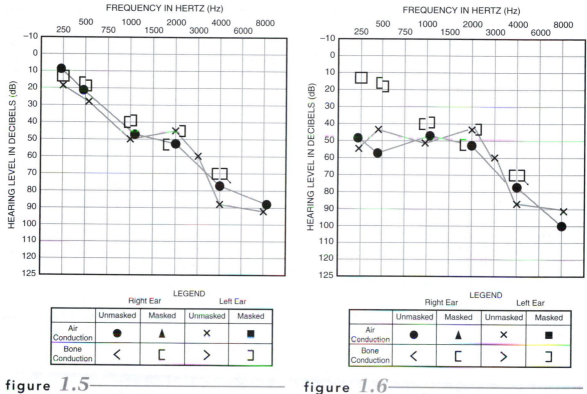

figure *1.5*

A bilateral, minimal sloping to profound sensorineural hearing loss.

figure *1.6*

A bilateral, moderate-to-profound mixed hearing loss.

correctable through medical intervention. On the audiogram, a sensorineural hearing loss is one in which some or all of the bone-conduction and air-conduction symbols are out of the range for normal hearing and no air-bone gaps are present. Figure 1.5 shows an audiogram of a bilateral, minimal sloping to profound sensorineural hearing loss. The arrow coming off of the left masked bone-conduction symbol (⌐) indicates no response from the patient.

Mixed hearing losses occur when a problem exists in both the conductive and sensorineural mechanisms. For example, a child with a moderately severe sensorineural hearing loss with otitis media and effusion may present with a mixed hearing loss on an audiologic evaluation. In most cases, problems in the conductive mechanism can be medically corrected, but problems in the sensorineural mechanism cannot. For example, the air-bone gaps may close up after the child has pressure equalization tubes placed in her eardrums. On the audiogram, mixed hearing loss is one in which some or all of both the air- and bone-conduction thresholds fall beyond the range of normal and there are air-bone gaps. Figure 1.6 shows an audiogram of a bilateral, moderate-to-profound mixed hearing loss.

Retrocochlear and **central hearing losses** are caused by congenital or acquired damage or disease (e.g., tumors) to the auditory nerve and its pathways, and reception and processing areas in the cortex. Patients who have these disorders may or may not have a loss of hearing sensitivity and other symptoms such as dizziness, ringing in the ears, and difficulty understanding speech. These disorders often present with **asymmetric audiometric results**, meaning that the results in each ear are different. Asymmetry in audiometric results and presence of the aforementioned symptoms are classic "red flags" indicating the need for further audiologic or medical evaluation. Customarily, these patients are scheduled for **auditory brainstem response testing** (ABR). An ABR is a nonbehavioral test (one that doesn't need patients to consciously respond to testing) that measures how the auditory nerve conducts impulses from the periphery to the auditory brainstem pathways in response to auditory stimuli. Some physicians prefer to forgo the ABR testing and schedule patients for radiographic studies, including **magnetic resonance imaging**. Magnetic resonance imaging is a diagnostic procedure in which radio waves are applied to the body so that the nuclear magnetic resonance of atoms produces images of internal organs and tissues on a computer (*Merriam-Webster's Medical Online Dictionary*, 2008). These losses are usually managed medically/surgically; traditional hearing aids are often not successful, especially after surgical removal of tumors.

Configuration of Hearing Loss

Configuration of the hearing loss describes the shape or direction the air-conduction threshold symbols in either the right and/or left ears assume when placed on an audiogram. Words like "downward-sloping," "upward-sloping," and "flat" are most often used to describe configuration of hearing loss and are shown in Figure 1.7, diagrams A, B, and C. Communication sciences and disorders students may also hear configurations called "corner," "cookie bite," or "reverse cookie bite" in audiograms; examples of these are shown in Figure 1.8, diagrams A, B, and C.

Pure-Tone Averages and Speech Audiometry

Audiograms also provide information on pure-tone averages (PTA) and results for speech audiometry. There are different types of pure-tone averages. **Pure-tone average 1** (PTA1) is the arithmetic average of the air-conduction thresholds for 500, 1000, and 2000 Hz in one ear. The frequencies of 500, 1000, and 2000 Hz are also known as the "speech frequencies," or the frequency region containing the most salient spectral energy for speech. **Pure-tone average 2** (PTA2) is the arithmetic average of the air-conduction thresholds taken at 1000, 2000, and 4000 Hz in one ear. PTA2 is considered when PTA1 is not particularly useful in indicating the patients' degree of hearing loss, such as when hearing thresholds are within normal limits up to 2000 Hz, but there is significant hearing loss in the higher frequencies. A **two-frequency pure-tone average** is obtained by averaging the two best air-conduction thresholds at 500, 1000, and 2000 Hz in one ear and is used when one of the thresholds is significantly below the other two (e.g., 20 dB HL at 500 Hz, 25 dB HL at 1000 Hz, and 70 dB HL at 2000 Hz).

Why are pure-tone averages important, and why do we need different types of them? Pure-tone averages are important for at least three reasons. First of all, pure-tone averages provide an overall descriptor of an audiogram; these averages are particularly useful when the audiogram is quite complex and requires at least a few sentences for a complete description. By using the pure-tone average, a single number summarizes the degree of hearing loss in critical frequency regions. Second, the pure-tone average is used to describe a patient's overall degree of hearing loss. For example, if a 60-year-old had pure-tone averages of 56 dB in the right ear and 59 dB in the left ear, his degree of hearing loss would be "moderate." Third, a pure-tone average is useful for cross-checking speech audiometry results. For example, PTA1 should be within +6 or −6 dB of the pure-tone average in the same ear (Stach, 2010).

The **speech recognition threshold** (SRT) is the softest hearing-threshold level that the patient can repeat back, or point to pictures on a board representing **spondee words**,

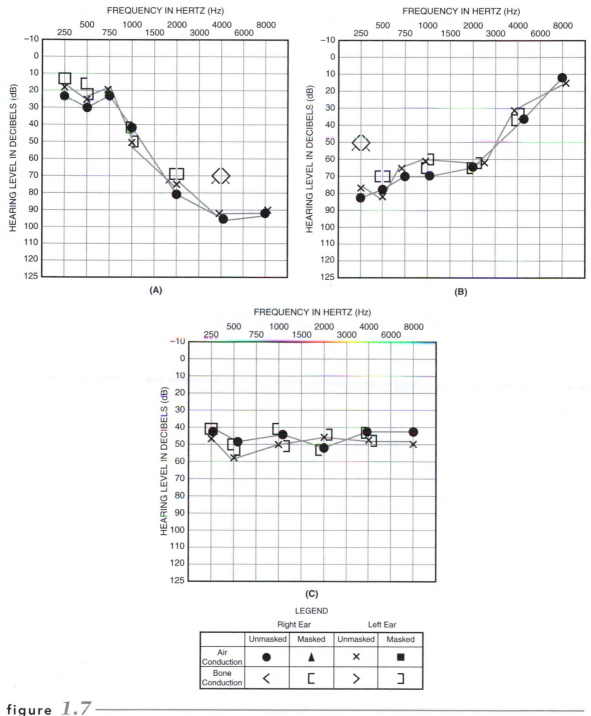

figure *1.7*

(A) Audiogram of a downward sloping sensorineural hearing loss; (B) Audiogram of a bilateral, upward sloping sensorineural hearing loss; (C) Audiogram of a bilateral, flat moderate sensorineural hearing loss.

15

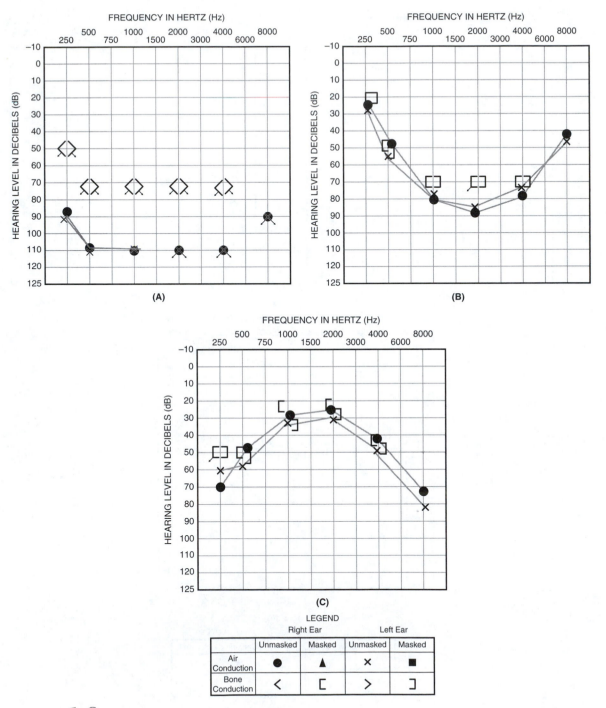

figure *1.8*

Audiogram showing configuration types. **(A)** Audiogram of a "corner" configuration; **(B)** Audiogram of a "cookie bite" configuration; **(C)** Audiogram of a "reverse cookie bite" configuration.

with 50% accuracy. Spondees are compound words consisting of two syllables that are of equal stress (e.g., baseball, hotdog, armchair). The SRT is a threshold test in which speech stimuli are presented at or around threshold. Similar to the SRT is the **speech awareness threshold** (SAT), which is the softest hearing level at which the patient can detect the presence of speech. The SAT is obtained on very young children or other patients who cannot respond appropriately for obtaining SRTs. Sometimes students confuse the SRT with the **speech recognition score**, which is the percent of words correctly repeated back when presented at suprathreshold level. **Suprathreshold levels** are levels that are above threshold and are usually presented at a comfortable level. Words for speech recognition testing are presented at about 35 dB above the SRT in the same ear, or 35 dB **sensation level** (SL). Sensation level refers to the number of decibels above a certain reference threshold that must be specified. For example, if a patient had a 25 dB HL SRT in the right ear, the words for obtaining the speech recognition score would be presented at 35 dB SL (re: SRT), which would be 60 dB HL on the audiometer dial (i.e., SRT of 25 dB HL + 35 dB = 60 dB HL). Other speech audiometry measures used in fitting hearing aids, such as most comfortable listening level and loudness discomfort level, are discussed in Chapter 6 on amplification.

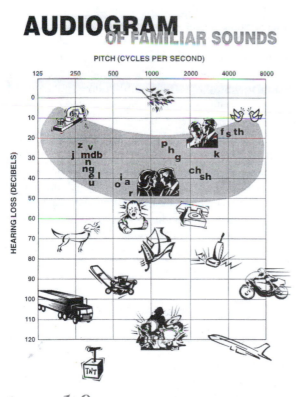

figure *1.9*

Familiar sounds on the audiogram.

Source: From *Hearing in Children* (5th edition, p. 18), by J. L. Northern and M. P. Downs, 2002. Baltimore, MD: Lippincott, Williams, and Wilkins. Reprinted with permission.

Tools for Explaining the Audiogram

Audiologists and speech-language pathologists need tools to explain the effects of a hearing loss to patients and their families. Two useful tools are the Familiar Sounds on the Audiogram (Northern & Downs, 2002) and the Count-the-Dot Audiogram (Lundeen, 1996; Mueller & Killion, 1990). Figure 1.9 shows the **Familiar Sounds on the Audiogram**, which is a tool consisting of an audiogram that has speech and other familiar sounds superimposed at the frequency and hearing level of their approximate spectral energy. For example, the /f/ and /s/ are located at approximately 20 dB HL at 4000 Hz, which indicates that they are soft, high-frequency sounds. Audiologists can draw the audiometric symbols of a patient with a moderate high-frequency sensorineural hearing loss to explain why he or she cannot hear these phonemes. Sounds that are below or softer than patients' audiometric thresholds cannot be heard. Alternatively, sounds above or louder than patients' pure-tone thresholds can easily be heard. The Familiar Sounds on the Audiogram tool is very helpful for understanding why patients can and cannot hear certain sounds.

The **Count-the-Dot Audiogram** is another useful tool graph that has 100 dots superimposed

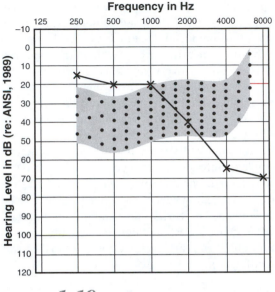

figure *1.10* ────────────────

Modified count-the-dot audiogram.

Source: Reprinted with permission from "Count-the-Dot Audiogram in Perspective," by C. Lundeen, 1996, *American Journal of Audiology* 5(58), copyright 1996 by American Speech-Language-Hearing Association. All rights reserved.

onto an audiogram for the purpose of calculating an Articulation Index for patients. The Articulation Index has also been called the Audibility Index. The **Articulation Index** is an estimation of the availability of speech energy expressed in percent ranging from 0%, no audibility, to 100%, complete audibility. Mueller and Killion (1990) developed a Count-the-Dot Audiogram, that has been widely used in diagnostic and rehabilitative audiology. In 1996, Lundeen modified that version to the one presented in Figure 1.10 for increased accuracy. Please refer to his article for a complete discussion of the topic.

The grey-shaded area represents the range of frequency and hearing level for conversational speech energy at a distance of one meter. Each dot represents 1% of speech audibility. Note that the density of the dots is greater in the higher frequencies than the lower frequencies because the former is more heavily weighted for intelligibility. To calculate an Audibility Index, audiologists must first superimpose patients' pure-tone air-conduction thresholds and connect them with straight lines (see lines superimposed on Figure 1.10). The number of dots falling below the audiometric thresholds (toward the bottom of the graph) is the Audibility Index. For instance, Figure 1.10 also provides an example of audiometric thresholds from a patient's left ear plotted on a Count-the-Dot Audiogram. By counting the number of dots below the audiometric thresholds, the patient has an unaided index of 50% for face-to-face conversational speech. Mueller, Johnson, and Carter (2007) stated that patients who have an unaided Audibility Index below 85% are candidates for amplification, if the hearing loss is causing difficulties with certain activities and interpersonal communication. Although someone may be a candidate for a hearing aid based on his or her audiometric profile, a patient may not accept that he or she has a problem. The Count-the-Dot Audiogram can be used to counsel patients regarding the audibility of speech when considering their degree of hearing loss.

EFFECTS OF HEARING LOSS

The impact of hearing loss on individuals and society is great. A child who is born with a profound sensorineural hearing loss may not learn how to use spoken language. An adult who suddenly acquires a hearing loss may not be able to perform the duties required in his or her job. An elderly person may become isolated from family and friends due to **presbycusis**, which is hearing impairment due to aging. In other chapters of this book, specific examples regarding the effects of hearing loss on different age groups will be explored in depth. However, we will discuss the effects of age of onset and degree of hearing loss in general terms here, prior to presenting a model for rehabilitation.

Age of Onset

The term **age of onset** refers to the chronological age of a patient when a hearing loss develops. A **congenital hearing loss** is one that is present at birth. For example, an expectant mother who was exposed to rubella during her first trimester of pregnancy likely will have a child who has a congenital sensorineural hearing loss in addition to other anomalies. A **prelingual hearing loss** is one that develops before the acquisition of speech and language or from birth to 2 years. A **perilingual hearing loss** is one that develops between ages 3 and 5 years, or during the period of the most rapid speech and language acquisition. A **postlingual hearing loss** is one that develops after the age of 5 or after speech and language development. The term **acquired hearing loss** is often used to describe hearing losses that develop after the age of 18, or the completion of schooling. The most important point to remember is that the earlier a hearing loss developed, the greater the impact on a child's speech and language development.

Effects of Degree of Hearing Loss

It is almost impossible to discuss the effects of age of onset of hearing impairment without also considering the degree and configuration of hearing loss. The segment of the population with hearing impairment can be divided into two groups—**hard of hearing** and **deaf**. Hard-of-hearing individuals are those who have PTAs or SRTs that are generally less than about 80 dB HL. Functionally many of these patients are able to understand speech without the use of visual cues, with assistance from hearing aids or devices known as cochlear implants. Deaf individuals are those who have PTAs or SRTs in excess of 80 to 90 dB HL. Generally, these individuals cannot use their residual hearing to understand speech without the use of visual cues even when wearing hearing aids. The audiogram is not the only tool used to classify a person with hearing impairment as hard of hearing or deaf. For example, a person who audiometrically should be considered hard of hearing, but who cannot use his or her residual hearing with amplification to understand spoken language, may be considered deaf. Alternatively, someone who is audiometrically deaf, but who has developed his or her residual hearing through early auditory habilitation efforts, may want to be considered hard of hearing. The best rule of thumb is to not classify patients on the basis of audiometric data and consider each patient as a unique individual.

A Model for Describing the Effects of Hearing Loss

Effects of hearing loss, like any other affliction, affect people all over the world. Models are needed for comparing the effects of illness and disability on people of various cultures. The **World Health Organization** (WHO) is the United Nations' specialized agency for health. It was established in April 1948 with the goal of improving health for all people in the world. **Health** is defined in WHO's Constitution as a state of complete physical, mental, and social well-being and not merely the absence of disease or illness. The WHO has established a classification system and model that provides a standard language and framework, the **International Classification of Functioning, Disability, and Health** (ICFDH) (WHO, 2001), for use in describing health and health-related states. The ICF can be used for many purposes in different health disciplines to provide health and health-related domains that help describe the following:

- Changes in body function and structure
- What a person can do in a standard environment (level of capacity)
- What a person can do in his or her day-to-day environment (level of performance)

These domains are classified from body, individual, and societal perspectives through the use of two lists: (1) body functions and structures, and (2) domains of activity and participation. In addition, in the ICF, the word **functioning** refers to all body functions, activities, and participation. The term **disability** is an umbrella term for impairments, activity limitations, and participation restriction. The ICF includes environmental factors that interact with all components of the model.

Several terms are important to know in understanding the application of the ICF and the use of its model for auditory rehabilitation (WHO, 2002). First, **body functions** are physiological functions of body systems (including psychological functions). For example, hearing is a body function in which the auditory system takes acoustic energy that, through a series of processes, results in the function of hearing. Second, **body structures** are anatomical parts of the body such as organs, limbs, and their components. The pinna, the external auditory canal, the tympanic membrane, and the basilar membrane are only a few of the body structures involved in the function of audition. Third, **impairments** are problems in body function or structure such as a significant deviation or loss. For example, an impairment of audition results from destruction (i.e., problems) in sensory hair cells (i.e., body structures) resulting in a permanent sensorineural hearing loss. Fourth, **activity** is the execution of a task or action of an individual that pertains to what the patient can do. For example, common activities of daily living include talking on the telephone and to the grocery clerk, friends, and neighbors. Fifth, **participation** is involvement in life situations. For example, involvement in life situations may include calling friends on the phone to catch up on the latest gossip, shopping at the grocery store, inviting friends over for dinner, and organizing a neighborhood watch program. Sixth, **activity limitations** are difficulties that an individual may have in executing tasks. Clinicians ask, "What can't the patient do because of his or her hearing loss?" For example, because of a hearing loss, a person may not be able to talk on the phone and may have difficulty in face-to-face interactions. Seventh, **participation restrictions** are problems an individual may experience, restricting involvement in life situations. Audiologists ask, "How is the patient's involvement with others affected by his or her hearing loss?" For example, because of a hearing loss, a person may not be able to keep in touch via telephone with friends and family who live out of state, or he or she may feel uncomfortable having company over. Eighth, **environmental factors** make up the physical, social, and attitudinal environment in which people live and conduct their lives.

The WHO stated that at least two models have been proposed for disability (Hnath-Chisolm & Abrams, 2008; WHO, 2002). The perspective of a **medical model** is that disability is a characteristic of a person or patient directly caused by disease, trauma, or other health condition requiring medical care provided by a professional. Using the medical model, a child with otitis media and mild conductive hearing loss may be treated successfully by a physician who prescribes antibiotics. However, a purely medical model does not account for the disabilities related to hearing loss because the large majority are sensorineural and are not amenable to medical treatment (Hnath-Chisolm & Abrams, 2008; WHO, 2002). The **social model** views disability as a socially created problem, not as an attribute of the person. For example, the social model would suggest that people with hearing losses do not have a problem; it is the problem of a society that is unaccommodating toward individuals who are deaf or hard of hearing. However, a purely social model will not work either because people with hearing loss own some responsibility for overcoming their disability in order to be capable and functioning members of society (Hnath-Chisolm & Abrams, 2008; WHO, 2002). Based on the limitations of the other two models, the WHO's ICF proposed another model of disability, the **biopsychosocial model**, which is based on an integration of the medical and social models

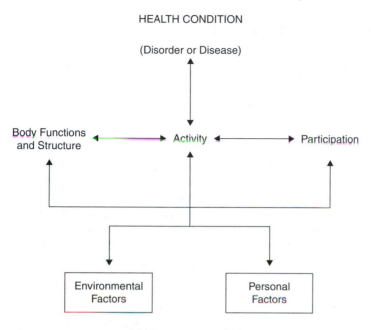

HEALTH CONDITION

(Disorder or Disease)

Body Functions and Structure ←→ Activity ←→ Participation

Environmental Factors

Personal Factors

CONTEXTUAL FACTORS

figure *1.11*

A biopsychosocial model of disability.

Source: From *Towards a Common Language for Functioning, Disability, and Health: ICF—the International Classification of Functioning, Disability, and Health,* by the World Health Organization, 2001, Geneva, from WHO/EIP/GPE/CAS/01.3; http://www.who.int/classifications/icf/training/icfbeginnersguide.pdf. Reprinted with permission.

(Hnath-Chisolm & Abrams, 2008; WHO, 2002). The model appears in Figure 1.11.

According to the biopsychosocial model, disability and functioning are outcomes of the interactions between health conditions (i.e., disorder or disease) and contextual factors (i.e., environmental factors and personal factors). Environmental factors can include elements such as:

- Social attitudes
- Architectural characteristics
- Legal and social structures
- Climate
- Terrain

Similarly, personal factors can include elements such as:

- Gender
- Age
- Coping styles
- Social background
- Education
- Profession
- Past and current experiences
- Behavioral patterns
- Character

The model has three levels of human functioning classified by the ICF: (1) functioning at the level of the body or body part, (2) the entire person (i.e., activity limitation), or (3) participation (i.e., participation restriction). Therefore, disability involves dysfunction at one or more of these levels. For example, an elderly person may have a high-frequency sensorineural hearing loss that affects his or her activity or ability to execute a task (e.g., hearing a speaker in a large room) and his or her participation or involvement in life situations (e.g., taking part in bingo games). However, the effect of the hearing loss cannot be determined without considering environmental factors and personal factors. For example, the effect of hearing loss on the person's ability to play bingo will depend on the acoustics of the bingo hall, the attitudes of the organization sponsoring the bingo game toward accommodating patrons with hearing loss, and so on. Similarly, the personal actions of the bingo player can determine the effect of his or her hearing loss on the experience. For example, will the person self-advocate by asking either the caller to speak clearly or the organization to install video monitors to show the called numbers? In conclusion, the effects of hearing loss involve a multidimensional model of factors that is highly variable from person to person and across different communication contexts. To understand how the principles of the ICF model apply, let's take a look at its use in an auditory rehabilitation model.

A MODEL FOR AUDITORY REHABILITATION

A strong theme of this textbook is a process-oriented approach to auditory rehabilitation within the context of the hearing healthcare continuum of identification, diagnosis, and intervention. Figure 1.12 shows a model for auditory rehabilitation (Boothroyd, 2006a; Lesner & Kricos, 1995; WHO, 2001). As discussed earlier, screening for or identification of hearing loss includes procedures by which patients are either referred for further testing or dismissed. Diagnosis of hearing loss includes a complete audiologic evaluation for determining type, degree, and configuration of hearing loss. Diagnosis of a hearing loss requires a physical examination of bodily structures and function to determine if the hearing loss can be ameliorated via medical management. Usually conductive and mixed hearing losses are partially or completely amenable to medical intervention. Loss of hearing sensitivity because of middle ear effusion is often reversible through antibiotics or placement of pressure equalization tubes. However, no treatments exist for most types of sensorineural hearing loss other than the use of sensory aids such as hearing aids, hearing assistive technology, and/or cochlear implants coupled with appropriate auditory rehabilitation. Management of sensorineural hearing loss requires assessment of patients' activity limitations and participation restrictions mediated by personal and environmental factors.

In our Casebook Reflection, Charles Smith presents with an acquired sensorineural hearing loss and may benefit from auditory rehabilitation. Management of his hearing impairment requires determination of what he can and cannot do (i.e., activity limitations), how his current status limits his interactions with others (i.e., participation restriction), and its effect on his quality of life. For example, we already observed that Charles had difficulty understanding speech in noisy situations, which interferes with having a stress-free meal with his wife at a restaurant.

What other difficulties is Charles having and how are they affecting his interactions with others and quality of life? Answering this question requires consideration of Charles's personal and environmental factors. Assessing personal factors requires a holistic approach to auditory rehabilitation and considers patients' (1) communication status (i.e., audiogram, visual/auditory perception of speech, and prior experience with sensory aids); (2) physical status (i.e., general health, visual status, and vestibular system); (3) psychological status (i.e., mental status, sense of well-being, motivation,

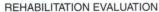

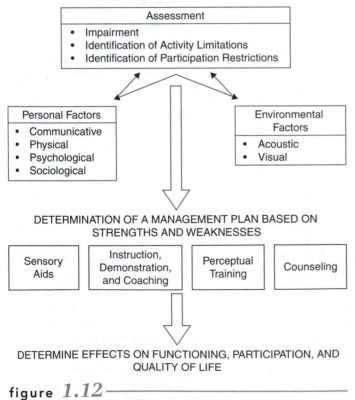

figure *1.12*

A model for auditory rehabilitation.

attitude, and expectations); and (4) sociological status (i.e., physical environment, social environment, and financial status) (Lesner & Kricos, 1995). Environmental factors may include the acoustic conditions and lighting of the places Charles likes to go (e.g., restaurants, lecture halls on campus, the Elks Lodge). The rehabilitation evaluation involves the active participation of the audiologists, speech-language pathologists, and patients and their families. Both Charles and Irene will identify and prioritize treatment goals with the audiologist who will design an individualized auditory rehabilitation plan.

Auditory rehabilitation involves four main areas: (1) sensory aids; (2) instruction, demonstration, and coaching; (3) perceptual training; and (4) counseling. The first step in most auditory rehabilitation programs is to fit the patient with sensory aid(s) in the form of hearing aids, cochlear implants, and/or hearing assistive technology. For example, fitting Charles with hearing aids is just the first part of the rehabilitation process. Patients also need instruction, demonstration, and coaching. Charles needs to learn about the care and use of his hearing aids and accompanying hearing assistive technology. Audiologists provide the initial instruction and demonstration of these devices. However, new hearing aid wearers may benefit from hearing aid orientation groups that involve coaching by peers about ways of addressing issues related to overcoming the effects of hearing loss. Mentoring by trained peers is emerging as a new model for coaching patients with hearing loss. Some patients may benefit from audiovisual perceptual training, including instruction on the importance of using good listening skills and the basics of speechreading. However, some may benefit from formal speechreading classes and/or use of self-paced, computerized auditory training programs provided by audiologists and speech-language pathologists. The fourth area of auditory rehabilitation is counseling in dealing with the diagnosis and psychosocial aspects of hearing loss. Counseling is generally of two types: (1) **informational counseling**, and (2) **personal adjustment counseling**. Charles and Irene will receive informational counseling from the audiologist in receiving explanation of the results of the audiologic evaluation. Moreover, they may need some personal adjustment counseling in minimizing the effects of Charles's hearing loss in their personal interactions.

At the end of treatment, reassessment occurs with active participation from patients and their significant others by addressing these issues: What can the patient do that he or she could not do before? How have the patient's interactions with others changed? And how has auditory rehabilitation ultimately affected the patients' and families' quality of life? For example, Charles, Irene, and his audiologist assess his progress, particularly in selected problematic communication situations. What can Charles do now that he could not do before? Can he understand his wife better when dining at their favorite restaurant? Do they eat out more often and with friends? Has auditory rehabilitation improved Charles and Irene's quality of life?

OTHER AREAS OF AUDITORY REHABILITATION

Most of the time when students consider auditory rehabilitation, they think about the impact of permanent sensorineural hearing loss, hearing aids, cochlear implants, and so on. However, auditory rehabilitation involves remediating other peripheral and central disorders besides hearing loss. In this section, readers are introduced to other areas of auditory rehabilitation involving (central) auditory processing disorders, tinnitus/hyperacusis, and vestibular and balance disorders.

(Central) Auditory Processing Disorders

Patients with (central) auditory processing disorders ([C]APD) usually have normal hearing sensitivity or a normal audiogram but have difficulty making sense out of what was heard, particularly when the message is compromised by other factors such as background noise or competing messages. The auditory nerve and pathways that transmit information are more than simply ways to get to the brain: they play a large role in the neural processing of that information before the cognitive and linguistic operations are performed in the cortex (Bellis, 2003).

Children with (C)APD may be referred to an audiologist for hearing testing because they have difficulty understanding what is being said in the classroom, cannot follow directions, or may have spelling or reading difficulties. (C)APD is suspected when such children are found to have normal hearing sensitivity. Bellis (2003) suggests that children undergo a multidisciplinary screening in order to identify those who need a comprehensive central auditory processing evaluation versus those who have other issues. A **multidisciplinary screening for central auditory processing disorders** identifies patients needing a comprehensive evaluation and reduces the need for unnecessary referrals. Other professionals involved may include speech-language pathologists, psychologists, reading specialists, and so on. Patients who fail the screening undergo a complete central auditory processing evaluation that often includes behavioral and nonbehavioral testing.

Once (C)APD has been diagnosed, audiologists, speech-language pathologists, and other professionals collaborate to design management strategies specifically targeted to meet the patients' needs. Intervention should occur as soon as possible to take advantage of **brain plasticity**, maximize treatment outcomes, and minimize any residual problems caused by the disorder (ASHA, 2005a, 2005b). Brain plasticity is the ability of the cortex to reorganize as a result of repeated experiences, such as auditory training. Specific therapeutic strategies may be classified as either "**bottom up**" or "**top down**." Bottom-up strategies aim to enhance the signal being heard through the use of technology and auditory training developing patients' perceptual skills (ASHA, 2005a, 2005b). Top-down strategies focus on the development of compensatory strategies to overcome processing problems by relying on patients' knowledge of language, memory, and attention (ASHA, 2005a, 2005b). Bellis (2003) stated that the approach for managing (C)APD should be viewed as a tripod of three approaches: (1) environmental modifications and teaching suggestions for maximizing patients' access to auditory information, (2) remediation techniques to enhance auditory processing, and (3) use of compensatory strategies on the part of the child or adult to maximize the use of auditory information. Chapter 10 discusses how audiologists and speech-language pathologists work together with other educational professionals in assisting children with (C)APD.

Tinnitus and Hyperacusis

Tinnitus is sounds or noises in the head (Davis & Rafaie, 2000). Some people have constant tinnitus, meaning that it is always there; others have intermittent tinnitus, meaning that it is there some of the time. Tinnitus may be in one ear or both and may be described as hissing, roaring, whistling, chirping, or clicking (American Tinnitus Association [ATA], 2009). It is difficult to determine the prevalence of tinnitus or the proportion of the population it affects due to a lack of agreement on a single definition of the condition and its variable effects across patients. The American Tinnitus Association estimates that of the 50 million people in the United States who have tinnitus, 12 million have it severely enough to be brought to the attention of a healthcare provider, and 2 million to the degree that it is debilitating (ATA, 2009). Many people with tinnitus also suffer from **hyperacusis**, or a hypersensitivity to the loudness of sounds. Tinnitus can affect people of all ages, although children are less likely to report tinnitus, particularly if they have experienced it since birth (Hegarty & Smith, 2000). Several known causes of tinnitus include impacted cerumen, ingestion of certain medications, ear/eye infections, jaw problems, cardiovascular disorders, tumors, noise exposure, head and neck trauma, and presbycusis (ATA, 2009; Davis & Rafaie, 2000). Although some tinnitus may be ameliorated through medical management, the majority of cases are incurable and permanent. Audiologists are involved in the evaluation of and treatment of tinnitus. For some, tinnitus has a strong psychological component negatively affecting health-related quality of life. In some cases, audiologists need to refer patients to mental health professionals for assistance in coping with tinnitus in their lives. We will be discussing more about audiologists' role in tinnitus management in Chapter 11.

Vestibular and Balance Disorders

With an expanding scope of practice, audiologists also assess and manage balance system disorders. Desmond (2001) stated that the primary function of our balance system is to permit us to interact and maintain contact with our surroundings in a safe and efficient manner. Our sense of balance requires gathering information from the visual, somatosensory, and vestibular senses that integrate in the brainstem for processing in the cortex (Desmond, 2001). **Somatosensory senses** involve providing information about the body's position using skin and muscle receptors. Equilibrium is possible if information coming from these sources is predictable and nonconflicting, enabling us to move about the environment with an automatic maintenance of balance (Desmond, 2001). Nonconflicting input means that similar data are received by matched pairs of sensory end organs for balance in each ear, such as the cristae ampullaris that are located in the ampulla of each of the semicircular canals, as well as the maculae as in the utricle and the saccule. Each of the following semicircular canals occupies a separate anatomical plane and is at right angles to each other: (1) superior canal (i.e., coronal plane), (2) posterior canal (i.e., sagittal plane), and (3) horizontal canal (i.e., transverse plane). The inner ear fluid, or endolymph, flows toward or away from the sensory organ with varying head movements and, if the response is the same in the canals in both sides of the head, balance is maintained (Desmond, 2001). However, when information is in conflict, the brainstem must reflexively adjust, which causes a sense of imbalance and a resulting sensation of **vertigo** and nausea (Desmond, 2001).

The prevalence of balance disorders increases with age. For example, an epidemiological study surveyed elderly people and found that the prevalence of balance disorders was 33% at 70 years of age and increased 40–50% for those around 90 years of age (Jönsson, Sixt, Landahl, & Rosenhall, 2004). Dizziness in the primary care setting represents a broad spectrum of diagnoses in the elderly population (Sloane, Dallara, Roach, Bailey, Mitchell, & McNutt 1994). However, **benign paroxysmal positional vertigo** (BPPV) is the most common form of vertigo and results from an asymmetrical fluid response due to a conflicting response to head movement in one of the semicircular canals. Audiologists are involved with the management of balance disorders such as BPPV, which will be discussed further in Chapter 11.

SUMMARY

This introductory chapter of *Introduction to Auditory Rehabilitation: A Contemporary Issues Approach* defined important terms and described specific roles of the complementary and overlapping roles of audiologists and speech-language pathologists who provide auditory rehabilitation in various service delivery sites. Readers reviewed the fundamentals of audiogram interpretation; types, degrees, and configurations of hearing loss; and a model for auditory rehabilitation. The foundations for practicing auditory rehabilitation, new horizons, and contemporary challenges facing clinicians were summarized, setting the stage for themes that will be further developed throughout the textbook.

LEARNING ACTIVITIES

Interview an audiologist and speech-language pathologist regarding the following:

- Their roles in auditory rehabilitation in their current positions
- Their opinions of the greatest challenges facing provision of auditory rehabilitation services
- Interview a person with hearing loss regarding their experiences with auditory rehabilitation. What types of services and hearing instruments did they receive? What aspects of the rehabilitation were successful? Which were not?

CHAPTER two

Psychosocial Aspects of Hearing Impairment and Counseling

LEARNING *objectives*

After reading this chapter, you should be able to:

1. Discuss Erikson's (1968) theory of personality development and the psychosocial impact of hearing loss and other auditory dysfunction across the life span.
2. Define different counseling approaches.
3. Describe different counseling techniques.
4. Explain how to deal with patients' resistance to getting help for hearing losses.

Hearing loss has psychological effects on patients and their significant others; it poses unique challenges at different points throughout a lifetime. Hearing loss at birth is more of an immediate psychological issue for parents than it is for the newborn. However, later on, hearing loss for a child may create barriers to forming relationships with peers. Adolescents with hearing loss may have identity issues and uncertainty about the future. A middle-aged man with a newly acquired hearing loss may have issues with his own mortality. An elderly woman with a severe sensorineural hearing loss may refuse to wear the hearing aids purchased by her adult children to protest her loss of independence. Hearing loss, whether congenital or acquired, has varying psychological and social implications across the life span. Let's check up on the Smiths and the Washingtons on their journeys with the diagnosis and management of hearing loss. As the opening vignette in Chapter 1 revealed, Charles Smith's hearing loss has become an issue with his family.

Casebook Reflection

Charles's Hearing Loss

"OK, we're all done with your hearing evaluation. I'll be in to remove the earphones," Kendra, a doctor of audiology student, said via the patient-talkback on the audiometer.

Charles, an energetic 70-year-old, was glad that he had just finished his audiologic evaluation. Charles had been dreading this appointment for weeks. He went only at the insistence of his wife, Irene. Charles reasoned that if he had an evaluation, his wife would get off of his back. Charles was a professor emeritus in the biology department at the local university, which had a speech and hearing clinic.

"Let's get these earphones off," said Kendra removing them. "Let me help you up and out of the booth and we will tell you what we've found out."

"Have a seat right here, Dr. Smith," offered Kendra with her clinical supervisor looking on. "This is your audiogram. Across the horizontal axis is frequency, or pitch. Along the vertical axis is intensity, or loudness. Those symbols represent the softest sounds that you can hear. The red circles are your right ear and the blue Xs are for the left ear. Remember we tested you with earphones and the bone oscillator?"

"Yes," Charles said.

"Well, the bone oscillator tested the inner ear directly by vibrating the bones of the skull, bypassing the outer and middle ear. The earphones sent the tones through the outer, middle, and then inner ear. Because we assessed your middle ear function and it was normal, *and* we got the same results by testing with the bone oscillator and earphones, our testing determined that you have a moderate to severe sensorineural hearing loss in both ears," Kendra explained and went on to discuss other test results.

"Do you have any questions?" Kendra asked.

"No, I don't," Charles answered.

"We believe that you're a good candidate for hearing aids," offered Kendra.

"Did my wife call you?" asked Charles smiling.

"No . . .," answered Kendra, looking at Dr. Weil for guidance.

"Why do you ask?" asked Dr. Weil.

"Well, I came in for an audiologic evaluation to please her. I don't have a problem, she does. You just tell me what hearing aids to buy and I'll be on my way."

"We'll go get some different styles of hearing aids to show you," Dr. Weil said.

Walking down the hall, Dr. Weil said, "Kendra, you let me handle this one. I need to talk to Dr. Smith about what's going on with his hearing loss, how he feels about it, and how it affects his family."

Whether Charles achieves a positive outcome depends on the acknowledgment of his loss and the management of his ambivalence toward receiving help for his problem. The situation is different in Joshua's case.

Casebook Reflection

Joshua's Hearing Loss

Debbie Washington anxiously had observed her son's auditory brainstem response test. She had been on pins and needles ever since bringing her baby home three weeks earlier, knowing he had been referred for audiologic testing following his newborn hearing screening. Joshua had slept while Dr. Elizabeth Trenoth, clinical audiologist, performed the ABR test. Debbie was concerned, as Dr. Trenoth appeared to be very serious when observing the computer screen.

"Well, we're all done. Let me remove these electrodes," Dr. Trenoth said. "Did your husband come with you?"

"Yes, he did. We were running a little late so he dropped us off at the front door to find a parking place. He must be out in the waiting room," Debbie explained.

"I'll tell the receptionist to ask him to come to my office," said Dr. Trenoth in a serious tone of voice.

"Good morning, Mr. Washington. I'm Elizabeth Trenoth. I'm your son's clinical audiologist," Dr. Trenoth said, shaking Leon's hand. "Please, have a seat."

Leon noticed the anxious look on his wife's face. He grasped her hand as he sat down.

"I performed an ABR test on Joshua today. Basically, I've looked in Joshua's ears and completed immittance testing, which checks out the conductive mechanism. The conductive mechanism is made up of the outer and middle ear. Joshua has no outer or middle ear problems," explained Dr. Trenoth.

At that moment, Debbie squeezed Leon's hand in relief as she looked over at her husband.

"I then performed an auditory brainstem response test. Basically, the earphones clicked sounds into your son's ears. The electrodes recorded how the clicks went through his auditory system, the outer, middle, and inner ear, stimulating the nerve for hearing that sends the signal up to the brain. I've repeated the test at least twice on each ear. I'm sorry, I have some difficult news, but the results indicate that your son has a severe to profound sensorineural hearing loss."

At that moment, Debbie released her hand from her husband's. It felt as if a lightning bolt had struck her body. Immediately her heart started to race, her mind went blank, and her eyes glassed over. Dr. Trenoth had seen this reaction before from parents who had received the same news for the first time.

Debbie Washington has just had a life-defining moment. From this moment on, the Washingtons' lives will never be the same. Much of who Joshua will become and how he feels about himself is affected by how his parents deal with the fact that their son has a hearing loss.

The knowledge and skills of the communication sciences and disorders professionals who serve Charles and Joshua and their families will also have an impact on the outcome of their stories. Serving patients with hearing loss and their families requires the knowledge of the psychosocial aspects of hearing loss. The purpose of this chapter is to provide a basic understanding of the psychosocial aspects of hearing loss and examples of appropriate counseling approaches to be used with patients of different ages, degrees/onset of hearing loss, and from diverse cultural backgrounds.

PSYCHOSOCIAL EFFECTS OF HEARING LOSS

The psychosocial effects of hearing loss impact personality development. Erik Erikson, a psychologist, theorized that personality develops over a lifetime and requires mastery of tasks unique to each stage of life. Hearing loss may be present at birth or may be acquired later in life, possibly impacting either development or maintenance of patients' self-concept. In addition, not only do patients have to address internal inadequacies exacerbated by hearing loss, but they must wear hearing aids, signaling their disability visibly to the public. To address these issues, we will now discuss the impact of hearing loss on personality development and the social stigma of wearing hearing aids.

Hearing Loss and Personality Development

Hearing loss may have a profound effect on patients and their family members. In Chapter 1, we discussed how the impact of hearing loss depends on degree, time of onset, and type of hearing loss. The following section presents a brief overview of how hearing loss may affect personality development. Greater detail is provided in subsequent chapters that discuss auditory rehabilitation across the life span.

Congenital Hearing Loss

The psychosocial effects of hearing loss may be understood through Erikson's model of personality development. Table 2.1 depicts Erikson's stages of personality development by age and description. According to Erikson (1968), life is a series of stages in which major tasks must be mastered, each with consequences for personality development. If a task is not mastered, then the person will have unresolved issues, negatively impacting his or her journey through life's stages. The stage for 0 to 12 months of age is Trust versus Mistrust. The major task of this stage is to learn to trust and feel secure in the world. If infants learn to trust, they have a greater likelihood of developing hopeful and self-confident personalities. If not, they may become anxious and doubtful individuals. Many factors can interfere with accomplishing a task for a particular stage in life. Neglectful parents may impact their child's ability to bond with them. The parent-infant bond sets the stage for future relationships with others. Failure to bond with caregivers may result in mistrust of the world and other people.

Congenital hearing loss, or a hearing loss that is present at birth, may also affect personality development. Even though caregivers may be out of direct sight, children with

table *2.1*   Erikson's (1968) Stages of Development

Ages	Erikson's Stage	Description
0–12 months	Trust versus Mistrust	Hopeful, self-confident versus mistrustful
1–3 years	Autonomy versus Shame and Doubt	Autonomous, proud versus self-doubt, self-consciousness
3–6 years (preschool)	Initiative versus Guilt	Creative, independent versus guilt and inhibition
6–12 years (school age)	Industry versus Inferiority	Productive, positive learning versus inadequacy, self-doubt, and inhibition
12–18 years (adolescence)	Identity versus Role/Identity Confusion	Inner solidarity, knowledge of oneself versus role confusion
18–35 years (young adulthood)	Intimacy versus Isolation	Trust, sharing versus distancing from others
35–60 years (middle age)	Generativity versus Stagnation	Mentoring, guiding new generations, nurturance versus self-absorption, preoccupation
Over 60 years (later life)	Integrity versus Despair	Sense of satisfaction, acceptance with oneself and station in life versus despair, anger

Source: Information from *Geriatric Audiology* (p. 44), by B. E. Weinstein, 2000, New York: Thieme. Copyright 2000 by B. E. Weinstein. Reprinted with permission.

normal hearing can hear when their parents are nearby. Alternatively, infants who are deaf may feel anxious when their parents are not visible. Therefore, infants with hearing loss may have more anxiety and may be mistrustful of the world. Similarly, parents of an infant who is deaf may be going through a grieving process affecting parent-infant bonding. Most parents experience an emotional reaction to the diagnosis of permanent hearing loss in their child consistent with the stages of grief, including shock, guilt, depression, anger, or anxiety (Kübler-Ross, 1969; Thibodeau, 1993). Parents may grieve for the loss of their hopes of having a perfect child. Having parents verbalize their feelings often helps them to accept their child's hearing loss (Johnson & Danhauer, 1997a). Failure to do so may result in **maladaptive behaviors**, which are destructive coping mechanisms that may interfere with parenting and auditory habilitation.

The period of 1 to 3 years old is the Autonomy versus Shame and Doubt stage. Toddlers who explore the world on their own develop autonomy and self-esteem. As a reaction to the diagnosis of hearing loss, parents may develop maladaptive behaviors and become overprotective, fearing for their child's safety and may discourage any attempts at their child's autonomy. Parents' disapproval of initial attempts at independence may elicit feelings of shame and doubt in their toddler. Dysfunctional parenting during these early years can have a snowball effect, negatively impacting the preschool years, or Initiative versus Guilt stage. Parents' overprotectiveness may create self-doubt and self-consciousness and inhibit their child's efforts in developing independence. Compounding these problems in the parent-child relationship may be an inability to communicate with each other. A willful preschool child who is deaf, with severely delayed receptive/expressive language skills, may frustrate his or her parents, who may feel that they have to rely on spanking to control behavior. The child may be punished frequently and never understand why, creating additional guilt and an inhibition of creativity and self-expression.

The child with congenital hearing loss may enter the school-age years with an enormous amount of distrust, self-doubt, guilt, and a low sense of self-esteem. From 6 to 12 years old, children go through the Industry versus Inferiority stage, growing mentally, phys-ically, and socially as well as forming attachments and identities within their peer groups (Erikson, 1968). School-age children with hearing loss and low self-esteem have language problems interfering with academic achievement and making friends. They may feel self-conscious about their hearing losses and wearing hearing aids and/or FM systems; some children may even be teased by their peers. Children with hearing loss fall farther behind their peers in academic and social development, magnifying their feelings of inad-equacy, self-doubt, and low self-esteem. They may even perceive themselves as less socially acceptable than their peers and may experience failure not only in school, but in therapy sessions with well-meaning speech-language pathologists (Cappelli, Daniels, Durieux-Smith, McGrath, & Neuss, 1995).

Children with hearing impairment and their parents enter adolescence, a turbulent pe-riod of development, at a severe disadvantage. Adolescence, ages 12 to 18 years, is difficult even for children with normal hearing and their parents. Erikson (1968) called adolescence the Identity versus Role/Identity Confusion stage during which teenagers yearn for peer approval and independence from their parents (Altman, 1996). For example, adolescents may shy away from their parents and other family members in favor of their peer groups to define themselves, developing their sense of self through the eyes of their friends. At times, teenagers may long for the security of earlier childhood, yet may want to strike out on their own without the supervision of their parents. Most teenagers emerge from adolescence with inner solidarity and self-knowledge, the necessary ingredients for the formation of in-timate relationships. Conversely, some teenagers with hearing loss enter adolescence with a low sense of self-esteem and may have difficulty finding a peer group. Teenagers who are deaf, who may not have identified with a peer group, may feel that they do not fit into the Hearing world or the Deaf world, feeling lonely and misunderstood. (*Hearing* and *Deaf* are capitalized here because they represent specific cultures in society.) Moderate sen-sorineural hearing losses are sometimes more problematic than severe to profound sen-sorineural losses because they put teenagers between two worlds, not entirely Hearing, and not entirely Deaf (Harvey, 1998). Teenagers with severe to profound hearing losses may sign and belong to a Deaf peer group. Teenagers who are hard of hearing may emerge from adolescence with role/identity confusion, not knowing where they belong.

Young adulthood, ages 18 to 35 years, encompasses the Intimacy versus Isolation stage (Erikson, 1968). Young adults are expected to seek a mate, marry, and settle down, requir-ing trusting others enough to share themselves to the extent necessary for forming intimate relationships. For young adults with a poor sense of self, this period of life may be difficult and overwhelming, especially for those who feel isolated from others. A low sense of self-esteem may prevent these individuals from reaching out, taking risks, and finding a life partner. Young adults with hearing loss also may have failed to develop their academic potential, limiting their occupational options. Therefore, auditory habitation must address more than early identification, diagnosis, and treatment of hearing loss; it should involve addressing the psychosocial needs of parents and their children with hearing loss. We will discuss the effect of congenital and *acquired* hearing loss (i.e., onset after the development of speech and language) on children and their families in Chapters 9 and 10.

Acquired Hearing Loss in Middle Age and Beyond

Acquired hearing loss in middle age presents different psychosocial effects than congenital hearing loss. With an acquired hearing loss, up until the loss develops, the adult, typically in middle age, has a well-formed sense of self as a hearing person. Adults are defined by their role in their families as husband or wife, father or mother; in the workplace; through their memberships in community organizations; their hobbies; and so on. During middle age, 35 to 60 years, adults are in the Generativity versus Stagnation stage (Erikson, 1968). The period is exemplified by peak performance levels in the workplace. The development of hearing loss is psychologically traumatic for the middle-aged individual because it represents a loss of self. It is not uncommon for these patients to go through a grieving process for the way they used to be because of the incongruence between their old reality and their current status with their hearing loss (Van Hecke, 1993). For example, a 50-year-old man who has a sudden hearing loss may perceive himself at the top of his game in life, but the painful reality of the situation may make him feel "old before his time." It is not uncommon for people in their 50s to fear being replaced at work by a 20-something young adult who is "fresh out of school." Development of a hearing loss may feed the middle-aged person's paranoia about being homeless at 60 years old. A sudden loss of function is traumatic at any time, but especially during middle age. An important accomplishment in middle age is to mentor, nurture, and guide new generations within their families, communities, and society. Development of a sudden hearing loss may result in self-absorption and a preoccupation with anxiety and doubt about the future. Patients with additional auditory dysfunction, such as tinnitus, may have even greater distress (Henry & Wilson, 2001). Gradual development of acquired hearing loss over time may also have psychosocial effects for middle-aged adults and for those in later life. Whereas acute, sudden-onset hearing loss represents a trauma, the insidious loss of hearing sensitivity over time often takes the individual by surprise. Frequently, middle-aged or older adults do not notice their loss of hearing sensitivity until it is mentioned by a friend or family member. Gradual hearing loss is problematic for the self-image of middle-aged individuals who also associate sensory impairments with old age.

Adults age 60 and up, which Erikson (1968) calls later adulthood, in the stage of Integrity versus Despair, also find hearing loss troubling. The goal of this stage is to be satisfied, accepting of one's self and station in life. Hearing loss, a chronic health condition in the elderly, can result in loss of independence. With old age comes a role reversal between parent and child. Older adults may have difficulty executing the tasks of daily living while struggling for personal dignity, and well-meaning adult children may overmanage their elderly parents. To the older adult, hearing loss and the resulting need for hearing aids are not only stigmatizing but representative of deeper issues. Battles regarding the purchase of hearing aids may be a symptom of a deeper struggle for independence by the elderly parent.

Hearing Loss and Hearing Aid Stigma

Devices to improve hearing have been used for hundreds of years. Today, they are the primary treatment for sensorineural hearing losses, although the stigma of wearing instruments—the **"hearing aid effect"**—is one of the main reasons people do not seek help. The media has contributed to the stigma by using hearing loss and hearing aids as a source of comedy. People do not like being laughed at. For nearly a century, the hearing aid industry has focused marketing campaigns on the miniaturization of companies' product lines. It has been hypothesized that the stigma was fueled by the hearing aid industry itself. As an introduction to further discussing hearing aid stigma, consider the exhibit described in the following Casebook Reflection.

Casebook Reflection

Deafness in Disguise

"Deafness in Disguise" is an online exhibit that resulted from collaboration between the Central Institute of the Deaf and the Washington University School of Medicine: Bernard Becker Medical Library in St. Louis, Missouri. The online exhibit focuses on how hearing devices were designed to be invisible or hidden by everyday objects. Visitors to the exhibit can trace technological development from the 19th century to present day and review how marketing has emphasized concealment of hearing aids. The exhibit is available at http://beckerexhibits.wustl.edu/did.

Despite technological advancements resulting in nearly invisible devices, stigma, or the hearing aid effect, is a major concern for patients and their families. Issues about the hearing aid effect may be symptoms of deeper psychosocial issues surrounding hearing loss. Parents who have not come to grips with a child's hearing loss may be overly concerned about the size of hearing aids. A teenager who has low self-esteem may not wear his or her hearing aids on a date. A middle-aged woman may not wear hearing aids at work for fear of appearing older to her boss who is downsizing the company. An important consideration, however, is the origin of stigma. Is it in the minds of patients and their families, the public, or both? A review of the research about the hearing aid effect helps to sort out these issues in an effort to guide audiologists and speech-language pathologists in providing appropriate counseling about hearing loss and hearing aids.

Early Studies

Early studies involving the hearing aid effect were done prior to the development of in-the-ear hearing aids (those that fit completely in the ear). These earlier studies used behind-the-ear and body hearing aids, which will be discussed more thoroughly in Chapter 6. Briefly, behind-the-ear hearing aids fit behind the pinna and are connected to the ear via an earmold with tubing. Body hearing aids are worn on the person and are connected to the ear via a cord, receiver, and earmold. Those studies found that the visual presence of hearing aids on an individual could elicit negative reactions from observers who had different backgrounds and experiences from those who had a hearing impairment. The observers in these studies rated photographic slides of persons with and without hearing aids. Each person in the slides was depicted in three identical photographic portraits (e.g., same facial expression and clothes), differing only in hearing aid condition (i.e., wearing no hearing aid, a behind-the-ear hearing aid, or body hearing aid). The slides were arranged into three groups in a way that each group (1) was in the same order, (2) showed each person only once and in a different hearing aid type from any other group of slides, and (3) contained the same number of slides of persons in each of the three hearing aid types.

Typically, the observers were randomly assigned to three different groups, each of which would view a different group of slides. Thus, each observer saw each subject only one time in only one hearing aid condition. The observers' task was to either rate the subject on scales (e.g., 7-point scales with a bipolar adjective at each end of a scale such as "beautiful"–"ugly") or answer open-ended questions about the person (e.g., "How old does this person look to you?"). Data collected from the studies were analyzed for significant differences among hearing aid conditions.

These earlier hearing aid effect studies concluded that some individuals may be rated more negatively on factors such as achievement, intelligence, personality, appearance, and socioeconomic status, as well as thought of as being older when wearing hearing aids than when not (Mulac, Danhauer, & Johnson, 1983). In addition, the size of the hearing aid affected ratings in that subjects were perceived more negatively when wearing a body hearing aid than when wearing a smaller behind-the-ear hearing aid or no hearing aid at all.

The hearing aid effect has been demonstrated among preschool children with normal hearing and speaking abilities who were rated by audiologists and speech-language pathologists (Danhauer, Blood, Blood, & Gomez, 1980); school-age hearing aid wearers when rated by their peers (Dengerink & Porter, 1984); school-age hearing aid wearers who had normal hearing, were hard of hearing, or deaf rated by college students (Blood, Blood, & Danhauer, 1978); and elderly persons rated by college students and their peers (Johnson & Danhauer, 1982; Johnson, Danhauer, & Edwards, 1982; Mulac et al., 1983). Observers in these studies had no prior knowledge of the individuals depicted in the slides. Therefore, their ratings were based solely on the presence and size of the hearing aids. The variety of observers used in the study showed that even speech-language pathologists and audiologists who know about hearing loss displayed negative impressions toward individuals wearing hearing aids. In conclusion, the results of these earlier studies showed that the hearing aid effect may originate in the minds of people who interact with those wearing hearing aids.

Later Studies

Even though advances in hearing aid technology have resulted in cosmetically appealing styles of hearing aids, only 20% of people with hearing loss have sought help for their disabilities (Kochkin, 1990, 1994; Kochkin & Rogin, 2001). The results of recent research were that people shy away from amplification because of how the hearing aids look or how the public may view the person wearing these devices (Johnson & Danhauer, 1997a). Kochkin (1991) interviewed 250 hearing healthcare professionals by telephone and asked, "Why don't people buy hearing instruments?" The three main reasons emerging from the survey were stigma, vanity, and cosmetics. These professionals also felt that their patients feared appearing weak, frail, handicapped, old, retarded, or ugly, or being made fun of when wearing hearing aids.

In still another study, Kochkin (1994) randomly assigned photographs of 13 styles of hearing aids that ranged in obtrusiveness from a large behind-the-ear hearing aid to a completely invisible hearing aid to 6,500 people who had a hearing loss. The respondents were asked to indicate likelihood for buying the hearing aid in the photograph and to rate it on items asking about image. Not surprisingly, people reported that they were more likely to buy the less noticeable hearing aid (e.g., high purchase intent). In addition, the smaller, less conspicuous hearing aids were rated as more technologically sophisticated than larger, more noticeable hearing aids. Kochkin concluded that in order for behind-the-ear hearing aids to reach their full market potential, the industry needed to improve the overall image of the larger instruments and that audiologists should emphasize what the hearing aids can do to improve communication rather than what they look like. Moreover, the industry should miniaturize signal processing circuitry to fit in smaller styles of hearing aids. These results indicate that the fear of hearing aid stigma affects patients' preferences for hearing aid style.

The hearing aid effect cannot be remedied only by changing public perception of hearing aids; patients' low self-esteem when wearing hearing aids must also be addressed. Doggett, Stein, and Gans (1998) surveyed older females' impressions of unaided and aided peers who read a short passage to them. Half of the respondents were told that their peer was wearing a hearing aid, and half were not. The respondents rated the aided peers more negatively on confidence, intelligence, and friendliness, but ratings were similar for the unaided and aided conditions for vocal intensity, reading time, age, and attractiveness. Furthermore, the negative ratings for the aided peers were consistent even for the respondents who did not know that their peers were wearing hearing instruments. The investigators hypothesized that the hearing aid effect in this study was attributable not only to the visual presence of hearing aids, but the negative image portrayed by the peers when wearing hearing instruments. In conclusion, the hearing aid effect may be the result of observers' negative impressions toward visual presence of a hearing aid and a poor self-image portrayed by hearing aid wearers.

Many patients may benefit from amplification, but for some reason do not want it. Obviously, many do not want others to know that they have a hearing loss, are concerned about the hearing aid effect, and so on. An integral part of an audiologist's job is to counsel patients with hearing loss on the acceptance of their disability and adjustment to possible negative attitudes from the public. Blood and Blood (1999) investigated communication partners' ratings of two male college students with hearing loss under two conditions. In one condition, the students openly acknowledged their hearing loss, spoke about adjustment, daily struggles, and so on. In the other condition, the students did not acknowledge their hearing impairment. Communicative partners rated the students more favorably on personality, employability, and adjustment when the students were open about their hearing loss than when not. Stigma about hearing loss and hearing aids may be reduced through counseling patients on acceptance of their disability and openness with others.

Patients' acceptance of their hearing loss and associated communication deficits may vary with age and the stages of life. Hearing loss may be more acceptable and even expected as people age. To test this hypothesis, Erler and Garstecki (2001) surveyed the degree of stigma related to hearing loss and hearing aid use in women from three different age groups of 35 to 45 years, 55 to 65 years, and 75 to 85 years. Women having hearing within normal limits for their ages read statements about peers and then rated the characteristics on 7-point scales that had adjectives with opposite meaning at either end (e.g., "young" versus "old"). They were told that placing a mark close to an adjective indicated their opinion for a particular statement. For example, if a mark was placed in response to the statement "She has to frequently ask for clarification of what was said" on the scale like this:

Old__ X __ ____ ____ ____ ____ ____ ____ Young,

then the respondent believed that frequently asking for clarification was a characteristic of an older person. The researchers found that stigma typically associated with hearing loss and hearing aid use declined with increasing age. In addition, all women associated hearing loss with more stigma than hearing aid use. The younger women seemed to feel more stigma with hearing loss and hearing aid use than did the older women. In other words, the older women may have felt that hearing aid use was a norm for their peer group. Similarly, Cienkowski and Pimental (2001) administered a version of the *Attitudes Towards Loss of Hearing Questionnaire* (Saunders & Cienkowski, 1996) to young adults and compared their responses to older adults with hearing loss. These investigators found that the young adults in their study did not associate hearing aids with aging or diminished cognitive functioning. However, the young adults were reticent about their own use of hearing aids if they were diagnosed with hearing loss.

In conclusion, over the past 35 years, the majority of hearing aid effect studies have demonstrated that the public tends to have negative impressions toward the visual presence of hearing aids. The finding was consistent for all ages of hearing aid wearers and observers. In addition, hearing aid wearers may feel self-conscious and portray a negative self-image that may contribute to the stigma experienced by the public (Doggett et al., 1998). Educating the public and counseling people with hearing loss and their significant others should reduce hearing aid stigma. Moreover, the stigma may also have been reduced by the recent popularity of ear-level Bluetooth® devices that resemble hearing aids.

COUNSELING

Audiologists and speech-language pathologists may have to unravel patients' and their families' issues regarding diagnosis and management of hearing loss. However, communication sciences and disorders professionals are not mental health professionals. Although audiologists and speech-language pathologists are not trained to provide psychological therapy to patients and their families, they may inform and counsel on matters directly related to their communication disorders. Sweetow (1999, p. 3) defines **counseling** as "the gathering of information through careful listening, the conveying of information, and the making of adjustments in one's strategies based on that knowledge." Therefore, it is important to understand different types and techniques for counseling appropriate in auditory rehabilitation.

General Types of Counseling

Two different types of counseling that audiologists and speech-language pathologists do are informational counseling and personal adjustment counseling. **Informational counseling** is providing information to patients and their family members, including describing how the auditory system works, explaining an audiogram, and summarizing the benefits derived from the use of amplification (English, 2002). Audiologists are successful with this technique when they meet patients' informational needs for understanding and coping with hearing loss. For instance, let's go back to the scenario involving the Washingtons, in session with Dr. Trenoth when discussing the nature of Joshua's hearing loss. Recall that the Washingtons were the young family introduced in Chapter 1 who were concerned when their son Joshua failed his newborn screening. They have just been told that Joshua has a hearing loss. The following table includes the parents' needs, conversation between Dr. Trenoth and the Washingtons, and the outcome of the exchange.

Parental Needs	Conversation	Outcome
To understand the nature of sensorineural hearing loss	**Leon:** "Dr. Trenoth, could you explain what a sensorineural hearing loss is?" **Dr. Trenoth:** "Sure, most often a sensorineural hearing loss is the result of the death of sensory hair cells. Hair cells are necessary to change hydrodynamic energy into neural impulses, which send information via the nerve to the brain, and affect hearing and balance."	MATCH: Audiologist's statement meets parents' informational need.

(Continued)

Parental Needs	Conversation	Outcome
To understand the cause of the sensorineural hearing loss	**Leon:** "What causes these types of hearing loss?" **Dr. Trenoth:** "In newborns, something may have happened during the pregnancy, particularly during the first trimester, such as a virus, the ingestion of drugs that may have been ototoxic . . ."	MATCH: Audiologist's statement meets parents' informational need.
To express fear that something she did caused her son's hearing loss	**Debbie:** "I'm a bad mother. I should have been more careful during my pregnancy." **Dr. Trenoth:** "Often, the cause of hearing loss is unknown."	MISMATCH: Audiologist's informational response does little to allay Debbie's fears.
To express deep sadness	**Debbie:** "What have I done? What have I done?" **Dr. Trenoth:** "Debbie, there's nothing about these results that suggests you're not a wonderful mother . . . What makes you think you caused Joshua's hearing loss?"	MATCH: Audiologist's use of an affective statement in reply to Debbie's statement shows that Debbie's feelings have been heard.

In the first two conversational exchanges, Dr. Trenoth's responses matched Leon's requests for information. These two incidents exemplify the concept of a **communication match** in that the needs of a patient's parents were expressed and heard in a professional interaction, then met by the explanation by the clinician (English, 2002). Clinicians' ability to meet patients' needs is a skill that must be developed over time. In the first example, Dr. Trenoth heard and met Leon's request for information. However, other patients' needs are not easily identified by clinicians and, therefore, may go unmet. A **communication mismatch** occurs when patients express needs, usually emotional, in professional interactions that are not identified and met by clinicians (English). Patients often express these needs using **affective statements** that convey their feelings about issues related to hearing loss. Identifying these statements requires a special skill known as **listening with the third ear** or the heart (English). More professionally, listening with the third ear is to be attentive to patients' affective statements that may signal social or emotional difficulties with hearing loss. These statements are rarely direct expressions of need and often go unnoticed by the clinician. Let's look at the third exchange in the previous table. Debbie's statement expressing her fear that she may have caused her son's hearing loss was not addressed by Dr. Trenoth, who responded that the causes of congenital hearing loss are often unknown. Clearly, a communication mismatch occurred, and Debbie's expressed need was not heard nor met by Dr. Trenoth.

At this point, the conversation could have gone one of two ways. It could have become one-sided, with Dr. Trenoth providing facts about congenital hearing loss and ignoring Debbie's feelings. Alternatively, Dr. Trenoth could have tuned into Debbie's needs and provided a more thoughtful response. Fortunately, Dr. Trenoth was a good listener and was able to match Debbie's second affective statement with a heartfelt response, signifying that she heard and understood Debbie's fear. **Personal adjustment counseling** is helping children cope with and solve problems caused by the secondary social and emotional effects of hearing loss. It involves patients' affective statements with appropriate affective responses showing that the clinician heard and addressed their needs (English). In this example, Dr. Trenoth switched from using informational counseling to personal adjustment counseling by matching Debbie's affective statement with an appropriate response. Effective clinicians such as Dr. Trenoth listen to their patients and respond appropriately. At this point, Dr. Trenoth can follow a process established by experienced counselors that assists patients and their families to identify, understand, and seek solutions to their problems related to hearing loss (Egan, 1998; English, 2002, pp. 8–9). The process consists of seven steps, as follows:

1. Help patients tell their stories.
2. Help patients clarify their problems.
3. Help patients challenge themselves in solving their problems.
4. Help patients set goals.
5. Help patients develop an action plan.
6. Observe patients as they implement their plans.
7. Help patients evaluate their plans.
   - Did the plans accomplish the patients' goals?
   - Is more consideration needed?
   - Did new goals emerge?

Counseling is not providing prescriptive solutions to patients' problems. Rather, it is an interactive process that occurs within the context of a professional relationship aimed at empowering patients to *recognize* and seek solutions to their own problems. The end result should be the development of patients' self-mastery over problems related to hearing loss. We will discuss this process in more detail in Chapter 10.

Another dichotomy to consider is the professional-centered versus client-centered approach to counseling. Using a **professional-centered approach**, the clinician asks the questions; is in control; has the role of diagnosing, reaching conclusions, and reporting; makes professional decisions regarding the needs of the patient and family; and leads in the decision-making process responsible for all decisions (Sweetow, 1999). The **client-centered approach**, however, is characterized by empathetic listening, unconditional positive regard, counselor congruence, and listening with concern (Sweetow, 1999). **Empathetic listening** is not only hearing what patients are saying, but being able to relate to their feelings. **Unconditional positive regard** is accepting patients and their values and decisions regardless of one's own background and values. English (2002) has commented that unconditional positive regard is accepting patients, "warts and all." It may be difficult for a young audiologist to understand why an elderly patient who survived the Great Depression feels that the cash outlay for hearing aids is not justified. Regardless of what clinicians think or feel about their patients, they should avoid expressing their negative impressions. Moreover, they should make an effort to have their verbal statements match their body language, which is known as **counselor congruence**. For example, audiologists who say to their patients that they are listening, but who look out their windows or at their watches, and ask questions that patients have already answered are not demonstrating counselor congruence.

Which type of counseling is best: informational or personal adjustment? Which approach is the best to use: professional-centered or client-centered? Unfortunately, there is not one correct answer to these questions. It depends on the situation. Each patient is different, each clinician is different, and each clinical encounter is different. In some situations, a professional-centered approach may be best. At the beginning of this chapter, Debbie and Leon Washington had just found out that their son Joshua had a profound sensorineural hearing loss. We saw how Debbie reacted with deep sadness and fear. Leon was in a state of shock. At that point, Dr. Trenoth used a professional-centered approach by taking control of the situation. She decided on what the Washingtons should do next, what referrals should be made, and so on. The professional-centered approach in this situation was very appropriate and even expected by these parents because they were immobilized by the diagnosis of their son's hearing loss, and they wanted to be told what to do, whom to see, and so on. In time, Dr. Trenoth will change to a more client-centered approach, especially when providing various treatment options for Joshua to the Washingtons.

At times, a client-centered approach is the most appropriate even if a patient wants to be told what to do. For example, Charles agreed to an audiologic evaluation at the insistence of his wife and adult children. Up until the audiologist's explanation of the results, Charles was in denial. After being shown the audiogram, Charles finally conceded to having a hearing loss but still felt that he did not have a problem. He wanted Dr. Weil to decide what type of hearing aids he should purchase, and so on. Irene was delighted with Charles's compliant attitude. Little did she know that Charles reasoned that the only way that his family would leave him alone would be if he purchased the hearing aids. In this scenario, the professional-centered approach was not appropriate because unless Charles was "on board," he would either consciously or subconsciously sabotage any auditory rehabilitation efforts, wasting everyone's time and his own resources. Effective clinicians know when to use informational versus personal counseling, when to use a professional-centered approach versus a client-centered approach, and when a referral to a mental health professional is needed.

As stated earlier, communication sciences and disorders professionals are *not* mental health professionals. Effective clinicians must know when professional counseling is needed for a patient or family. English (2002) defined **professional counseling** as mental health professionals (e.g., psychiatrists, psychologists, social workers) using their knowledge and skills to help people solve pervasive life problems. Professional counseling often involves psychotherapy and medical treatment of mental or emotional disorders. Psychotherapists may work with patients in searching for the origin of their problems by delving into their pasts and focusing on such things as familial relationships and past trauma. Alternatively, psychiatrists are physicians and mental health professionals who seek to determine medical reasons for mental or emotional disorders. Clearly, professional counseling is not within the scope of practice for either audiologists or speech-language pathologists. **Nonprofessional counseling** involves providing information and support for emotional crises that involve discipline-specific issues (English). See Table 2.2 for characteristics of nonprofessional and professional counseling.

table *2.2*   Characteristics of Nonprofessional and Professional Counseling

Nonprofessional Counseling	Professional Counseling
• Audiologist or speech-language pathologist	• Mental health professionals
• Discipline-specific	• Involves psychotherapy and/or prescription medications
• Focus on here and now	• Focuses on past experiences
• No search for causes or etiologies	• Searches for causes/etiologies
• Focuses on problem solving	• Focuses on restructuring personality

Source: Information from *Counseling Children with Hearing Impairment and Their Families* by K. M. English, 2002, Boston, MA: Allyn & Bacon.

For auditory rehabilitation, nonprofessional counseling is providing information and support for emotional issues that involve hearing loss. Audiologists and speech-language pathologists must know where their professional scope of practice ends and that of mental health professionals begins. For example, Dr. Weil may provide information on effective communication strategies for Irene to use with Charles. However, she should not provide an analysis of the Smiths' family dynamics. Similarly, Dr. Trenoth may lend a sympathetic ear to Debbie Washington, but she is professionally obligated to refer Mrs. Washington to a mental health professional for counseling should she suspect symptoms of clinical depression.

Nonprofessional counseling in communication sciences and disorders is done by non–mental health professionals (e.g., audiologists/speech-language pathologists), is discipline specific, is in the here and now, does not search for causes/etiologies, and focuses on problem solving. In other words, the focus should be on current issues directly related to hearing loss and some immediate solutions to problems. On the other hand, professional counseling is done by mental health professionals, involves psychotherapy or prescription medications, may delve into past experiences in searching for causes/ etiologies, and focuses on restructuring the personality. Clearly, audiologists and speech-language pathologists must respect professional boundaries and remain within their scope of practice.

In Chapter 4, we will discuss cross-professional competence in providing services to patients with hearing losses and their families. **Cross-professional competence** is the ability to competently execute services within one's scope of practice to a diverse patient population in a wide variety of service delivery sites in collaboration with other professionals toward positive patient outcomes. Cross-professional competence is critical for communication sciences and disorders in counseling their patients. If there is any doubt, patients with psychological and significant personal adjustment issues should be referred to a mental health professional, particularly patients who may engage in self-destructive behavior or contemplate suicide. English (2002) recommended that clinicians have a referral list available *before* patients and their families are in crisis.

It is difficult to envision how hearing loss or a related auditory disorder could lead patients to consider suicide as a solution for, or the only way out of, their problems. One such related auditory disorder is *tinnitus*, or ringing in the ears, discussed in Chapter 1. The best estimates of prevalence for patients who have frequent tinnitus range from 10.1% to 14.5% of the population (Davis & Rafaie, 2000). Erlandsson (2000) explained that tinnitus patients who believe that no one understands their illness and its annoyance are at a much higher risk for developing depression that may lead to suicide (Lewis, Stephens, & Huws, 1992). In a series of case studies involving suicide, five out of six of the patients had a specific type of the disorder, **pulsatile tinnitus**, a noise in the head that pulsates, similar to a heartbeat, and is usually vascular in origin. Audiologists who work with tinnitus patients are advised to be sensitive for signs of depression and be ready to make referrals to qualified medical professionals when necessary. And again, clinicians should have referral sources ready for immediate use.

Also important for counseling is **cross-cultural competence**, which is the ability to serve a diverse patient population and their family members in providing intervention that is both relevant to their culture yet functional in the mainstream of society. It is sometimes difficult to counsel patients from cultural backgrounds other than one's own. In some cases, patients and their family members may not feel comfortable sharing personal information with clinicians who are different from them. In this case, what can a clinician do? The best approach is to treat all patients with unconditional positive regard and accept the fact that cultural barriers may affect the rehabilitation process. Clinicians must be curious and display a genuine willingness to learn about patients' cultural backgrounds. Patients will sense the openness and may begin to develop trust, which may lead them to share their thoughts, feelings, and struggles with hearing loss with their clinicians. When necessary, audiologists and speech-language pathologists should refer patients from diverse backgrounds to mental health professionals experienced in dealing with cultural-specific issues. For example, dysfunctional family dynamics involving a teenager who is deaf and born to hearing parents should be brought to the attention of a mental health professional sensitive to issues of the Deaf culture. In the coming chapters, we will discuss cross-cultural competence required to serve diverse patient populations of different ages. In spite of these challenges, audiologists and speech-language pathologists may find the following counseling techniques helpful in facilitating clinician-patient relationships.

Examples of Counseling Techniques

Throughout the textbook, we will be discussing counseling in reference to patients of different ages in a variety of scenarios across service delivery sites. The following section provides a few examples of counseling techniques to be used with patients and/or significant others at the start of the auditory rehabilitation process.

Techniques for Informational Counseling

Do you remember everything that your physician tells you? Or do you find yourself struggling to remember details about lab results and so forth? If so, you are not alone. Margolis (2004) estimated that patients retain about 50% of the information provided to them by healthcare professionals and that 40% to 80% is immediately forgotten. Patients who retain this information are more satisfied, adhere to healthcare professionals' recommendations, and achieve better outcomes than patients who do not remember (Margolis, 2004). For example, patients' accurate recall results in lower anxiety, reduced treatment time, and lower healthcare costs (Margolis, 2004). Therefore, hearing healthcare professionals should try to maximize patients' retention of relevant information. Table 2.3 displays patient characteristics, mode of presentation, and clinician factors that can either enhance or hinder information recall.

   Patients who have some familiarity with hearing loss will retain more information than those patients with no prior experience with hearing loss. For example, a middle-aged baby boomer is more apt to remember details about the results of his own audiologic evaluation if he had accompanied an elderly parent to a similar appointment in the past. Second, patients are more likely to retain expected information rather than news that comes as a surprise. In addition, patients are more likely to remember details when in a similar mood as when they initially heard the information. For example, parents when in a sad mood may be able to remember almost everything that was said during the sorrowful day when receiving diagnosis of hearing loss in their child. Third, patients who are younger may be able to recall more information than older persons. A middle-aged son may retain more information from a family counseling session than his elderly parent retains. Fourth, patients learn more when receiving information in a moderately anxious state than in a calm or high anxiety state. Patients and their family members who are somewhat anxious may be more motivated to remember test results than those who are calm or indifferent. On the other hand, patients and family members who are in a state of high anxiety may be too stressed

table *2.3*   Factors Affecting Patient Retention of Information

	Patient Characteristics	Mode of Presentation	Clinician Factors
Assists in Retention	• Familiarity with hearing loss • Prior expectation of results • Positive results (hearing loss) • Similar emotional state when receiving information when recalling information • Younger age • Moderate anxiety level • Acknowledgement of hearing loss	• Simple, easy-to-understand format • Small amount of information • Information presented first • Categorization of information • Verbal and written information presented together • Specific information provided	• Use of simple vocabulary and sentence structure • Knowledge of patient's interests and level of understanding • Calm manner • Underscoring of important points • Sensitivity to cues signaling patient lack of understanding
Hinders Retention	• No prior experience with hearing loss • Unexpected results • Negative results (normal) • Different emotional state when receiving information than when recalling information • Older age • Stress or high anxiety • Denial	• Complex format • Large amount of information • Information that is presented last • Non-categorization of information • Presentation of information verbally or in written form only • General information provided	• Use of scientific jargon and complex sentence structure • Lack of awareness of patients' interests and level of understanding • Over-anxious manner • No underscoring of important points • Lack of sensitivity to cues regarding patients' understanding
No Affect on Retention	• Intelligence		

Source: Information from "Boosting Memory with Informational Counseling: Helping Patients Understand the Nature of Disorders and How to Manage Them," by R. Margolis, August 3, 2004, *The ASHA Leader.*

out to remember anything said by audiologists. Margolis explained that high stress causes "attention narrowing" (Kessels, 2003). Fifth, patients who are more apt to acknowledge their hearing losses remember more of what audiologists say than those who are in denial of their problems. Obviously, patients who believe what the audiologist says are more apt to remember the information than patients who do not believe that they have a hearing loss.

The manner in which information is presented may have an effect on patients' retention. Margolis (2004) has also recommended tips on the delivery of information that may increase the likelihood of patient recall. First, simple and easy-to-understand information is better remembered than material that is too complex. Second, patients retain more when small bits are presented as compared to large amounts of information. Third, patients recall information that is presented first more readily than that which is presented last. Therefore, audiologists and speech-language pathologists should present the most important information first. Fourth, patients learn more easily when facts are grouped into meaningful categories (e.g., recommendations, diagnosis, test results) than when presented in an unorganized fashion.

Margolis (2004) recommends using the **method of explicit categorization**, or defining for patients and presenting information with the topics presented in the following order:

- "We are going to go over *recommendations*;
- Then we will talk about your specific hearing problem (*diagnosis*);
- Then we will go over specific *test results*;
- We will then talk about long-term expectations or *prognosis*."

Because information that is presented first tends to be better recalled, recommendations are presented before anything else because intervention requires patients' adherence to clinicians' directives. Furthermore, briefly providing an introduction to the manner of presentation prior to delivery helps to prepare patients and their families for receiving important information. Fifth, patients remember more information when it is presented verbally *and* in written form, or possibly in pictorial form, rather than in just one format. Sixth, patients retain more when specific information is presented rather than when it is more general.

The presentation style of the clinician also may affect the amount of information retained by patients. First, information is more readily retained when presented by clinicians who use simple vocabulary and sentence structure, rather than those who use jargon and complex utterances. Second, information is more easily remembered when clinicians take into consideration patients' interests and level of understanding. Effective presentation requires gauging information so it matches patients' immediate concerns and level of understanding, but not so simple that it may seem demeaning or patronizing. Third, patients recall information more easily when presented by clinicians who are calm and who underscore important points than by those who are anxious and speak in a monotone. In summary, clinicians may improve recall of information by carefully considering factors relating to patients and their families, and adjusting their manner and style of presentation.

Techniques for Personal Adjustment Counseling

Purchasing and using hearing aids may represent a big change for a patient. Getting hearing aids may be as big a step for patients as losing weight or quitting smoking is for others. Audiologists may face the same obstacles in working with their patients as physicians do in convincing their patients that obesity and smoking are detrimental to their quality of life. Until a patient is ready to change, he or she won't get a hearing aid, lose weight, or quit smoking. No amount of badgering or persuasion will change ambivalent patients; it only makes them more resistant to change. In the previous scenario, Charles is ambivalent about getting hearing aids. The more Irene insists on her husband purchasing hearing aids, the more Charles resists, creating a vicious cycle (Harvey, 2004; Miller & Rollnick, 2002).

Harvey (2004) believes that communication sciences and disorders professionals need a psychological model of how people change in order to understand ways that clinicians can facilitate that process. He suggested that the following "wheel of change model" (Norcross & Prochaska, 2002; Prochaska, Norcross, & DiClemente, 1992), which describes stages through which patients go in solving a problem requiring change, could be helpful:

- **Precontemplation:** the stage in which patients are still in denial about their problems
- **Contemplation:** the stage in which patients are ambivalent in that they acknowledge the problem but are resistant to change
- **Determination:** the stage in which patients are more open to change than they are resistant to change
- **Action:** the stage in which patients take steps to change

- **Maintenance:** the stage in which patients must sustain their efforts to change
- **Relapse:** the stage in which patients choose not to continue the effort to change, and return to the original state

Let's take a look at how these stages apply to Charles. Before going to the audiologist, Charles was in the precontemplation stage because he was in denial about the existence of his hearing loss and communication problems. Having had an audiologic evaluation and being counseled about the type and degree of hearing loss, Charles has transitioned to the contemplation stage in which he now must acknowledge the problem, even though he still does not want to change. The more that Irene and Dr. Weil, Charles's audiologist, provide reasons why he should get hearing aids, the more ambivalent he will be toward getting amplification.

Harvey (2004) suggested using the **motivational interviewing protocol** (Miller & Rollnick, 2002) to elicit self-motivational statements from ambivalent patients who may be encouraged to change. Undoubtedly, Charles will not purchase and use hearing aids simply because his wife wants him to. Charles will not change until he is ready to do so. People cannot be externally motivated to make a permanent change; they must be internally motivated to do so. Self-motivational statements enhance patients' perception that they are using their own free will in deciding to change. Audiologists' goal should be to elicit self-motivational statements from ambivalent patients. The following four types of self-motivational statements are examples of how Dr. Weil may elicit them from Charles after showing him his audiogram (Harvey, 2004; Miller & Rollnick, 2002):

- **Problem recognition:** Signifies acknowledgement that a significant issue exists

   EXAMPLE:
   - Dr. Weil: "What problems do you seem to be having?"
   - Charles: "I didn't realize that I had that much of a hearing loss."

- **Expression of concern:** Indicates uneasiness about a particular condition

   EXAMPLE:
   - Dr. Weil: "What concerns do you have about your hearing loss and how has it affected your relationships?"
   - Charles: "I'm worried about how I argue with my wife over these issues."

- **Intention to change:** Indicates a desire to change

   EXAMPLE:
   - Dr. Weil: "If you did get hearing aids and were 100% successful, what do you think would change?"
   - Charles: "I'd really like to reduce the tension between me and my family."

- **Degree of self-efficacy:** Expresses a belief in one's ability to accomplish a goal

   EXAMPLE:
   - Dr. Weil: "What are your options for improving the relationship between you and your wife?"
   - Charles: "I believe that using hearing aids will help solve the problem."

Harvey (2004) also recommended other strategies such as using open-ended questions, reflective listening, affirmation, and circular questioning. Using **open-ended questions** allows patients to tell their story and ask for explanations rather than for answers from a select group of options (e.g., yes or no). For example, Dr. Weil may say to Charles, "Tell me what you think the problem is. . . ." **Reflective listening** is a strategy by which professionals take a guess at what the patient means by using a statement that contains the word "you" and rephrasing what the patient has already said. **Affirmations** include statements of appreciation, understanding, and compliments that validate patients. Below are some examples of uses of these strategies.

Conversation	Strategy
Dr. Weil: "Did you think your hearing loss was that bad?"	
Charles: "No, I didn't. . . ."	
Dr. Weil: "Because you came for the hearing evaluation today, do you have some issues with your hearing?"	
Charles: "Yes . . . I seem to be annoying my family, in particular my wife. She gets angry with me, but I think she purposely mumbles. . . ."	
Dr. Weil: "Let me see if I understand what you're saying.	Reflective Listening
You feel that your hearing loss annoys your wife.	
That sounds like a source of contention between the two of you. How does that make you feel?"	Open-ended Question
Charles: "It makes me feel terrible. It ruins our whole day sometimes. Just the other night, we went out to dinner. . . . I didn't hear her, misunderstood the server, and she made a big deal out of it. . . .	
I was so embarrassed. I think she sets me up so she can prove a point."	
Dr. Weil: "You look angry. Tell me about how you feel."	Affirmation/Open-ended Question
Charles: "I feel humiliated. I feel like an idiot when she does that to me. She mumbles."	
Dr. Weil: "Let me see if I understand what you're feeling.	Reflective Listening
You say that you feel humiliated when she does this in public. Your feelings are understandable. Do you really think that she 'sets you up' or do you have difficulty hearing others too?"	Affirmation
Charles: "Well, I did have difficulty understanding the server too."	

Harvey (2004) suggested another technique called **circular questioning** that probes the role of the relevant significant others in the patient's life (Palazzoli, Boscolo, Cecchin, & Prata, 1977). Harvey stated that circular questioning provides the clinician with an understanding of the family dynamics surrounding the patient and his or her auditory rehabilitation program. For example, in the Casebook Reflection on the next page, Dr. Weil uses circular questioning to find out whether others in Charles's family also have issues with his hearing loss.

Dr. Weil used circular questioning to find out about the family dynamics surrounding Charles and his hearing loss. By probing, Dr. Weil was able to learn about the underlying tensions in the family and Charles's ambivalence toward getting hearing aids. Charles's identity is that of breadwinner and head of the household. For as long as he can remember, he has been the one whom his wife, son, and daughter looked up to. Charles feels a loss of identity when his wife points out his weaknesses and his son goes to his mother for advice.

Use of Circular Questioning

Dr. Weil: "You mentioned that you're annoying your family. Who else, besides Irene, seems to be annoyed with you?"

Charles: "My son, Bob."

Dr. Weil: "Tell me about how you seem to be annoying them."

Charles: "Well, Bob only joins in after Irene starts harping about my hearing loss. Carol, my daughter-in-law, seems to be the one who tells them to lay off. I appreciate that."

Dr. Weil: "How would you feel about Irene, Bob, and Carol coming to your next appointment?"

Charles: "I really don't want them here."

Dr. Weil: "Why?"

Charles: "Irene will just make a big deal out of my hearing loss. She'll say, 'I told you so. . . . Now, let's get you some hearing aids.' Bob, will say, 'Yeah, Dad, time for you to get some help.'"

Dr. Weil: "You look really angry!"

Charles: "I am! I am a Vietnam War veteran! I'm the head of the family! I don't like being thought of as needing help. My wife and son used to come to me for help! Now, they say I need it! Bob asks Irene for advice now."

Dr. Weil: "How does that make you feel?"

Charles: "Like an old goat! With hearing aids, everyone can see I'm an old goat!"

Use of a Decisional Balance Sheet

Dr. Weil: "Charles, I believe that hearing aids could help your situation. However, I understand how you feel. Let's weigh the pros and cons of getting hearing aids. Let's write them down on this chart. On the top of the chart, let's write, 'No Hearing Aids' and 'Get Hearing Aids.' Over here, let's put 'Pros' here and the 'Cons' in this column. What are the advantages of not getting hearing aids?"

Charles: "I don't have to spend any money. People won't think I'm an old goat. I don't have to mess with them. Irene, my wife, can't say 'I told you so'!"

Dr. Weil: "Anything else?"

Charles: "No, that's about it."

Dr. Weil: "OK, what about the pros of getting hearing aids?"

Charles: "I'd hear better. Irene and Bob would leave me alone. I wouldn't miss out on conversations."

Dr. Weil: "OK, good. Anything else?"

Charles: "No."

Dr. Weil: "OK, now let's talk about the cons of not getting hearing aids."

Charles: "My wife and son would continue to be annoyed with me. I'd feel guilty about the tension I'm causing. I would miss out on a lot of what's going on."

Dr. Weil: "Anything else?"

Charles: "No."

Dr. Weil: "OK, now the cons of getting hearing aids."

Charles: "I'd have to spend some money. I'd have to buy batteries. I'd look like an old goat. Irene and my son would have 'won.'"

Dr. Weil: "Anything else?"

Charles: "No, that's it."

table *2.4*   Decisional Balance Sheet

	No Hearing Aids	Get Hearing Aids
Pros (Benefits)	1. No cash outlay 2. No stigma 3. Wife can't say "I told you so."	1. Better hearing 2. No more family hassle 3. Better conversations
Cons (Costs)	1. Family hassle 2. Guilt about prolonging tension 3. Miss out 4. Must concede defeat to Irene	1. Cash outlay 2. Cost of upkeep (e.g., battery) 3. Stigma

Source: Information from *Psychosocial Aspects of Hearing Loss,* by M. Harvey, 2004, Elkins Park, PA: Pennsylvania College of Optometry (currently Salus University).

Hearing aids represent old age and feebleness to Charles. Getting hearing aids signifies to Charles that he is an old man and no longer his wife, daughter, and son's hero.

In a sense, circular questioning had provided Dr. Weil a window to the family dynamics surrounding Charles's hearing loss and his ambivalence toward seeking help. In addition, Charles was provided an opportunity to voice his anger and fear. Charles has let Dr. Weil into his world. Now, they could try to sort out the issues surrounding his ambivalence in a collaborative manner. Harvey (2004) recommended using a **decisional balance sheet**, which is a chart that assists audiologists and patients to sort out ambivalent feelings toward change by listing the advantages and disadvantages of a decision. Table 2.4 shows a decisional balance sheet that Charles and his audiologist made from the Casebook Reflection on the previous page.

Dr. Weil and Charles have completed the matrix; now they can weigh the pros and cons of getting hearing aids. Recall that Charles is in the contemplation stage. If the pros of getting hearing aids outweigh the cons, and the cons of not getting hearing aids outweigh the pros, Charles may move into the determination stage and start auditory rehabilitation.

Techniques for Codependency Issues

We have discussed Charles's reluctance to pursue amplification. However, rarely is the spouse of the person with hearing impairment encouraged to reflect on how he or she may be contributing to his or her loved one's refusal to seek help. Irene, Charles's spouse, should consider how she may in fact be enabling Charles to not deal with the realities of his hearing loss. For example, Irene may be codependent in Charles's communication problem by constantly repeating herself or raising her voice, or being the conduit for their communication with the outside world by talking on the telephone for her husband (Carmen, 2009). By resisting the temptation to rescue her husband, Irene may help Charles recognize his need for seeking treatment for his hearing loss. Significant others must understand their reactions to hearing loss and any resentment toward their loved ones. Carmen developed a series of

INSTRUCTIONS: *The following questionnaire may help you gain clarity on your own feelings. Answer "yes" or "no" to each question.*

1. Do you feel angry that your loved one is not getting help?

    Yes   No

2. Do you think you contribute to the problem by your upset?

    Yes   No

3. Does it upset you when you have to repeat yourself?

    Yes   No

4. Do you "fill in the gaps" your loved one doesn't hear?

    Yes   No

5. Do you resent filling in these gaps?

    Yes   No

6. Do you sometimes comply with your loved one's request to avoid certain social situations because of the hearing loss, and as a result, do you resent this?

    Yes   No

7. Do you feel your loved one is vain?

    Yes   No

8. Do you believe your loved one's self-image (vanity) is more important than his need to hear?

    Yes   No

9. Do you resent this?

    Yes   No

10. Do you think your loved one feels it is more important to maintain the illusion of hearing normally rather than taking positive action to do something about it?

    Yes   No

11. Do you find yourself arguing with your loved one over issues of not hearing?

    Yes   No

12. Do you get frustrated socially when your loved one engages in conversations that result in obvious hearing problems?

    Yes   No

figure *2.1*———————————————————————

Exploring issues related to a loved one's resistance to getting help for a hearing loss.

Source: From *How Hearing Loss Impacts Relationships—Motivating Your Loved One,* by R. Carmen, pp. 52–53, Auricle Ink Publishers, retrieved from www.betterhearing.org/ aural_education_ and_counseling/articles_tip_sheets_and guides/hearing_loss_and_a_loved_ one_detail.cfm. Reprinted with permission.

questions significant others may use to examine their reactions to their loved ones' resistance to change (see Figure 2.1).

The questions focus on significant others' repetition of missed information, filling in the gaps in a conversation, and avoidance of social situations in order to rescue loved

1. Stop supporting a system of communication that does not work.

2. Set new boundaries by changing your priority in communication from needing to help him hear to managing only your own communication needs.

3. Accept the probability that he will fail in communication and that's okay because it's part of a process toward treatment.

4. If you do not remain his ears, he may find someone else to lean on. That's okay. Just don't make it wrong for him.

5. Trust yourself, maintaining your own high self-esteem without having to fall back into a cycle of hearing for him just because he expects it.

6. Control your fear—you cannot use your own fear of conflict with him as an excuse to avoid making changes that will benefit you both (because you already have conflict!).

7. Be truthful with yourself AND start being truthful with him on how his hearing problem impacts you, speaking from your heart, not from anger.

8. Give him choices, options, and helpful alternatives, but do not give him demands, threats, and consequences.

9. Be sensitive with your loved one in the way you broach the topic of seeking treatment.

10. Accept no excuses, but realize that no matter what you do, he may not change and it's not your fault.

figure *2.2*

Ten steps toward your loved one's hearing independence.

Source: From *How Hearing Loss Impacts Relationships—Motivating Your Loved One,* by R. Carmen, pp. 52–53, Auricle Ink Publishers, retrieved from www.betterhearing.org/ aural_education_ and_counseling/articles_tip_sheets_and guides/hearing_loss_and_a_loved_one_ detail.cfm. Reprinted with permission.

ones and placate their vanity and need to appear "normal." In addition, significant others are further probed regarding any resentment toward their loved ones. If significant others answer "yes" to a majority of these questions, they have significant issues to address with their loved ones. By recognizing their contributions to and their negative reactions toward the problem, significant others can help their loved ones toward independent hearing.

Significant others may need additional support in disentangling from the codependent situation. To assist with this process, Carmen (2009) suggested 10 steps for significant others to take toward encouraging a loved one's hearing independence (see Figure 2.2). The 10 steps focus on the establishment of boundaries and the need to step back from the situation to allow for the other person to fail and then grow toward finding his or her own solutions to communication problems. Significant others must resist the temptation of participating in codependent patterns of behavior and allow their partners to "hit rock bottom" if necessary. The enabler must be reminded to stand his or her ground and trust his or her own instincts and not fear conflicts arising from expectations of maintaining the status quo. The realization that people can control only their own behaviors allows enablers to eliminate their participation in codependent situations. This frees the enabler to change, regardless of what others may do. Above all, the people involved should treat each other and their decisions to change or not to change with respect. Other psychosocial aspects of hearing loss are discussed in chapters on intervention across the life span.

SUMMARY

The chapter has discussed the effect of hearing loss on personality development throughout the life span. Psychosocial issues regarding hearing loss and auditory rehabilitation have different effects for congenital versus acquired hearing loss and for patients who are hard-of-hearing versus deaf and their families. Communication sciences and disorders professionals often find themselves in the role of counselor. This chapter has compared and contrasted informational versus personal adjustment counseling, patient-centered versus professional-centered counseling, and nonprofessional versus professional counseling. In addition, the importance of cross-professional and cross-cultural competence in counseling was discussed. The chapter presented some basic counseling techniques that clinicians may find helpful when working with patients who have hearing impairment and their families as they work through some issues. In addition, some considerations were presented for how significant others can recognize and deal with their contribution to and reactions toward their loved ones' resistance to seeking treatment for their hearing losses.

LEARNING ACTIVITIES

- Develop scripted clinical scenarios in which students assume the roles of clinician and client. Have class members make cards that say "communication match" on one side and "communication mismatch" on the other side. Have them hold up the appropriate classification for each conversational turn.
- Interview an audiologist or a speech-language pathologist regarding counseling techniques the professional uses with patients who have hearing loss and their families.

CHAPTER three

Multicultural Issues in Auditory Rehabilitation

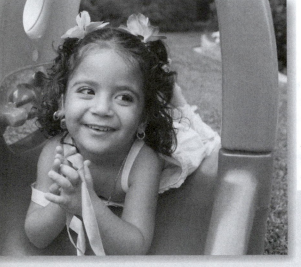

LEARNING *objectives*

After reading this chapter, you should be able to:

1. Describe the incidence and prevalence of hearing loss for persons of culturally and linguistically diverse backgrounds.
2. Describe ways that multiculturalism affects auditory rehabilitation.
3. Define important terms for cultural competence.
4. Discuss the importance of cross-cultural competence in communication sciences and disorders professionals.
5. Consider ways of developing cross-cultural competence with members of the Deaf community and other cultural and ethnic minorities.
6. Implement practices for cross-cultural competence in auditory rehabilitation.

We live in a multicultural society, and that trend is expected to increase. **Multiculturalism** is the acknowledgement that society is composed of many different groups, or **cultures**. A culture is a group of people who share a common characteristic involving race, ethnicity, gender, sexual orientation, religion, or geographic region in addition to beliefs, behaviors, traditions, and mores. Figure 3.1 shows aspects of multiculturalism.

The number of patients of culturally and linguistically diverse backgrounds requiring auditory rehabilitation is expected to grow in the coming years. The National Institutes of Health Office of Management and Budget (OMB, 1997) Directive 15 provided standards for researchers for describing participants' race and ethnicity in federally funded scientific studies, including those in auditory rehabilitation (National Institutes of Health, 2001). Minimally, scientists should define those who participate in research studies as belonging to one of two ethnic groups, Hispanic/Latino or Non-Hispanic/Latino, and one or more of five racial groups of American Indian/Alaskan Native, Asian Americans, Black/African American, Native Hawaiian/other Pacific Islander, and/or White. Remember, these are minimums, and patients and families requiring auditory rehabilitation may be much more diverse.

It is estimated that there are 308.7 million people in the United States (U.S. Census Bureau, 2010). The Hispanic/Latino population, the largest minority group, with 50.5 million people, is 16.3% of the population (U.S. Census Bureau, 2010). The Black/African American segment of the population is the next largest minority group, with 39 million members, constituting 12.6% of the population (U.S. Census Bureau, 2010). The third largest minority group is expected to be Asian Americans, with 14.7 million people, or 4.8%, of the population (U.S. Census Bureau). It is estimated that 47 million Americans speak a language other than English in their homes, and 21.4 million of the individuals have limited proficiency with the dominant language (U.S. Census Bureau, 2010). Population experts predict that by the year 2050, nearly half of the U.S. population will be composed of individuals from culturally and linguistically diverse backgrounds, of whom an estimated 6.2 million will have a communication disorder (Battle, 2002).

So when you encounter others different from yourself, do you have preconceived notions about who they are and what they are like? I think we all do. Our initial impressions of someone may be based on what someone wears, the car he or she drives, and how he or she walks, talks, and so on. We may not

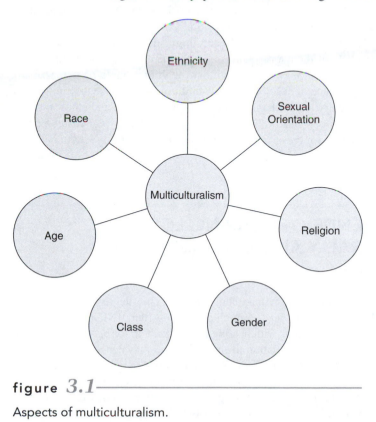

figure *3.1*

Aspects of multiculturalism.

consciously know exactly what it is that causes us to judge an individual that we have not even met yet. When we negatively judge someone without adequate knowledge or reason, we are exercising **prejudice**. Our prejudices may be based on our previous experiences or even what our parents might have told us. Some prejudice is based on strong views about the superiority of one group of people over another. **Racism** is the belief that one race is superior to another; **sexism** is the belief that one gender is superior to the other. **Ageism** is discrimination against people on the basis of their age, usually against the elderly. A less familiar prejudice is **heterosexism**, which is the belief that love relationships between a man and a woman are superior to homosexual partnerships. Most people have some prejudice; it is just part of being human. Some people can recognize their biases and ensure that those beliefs do not affect their interactions with others. When prejudice results in differential treatment of a group of people, it is called **discrimination**.

Having preconceived notions about persons who are members of racial or other ethnic minority groups and the way they communicate interferes with appropriate diagnosis and management of hearing loss. One way to overcome prejudice is to develop **cultural sensitivity**, or a willingness to learn about and address the needs of *every* patient. However, cultural sensitivity is paradoxical in that when we interact with a group of people differently based on their ethnicity, for example, we are reacting on the basis of stereotypes, even if it is with the best of intentions. A **stereotype** is a collection of characteristics attributed to a particular group. Stereotyping can be minimized by defining a **culturally and linguistically diverse patient** as *every* patient who has a distinct culture and who is influenced by gender, geographic location, age, language ability, sexual orientation, and gender identification (American Speech-Language-Hearing Association [ASHA], 2004a). However, in this textbook, we will refer to people of culturally and linguistically diverse backgrounds as those who are not members of the mainstream Anglo-European American culture.

This chapter covers multicultural aspects of auditory rehabilitation. In particular, readers will understand the importance of developing cross-cultural competence in dealing with members of the Deaf community and with persons who belong to racial and ethnic minorities. Cultural aspects of auditory rehabilitation will be presented using contemporary examples, and specific practices for cross-cultural competence will be provided for auditory rehabilitation.

INCIDENCE AND PREVALENCE OF HEARING LOSS FOR PERSONS OF CULTURALLY AND LINGUISTICALLY DIVERSE BACKGROUNDS

Approximately 17% (36 million) of American adults report some degree of hearing loss (National Institute on Deafness and Other Communication Disorders [NIDCD], 2010). As stated elsewhere, only about 1 in 5 adults with hearing loss seeks help for his or her problem. Some of the research has indicated a variation of incidence and prevalence of hearing loss based on race and ethnicity. Recall that *incidence* is the number of new cases of a disability per a given time period; *prevalence* is the number of persons afflicted per segment of the population. Countries may differ in the varieties of genetic disorders and diseases that cause hearing loss (Arlinger, 2000). It has been estimated that 14.3% of non-Hispanic White adults reported some hearing difficulties as compared with 6.1% of non-Hispanic Black and 13.9%

of Hispanic adults (Caban, Lee, Gómez-Marin, Lam & Zheng, 2005). About 2 to 3 out of every 1,000 children in the United States are born deaf or hard of hearing (NIDCD, 2010).

It has been found that 8.9% of children who are deaf or hard of hearing come from homes in which more than one language is spoken, and 10.3% are from monolingual Spanish-speaking homes (Ramkisson & Khan, 2003). The prevalence of bilateral hearing loss, including minimal degrees of loss for children, was 1.7% for African Americans, 6.8% for Cuban Americans, 2.8% for Mexican Americans, 5.8% for Puerto Ricans, and 1.5% for non-Hispanic Whites (Lee, Gómez-Marin, & Lee, 1996). For the school year 2007–2008, the Gallaudet Research Institute estimated that over 50% of deaf or hard-of-hearing children in elementary or secondary schools were from culturally and linguistically diverse populations. Approximately 30% of the children were Hispanic/Latino, 16% from Black/African American families, and 4% were of Asian backgrounds (Gallaudet Research Institute, 2009). Not only do these groups differ in what proportions have hearing loss, but also in their access to healthcare—particularly those who are from impoverished backgrounds. Many do not have access to basic healthcare when they are ill, so hearing healthcare may be a low health priority for families struggling to survive.

MULTICULTURAL INFLUENCES ON THE AUDITORY REHABILITATION PROCESS

When audiologists and speech-language pathologists enter into a clinical relationship with patients and their families, it is only natural to have some preconceived notions. Before patients arrive, clinicians may have some prejudices toward patients based merely on the name of the referral source, the patient's surname, or the location of the patient's residence. Alternatively, clinicians must realize that patients from culturally and linguistically diverse backgrounds may have no idea why they are being referred or what exactly audiologists and speech language pathologists do.

Prejudices may also develop during initial encounters between clinicians and patients. A speech-language pathologist may talk down to a family dressed in old clothing, making the assumption that they are poor and uneducated. An Asian American family may be offended by the casual dress and "laid-back" demeanor of a young Anglo-European American clinician, preferring an older, more seasoned audiologist (Greer Clark & English, 2002). Professional services and clinical outcomes may or may not be affected by these prejudices. The family may, in fact, be highly educated and offended by the patronizing clinician and go elsewhere for services. The Asian family may discount the young clinician and fail to follow through with her recommendations. Clinicians have control only over their own thoughts, feelings, and actions, and must realize that various aspects of culture such as common history, beliefs/values, customs, material culture, learning style, language, social interaction style, social organization, and so on may influence the cycle of activities in a therapeutic relationship. The cycle of activities is defined as follows and shown in Figure 3.2 (Stockman, Boult, & Robinson, 2004):

- **Referring:** providing access to clinical services
- **Scheduling:** selecting the time for a patient to receive clinical services
- **Gathering information:** obtaining patients' pertinent background information
- **Assessing:** determining the nature of a patient's hearing loss and/or balance disorder
- **Recommending:** advising and/or counseling the patient about potential treatment plans

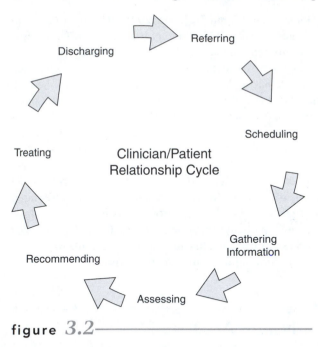

Discharging

Referring

Treating

Scheduling

Clinician/Patient Relationship Cycle

Recommending

Gathering Information

Assessing

figure 3.2

Cycle of a therapeutic relationship.

Source: Based on "Multicultural Issues in Academic and Clinical Education: A Cultural Mosaic," by I. J., Stockman, J. Boult, and G. Robinson, July 20, 2004, *The ASHA Leader.*

- **Treating:** ameliorating or lessening the impact of the patient's hearing loss and/or balance disorder
- **Discharging:** terminating the therapeutic relationship

Referral for Services

The opportunity for referral for hearing health-care services varies across the life span and for patients from culturally and linguistically diverse backgrounds. Generally speaking, access to hearing healthcare has been more restricted for them than for members of the mainstream culture. However, more than 45 states mandate universal newborn hearing screening for all babies before they are discharged from the birthing hospital as part of early hearing detection and intervention (EHDI) programs. The Joint Committee on Infant Hearing (JCIH) Year 2007 Position Statement (JCIH, 2007) recommended that hearing screening for all children should occur by 1 month of age, diagnosis of hearing loss should occur by 3 months of age, and formal intervention should be started by 6 months of age. Moreover, hearing aids are to be fit on children within one month of diagnosis. Even with these programs in place, cultural and linguistic barriers often prevent young children from getting the help they need, particularly when parents do not understand the purpose of screening, the effects of untreated hearing loss, and the importance of follow-up on referrals to appointments with audiologists and physicians. Information about EHDI programs needs to be provided to parents in their native languages at a level that is understandable. In addition, referral sources must be prepared to serve and communicate with patients from culturally and linguistically diverse backgrounds.

Appendix 3.1 contains the Program Checklist for the *Cultural Competence with Early Hearing Detection and Service Delivery Systems* that heightens awareness of agencies working with families from culturally and linguistically diverse backgrounds. In addition to linguistic barriers, other reasons that parents do not follow through with referrals include a lack of health insurance, a young age of the mother, a family with more than two children at home, and a late delivery of prenatal care (National Center on Birth Defects and Developmental Disabilities, 2006). It has been found that addressing childcare issues and transportation needs of families may improve parental compliance in newborn hearing screening programs (Isaacson, 2000).

For older children, a referral for audiologic services may begin with a failed hearing screening at school or a report from a teacher who may have noticed that a child is not attending well or is unable to follow directions. School personnel may have difficulty conveying concerns about culturally diverse children's hearing losses to parents who do not speak English. School systems should have a way of communicating with parents, including having personnel who may contact families and provide informational materials about hearing loss in the families' native languages. Many of these children live in poverty and do not have consistent access to routine medical care through a pediatrician who may also screen for hearing loss and refer to an audiologist when necessary.

Referral for hearing healthcare services for adults who are culturally and linguistically diverse may be unlikely, especially for those who do not have access to basic healthcare services. It has been estimated that nearly one-third of Hispanic/Latino and Black/African American adults have no form of health insurance (National Center for Health Statistics, 2009). Many adults forgo seeking help when they are ill, let alone when they don't hear well. Hearing loss seems to be something they are likely to cope with. One possible avenue to necessary hearing healthcare for adults who work in industry is **hearing conservation programs** designed to prevent noise-induced hearing losses. In these programs, workers have their hearing assessed every year and are referred for auditory rehabilitation if they develop noise-induced hearing loss. Workers participating in hearing conservation programs routinely are counseled on the importance of correctly wearing hearing protection devices to prevent hearing loss when in noisy environments. Rabinowitz and Duran (2001) found that workers whose first language was not English, were in non-English-speaking homes, or who were not literate in their native language or in English had a greater prevalence of incorrectly using hearing protection devices. It is important that hearing conservation programs make materials accessible and understandable to all to prevent noise-induced hearing loss. In addition, many older adults from culturally and linguistically diverse backgrounds may not have access to consistent medical care or have opportunities to have their hearing screened. Frequently, hearing screenings are conducted in long-term residential care facilities. However, fewer than 10% of residents of these facilities are of culturally or linguistically diverse backgrounds.

Scheduling Appointments

A referral usually results in scheduling an appointment with a hearing healthcare professional. Hospital staff may schedule children who fail their newborn hearing screening for appointments with audiologists before families leave the hospital. Again, parents from culturally and linguistically diverse backgrounds may not follow through if they do not know the reason for the appointment. The chances for kept appointments are better for hospital-based programs in which parents return to the same facility for the audiologic evaluation. However, many regional hospitals have community-based programs that rely on local audiologists to conduct the audiologic evaluations on babies who fail their newborn hearing screening. Hospital nurses may have difficulty scheduling these families because the hospital records do not reflect the families' current addresses or accurate telephone numbers. Danhauer, Pecile, Johnson, Mixon, and Sharp (2008) found that contact information of Spanish-speaking migrant farm workers whose babies were referred for diagnostic testing was often inaccurate, possibly due to the transient nature of this segment of the population. Moreover, these families may be fearful of returning calls in response to messages left by unfamiliar, English-speaking individuals. Danhauer and colleagues commented that hiring a bilingual receptionist improved the scheduling for Spanish-speaking patients.

Families of culturally and linguistically diverse backgrounds may value punctuality differently than mainstream culture and may be late to their scheduled appointments. Western culture values punctuality more than Hispanic/Latino, American Indian/Alaskan Native and Black/African American cultures do (Greer Clark & English, 2004). Clinicians should exercise unconditional positive regard and consider that tardiness to appointments may be due to differences in cultural viewpoints, rather than apathy or a lack of respect for the healthcare professional. Furthermore, members of extended Hispanic/Latino or American Indian families frequently attend appointments and participate in decision-making. It is not uncommon for members of the extended family to participate in caregiving, which may make determination of responsible parties difficult and may compromise patient confidentiality (Moxley, Mahendra, & Vega-Barchowitz, 2004). Also, with Western cultures, the length of a session is more clock-time oriented, lasting for a specified period of time, whereas other cultures may have more event-time orientation, with an expectation for a session to last for however long it takes to accomplish an objective or process (Moxley et al., 2004).

Gathering Information

Gathering information for the **case history** may be a challenge, particularly if patients do not have command of the English language. A case history is a form used for collecting relevant patient information in an organized fashion, which assists in planning diagnostic evaluations. Having case history forms available in Spanish and other languages that are spoken by the local community may help. However, even if the forms are in patients' native languages, the families may not be able to read or write. Another cultural barrier may be patients' reluctance to discuss personal information with professionals. Asian Americans and Hispanic Americans may be less apt to disclose personal information to strangers who may be of a different culture than their own.

Assessing

Assessment may be difficult for patients, particularly for those who do not know who audiologists or speech-language pathologists are or what they do. Patients from diverse populations may find sitting in a sound-treated booth, wearing earphones, and listening to unfamiliar stimuli a threatening experience. Unless the instructions for an audiometric evaluation are understood by the patient, the odds of obtaining a valid audiogram are poor. Obviously, patients cannot respond appropriately if they do not know what to do. Use of an **interpreter** in these instances is recommended. An interpreter is a person who serves as a conduit for communication between individuals who use different languages. We will discuss use of interpreters later in the chapter. If interpreters are not available, family members can often assist with communication. Many audiologists may find that a significant proportion of their caseload is Spanish speaking. Appendices 3.2 and 3.3 contain English-to-Spanish and Spanish-to-English translations of common words in audiology (Northrup, 2009) that may be helpful to use.

Another important part of the audiologic evaluation is speech audiometry, which includes obtaining speech recognition thresholds and scores discussed in Chapter 1. It is important to use test materials in patients' native languages for valid results. Crandell and Smaldino (2004) have labeled non-native speakers of English as "special listeners" who perform more poorly than their English-speaking peers on speech recognition tests when presented orally. Therefore, it is important to consider that poorer performance may be due to linguistic factors rather than to inherent deficits caused by hearing losses or auditory processing problems. Appendix 3.4 has the contact information for Auditec of St. Louis, which provides test materials for speech audiometry in multiple languages.

Recall that the audiologic evaluation primarily determines the type, degree, and configuration of hearing loss. In Chapters 6 and 12, we will discuss other evaluation procedures that include the impact of hearing loss through the use of **self-assessment scales** or questionnaires filled out by patients and significant others that are designed to measure the impact of hearing loss in various areas of life. These scales should be in patients' native languages so that they may clearly understand each question and provide appropriate responses. Because different cultures value communication and various activities in different ways, patients' scores on these scales should be compared with their peer groups. Dr. Robyn Cox, who heads the Hearing Aid Research Laboratory in the School of Audiology and Speech-Language Pathology at the University of Memphis, has made several of the self-assessment tools that she and her colleagues have developed available in multiple languages (see contact information appearing in Appendix 3.4).

Recommending, Advising, and Counseling

Recommending includes advising and counseling patients and families about diagnostic results and potential treatment plans (Stockman et al., 2004). Chapters 2 and 9 discuss the impact of a diagnosis of hearing loss in a child and how it affects families. Most of the research on how to break the news to parents has not involved parents from culturally and linguistically diverse backgrounds. For families who do not speak English, common sense indicates that doing so should involve audiologists who either speak their language or who use a skilled interpreter. Until research indicates otherwise, audiologists should follow the same suggestions provided by English (2002) for breaking the news of diagnosis of hearing loss in a child as discussed in Chapter 9. Briefly, audiologists should select a quiet place, schedule ample time, avoid any interruptions, and be responsive to parents' needs when breaking the news. They should follow the parents' lead in what and how much information to provide. Parents are apt to be in shock, and reactions to stress vary greatly among different cultural groups.

Regarding counseling adult patients, it is probable that patients from culturally and linguistically diverse backgrounds remember even less than 50% of what audiologists tell them if the information is presented in their non-native language. Therefore, clinicians should be more diligent in following Margolis's (2004) tips for informational counseling provided in Chapter 2. Avoiding jargon, using simple structure, and checking comprehension can go a long way in evaluating whether patients have enough information to be able to comply with recommendations for treatment.

Audiologists should be advised that individuals from culturally and linguistically diverse populations may not follow recommendations in a timely manner or even at all. Audiologists may strongly recommend to parents that their infants diagnosed with sensorineural hearing loss be fit with amplification within one month of diagnosis. Hispanic/Latino or American Indian/Alaskan Native parents may not feel the same sense of urgency for habilitation, or may even prefer to use alternative healing systems (Moxley et al., 2004). Audiologists may also be more mystified when parents do not follow through even when the parents seemed to be in complete agreement with recommendations during the counseling session. Some Asian and Hispanic/Latino cultures hold healthcare professionals, such as audiologists, in such high regard that they consider disagreeing with the professional disrespectful (Moxley et al., 2004).

Treating

In Chapter 1, the auditory rehabilitation model introduced four areas of auditory rehabilitation to include sensory aids; instruction, demonstration, and coaching; perceptual training; and counseling. Sensory aids include devices such as hearing aids, hearing assistive technology, and cochlear implants, which may be affected by culture in a number of ways. Patients who are members of minority groups may not have had as much exposure to hearing aids or hearing assistive technologies as members of the mainstream culture. Minority patients are less likely to have had a family member or friend who has used these devices (Wolf, 2004). Moreover, members of some cultural groups may feel that hearing loss does not need treatment because it is a normal part of aging (Wolf, 2004). African Americans and Hispanic/Latino Americans are less likely to use hearing aids and hearing assistive technology than Anglo-European Americans (Lee, Carlson, Lee, Ray, & Markides, 1991; Lee, Gómez-Martin, & Lee, 1996; Kaye Yaeger, & Reed, 2008). Black/African Americans are less likely to stigmatize their peers who wear hearing aids than their Anglo-European American counterparts (Davis, Jackson, Smith, & Cooper, 1999). Some cultures may view purchasing hearing assistive technology for watching television a waste of money. Other cultures may value independence and may view use of hearing assistive technology as a sign of weakness and stigma. Public health campaigns should be directed toward these groups about the insidious effects of untreated sensorineural hearing loss and the benefits from amplification (Chisolm et al., 2007). Moreover, patients who do not speak English need to be counseled and receive written information about the pros and cons of cochlear implants in their native languages. Patients cannot provide informed consent unless they fully understand the risks and benefits of treatment. Another cultural issue regarding cochlear implants is acknowledging the feelings of the Deaf community toward these devices for children. We will discuss more of this issue later in the chapter.

Instruction about, demonstration of, and coaching for the use of hearing aid and hearing assistive technology may be compromised if the delivery of those devices is not in the native language of patients and their families. Culture may also influence group hearing aid orientation sessions, mentoring, and counseling dynamics because patients of culturally and linguistically diverse populations differ in their willingness to discuss personal issues with strangers. Individuals of Asian backgrounds and their families may not feel comfortable discussing communication issues with others. Moreover, perceptual training may need to be conducted by clinicians who are native speakers because each language differs in its understandability by persons with hearing impairment (Arlinger, 2000). Audiologists may need to recommend patients from diverse backgrounds to other professionals for culturally specific and appropriate standards of care.

Discharging

Discharging is terminating the therapeutic relationship. Ideally, discharging is the result of patients and their family members achieving their goals through auditory rehabilitation. Discharging technically does not terminate the relationship permanently because patients with hearing loss need annual reevaluations and hearing aid checks. It is important to note, though, that patients from culturally and linguistically diverse backgrounds may have different expectations and goals than those recommended by the audiologist or speech-language pathologist. Some skills necessary for the mainstream culture may not be relevant in others. Clinicians should not be offended if these patients do not take part in or continue with all recommended treatment sessions for cultural reasons. For example, an elderly Asian American woman's adult children may feel that those hearing aid orientation sessions teaching their mother how to take care of her hearing aids are not necessary because the mother lives with her extended family, who attends to her every need.

DEVELOPING CROSS-CULTURAL COMPETENCE

Unfortunately, more often than not, clinician/patient relationships are affected by **egocentrism**, or the negative attitudes that arise when a person's culture is compared with someone else's. Egocentric individuals believe that the beliefs, behaviors, traditions, and mores of their own culture are the standard by which all others are to be compared. Egocentrism on the part of the clinician or patient can affect clinical outcomes, but may be overcome with a willingness to develop cultural sensitivity, or a willingness to learn about other people and their culture. An openness to others different from oneself is the first step toward **cross-cultural competence**, or the ability to understand the origin of one's bias (e.g., personal history), but yet establish a common ground with patients from diverse backgrounds.

Lynch and Hanson (1997) believed that the development of cross-cultural competence requires five basic tasks. Clinicians first must develop an understanding of their own cultural, ethnic, and linguistic backgrounds in addition to their presuppositions about others who are different from themselves. That is, insightful clinicians must develop a keen self-awareness of their biases and how they impact interactions with others. Second, clinicians must realize that although everyone is influenced by their cultural, ethnic, and linguistic backgrounds, those conditions do not fully define the individual. Effective clinicians know that each patient is a unique human being, unlike anyone else. Third, clinicians must acknowledge that culture is dynamic and always changing at local, state, and national levels, requiring a proactive approach in meeting the needs of an ever-changing diverse patient population. This requires that clinicians expand their knowledge and skills to meet the changing demographics of the patient population. Fourth, clinicians must meet two responsibilities to their patients. One is to transcend cultural boundaries to understand what strategies and solutions are appropriate within the patient's culture. The second responsibility is to assist the patient and his or her family members to negotiate the mainstream culture, which may be new and threatening to them. Fifth, clinicians must recognize that all interactions and interventions take place in a larger sociopolitical context. Cross-cultural competence requires keeping up-to-date with multicultural issues in healthcare and auditory rehabilitation.

The development of cross-cultural competence is often met with five obstacles cited by Lynch (1997a, 1997b) as stated by Guthrie (1975). First, understanding of a person's first culture occurs in early childhood and is established by age 5. Old habits and ways of thinking are hard to change. Clinicians may find it difficult to overcome long-standing prejudices learned in childhood; patients and their families who have recently immigrated to the United States may find it difficult to adapt to the dominant culture. Second, children adapt to and learn new cultural patterns more easily than adults. For example, children may easily acquire the language of their new country while their parents struggle with even the simplest words and phrases. Third, a person's values are determined by his or her first cultural experiences and may need to be changed to be effective in a second culture. This could explain why children might easily adapt to school in their new country while their parents might have difficulty establishing relationships with others at work. Fourth, ideas about a person's first culture introduce bias in interpreting a second culture, necessitating challenging previously held stereotypes in order to effectively serve members of minority groups and their families. Fifth, a person's long-standing behavior patterns are used to express his or her deepest values, requiring insight into knowing how their backgrounds influence their thoughts, beliefs, and interactions with persons from other cultures.

Clinicians serving diverse patient populations may experience **"culture shock,"** which has been defined as a series of disorienting encounters when a person's basic values, beliefs, and patterns of behavior are challenged by another culture (Lynch, 1997a, 1997b). Americans often experience culture shock when visiting a foreign country for the first time where the people may speak only inches away from their communicative partner's face. Even traveling to another part of the United States (e.g., a New Yorker visiting Memphis) or to a different neighborhood in one's city (e.g., a native San Franciscan visiting Chinatown) may result in culture shock. Similarly, providing services to members of cultures other than one's own can result in culture shock.

Some healthcare professions require more cross-cultural competence than others. Communication sciences and disorders specialists require a greater degree of cross-cultural competence than optometrists who assess visual acuity, prescribe and fit eyeglasses, and send the patient home, often without need for extensive follow-up. Audiologists and speech-language pathologists, on the other hand, assess and remediate patients' communication abilities, which are deeply rooted in their native cultures. Similarly, psychologists, assisting patients with adjustment issues and interpersonal relationships, comprise another group of professionals requiring cross-cultural competence. Students may ask, "How do I develop cross-cultural competence?" The professional odyssey of Dr. Michael Harvey, psychologist, described in the following Casebook Reflection, is an excellent example of the development of cross-cultural competence required to work with patients from different cultures.

Casebook Reflection

Meet Dr. Michael Harvey

Dr. Michael Harvey is a clinical psychologist with a private practice in Framingham, Massachusetts, specializing in serving patients having hearing loss whose primary culture may be hearing, Deaf, or both. He has written three books on the psychosocial aspects of hearing loss. In his work, Dr. Harvey describes people with hearing loss from the hearing world as having acquired hearing loss, or as being hard of hearing, deafened, hearing impaired, or deaf. On the other hand, he describes those who are members of the Deaf culture as being born deaf, or culturally deaf, and as using American Sign Language.

Dr. Harvey's interest in the Deaf community began when he enrolled in an American Sign Language (ASL) course as a hobby. His interactions within the Deaf world were similar to beaming down to another planet that was very different from his own. He experienced culture shock that challenged his basic values, beliefs, and patterns

of behaviors as a hearing person. Dr. Harvey's development of cross-cultural competence began with an understanding of the history of oppression of deaf people manifested by job discrimination, bigotry, negative stereotyping, and humiliation by the mainstream culture. Furthermore, he used his cultural background of being Jewish as a conduit for reaching a common ground with the Deaf community. Although having never experienced any significant degree of oppression, Dr. Harvey had indirectly been affected by the Holocaust and anti-Semitism. He questioned what the Jews and Germans, their oppressors, needed from each other to go on in peace. He surmised that Jews needed empathy and an emotional validation, or acknowledgement, of the pain they had endured at the hands of Germans. On the other hand, the Germans needed the Jews to understand that not all of their countrymen were responsible for the Holocaust. Similarly, Dr. Harvey believes that members of the Deaf community need similar understanding from the members of the hearing community in order to heal their emotional wounds. Likewise, members of the Deaf community should not hold all hearing persons responsible for the oppression experienced in the mainstream culture. By developing cross-cultural competence, Dr. Harvey effectively counsels persons with hearing loss who are "caught between two worlds" of the hearing and Deaf communities.

Communication sciences and disorders professionals must develop cross-cultural competence to provide relevant interventions for patients and their families who are functional both in their primary and mainstream cultures. Cultural competence includes recognizing racial, ethnic, and/or linguistic effects on service delivery and being knowledgeable of those differences, but yet responsive to the varied needs of a diverse patient population (ASHA, 2004a). In particular, effective auditory rehabilitation requires clinicians to develop cross-cultural competence with both the Deaf community and with members of different racial and ethnic groups.

Developing Cross-Cultural Competence With the Deaf Community

Students in communication sciences and disorders approach the pursuit of providing services to the 30 million Americans with hearing loss with the best of intentions. The majority of those with hearing loss, and their families, welcome the habilitative and rehabilitative efforts of audiologists and speech-language pathologists. However, note the dismay of a young audiologist counseling the deaf parents of a newborn with profound hearing loss in the following Casebook Reflection.

Casebook Reflection

A Puzzled Audiologist

Husband and wife George and Wilma Jeffcoat are deaf and use American Sign Language (ASL). They met as teenagers at the state school for the deaf and blind. They fell in love and married after George completed his studies at Gallaudet University. Mr. and Mrs. Jeffcoat had made an appointment at Dr. Gloria Garcia's audiologic practice for follow-up testing for an audiologic evaluation of their son, William. The Jeffcoats had been accompanied by an oral interpreter. The discussion that follows is through the interpreter. Dr. Garcia had just completed the testing of William, who slept in his car seat while his parents sat in a room nearby. After analyzing the results of the evaluation, Dr. Garcia took a deep breath and asked the Jeffcoats to join her in her office with their interpreter.

"Mr. and Mrs. Jeffcoat, I'm afraid I have some difficult news. The results of testing revealed that your son has a severe to profound hearing loss," explained Dr. Garcia, who was ready with a box of tissues.

The Jeffcoats smiled at each other and at William, who was fast asleep in his mother's arms. "We couldn't be more proud of him! Thank you, Dr. Garcia, for your help. We'll be leaving now," said Mr. Jeffcoat as he gathered the family's belongings.

"Mr. Jeffcoat, do you have any questions? I'd like to schedule a follow-up appointment to discuss an intervention plan for William including the use of hearing aids and early intervention services," explained Dr. Garcia.

"No, thank you. Our son is deaf and we will not need your services right now. He will learn to use sign language," insisted Mr. Jeffcoat. "We would like to pay our bill and go home. Thank you again."

Dr. Garcia stood in the hallway as the Jeffcoats paid their bill, waved good-bye, and left calmly, even happy with the diagnostic outcome. Dr. Garcia wondered what kind of struggles the Jeffcoats had faced in their lives due to their deafness. How do they feel about their son facing those same obstacles? Why were they not interested in learning about communication options for their child?

Indeed, Dr. Garcia had no idea why William's parents did not seem concerned about the results of the audiologic evaluation and were not interested in her recommendations of amplification and early intervention.

The Jeffcoats, like some members of the Deaf community, believe that communication sciences and disorders professionals have a two-fold agenda to (1) mitigate a disability and (2) eradicate Deaf culture (Lane, Hoffmeister, & Bahan, 1996). Some members of the Deaf community believe that audiologists and speech-language pathologists view persons with hearing loss as having a disability that presents obstacles to employment and full participation in a hearing society (Lane et al., 1996). Communication sciences and disorders professionals, pediatricians, special educators, welfare workers, and other professionals lobby on behalf of persons with hearing impairment at local, state, and federal governments for funds to help mitigate the disability of hearing loss. However, the Deaf community rejects the **medical model of deafness**, which classifies those with hearing loss as "sick" individuals trying to get well. Furthermore, some individuals believe that efforts to prevent hearing loss through genetic counseling and the cochlear implantation of young deaf children are methods used for eradication of the Deaf culture (Lane et al., 1996).

The cultural and linguistic minority of the Deaf world, organizations of culturally Deaf adults in the United States and abroad, as well as the World Federation of the Deaf believe that the benefits of pediatric cochlear implantation are unproven, and that psychological, social, and linguistic risks have not been fully assessed in clinical trials (Lane & Bahan, 1998). Furthermore, in 2000, the National Association of the Deaf (NAD) published a position paper that focuses on preserving the psychosocial integrity of adults who are hard of hearing or deaf. The aim of the position statement was for hearing loss to be viewed from a **"wellness model of deafness,"** and not as an impairment to be treated, and as a different culture, rather than as a group with a disability.

The beliefs and indifference experienced by Dr. Garcia are shocking to audiologists and speech-language pathologists when they first encounter them. Indeed, Dr. Garcia experienced a heavy dose of culture shock when counseling William's parents. However, if clinicians seek to understand the Deaf community, a common ground may be achieved in meeting the needs of deaf children and their families. Understanding begins with learning about the history of the oppression of the Deaf by mainstream society. Knowledge of these injustices can assist hearing healthcare professionals to be empathetic to the initial suspicions of members of the Deaf community and their need for medical professionals, including speech-language pathologists and audiologists, to view Deaf culture as a viable option for children with deafness and their families. For example, NAD (2000) recommended that members of the medical community refer these families to "qualified experts" in deafness to be exposed to role models and receive information about the history of deafness and deaf people. Furthermore, communication sciences and disorders training programs should educate future professionals on a "wellness" model of deafness, rather than one of disability.

Developing Cross-Cultural Competence With Racial and Ethnic Minorities

The majority of speech-language pathologists and audiologists have Anglo-European roots despite strong efforts of the American Speech-Language-Hearing Association and the American Academy of Audiology to increase the racial and ethnic diversity of the professions. As stated earlier, cultural sensitivity begins with a willingness to learn about others. It is impossible to learn everything there is to know about other cultures, but it may help to compare and contrast cultures on general aspects of interpersonal relationships such as greetings and tips for visiting someone's home. Table 3.1 compares and contrasts the manner of greeting and tips for visiting the homes of patients of

table *3.1*   Greetings and Customs for Interacting Among Various Racial and Ethnic Groups

Ethnic or Racial Group	Greetings	Customs for Interaction or Visiting
Anglo-European American	• Warm, firm handshakes with direct eye contact is expected. • An arm's length is considered one's personal space that should not be violated. • Males usually shake hands with males, although there are no rules against women shaking hands with men or young persons shaking hands with the elderly. • Turn-taking during conversation is important. • Personal topics, personal self-disclosure, and controversial issues are avoided.	• Punctuality is expected. • Direct, face-to-face communication is expected. • Personal opinions are expressed openly.
African American	• Address by surnames and title (e.g., Mr., Mrs., Miss, etc.) unless permission is granted to use first names.	• Avoid telling the family that they are touchy about racial issues. • Avoid racial jokes even about one's own culture. • Avoid stereotyping African American families. • Don't talk with coworkers about personal matters. • Don't judge family function by socioeconomic status.

(Continued)

table *3.1* (Continued)

Ethnic or Racial Group	Greetings	Customs for Interaction or Visiting
Asian American	• Address by surname. • Avoid prolonged eye contact. • Avoid physical touching. • Greet family members from oldest to youngest. Handshaking • Only males shake hands. • Youngsters do not shake hands with elders.	• Avoid personal questions during initial contact. • Remove shoes when entering the home. • Sit with feet flat on the floor and hands folded in your lap. • Accept food or drink if offered. • Demonstrate emotional restraint.
Latin American	• Speak to husband before the wife if both are present. • Use a calm tone of voice. • Initial "small talk" is important for establishing rapport. • Provide background about what can be expected in future interactions.	• Respect cultural artifacts/rituals and their importance to the family. • Don't rush or be impatient, which shows disrespect. • Don't be too direct. • Build interpersonal relationships. • Sit with good posture. • Avoid the term "illegal alien"; use the term "undocumented immigrant" instead.
Middle-Eastern American	• Personal space or social distance is shorter than for Anglo-European Americans. • Men may kiss other men on the cheek upon greeting. • Women may exchange hugs and/or kisses upon greeting. • Avoid direct or assertive communication.	• Remove shoes when entering the home unless family does not. • Accept food and/or drink if offered and partake in the hospitality. • Do not sit with your back to an adult who is present. • Sit with legs up or crossed in front. • Stand when new guests arrive, particularly the elderly.
Native American	• Initial "small talk" is important for establishing rapport. • Provide background about what can be expected in future interactions.	• May not answer knocks at the door or doorbell. • Ask whether an appointment is convenient (scheduling a time may not be as good). • Ask family where they would like you to sit. • Family members may come and go from the home. • Confidential topics may best be handled in the office. • Accept food and/or drink and partake in the hospitality. • In rural areas, unscheduled visits should be signaled by a honking of a car horn.

Source: Information from *Developing Cross-cultural Competence: A Guide for Working with Children and Their Families* (2nd edition), by E. W. Lynch and M. J. Hanson, 1997, Baltimore, MD: Brookes.

Anglo-European descent with those of other racial and ethnic backgrounds. For example, Anglo-European Americans typically greet each other warmly with a firm handshake and strong eye contact with no particular order regarding persons to be acknowledged first (Hanson, 1997). Alternatively, members of other racial and/or ethnic groups may be offended by the Anglo-European American style. Asian Americans acknowledge persons in order of age (i.e., oldest to youngest), by appropriate title (e.g., Mr., Mrs., Miss, etc.), with men shaking hands only with men, and youngsters not shaking hands with elders, preceded with a slight bow and avoidance of direct eye contact (Chan, 1997).

Developing cross-cultural competence is paradoxical in that placement of groups of people into broad racial and/or ethnic categories in Table 3.1 promotes stereotyping and the notion that people can be placed into six categories of Anglo-European American, African American, Asian American, Latin American, Middle-Eastern American, or Native American. Although characteristics of these groupings may be accurate, they rarely apply completely to an individual patient (Moxley et al., 2004). Readers should be advised that within each category is rich diversity. For example, African Americans as a group have great diversity in their values, lifestyles, and cultural preferences and constitute a community of three distinct ethnic groups: (1) those born in America, (2) those born in the Caribbean, and (3) those born in Africa (Willis, 1997).

The other categories represent even more diverse groups. For example, Asian Pacific Americans, the fastest growing ethnic group in the United States, includes more than 60 separate groups, with the vast majority originating from three different immigrant groups: (1) East Asia (i.e., China, Japan, and Korea), (2) Southeast Asia (i.e., Burma, Cambodia, Indonesia, Laos, Malaysia, the Philippines, Singapore, Thailand, and Vietnam), and (3) South Asia (i.e., Bangladesh, Bhutan, India, Pakistan, Nepal, and Sri Lanka) (Chan, 1997). Similarly, the Latin American population is extremely diverse and includes persons of Mexican, Puerto Rican, Cuban, Central American (e.g., Salvadoran, Guatemalan, Nicaraguan, Honduran, Panamanian), South American (e.g., Brazilian, Colombian, Ecuadorian, Peruvian), and Caribbean origins (Zuniga, 1997). Middle-Eastern Americans are difficult to define because they consist of a complex combination of historical, religious, linguistic, racial characteristics, and geographical origins in Asia and Africa including Lebanon, Syria, Israel, Palestine, Bahrain, Egypt, Iran, Jordan, Kuwait, Oman, Qatar, Saudi Arabia, Sudan, Turkey, the United Arab Emirates, and Yemen (Sharifzadeh, 1997). In addition, the term "Middle East" is a cultural term used to describe society and civilization found in segments of countries adjacent to the preceding geographical areas such as Afghanistan, Algeria, Cyprus, Libya, Morocco, Pakistan, and Tunisia; countries of Central Asia (e.g., Kazakhstan, Kyrgyzstan, Tajikistan, Turkmenistan, and Uzbekistan); and the newly independent countries of Armenia, Azerbaijan, and Georgia in the Caucasus region (Sharifzadeh). Finally, Native Americans reside in every state and in most major American cities in the United States and comprise more than 500 distinct tribal groups and villages, which are frequently grouped regionally (e.g., Northeastern and Southwestern) and are quite diverse (Joe & Malach, 1997). In summary, the United States is a melting pot of diverse cultures, each of which has its own geographical and historical origins that influence contemporary life. The racial and ethnic backgrounds of communication sciences and disorders professionals and those of patients and their families can and do affect service delivery in auditory rehabilitation.

TOWARD CROSS-CULTURAL COMPETENCE IN AUDITORY REHABILITATION

Are there any guidelines for audiologists, speech-language pathologists, and other healthcare providers in working with patients from culturally and linguistically diverse backgrounds? The Office of Minority Health of the U.S. Department of Health and Human Services developed National Standards on Culturally and Linguistically Appropriate Services (CLAS) for health management organizations. The principles of that document appear in Appendix 3.5 and can serve as a guideline for audiologists and speech-language pathologists who serve patients from culturally and linguistically diverse backgrounds. Note that the recommendations are not just for clinicians providing services, but everyone within a healthcare facility interacting with patients and families. So principles of cross-cultural competence extend to the front office staff of a private practice, to nurses in a hospital. Obviously, healthcare providers cannot meet these standards for all patients, but they should try for at least significant proportions of the local community. In many areas of the country, a significant proportion of the population is Spanish speaking, and many clinicians are unable to provide services competently to these patients and their families. Quite some time ago, Flores, Martin, and Champlin (1996) surveyed audiologists in Arizona, California, Colorado, New Mexico, and Texas and found that 52% were unable to provide services in Spanish using their own linguistic abilities. The majority of these audiologists used interpreters in some clinical situations. Interpreters can be family members, office staff, or audiology or speech-language pathology assistants. Use of interpreters may assist in information gathering, giving instructions, and relaying test findings to patients and their family members (Ramkissoon & Khan, 2003). Moreover, the use of interpreters provides additional nontangible benefits such as sharing patients' cultural and/or ethnic backgrounds and facilitation in establishing trust in the clinical interaction (Ramkissoon & Khan, 2003).

Successful utilization of an interpreter requires adequate preparation prior to the patient's arrival such as selecting the interpreter, meeting prior to the session, and reviewing postsession issues. Figure 3.3 has suggestions for each stage of the process. Selection of an interpreter requires consideration of multiple factors. First, interpreters should be selected on the basis of their proficiency of English and the minority language. The interpreter needs to be able to accurately describe the type, degree, and configuration of a hearing loss, and audiologists' recommendations. Alternatively, for example, the interpreter should relay parents' concerns regarding their child's hearing loss. Second, clinicians should consider the interpreter's educational background and prior experiences. Has the interpreter had any educational background in health sciences or experience translating in similar situations? Third, clinicians should contrast interpreters' communication styles with their own. Do they feel comfortable and at ease working with the prospective interpreter? Will patients and their family members feel the same way? Once an effective interpreter has been selected, it is advisable to use his or her services on a long-term basis to establish rapport and increase the efficiency of information transmission. Please refer to Appendices 3.2 and 3.3 at the end of the chapter for common phrases used during audiologic evaluations translated from English to Spanish and Spanish to English, respectively.

Fourth, audiologists and speech-language pathologists should plan well in advance of the session and meet with interpreters, particularly those who may require extra time

Selecting an Interpreter

- Determine the interpreter's level of proficiency in English and the minority language.
- Assess the interpreter's educational background and experience.
- Be aware of the interpreter's communication style.
- Try to use the same interpreter for multiple assignments so that you may establish a familiar working relationship.

Prior to the Session

- Meet with the interpreter in advance to allow adequate preparation time.
- Review the goals and procedures of the test and/or treatment materials.
- Ensure that the interpreter understands your confidentiality policies.
- Explain that the oral interpreter will need to limit nonverbal cues, such as hand gestures and vocal variation, that may impact assessment results.
- Review test validity and reliability to ensure that the interpreter understands the need to avoid unnecessary rewording of testing prompts.
- Establish a rapport with the interpreter.
- Remind the interpreter to take notes on the patient's responses.
- Learn greetings and the appropriate pronunciation of names in the family's primary language or signs.

During the Session

- Introduce yourself (as the speech-language pathologist or audiologist) and the interpreter in the patient's native language if possible.
- Describe your roles and clarify expectations.
- Ensure that the interpreter is taking notes.
- Use short, concise sentences.
- Pause frequently to allow the interpreter to translate information.
- Allow enough time for the interpreter to organize the information for effective translation.
- Periodically check with the interpreter to see if your speech is too fast or too slow, too soft, or unclear.
- Understand that words of feeling, attitude, and qualities may not have the same meaning when directly translated.
- Talk directly with your patient.
- Be aware of nonverbal body language and gestures that may be offensive to the family's culture.
- Avoid oversimplification of important explanations.
- Provide written materials in the family's native language whenever possible.
- Build in extra time for the session.

After the Session

- Review the patient's errors.
- Ensure that the interpreter reports the patient's response as well as the anticipated response.
- Avoid use of professional jargon.
- Discuss any difficulties in the testing process.
- Discuss any difficulties in the interpretation process.

figure *3.3*

Suggestions for using an interpreter.

Source: From *Tips for Working with Interpreters,* by the American Speech-Language-Hearing-Association, 2006, retrieved from www.asha.org/practice/multicultural/issues/interpret.htm. Reprinted with permission.

understanding the nature of the testing or subtle nuances of a particularly complicated case. Clinicians should review the goals and objectives of the evaluation or treatment session with interpreters and remind them, for example, not to ask leading questions when interviewing parents. Fifth, interpreters need to understand that any information or communications that occur in the clinical milieu are strictly confidential. If interpreters are involved in testing, they should be reminded to minimize nonverbal cues (e.g., hand gestures and/or vocal variations) that may impact assessment results. Sixth, clinicians should review the importance of validity and reliability of specific tests necessitating the need for following specific protocols. Interpreters may be more cooperative if they know the rationale behind having to comply with detailed instructions. Seventh, because interpreters are often family members or may even be volunteers, it is important to establish a comfortable rapport with them so that they may be more apt to go the extra mile such as taking notes of patients' responses. Alternatively, clinician-interpreter relationships are based on give-and-take; clinicians must also reach out to interpreters by learning greetings and the correct pronunciation of patients' and their family members' names. Adequate preplanning should increase the likelihood of having a successful session.

At the beginning of the session, the clinician should introduce him- or herself and the interpreter in the patient's native language. It is important to clarify the roles and expectations of the clinician and the interpreter. The clinician is the professional, and the interpreter is the conduit for information transmission. Clinicians' style of communication should include use of short, concise sentences, pausing frequently for an organized translation of information. Periodically, clinicians should unobtrusively check on the appropriateness of their use of words and rate of speaking and make adjustments accordingly. Clinicians should speak directly to patients and their family members avoiding any body language and/or gestures that may be culturally offensive. It is important for clinicians not to be patronizing by oversimplifying information or explanations. And as usual, these patients and their families are not going to remember everything that has been said. Interpreters should be encouraged to follow Margolis's (2004) suggestions for improving patients' recall of information, which we reviewed in Chapter 2 (see Table 2.3), in addition to providing written materials summarizing important information in the patients' native languages.

After the session, clinicians should review with interpreters what they thought went well, what could have been better, and suggestions for future sessions. Likewise, interpreters should be encouraged to provide the same feedback to clinicians, particularly suggestions for facilitation of translation of information. Clinicians should ask interpreters their impressions of patients' responses during testing and how difficulties during the procedure may have affected the validity or reliability of results. As always, clinicians should avoid the use of jargon. In summary, the success of the session requires careful planning and teamwork on the part of clinicians and their interpreters.

Although some audiologists and speech-language pathologists may not have the luxury of using an interpreter, they can take several steps to increase the likelihood of accurate information transmission (Newman-Ryan, Northrup, & Villarreal-Emery, 1996; Northrup, 1985; Randell-David, 1989). First, determine any linguistic barriers to communication before any type of assessment by asking patients' preferences and who will accompany the patient to the appointment. Second, be aware of limitations of and techniques for obtaining a case history from the patient and his or her significant others. Clinicians may enlist the help of a bilingual colleague for difficult-to-convey or delicate areas of questioning. Above all clear and concise instructions should be provided supplemented with gestures and pantomime may be all that is needed to elicit appropriate responses in audiometry. Fourth, the use of instruction cards in patients' native languages should be available for those who can read. Fifth, explain that assessment procedures will not be harmful, and indicate when testing begins. Some of the equipment used for vestibular testing may frighten patients, and reassurance may be all that is needed to put them at ease. Sixth, clinicians should investigate the complexity of patients' linguistic environments and healthcare service delivery systems by determining answers to the following questions (ASHA, 2006a):

- What language(s) is/are used at home, at school, and/or at work?
- What language(s) does the family use?
- Who is responsible for the healthcare of the patient?
- What forms of medicine or healthcare service delivery are used by the patient and his or her family?

Last, clinicians should know bilingual healthcare professionals in their areas, especially otolaryngologists and neurologists, who may best serve the needs of a diverse patient population.

SUMMARY

This chapter discussed multicultural aspects of auditory rehabilitation. In particular, readers considered the importance of developing cross-cultural competence, particularly in dealing with members of the Deaf community and with persons who belong to racial and cultural minorities. Cultural aspects of auditory rehabilitation were presented and highlighted using contemporary examples. The use of interpreters was explored in encouraging students to develop cross-cultural competency in treating diverse patient populations with hearing impairment.

LEARNING ACTIVITIES

- Interview a person with a hearing loss who is of a cultural or ethnic background different from your own. What similarities do you share in feelings about hearing loss and the use of hearing aids?
- Explore the consumer pages on the websites of the American Speech-Language-Hearing Association (www.asha.org) and the American Academy of Audiology (www.audiology .org). Is the information appropriate for a diverse consumer population? Why or why not?

APPENDIX 3.1

Cultural Competence With Early Hearing Detection and Intervention Service Delivery Systems

Program Checklist

This checklist can be used to heighten awareness of your agency's policies and procedures when working with culturally and linguistically diverse populations.

- My agency or program incorporates cultural competence in its mission, goals, and values.
- My agency or program has a policy for handling inappropriate language or behaviors by staff members that are based on race, ethnicity, sex, ability, or sexual orientation.
- My agency or program has policies that ensure that the cultural and linguistic backgrounds of the patients it serves are taken into consideration when providing services.
- My agency or program actively recruits employees from diverse cultural and linguistic backgrounds.
- My agency or program collects Early Hearing Detection and Intervention (EHDI) data on races, ethnicities, and languages spoken at home.
- My agency or program has a list of agencies and health care providers (audiologists, speech language pathologists, pediatricians, etc.) who are qualified to work with the diverse cultural and linguistic communities in my state.
- My agency or program has a list of available certified interpreters.
- My agency or program facilitates meaningful participation of diverse consumers and communities in planning, delivery, and evaluation of services.
- My agency or program supports ongoing professional development and in-service training (at all levels) for awareness, knowledge, and skills in the areas of cultural and linguistic competence.
- My agency or program ensures new staff members are provided with training, technical assistance, and other supports necessary to work within culturally and linguistically diverse communities.
- My agency or program ensures culturally competent bilingual staff members are provided with training, technical assistance, and other support necessary to provide patients with appropriate information about the EHDI process.
- My agency or program has written materials or information that meets the cultural and linguistic needs of the communities it serves.
- My agency or program has a toll-free number staffed by qualified employees who speak the native languages of the communities it serves.

Source: From *Bringing Early Hearing Detection and Intervention Programs to Minorities,* by the Office of Minority Health, U.S. Department of Health and Human Services, National Center on Birth Defects and Disabilities, 2009, retrieved from www.cdc.gov/ncbddd/ehdi/documents/Minority_Tips.pdf.

APPENDIX 3.2
English-to-Spanish Translations of Common Words Used in Audiology

English	Spanish
acoustic neuroma	neurinoma del acústico
acoustic reflex	reflejo acústico
acoustic reflex decay	fatiga del reflejo acústico
air conduction	conducción o vía aérea
alerting/signaling devices	dispositivos de alerta o señalización
American Academy of Audiology	Academia Americana de Audiología
amplification	amplificación
amplifier	amplificador
amplitude values	valores de amplitud
analog	analoga
anxiety	ansiedad
assistive devices for the hearing impaired	dispòsitivos de ayuda para personas hipoacúsicas o sordas
assistive technology	tecnología de asistencia
attenuation	amortiguación (o atenuación)
audiogram	audiograma
audiologist	audiólogo (male) audióloga (female)
audiometer	audiómetro
auditory brainstem response (ABR)	respuesta auditiva a nivel del tronco/tallo cerebral
auditory closure	cierre auditivo
auditory evoked potentials	potenciales evocados auditivos
auditory figure ground	capacidad auditiva en ruido de fondo
auditory fusion	fusión auditiva
auditory integration training	entrenamiento de integración auditiva
auditory memory	memoria auditiva
auditory training	entrenamiento auditivo
aural rehabilitation	reeducación (o rehabilitación) auditiva
automatic gain control (AGC)	automático de ganacia
averaging	promediación
background noise	ruido de fondo
battery	pila (o batería)
battery door	portapilas (o compartimento de la batería)
beep	bip
bilateral	bilateral
binaural summation	sumación binaural
body aid	audífono de caja
bone conduction	conducción o vía ósea
bone oscillator	vibrador óseo
borderline	limítrofe

English	Spanish
BTE	retro-auricular
central auditory processing	trastorno de procesamiento auditivo central
cerumen	cerumen
CIC (see *completely-in-the-canal*)	
clicks	clics
cochlea	cóclea
cochlear implant	implante coclear
code	código
cognitive	cognitivo
completely-in-the-canal (CIC)	completamente dentro del oido
compression	compresión
conductive hearing loss	hipoacusia conductiva
contralateral routine of signals (CROS)	sistema cros
deaf	sordo
deafness	sordera
decibel (db)	decibelio (o decibel)
dichotic digits	números dicóticos
dichotic listening	audición dicótica
direct audio input (DAI)	ingreso o entrada directa de audio
disability	discapacidad
discrimination	discriminación
disorder	desorden, trastorno
distortion-product otoacoustic emissions (DPOAE)	emisiones otoacústicas por producto de distorsión
dizziness	mareo, vahío
ear	oído
ear/hearing protection	protección auditiva/del oído
ear canal	canal auditivo
ear canal resonance	resonancia del canal auditivo
ear canal volume	volúmen del canal auditivo
eardrum	membrana timpánica, tímpano
earhook	codo, gancho plástico
earlobe	lóbulo de la oreja
earmold	molde de oído
earphone	auricular
earwax	cerumen
EcoG (see *electrocochleography*)	
effective masking	enmascaramiento efectivo
electroacoustic	electroacústico
electrocochleography (EcoG)	electrococleografía
electrodes	electrodos
electronystagmography (ENG)	electronistagmografía
etiology	etiología
evoked otoacoustic emissions	emisiones otoacústicas evocadas
evoked potentials	potenciales evocados
eyeglass hearing aid	gafas auditivas
fax	facsímil

English	Spanish
feedback	silbido de retroalimentación
filter	filtro
flat	plano/llano/liso
FM (frequency modulated) system	sistema de radio FM
frequency	frecuencia
frequency range	rango de frecuencias
gain	ganancia
graphs	gráficos
hair cells	células ciliadas
handicap	desventaja (desventaja)
harmonic distortion	distorsión armónica
head trauma	traumatismo craneal
hearing	audición
hearing aid	audífono, aparato de oir, prótesis auditiva, auxiliar auditivo
hearing aid fitting	adaptación de audífonos
hearing impaired	hipoacúsico
hearing level	umbral auditivo (umbral auditivo)
hearing loss	pérdida auditiva
hearing screening	barridas audiométricas (barrida/tamizaje auditivo)
hearing test	examen audiométrico, prueba auditiva, examen de audición
high frequency	frecuencias agudas
immittance testing	examen impedanciométrico
impairment	impedimento, deterioro
incus	yunque
infrared system	sistema de rayos infra-rojos
inner ear	oído interno
insert earphones	auriculares de insersión
insertion	insersión
intensity-latency function	función intensidad-latencia
in-the-canal (ITC)	intra-canal
in-the-ear (ITE)	intra-auricular
intra-canal	intra-canal
ISO (International Standards Organization)	Organización Internacional de Estándares
ITC (see *intra-canal*)	
ITE (see *in-the-canal*)	
late/early potencials	potenciales tardíos/tempranos
left ear	oído izquierdo
lipreading/speechreading	lectura labio-facial
listen	escuche, oiga
low frequency	frecuencias graves
malleus	martillo
masking	ruido enmascarante, ensordecimiento
Meniere's disease	enfermedad de meniere
meningitis	meningitis
microphone	micrófono
middle ear	oído medio

English	Spanish
middle ear infection	infección del oído medio
middle latency evoked response (MLR)	potenciales evocados de latencia media
mild	leve
minimal response level	nivel de respuesta mínimo
minimum masking level	nivel de enmascaramiento mínimo
mixed hearing loss	sordera mixta
moderate	moderada
monaural	monaural
most comfortable level (MCL)	nivel de comodidad
narrow band noise	ruido de banda angosta
neckloop	lazo magnético alrededor del cuello
newborn	recien nacido
noise	ruido
normal	normal
normal hearing range	campo (rango) auditivo normal
off switch	interruptor de apagado
oral communication	comunicación oral
ossicular chain	cadena oscicular
OTM switch	interruptor
otoacoustic emissions (OAE)	emisiones otoacústicas
otosclerosis	otoesclerosis
otoscope	otoscopio
ototoxic	ototóxico
outer ear	oído externo
patent	abierto (permeable)
pressure equalization (PE) tube	tubo de ventilación
peak amplitude	cresta de amplitud (o pico de amplitude)
percentage	porcentaje
perforation	perforación
phonemes	fonemas
phoneme transition	transición fonémica
pinna	oreja (o pabellón auricular)
pitch	tono
plateau	meseta
presbycusis	presbiacusia
prescription	prescripción, receta
probe microphone measurement	medición de amplificación de inserción
programmable hearing aids	audífonos programables
profound	profunda
pulsed tones	tonos pulsados
pure tone testing	audiometría tonal
recruitment	reclutamiento
remote control	control remoto
repeat	diga, repita
retrocochlear pathology	patología retrococlear
reverberation	reverberación, eco

English	Spanish
right ear	oído derecho
SAT	umbral de detectabilidad del lenguaje
sedative	sedación
semicircular canals	conductos semicirculares
sensation level	umbral sensitivo
sensitivity	sensibilidad
sensorineural hearing loss	sordera neurosensorial (o sensorineural)
severe	severa
sign language	lenguaje manual/de señas (o lenguaje gestual)
signal/noise	relación señal ruido
sound	sonido
sound booth	cabinas audiométricas (o cabina sonoamortiguada)
sound field	campo libre
sound pressure level (SPL)	nivel de presión sonora
special test	examen especial
speakers (in the booth)	alto parlantes, bocinas
speech audiometry	logoaudiometría
speech discrimination	discriminación del habla
speech language pathologist	fonoaudiólogo/a (terapueta de lenguaje)
speech processor	procesador del lenguaje
speech understanding	comprensión del habla/lenguaje
SPL (see *sound pressure level*)	
spondee threshold (or SRT)	umbral de captación o recepción (. . . de palabras espondaicas)
spontaneous otoacoustic emissions (SOAE)	emisiónes otoacústicas espontáneas
stapedius reflex	reflejo estapedial
static compliance	compliancia estática
stirrups	estribos
stress	estrés (tensión)
sudden hearing loss	pérdida auditiva súbita
target	objetivo
T-coil (telephone coil)	bobina telefónica
TDD (telecommunications devices for the deaf)	ayudas de telecomunicación para personas sordas (sistema de . . .)
telephone amplifier	amplificador telefónico
temporal processing	procesamiento temporal
TEOAE (see *transient evoked otoacoustic emissions*)	
threshold	umbral
tinnitus	acúfeno, zumbidos en el oído, tínitus
tinnitus masker	(dispositivo) de enmascaramiento del tínitus
transient evoked otoacoustic emissions (TEOAE)	emisiónes otoacústicas (por transitorios)
transmitter	transmisor
tubing	tubo
tumor	tumor
tuning fork	diapasón
TV decoder	descodificador para TV

English	Spanish
tympanic membrane	membrana timpánica
tympanometry	timpanometría
uncomfortable loudness level (ULL)	umbral de molestia/de incomodidad
vent	taladro, abertura, agujero, vent
vertigo	vértigo
volume control	potenciómetro, control de volúmen
warbled tone	tono modulado
wave	onda
WDRC	compresión de rango dinámico amplio
whisper	susurro
white noise	ruido blanco
word recognition	reconocimiento de palabras

Source: From *English-Spanish Translations of Common Words Used in Audiology*, by B. Northrup, 2009, Dallas, TX: Author. Reprinted with permission.

APPENDIX 3.3

Spanish-to-English Translations of Common Words Used in Audiology

Spanish	English
abierto (permeable)	patent
Academia Americana de Audiología	American Academy of Audiology
acúfeno, zumbidos en el oído, tínitus	tinnitus
adaptación de audífonos	hearing aid fitting
alto parlantes, bocinas	speakers (in the booth)
amortiguación (o atenuación)	attenuation
amplificación	amplification
amplificador	amplifier
amplificador telefonico	telephone amplifier
analoga	analog
ansiedad	anxiety
audífono, aparato de oir, prótesis auditiva, auxiliar auditivo	hearing aid
audición	hearing
audición dicótica	dichotic listening
audífono de caja	body aid
audífonos programables	programmable hearing aids
audiometría tonal	pure tone testing
audiograma	audiogram
audiólogo, audióloga	audiologist
audiómetro	audiometer
auricular	earphone
auriculares de insersión	insert earphones
ayudas de telecomunicación para personas sordas (sistema de . . .)	TDD (telecommunications devices for the deaf)
barridas audiométricas (barrida/tamizaje auditivo)	hearing screening
binaural	binaural
bilateral	bilateral
bip	beep
bobina telefónica	T-coil (telephone coil)
cabinas audiométricas (o cabina sonoamortiguada)	sound booth
cadena osicular	ossicular chain
campo libre	sound field
canal auditivo	ear canal
capacidad auditiva en ruido de fondo	auditory figure ground
células ciliadas	hair cells
cerumen	cerumen, earwax
cierre auditivo	auditory closure
clics	clicks
cóclea	cochlea
código	code
codo, gancho plástico	earhook
cognitivo	cognitive
completamente dentro del oido	completely-in-the-canal (CIC)

Source: From *Spanish-to-English Translations of Common Words Used in Audiology*, by B. Northrup, 2009, Dallas, TX: Author. Reprinted with permission.

Spanish	English
compliancia estática	static compliance
compresión	compression
compresión de rango dinamico amplio	WDRC
comprensión del habla/lenguaje	speech understanding
comunicación oral	oral communication
conducción o vía aérea	air conduction
conducción o vía ósea	bone conduction
conductos semicirculares	semicircular canals
control automático de ganacia	automatic gain control (AGC)
control remoto	remote control
cresta de amplitud (o pico de amplitud)	peak amplitude
decibelio (o decibel)	db (decibel)
descodificador para tv	TV decoder
desorden, trastorno	disorder
desventaja/descapacidad	handicap
diapasón	tuning fork
diga, repita	repeat
digital	digital
discapacidad	disability
discriminación	discrimination
discriminación del habla	speech discrimination
dispositivos de alerta o señalización	alerting/signaling devices
dispósitivos de ayuda para personas hipoacúsicas o sordas	assistive devices for the hearing impaired
(dispositivo) de enmascaramiento del tínitus	tinnitus masker
distorsión armónica	harmonic distortion
electroacústico	electroacoustic
electrococleografía	electrocochleography (EcoG)
electrodos	electrodes
electronistagmografía	electronystagmography (ENG)
emisiones otoacústicas	otoacoustic emissions (OAE)
emisiones otoacústicas espontáneas	spontaneous otoacoustic emissions (SOAE)
emisiones otoacústicas evocadas	evoked otoacoustic emissions
emisiones otoacústicas por producto de distorsión	distortion-product otoacoustic emissions (DPOAE)
emisiones otoacústicas por transitorios	transient evoked otoacoustic emissions (TEOAE)
enfermedad de meniere	Meniere's disease
enmascaramiento efectivo	effective masking
ensordecimiento/ruido enmascarante	masking
entrenamiento auditivo	auditory training
entrenamiento de integración auditiva	auditory integration training
escuche, oiga	listen
estrés/tensión	stress
estribos	stirrups
etiología	etiology
examen audiométrico, prueba auditiva, examen de audición	hearing test
examen especial	special test
examen impedanciométrico	immittance testing
facsímil	fax
fatiga auditiva	acoustic decay

Spanish	**English**
fatiga del reflejo acústico	acoustic reflex decay
filtro	filter
figura/fondo auditivos OR capicidad auditiva en ruido de fondo	auditory figure ground
fonemas	phonemes
fonoaudiólogo/a (terapueta de lenguaje)	speech language pathologist
frecuencia	frequency
frecuencias agudas	high frequency
frecuencias graves	low frequency
función intensidad-latencia	intensity-latency function
fusión auditiva	auditory fusion
gafas auditivas	eyeglass hearing aid
ganancia	gain
gráficos	graphs
hipoacusia conductiva (or sordera conductiva)	conductive hearing loss
hipoacúsico	hearing impaired
impedimento, deterioro	impairment
implante coclear	cochlear implant
infección del oído medio	middle ear infection
ingreso o entrada directa de audio	direct audio input (DAI)
insersión	insertion
interruptor	OTM switch
interruptor de apagado	off switch
intra-auricular	in-the-ear (ITE)
intra-canal	in-the-canal (ITC)
lazo magnetico alrededor del cuello	neckloop
lectura labio-facial	lipreading/speechreading
lenguaje manual/de senas (o lenguaje gestual)	sign language
leve	mild
limítrofe	borderline
lóbulo de la oreja	earlobe
logoaudiometría	speech audiometry
mareo, vahío	dizziness
martillo	malleus
medición de amplificación de inserción	probe microphone measurement
membrana timpánica, tímpano	tympanic membrane, eardrum
memoria auditiva	auditory memory
meningitis	meningitis
meseta	plateau
micrófono	microphone
moderada	moderate
molde de oído	earmold
monaural	monaural
neurinoma del acústico	acoustic neuroma
nivel de comodidad	most comfortable level (MCL)
nivel de enmascaramiento mínimo	minimum masking level
nivel de presión sonora	sound pressure level (SPL)
nivel de respuesta mínimo	minimal response level
nivel/umbral auditivo	hearing level
normal	normal
números dicóticos	dichotic digits

Spanish	English
objetivo	target
oído	ear
oído derecho	right ear
oído externo	outer ear
oído interno	inner ear
oído izquierdo	left ear
oído medio	middle ear
onda	wave
oreja (o pabellón auricular)	pinna
Organización Internacional de Estándares	International Standards Organization (ISO)
otoesclerosis	otosclerosis
otoscopio	otoscope
ototóxico	ototoxic
patología retrococlear	retrocochlear pathology
pérdida auditiva	hearing loss
pérdida auditiva súbita	sudden hearing loss
perforación	perforation
pila (o batería)	battery
plano/llano/liso	flat
porcentaje	percentage
portapilas/(compartimento de la batería)	battery door
potenciales evocados	evoked potentials
potenciales evocados auditivos	auditory evoked potentials
potenciales evocados de latencia media	middle latency evoked response (MLR)
potenciales tardíos/tempranos	late/early potentials
potenciómetro, control de volúmen	volume control
presbiacusia	presbycusis
prescripción, receta	prescription
procesador del lenguaje	speech processor
procesamiento temporal	temporal processing
profunda	profound
promediación	averaging
protección auditiva/del oído	ear/hearing protection
rango/campo auditivo	normal hearing range
rango de frecuencias	frequency range
recien nacido	newborn
reclutamiento	recruitment
reconocimiento de palabras	word recognition
reeducación (o rehabilitación) auditiva	aural rehabilitation
reflejo acústico	acoustic reflex
reflejo estapedial	stapedius reflex
relación señal ruido	signal/noise
repita	repeat
resonancia del canal auditivo	ear canal resonance
respuesta auditiva a nivel del tronco/tallo cerebral	auditory brainstem response (ABR)
retro-auricular	BTE
reverberación, eco	reverberation
ruido	noise
ruido blanco	white noise
ruido de banda angosta	narrow band noise
ruido de fondo	background noise

Spanish	English
ruido enmascarante, ensordecimiento	masking
sedación	sedative
sensibilidad	sensitivity
severa	severe
silbido de retroalimentación	feedback
sistema cros	contralateral routing of signals (CROS)
sistema de radio FM	FM (frequency modulated) system
sistema de rayos infra-rojos	infrared system
sonido	sound
sordera	deafness
sordera mixta	mixed hearing loss
sordera neurosensorial o sensorineural	sensorineural hearing loss
sordo	deaf
sumación binaural	binaural summation
susurro	whisper
taladro, abertura, agujero, vent	vent
tecnología de asistencia	assistive technology
timpanometría	tympanometry
tono	pitch
tono modulado	warbled tone
tonos pulsados	pulsed tones
transición fonémica	phoneme transition
transmisor	transmitter
trastorno de procesamiento auditivo central	central auditory processing disorder
traumatismo craneal	head trauma
tubo	tubing
tubo de ventilación	pressure equalization (PE) tube
tumor	tumor
umbral	threshold
umbral auditivo (umbral auditivo)	hearing level
umbral de captación o recepción (. . . de palabras espondaicas)	spondee threshold (or SRT)
umbral de detectabilidad del lenguaje	SAT
umbral de molestia/de incomodidad	uncomfortable loudness level (ULL)
umbral sensitivo	sensation level
valores de amplitud	amplitude values
vértigo	vertigo
vibrador óseo	bone oscillator
volúmen del canal auditivo	ear canal volume
yunque	incus

APPENDIX 3.4

Multicultural Speech Recognition Testing Materials and Self-Assessment Tools

Speech Recognition Testing Materials in Multiple Languages

Auditec Inc.
2515 South Big Bend Blvd.
St. Louis, MO 63143
Phone: (800) 669-9065
or (314) 781-8890
Fax: (314) 781-4946
E-mail: auditecinfo@auditec.com
www.auditec.com

Multicultural Self-Assessment Tools

Dr. Robyn Cox
Hearing Aid Research Laboratory
807 Jefferson Ave.
Memphis, TN 38105
Phone: (901) 678-5858
www.memphis.edu/ausp/harl/index.htm

APPENDIX 3.5

National Standards on Culturally and Linguistically Appropriate Services (CLAS)

Standard 1. Health care organizations should ensure that patients/consumers receive from all staff members effective, understandable, and respectful care that is provided in a manner compatible with their cultural health beliefs and practices and preferred language.

Standard 2. Health care organizations should implement strategies to recruit, retain, and promote at all levels of the organization a diverse staff and leadership that are representative of the demographic characteristics of the service area.

Standard 3. Health care organizations should ensure that staff at all levels and across all disciplines receive ongoing education and training in culturally and linguistically appropriate service delivery.

Standard 4. Health care organizations must offer and provide language assistance services, including bilingual staff and interpreter services, at no cost to each patient/consumer with limited English proficiency at all points of contact, in a timely manner during all hours of operation.

Standard 5. Health care organizations must provide to patients/consumers in their preferred language both verbal offers and written notices informing them of their right to receive language assistance services.

Standard 6. Health care organizations must assure the competence of language assistance provided to limited English proficient patients/consumers by interpreters and bilingual staff. Family and friends should not be used to provide interpretation services (except on request by the patient/consumer).

Standard 7. Health care organizations must make available easily understood patient-related materials and post signage in the languages of the commonly encountered groups and/or groups represented in the service area.

Standard 8. Health care organizations should develop, implement, and promote a written strategic plan that outlines clear goals, policies, operational plans, and management accountability/oversight mechanisms to provide culturally and linguistically appropriate services.

Standard 9. Health care organizations should conduct initial and ongoing organizational self-assessments of CLAS-related activities and are encouraged to integrate cultural and linguistic competence-related measures into their internal audits, performance improvement programs, patient satisfaction assessments, and outcomes-based evaluations.

Standard 10. Health care organizations should ensure that data on the individual patient's/consumer's race, ethnicity, and spoken and written language are collected in health records, integrated into the organization's management information systems, and periodically updated.

Standard 11. Health care organizations should maintain a current demographic, cultural, and epidemiological profile of the community as well as a needs assessment to accurately plan for and implement services that respond to the cultural and linguistic characteristics of the service area.

Standard 12. Health care organizations should develop participatory, collaborative partnerships with communities and utilize a variety of formal and informal mechanisms to facilitate community and patient/consumer involvement in designing and implementing CLAS-related activities.

Standard 13. Health care organizations should ensure that conflict and grievance resolution processes are culturally and linguistically sensitive and capable of identifying, preventing, and resolving cross-cultural conflicts or complaints by patients/consumers.

Standard 14. Health care organizations are encouraged to regularly make available to the public information about their progress and successful innovations in implementing the CLAS standards and to provide public notice in their communities about the availability of this information.

Source: Information from *National Standards on Culturally and Linguistically Appropriate Services* (CLAS), Office of Minority Health, U.S. Department of Health and Human Services, 2009, retrieved from http://minorityhealth.hhs.gov/templates/browse.aspx?lvl=2&lvlID=15.

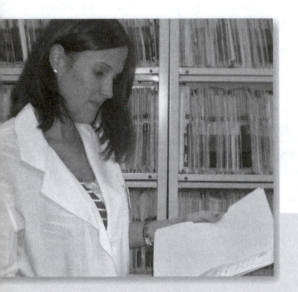

CHAPTER *four*

Professional Issues in Auditory Rehabilitation

LEARNING *objectives*

After reading this chapter, you should be able to:

1. Define cross-professional competence in working within various models of teaming for auditory rehabilitation.

2. Describe events leading to the development of the professional doctorate in audiology.

3. Compare and contrast the knowledge and skills required for the provision of auditory rehabilitation services by audiologists and speech-language pathologists.

4. Explain the multidimensional model of regulatory influences on auditory rehabilitation.

5. Discuss contemporary professional issues of reimbursement, evidence-based practice, and ethics in auditory rehabilitation.

A udiologists, speech-language pathologists, and other professionals work together to provide auditory rehabilitative services. Working together means teamwork. Understanding others and working with them in a harmonious fashion requires sensitivity to professional boundaries and touchy issues. This chapter introduces students to the concept of cross-professional competence and the importance of teamwork in auditory rehabilitation. The chapter underscores the importance of developing clinical competence by presenting a model of professional practice and the complementary yet overlapping roles of audiologists and speech-language pathologists in providing auditory rehabilitative (AR) services across service delivery sites. Moreover, readers will consider the contemporary professional issues of reimbursement, evidence-based practice, and ethics in auditory rehabilitation.

DEVELOPING CROSS-PROFESSIONAL COMPETENCE

What is "cross-professional competence" and why is it important for auditory rehabilitation? As defined in Chapter 2, *cross-professional competence* is the ability to competently execute services within one's scope of practice to a diverse patient population in a wide variety of service delivery sites, in collaboration with other professionals in order to achieve positive outcomes. Understanding this definition requires explanation and examples of some terms. First, each profession has a *scope of practice*, which, as defined in Chapter 1, specifically states what services members of a profession can or cannot provide. The American Speech-Language-Hearing Association (ASHA) has published scopes of practice for both audiologists (ASHA, 2004b) and speech-language pathologists (ASHA, 2007). Second, *service delivery site*, as defined earlier, is where auditory rehabilitation services are provided, such as in a private practice, speech and hearing center, public school, a hospital, rehabilitation, or long-term care facility. Third, *working in collaboration with other professionals* requires collegiality and an esprit de corps between and among audiologists, speech-language pathologists, allied-health professionals, educators, and physicians. In Chapter 1, we mentioned that a team approach sometimes is the most effective method of meeting the needs of many patients with hearing impairment and their families. This textbook presents multiple examples of how teaming and collaboration are key to rehabilitating patients of all ages with hearing loss and balance disorders.

In the rehabilitation field, several models of teaming have been proposed. Traditionally, rehabilitation teams have been thought of as *multidisciplinary* or *interdisciplinary* (ASHA, 1996). **Multidisciplinary teams** utilize discipline-specific skills of each member, and view rehabilitation efforts as the combined individual efforts of each discipline involved in a particular case (ASHA, 1996). For example, early intervention teams working with infants and toddlers are often multidisciplinary in their assessments in that each member performs his or her own battery of tests to provide an overall level of functioning of the patient and his or her family. The assessments, in this case, may be performed in different settings and on different days.

Interdisciplinary teams, on the other hand, involve specialists from different professions who possess discipline-specific skills, plus the ability to contribute to a team effort in accomplishing goals (ASHA, 1996). For instance, interdisciplinary assessment may occur during a cleft palate team meeting in which otolaryngologists, otologists, and audiologists perform their assessments in determining if a child with unilateral congenital atresia may benefit from a bone-conduction hearing aid or bone-anchored hearing aid. And **transdisciplinary teaming** is different yet, in that it involves breaking down boundaries between and among disciplines so that members of one profession may assist in providing cross-disciplinary services to patient populations who may be unserved or underserved. For example, audiologists may have to delegate the task of performing daily visual and listening checks on children's hearing aids to nurses and classroom teachers because American public schools have five times fewer audiologists than are needed to serve the hearing healthcare needs of school-aged children (Johnson, Benson, & Seaton, 1997). All three types of teaming are appropriate for auditory rehabilitation. Other types of teams found in auditory rehabilitation include the following:

- Balance assessment and management team
- Central auditory process screening, evaluation, and management team
- Cleft palate team
- Cochlear implant team
- Early hearing detection and intervention team
- Early intervention team
- Hearing conservation team
- Individualized education plan team
- Individualized family services plan team

Is a team approach of auditory rehabilitation widely accepted by audiologists and speech-language pathologists? For the most part, the answer is yes. Often, the success of a team requires that clinicians provide ongoing education to other professionals about the identification, diagnosis, and management of communication disorders, and in particular, hearing loss and balance disorders. Successful auditory rehabilitation requires ongoing informational outreach programs to the medical community. However, in some situations a team concept in auditory rehabilitation may be a sensitive topic for audiologists. The profession of audiology is currently going through a period of rapid change in its quest for autonomy as a doctoring profession. Audiologists may feel very protective about what they do and what professions should share in those responsibilities. The following Casebook Reflection provides a recent history of the professional doctorate in audiology.

Casebook Reflection

Recent History of the Professional Doctorate in Audiology

In 1978, the ASHA Task Force on Science discussed the need for a professional doctorate to ensure that programs offering the Ph.D. kept the degree aimed at training university professors and researchers. In 1983, ASHA underwrote a study that concluded that the master's degree did not provide adequate professional preparation for audiologists, and in 1984 an ASHA task force recommended requiring a professional doctorate. In 1986, the ASHA Audiology Task Force recommended that the Doctor of Audiology, Au.D., become the entry-level degree by 1998. In 1988, the Academy of Dispensing Audiologists (ADA) sponsored the first Conference on Professional

Education for Audiology, which called for audiology training to move to a doctoral level. In 1989, the ADA formed the Audiology Foundation of America (AFA) with a charge to "transform Audiology to a doctoral profession with the Au.D. as its distinctive designator." In the same year, an ASHA task force recommended that "ASHA should strongly endorse the concept of the professional doctorate." In the period from 1990 to 1992, six independent surveys reported that the majority of audiologists supported the Au.D. degree. In 1992, the ASHA Ad Hoc Committee on Professional Education recommended the Au.D. as the entry-level degree to practice, setting 2001 as the target year for implementation. However, the ASHA Executive Board voted against the recommendation, and its Legislative Council tabled the resolution. Several audiology-related professional organizations called for ASHA to facilitate Au.D. degree development and implementation.

In 1994, AFA awarded a $25,000 grant to Baylor College of Medicine for establishing the first Au.D. program. In 1995, AFA sponsored the Au.D. "Standards and Equivalency (S&E) Conference." Numerous audiology organizations participated, including the ADA. The goal of the S&E Conference was to develop mechanisms to recognize the experiential equivalency of current practitioners and to develop standards of education for the Au.D. degree programs. In 1995, ASHA recommended a doctoral degree (but not necessarily the Au.D.) for entry level to practice audiology. However, in 1997, ASHA postponed the transition to a doctoral degree as entry level to the year 2012. In 1997, ADA helped AFA sponsor fellowships for Au.D. students in four universities. By 1998, six residential Au.D. programs were available. In 1999, Nova Southeastern University in Florida began the first distance learning Au.D. program for practicing audiologists. Shortly following, the University of Florida, Central Michigan University, Pennsylvania College of Optometry, and the Arizona School of Health Sciences opened up other distance learning programs for practicing audiologists. Today, there are over 70 Au.D. programs in the United States.

Based on *Au.D. History and Timeline*, by the Academy of Doctors of Audiology, 2010, retrieved from http://www.audiologist.org/aud-history.html.

Transitioning to a doctoral-level entry degree was just one vision audiologists had for their profession. Another was establishing their own professional organization, the American Academy of Audiology (AAA), run by and for audiologists, an organization model that some believe best represents the interests of and is most able to determine the course of an autonomous profession. Together with ASHA, AAA champions access to hearing healthcare, particularly auditory rehabilitation for those with hearing losses and balance disorders. Another vision was for future Au.D. degree-holding audiologists to open their own private practices as the recognized leaders in the provision of auditory rehabilitation. Still another vision was establishment of the American Board of Audiology (ABA, 2005) to develop and enhance audiologic services to the public by establishing recognized standards in professional practice (ABA, 2005). Board certification in audiology is a voluntary credentialing program committed to high professional standards, ethical practices, and continued professional development aimed at formalizing the status of audiologists to consumers, employers, institutions, and public and private agencies (ABA, 2005). Moreover, the ABA has developed certification in specialty areas signifying high standards in areas involving auditory rehabilitation. For example, specialty certification in cochlear implants elevates the status of those who specialize in this area and may be valuable because it provides the following benefits (ABA, 2007, 2010):

- Standardizes training and knowledge of cochlear implant audiologists; specialty certification identifies the knowledge required to promote better patient outcomes.

- Verifies professional experience to employers and helps identify individuals who are qualified to fulfill a job description related to the cochlear implant population.
- Provides consumers a method of identifying audiologists with expertise in cochlear implants and increases confidence in consumers' view of the audiologist's level of expertise.
- Describes a training plan for individuals interested in specializing in cochlear implants.
- Helps individual audiologists identify themselves as experts; increases professional self-esteem.
- Assists the profession in defining audiologists' scope of practice.
- Increases the possibility of a heightened standard of living through appropriate salaries, provides a basis of career advancement, and maintains an adequate number of audiologists working with cochlear implants.

Some experts believe that specialty certification in auditory rehabilitation should be developed in many areas of practice (Hanavan, Greer Clark, & Abrahamson, 2006). Readers should also be aware of the Certificates of Clinical Competence in Audiology (CCC-A) and Speech-Language Pathology (CCC-SLP) granted by ASHA, two credentials that also signify high levels of expertise in providing services.

Despite changes within the professions of audiology and speech-language pathology, communication sciences and disorders students must develop cross-professional competence in collaborating with each other as well as with other professionals to provide greater access to hearing healthcare services to the 30 million Americans with hearing loss. Audiologists must acknowledge that speech-language pathologists work in settings in which the significant proportion of patients has no access to audiologists. Partnering with speech-language pathologists will be critical in meeting the hearing healthcare needs of the elderly, whose numbers are expected to grow tremendously in the next few decades. Both audiologists and speech-language pathologists must have the necessary knowledge and skills to be clinically competent to provide auditory rehabilitation.

DEVELOPING CLINICAL COMPETENCE

The ASHA scope of practice documents for audiology and speech-language pathology include services for auditory rehabilitation (ASHA, 2001). In no other area of professional practice do audiologists and speech-language pathologists share complementary, interrelated, and sometimes overlapping roles in the provision of auditory (re)habilitative services to children and adults with hearing loss. A document entitled "Knowledge and Skills Required for the Practice of Audiologic/Aural Rehabilitation" was prepared by the Working Group on Audiologic Rehabilitation (ASHA, 2001) to provide a description of the knowledge and skills audiologists and speech-language pathologists must demonstrate to enhance the delivery of services by members of both professions and the collaborative nature of auditory rehabilitation. Basic areas of knowledge required of both audiologists and speech-language pathologists are shown in Figures 4.1 and 4.2. Specialty knowledge and skills for audiologists and speech-language pathologists are also provided in Figures 4.1 and 4.2.

Basic Areas of Knowledge

Audiologists who provide AR services demonstrate knowledge in the basic areas that are the underpinnings of Communication Sciences and Disorders. These include the following:

  I. General Knowledge
  A. General psychology; human growth and development; psychosocial behavior; cultural and linguistic diversity; biological, physical, and social sciences; mathematics; and qualitative and quantitative research methodologies.

 II. Basic Communication Processes
  A. Anatomic and physiologic bases for the normal development and use of speech, language, and hearing (including anatomy, neurology, and physiology of speech, language, and hearing mechanisms);
  B. Physical bases and processes of the production and perception of speech and hearing (including acoustic or physics of sound, phonology, physiologic and acoustic phonetics, sensory perceptual processes, and psychoacoustics);
  C. Linguistic and psycholinguistic variables related to the normal development and use of speech, language, and hearing (including linguistics [historical, descriptive, sociolinguistics, sign language, second language usage], psychology of language, psycholinguistics, language and speech acquisition, verbal learning and verbal behavior, and gestural communication);
  D. Dynamics of interpersonal skills, communication effectiveness, and group theory.

Special Areas of Knowledge and Skills: Audiologists

Audiologists who provide AR have knowledge in the following special areas and demonstrate the itemized requisite skills in those areas:

III. Auditory System Function and Disorders
  A. Identify, describe, and differentiate among disorders of auditory function (including disorders of the outer, middle, and inner ear; the vestibular system; the auditory nerve and the associated neural and central auditory system pathways and processes).

 IV. Developmental Status, Cognition, and Sensory Perception
  A. Provide for the administration of assessment measures in the client's preferred mode of communication;
  B. Verify adequate visual acuity for communication purposes;
  C. Identify the need and provide for assessment of cognitive skills, sensory perceptual and motor skills, developmental delays, academic achievement, and literacy;
  D. Determine the need for referral to other medical and nonmedical specialists for appropriate professional services;
  E. Provide for ongoing assessments of developmental progress.

  V. Audiological Assessment Procedures
  A. Conduct interview and obtain case history;
  B. Perform otoscopic examinations and ensure that the external auditory canal is free of obstruction, including cerumen;
  C. Conduct and interpret behavioral, physiologic, or electrophysiologic evaluations of the peripheral and central auditory system;
  D. Conduct and interpret assessments for auditory processing disorders;
  E. Administer and interpret standardized self-report measures of communication difficulties and of psychosocial and behavioral adjustment to auditory dysfunction;
  F. Identify the need for referral to medical and nonmedical specialists for appropriate professional services.

figure *4.1* ———————————————————————————————

Knowledge and skills required for the practice of audiologic/aural rehabilitation: audiologists.

Source: Reprinted with permission from *Knowledge and Skills Required for the Practice of Audiologic/Aural Rehabilitation* [Knowledge and skills]. From www.asha.org/policy. Copyright 2001 by American Speech-Language-Hearing Association. All rights reserved.

(Continued)

VI. Speech and Language Assessment Procedures
   A. Identify the need for and perform screenings for effects of hearing impairment on speech and language;
   B. Describe the effects of hearing impairment on the development of semantic, syntactic, pragmatic, and phonologic aspects of communication, both in terms of comprehension and production;
   C. Provide for appropriate measures of speech and voice production;
   D. Provide for appropriate measures of language comprehension and production skills and/or alternate communication skills (e.g., signing);
   E. Administer and interpret appropriate measures of communication skills in auditory, visual, auditory-visual, and tactile modalities.

VII. Evaluation and Management of Devices and Technologies for Individuals With Hearing Impairment (e.g., hearing aids, cochlear implants, middle ear implants, implantable hearing aids, tinnitus maskers, hearing assistive technologies, and other sensory prosthetic devices)
   A. Perform and interpret measures of electroacoustic characteristics of devices and technologies;
   B. Describe, perform, and interpret behavioral/psychophysical measures of performance with these devices and technologies;
   C. Conduct appropriate fittings with and adjustments of these devices and technologies;
   D. Monitor fitting of and adjustment to these devices and technologies to ensure comfort, safety, and device performance;
   E. Perform routine visual, listening, and electroacoustic checks of clients' hearing devices and sensory aids to troubleshoot common causes of malfunction;
   F. Evaluate and describe the effects of the use of devices and technologies on communication and psychosocial functioning;
   G. Plan and implement a program of orientation to these devices and technologies to ensure realistic expectations; to improve acceptance of, adjustment to, and benefit from these systems; and to enhance communication performance;
   H. Conduct routine assessments of adjustment to and effective use of amplification devices to ensure optimal communication function;
   I. Monitor outcomes to ensure professional accountability.

VIII. Effects of Hearing Impairment on Functional Communication
   A. Identify the individual's situational expressive and receptive communication needs;
   B. Evaluate the individual's expressive and receptive communication performance;
   C. Identify environmental factors that affect the individual's situational communication needs and performance;
   D. Identify the effects of interpersonal relations on communication function.

IX. Effects on Hearing Impairment on Psychosocial, Educational, and Occupational Functioning
   A. Describe and evaluate the impact of hearing impairment on psychosocial development and psychosocial functioning;
   B. Describe systems and methods of educational programming (e.g., mainstream, residential) and facilitate selection of appropriate educational options;
   C. Describe and evaluate the effects of hearing impairment on occupational status and performance (e.g., communication, localization, safety);
   D. Identify the effects of hearing problems on marital dyads, family dynamics, and other interpersonal communication functioning;
   E. Identify the need and provide for psychosocial, educational, family, and occupational/vocational counseling in relation to hearing impairment and subsequent communication difficulties;
   F. Provide assessment of family members' perception of and reactions to communication difficulties.

X. AR Case Management
   A. Use effective interpersonal communication in interviewing and interacting with individuals with hearing impairment and their families;
   B. Describe client-centered, behavioral, cognitive, and integrative theories and methods of counseling and their relevance in AR;

figure *4.1*

(*Continued*)

C. Provide appropriate individual and group adjustment counseling related to hearing loss for individuals with hearing impairment and their families;

D. Provide auditory, visual, and auditory-visual communication training (e.g., speechreading, auditory training, listening skills) to enhance receptive communication;

E. Provide training in effective communication strategies to individuals with hearing impairment, family members, and other relevant individuals;

F. Provide for appropriate expressive communication training;

G. Provide appropriate technological and counseling intervention to facilitate adjustment to tinnitus;

H. Provide appropriate intervention for management of vestibular disorders;

I. Develop and implement an intervention plan based on the individual's situational/environmental communication needs and performance and related adjustment difficulties;

J. Develop and implement a system for measuring and monitoring outcomes and the appropriateness and efficacy of intervention.

XI. Interdisciplinary Collaboration and Public Advocacy

A. Collaborate effectively as part of multidisciplinary teams and communicate relevant information to allied professionals and other appropriate individuals;

B. Plan and implement in-service and public-information programs for allied professionals and other interested individuals;

C. Plan and implement parent-education programs concerning the management of hearing impairment and subsequent communications difficulties;

D. Advocate implementation of public law in educational, occupational, and public settings;

E. Make appropriate referrals to consumer-based organizations.

XII. Hearing Conservation/Acoustic Environments

A. Plan and implement programs for prevention of hearing impairment to promote identification and evaluation of individuals exposed to hazardous noise and periodic monitoring of communication performance and auditory abilities (e.g., speech recognition in noise, localization);

B. Identify need for and provide appropriate hearing protection devices and noise abatement procedures;

C. Monitor the effects of environmental influences, amplification, and sources of trauma on residual auditory function;

D. Measure and evaluate environmental acoustic conditions and relate them to effects on communication performance and hearing protection.

figure *4.1*

(Continued)

Communication sciences and disorders students learn the prerequisite knowledge and skills in their undergraduate and their graduate/professional training. However, effective auditory rehabilitation service provision requires an application and execution of this knowledge and these skills within a context of a multidimensional model that includes the regulatory influences on the practice of auditory rehabilitation shown in Figure 4.3.

Regulatory Influences on the Practice of Auditory Rehabilitation

Audiologists and speech-language pathologists must acknowledge the various federal/state laws, regulations, and practice guidelines that affect the delivery of auditory rehabilitative services. The model is hierarchical, multidimensional, dynamic, and context specific. The model is hierarchical because the spheres of influence descend from the broad and general (e.g., federal and state laws) to the narrow and specific (e.g., practice guidelines). The model is multidimensional in that multiple regulatory spheres of influence guide the provision of services. The model is dynamic in that activities at the top affect service provision at the bottom and vice versa. For example, laws affect audiologists' and speech-language

Basic Areas of Knowledge: Speech-Language Pathologists

Speech-language pathologists who provide AR services demonstrate knowledge in the basic areas that are the underpinnings of communication sciences and disorders. These include the following:

I. General Knowledge
   A. General psychology; human growth and development; psychosocial behavior; cultural and linguistic diversity; biological, physical, and social sciences; mathematics; and qualitative and quantitative research methodologies.

II. Basic Communication Processes
   A. Anatomic and physiologic bases for the normal development and use of speech, language, and hearing (including anatomy, neurology, and physiology of speech, language, and hearing mechanisms);
   B. Physical bases and processes of the production and perception of speech and hearing (including acoustics or physics of sound, phonology, physiologic and acoustic phonetics, sensory perceptual processes, and psychoacoustics);
   C. Linguistic and psycholinguistic variables related to the normal development and use of speech, language, and hearing (including linguistics [historical, descriptive, sociolinguistics, sign language, second language usage], psychology of language, psycholinguistics, language and speech acquisition, verbal learning and verbal behavior, and gestural communication);

Special Areas of Knowledge and Skills: Speech-Language Pathologists

Speech-language pathologists who provide AR have knowledge in the following special areas and demonstrate itemized requisite skills in those areas:

III. Auditory System Function and Disorders
   A. Describe the impact of various disorders of auditory function on communication (including disorders of the outer, middle, and inner ear, and the auditory nerve and the associated neural and central auditory system pathways and processes).

IV. Developmental Status, Cognition, and Sensory Perception
   A. Provide for the administration of assessment measures in the client's preferred mode of communication;
   B. Verify adequate visual acuity for communication purposes;
   C. Identify the need for assessment of cognitive, sensory perceptual and motor skills, developmental delays, academic achievement, and literacy;
   D. Determine the need for referral to other medical and nonmedical specialists for appropriate professional services;
   E. Provide for ongoing assessments of developmental progress.

V. Audiological Assessment Procedures
   A. Conduct audiologic screening as appropriate for initial identification and/or referral purposes;
   B. Describe type and degree of hearing loss from audiometric test results (including pure tone thresholds, immittance testing, and speech audiometry);
   C. Refer to and consult with an audiologist for administration and interpretation of differential diagnostic procedures (including behavioral, physiological, and electrophysiological measures).

VI. Assessment of Communication Performance
   A. Provide for assessment measures in the client's preferred mode of communication;
   B. Identify and perform screening examinations for speech, language, hearing, auditory processing disorders, and reading and academic achievement problems;
   C. Identify and perform diagnostic evaluations for the comprehension and production of speech and language in oral, signed, and written or augmented form;
   D. Provide diagnostic evaluations of speech perception in auditory, visual, auditory-visual, or tactile modalities;
   E. Identify the effects of hearing loss on speech perception, communication performance, listening skills, speechreading, communication strategies, and personal adjustment;
   F. Provide for clients' self-assessment of communication difficulties and adjustment of hearing loss;
   G. Monitor developmental progress in relation to communication competence.

figure *4.2*

Knowledge and skills required for the practice of audiologic/aural rehabilitation: speech-language pathologists.

Source: Reprinted with permission from *Knowledge and Skills Required for the Practice of Audiologic/Aural Rehabilitation* [Knowledge and skills]. From www.asha.org/policy. Copyright 2001 by American Speech-Language-Hearing Association. All rights reserved.

VII. Devices and Technologies for Individuals With Hearing Loss (e.g., hearing aids, cochlear implants, middle ear implants, implantable hearing aids, hearing assistive technologies, and other sensory prosthetic devices)
  A. Describe candidacy criteria for amplification or sensory-prosthetic devices (e.g., hearing aids, cochlear implants);
  B. Monitor clients' prescribed use of personal and group amplification systems;
  C. Describe options and applications of sensory aids (e.g., assistive listening devices) and telephone/telecommunication devices;
  D. Identify the need and refer to an audiologist for evaluation and fitting of personal and group amplification systems and sensory aids;
  E. Implement a protocol, in consultation with an audiologist, to promote adjustment to amplification;
  F. Perform routine visible inspection and listening checks of clients' hearing devices and sensory aids to troubleshoot common causes of malfunctioning (e.g., dead or corroded batteries, obstruction or damage to visual parts of the system);
  G. Refer on a regularly scheduled basis clients' personal and group amplification systems, other sensory aids, and assistive listening devices for comprehensive evaluations to ensure that instruments conform to audiologists' prescribed settings and manufacturers' specifications;
  H. Describe the effects of amplification use on communication function;
  I. Describe and monitor the effects of environmental factors on communication function.

VIII. Effects of Hearing Loss on Psychosocial, Educational, and Vocational Functioning
  A. Describe the effects of hearing loss on psychosocial development;
  B. Describe the effects of hearing loss on learning and literacy;
  C. Describe systems and methods of educational programming (e.g., mainstream, residential) and facilitate selection of appropriate educational options;
  D. Identify the need for and availability of psychological, social, educational, and vocational counseling;
  E. Identify and appropriately plan for addressing affective issues confronting the person with hearing loss;
  F. Identify appropriate consumer organizations and parent support groups.

IX. Intervention and Case Management
  A. Develop and implement a rehabilitative intervention plan based on communication skills and needs of the individual and family or caregivers of the individual;
  B. Provide for communication and counseling intervention in the client's preferred mode of communication;
  C. Develop expressive and receptive competencies in the client's preferred mode of communication;
  D. Provide speech, language, and auditory intervention (including but not limited to voice quality and control, resonance, phonologic and phonetic processes, oral motor skills, articulation, pronunciation, prosody, syntax/morphology, semantics, pragmatics);
  E. Facilitate appropriate multimodal forms of communication (e.g., auditory, visual, tactile, speechreading, spoken language, Cued Speech, simultaneous communication, total communications, communication technologies) for the client and family;
  F. Conduct interviews and interact effectively with individuals and their families;
  G. Develop and implement a system to measure and monitor outcomes and the efficacy of intervention.

X. Interdisciplinary Collaboration and Public Advocacy
  A. Collaborate effectively as part of multidisciplinary teams and communicate relevant information to allied professionals and other appropriate individuals;
  B. Plan and implement in-service and public-information programs for allied professionals and other interested individuals;
  C. Plan and implement parent-education programs concerning the management of hearing loss and subsequent communication problems;
  D. Plan and implement interdisciplinary service programs with allied professionals;
  E. Advocate implementation of public law in educational, occupational, and public settings;
  F. Refer to consumer-based organizations.

XI. Acoustic Environments
  A. Provide for appropriate environmental acoustic conditions for effective communication;
  B. Describe the effects of environmental influences, amplification systems, and sources of trauma on residual auditory function;
  C. Provide for periodic hearing screening for individuals exposed to hazardous noise.

figure *4.2*

(*Continued*)

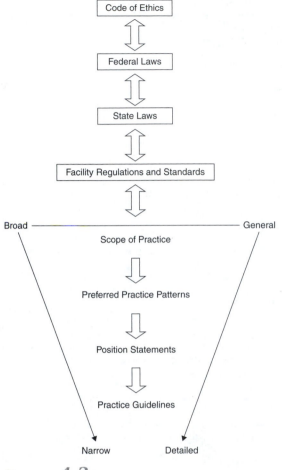

figure *4.3*

Multidimensional model of the regulatory influences on the practice of auditory rehabilitation.

Source: Scope of Practice in Audiology [Scope of Practice]. Available from www.asha.org/policy. Copyright 2004 by American Speech-Language-Hearing Association; JOHNSON, *Guidebook for Support Programs in Aural Rehabilitation*, 1E. © 1999 Delmar Learning, a part of Cengage Learning, Inc. Reproduced by permission. www.cengage.com/permissions.

pathologists' service delivery (i.e., top-down influence), but communication sciences and disorders professionals can lobby to change laws for increased funding enabling the delivery of adequate services to children in the schools (i.e., bottom-up influence). The model is context specific, meaning that service delivery sites ultimately determine applicable laws, rules, and regulations for service provision.

The codes of ethics for audiologists and speech-language pathologists are at the pinnacle of the model. The American Speech-Language-Hearing Association (ASHA) Code of Ethics (ASHA, 2010) provides guidelines for ethical practices in the professions. The situation can become more complicated when audiologists, for example, belong to several professional organizations with their own code of ethics. The American Academy of Audiology has published its own code of ethics that specifies guidelines for ethical practice for audiologists (AAA, 2009a). Occasionally, a professional organization will publish additional guidelines detailing ethical considerations in specific areas of practice. For example, the American Academy of Audiology published *Guidelines for Ethical Practice in Research for Audiologists* (Sininger, Marsh, Walden, & Wilber, 2003) written by the Task Force on Ethics in Audiology Research. Furthermore, the American Academy of Audiology board of directors accepted the recommendation of the Ethical Practices Board that the code of ethics be modified to include guidelines for researchers. Some ethical issues pertaining to auditory rehabilitation are discussed later in this chapter.

At the next level, audiologists and speech-language pathologists should be aware of federal and state laws affecting their practice. In December 2004, President George W. Bush signed into law the reauthorization of the Individuals with Disabilities Education Act (IDEA) with the Individuals with Disabilities Education Improvement Act (IDEIA) in accordance with the No Child Left Behind (NCLB) Act. The IDEA authorizes the federal government to release resources from the federal treasury to ensure that children with disabilities, including those who are deaf or hard of hearing, have access to a free and appropriate public education in the least restrictive environment (see Chapter 10). The changes in this federal law affect auditory rehabilitation service provision to school-age children having hearing loss. Another important law protecting the rights of persons with disabilities is Section 504 of the Rehabilitation Act of 1973 that states that no otherwise qualified individual with a disability is to be *"be excluded from the participation in, be denied the benefits of, or be subjected to discrimination under any program or activity receiving Federal financial assistance"* based solely on that disability. Another federal law that may impact auditory rehabilitation is the Americans with Disabilities Act (ADA) of 1990 that forbids discrimination on the basis of a disability (including hearing loss) in employment, in state and local government, public accommodations, commercial facilities, transportation, and telecommunications. A key element of this legislation is accessibility of those with disabilities to various aspects of American life through reasonable accommodations. For people with hearing loss, accommodations are frequently provided through hearing assistive technology. Another federal law is the Health Insurance Portability and Accountability Act (HIPAA) of 1996 (PL 104-191) that has far-reaching implications for healthcare in such areas as fraud and abuse, insurance portability, administrative simplification, and security of patient information. For example, the law states that patients have a right to determine where their healthcare information is sent. The information is to be used primarily for healthcare purposes. Violations of the privacy regulations can range from $100 for errors to up to $250,000 and 10 years in prison for malicious use of patient information. Audiologists and speech-language pathologists need to become familiar with HIPAA when providing services to patients with hearing impairment and their families.

At the next level of the model are state laws that may affect the provision of auditory rehabilitative services. Although the IDEA is a federal law, ultimately the special education laws of individual states determine its implementation. Other examples of state laws include those for licensure overseen by a board that consists of audiologists, speech-language pathologists, and consumers. For example, the Alabama Board of Examiners for Speech-Language Pathology (ABESPA) helps to ensure the highest quality of services to the citizens of the state of Alabama, including auditory rehabilitation. The intent of the licensure law is to (ABESPA, 2010):

1. Require educational training and licensure of any person who engages in the practice of speech-language pathology and/or audiology.
2. Encourage better educational training programs.
3. Prohibit the unauthorized and unqualified practice of speech-language pathology and audiology.
4. Prohibit the unprofessional conduct of persons licensed to practice speech-language pathology and/or audiology.

At the next level, accrediting bodies of healthcare organizations, such as The Joint Commission (formerly the Joint Commission on the Accreditation of Healthcare Organizations [JCAHO]), regulate the practice of healthcare providers, including audiologists and speech-language pathologists who provide auditory rehabilitation in medical facilities. In its 2010 Portable Comprehensive Accreditation Manual for Hospitals (CAMH), the official Handbook, the Joint Commission specifies dimensions of performance with regard to efficacy, appropriateness, availability, timeliness, effectiveness, continuity, safety, efficiency, respect, and caring. Each healthcare entity will have its own operating procedures that will influence the implementation of auditory rehabilitation in long-term residential care facilities for the elderly, for example, the number of these facilities will continue to increase to accommodate the expected growth in the number of persons over 65 years of age in the United States.

At the next level, Scopes of Practice in Audiology (ASHA, 2004b) and Speech-Language Pathology (ASHA, 2007): (1) describe the services provided by communication sciences and disorders professionals; (2) serve as a reference for healthcare, education, and other professionals, as well as for consumers, members of the general public, and policy makers concerned with legislation, regulation, licensure, and third-party reimbursement; and (3) inform members of ASHA, certificate holders, and students of the activities for which certification is required in accordance with the ASHA Code of Ethics (ASHA, 2010). In addition, AAA had a scope of practice document for its members, too (AAA, 2004a). The Scopes of Practice for Audiology and Speech-Language Pathology can assist communication sciences and disorders professionals in determining appropriate auditory rehabilitative services to be provided by each profession. Scope of practice documents are not static, but change and expand for both professions. For example, the rehabilitation of balance disorders is now within the scope of practice for audiologists.

Because the scopes of practice for audiology and speech-language pathology are rather broad, communication sciences and disorders professionals can rely on preferred practice patterns, position statements, and guidelines for clinical practice published by ASHA and AAA. **Preferred practice patterns** are statements that define universally applicable characteristics of specific clinical activities, including definitions, expected outcomes, clinical indications, clinical processes, setting and equipment specifications, and documentation, as well as specify which professionals perform the procedures (ASHA, 2006b). Preferred Practice Patterns for Audiology and Speech-Language Pathology are not official standards, but offer guidance for enhancing the quality of professional services to consumers (Grantham, 1996). Preferred practice patterns must be revised and updated to account for new technology and expanding scopes of practice.

Position statements, practice guidelines, task forces, and reports also assist audiologists and speech-language pathologists to provide quality auditory rehabilitative services to patients having hearing impairment. **Position statements** are documents on timely topics supported by available scientific evidence and/or expert opinion put forth by professional organizations consistent with intrinsic and/or extrinsic goals and objectives (AAA, 2009b). **Practice guidelines** are a systematically defined set of recommended procedures that are based on scientific evidence and/or expert opinion that have been designed to lead to well-defined outcomes (AAA, 2009b). **Task forces** are teams of experts recruited by professional organizations to assess and/or determine appropriate strategies for issues affecting professional practice and pertaining to the recognized areas of practice (AAA, 2009b). **Reports** are testimonies or accounts of factual information related to professional issues identified by a professional organization (AAA, 2009b). Throughout this textbook, we will review several types of documents pertaining to auditory rehabilitation.

PROFESSIONAL ORGANIZATIONS AND AUDITORY REHABILITATION

Professional organizations such as AAA and ASHA influence auditory rehabilitation in a variety of ways. For example, we already discussed how AAA has developed clinical practice guidelines, and later in this chapter we will discuss how both organizations are promoting evidence-based practice (EBP) in auditory rehabilitation. In addition, ASHA has published preferred practice patterns, position statements, practice guidelines, and practice standards related to the auditory rehabilitation of children and adults. ASHA has also developed **special interest divisions** for members to focus on different areas of expertise such as auditory rehabilitation. For example, the mission of the Aural Rehabilitation and Its Instrumentation Special Interest Division is to facilitate the ability to minimize or prevent, across the life span, the limitations and restrictions that auditory dysfunctions can impose on well-being, and on communicative, interpersonal, psychosocial educational, and vocational functioning (ASHA, 2006c).

Through their political action committees (PACs), both AAA and ASHA work hard to represent the issues of concern on Capitol Hill for the professions and for people with hearing impairments. For example, the AAA PAC promotes better understanding among elected officials regarding the importance of providing access to high-quality hearing healthcare services to patients with hearing impairment (AAA, 2006a). Both AAA and ASHA have been instrumental in lobbying for legislation on direct access and hearing aid tax credits. The idea of direct access is to eliminate the need for Medicare patients to obtain a physician referral prior to seeing an audiologist. The hearing aid tax credit legislation seeks to provide some persons a $500 tax credit toward the purchase of a hearing aid once every five years.

Some smaller professional organizations are focused solely on auditory rehabilitation. The **Academy of Rehabilitative Audiology** (ARA) has a goal of promoting excellence in hearing care through the provision of comprehensive rehabilitative and habilitative services by providing the following services (ARA, 2010):

1. Providing a forum for the exchange of ideas, knowledge, and experiences with the audiologic habilitative, and rehabilitative components of hearing care.
2. Fostering and stimulating education, research, and interest in habilitation and rehabilitation for persons who are hearing impaired.
3. Expanding and improving delivery of services to and on behalf of individuals with hearing impairment.
4. Receiving, holding and using gifts, bequests, and endowments for the organization to achieve its purposes.
5. Serving as a public policy advocate for audiologic rehabilitative and habilitative services.

These organizations may be contacted at the following addresses:

Academy of Rehabilitative Audiology
Association Coordinator
P.O. Box 2323
Albany, NY 12220-0323
Fax: (866) 547-3073
E-mail: ara@audrehab.org
www.audrehab.org

American Academy of Audiology
11730 Plaza America Drive
Suite 300
Reston, VA 20190
Phone: 1(800) AAA-2336
Fax: (703) 790-8631
www.audiology.org

American Speech-Language-Hearing Association
2200 Research Boulevard
Rockville, MD 20850-3289
Phone:
  Members: 1(800) 498-2071
  Nonmembers: 1(800) 638-8255
TTY (Text Telephone Communication Device): (301) 296-5650
E-mail: actioncenter@asha.org
www.asha.org

Other professional organizations within the professions that affect the provision of auditory rehabilitative services include the Educational Audiology Association, the National Hearing Conservation Association, and the Military Audiology Association, among others. Moreover, numerous physicians' professional organizations impact auditory rehabilitation, such as the American Medical Association, the American Academy of Pediatrics, and the American Academy of Otolaryngology, Head, and Neck Surgery.

CONTEMPORARY PROFESSIONAL ISSUES IN AUDITORY REHABILITATION

It is not possible to explore all professional issues related to auditory rehabilitation in a single chapter. However, readers may gain an appreciation through the following three examples: reimbursement, evidence-based practice, and ethics in auditory rehabilitation.

Reimbursement

Communication sciences and disorders professionals, especially those in private practice, need to be paid or reimbursed for services provided. Moreover, many patients cannot afford to pay out-of-pocket for auditory rehabilitation. Therefore, professional organizations such as ASHA and AAA work hard to strengthen the positioning of the professions within the healthcare arena so that audiologists and speech-language pathologists are paid for their services and more and more Americans have access to auditory rehabilitation.

What is a **third-party payer**? A third-party payer is an entity other than the healthcare provider or patient who reimburses for procedures performed, diagnoses made, and certain devices, supplies, and/or other equipment for patients (ASHA, 1996). Examples of third-party payers include private healthcare plans, Medicare, and Medicaid. Third-party payers require healthcare providers to submit claims for reimbursement using healthcare services coding systems. Third-party payers are extremely important because the majority of patients requiring auditory rehabilitation cannot afford to pay out-of-pocket for these services. Coverage for these services increases the public's accessibility to necessary hearing healthcare. For audiologists and speech-language pathologists, reimbursement of services is critical for meeting overhead and funding viable clinical programs. Audiologists, in particular, are trying to achieve adequate reimbursement for the auditory rehabilitative services they provide. Reimbursement for these services has been complex because of the large number of third-party payers and the variations in how they classify and reimburse for auditory rehabilitation. One obstacle has been that because Medicare had viewed audiologic services as diagnostic, other third-party payers do, too; this has limited the amount of reimbursement for auditory rehabilitation. In Chapter 1, we explained how the ASHA Health Care Economics Committee recommended and had the term "aural rehabilitation," associated with speech-language pathology, replaced with the more professionally neutral term of **auditory rehabilitation** for use in coding to increase the likelihood of reimbursement for services provided by audiologists (White, 2006, 2009). Three healthcare coding systems that are important to audiologists and speech-language pathologists are briefly described here. However, detail regarding how to use these coding systems is beyond the scope of this textbook. For more information, readers should see Hosford-Dunn Roeser and Valente (2008).

The *Current Procedural Terminology* (CPT), maintained by the American Medical Association, uses a five-digit code (e.g., 92553) to report healthcare procedures or services rendered to patients. For example, the CPT code for pure-tone air- and bone-conduction testing is 92553. CPT codes are a recognized and reliable vehicle for nationwide communications among various stakeholders in healthcare (e.g., physicians, patients, audiologists, speech-language pathologists, third-party payers, and so on) (AAA, 2009c). The Department of Health and Human Services stated that the CPT code set is the national standard for healthcare services and procedures under HIPAA and must be used if electronic transactions are to be processed (AAA, 2009c). The potential for choosing the appropriate code is increased when healthcare providers follow these guidelines (AAA, 2009c):

- Choose codes that actually reflect what was done.
- Choose the most comprehensive code that "bundles" other coded procedures under one procedure.
- Choose a correct modifier, consisting of two codes, that is tacked on to supply additional information.

Modifiers provide additional information about a procedure. For example, the modifier -52 is used to indicate reduced services, such as when an audiologist performs pure-tone air- and bone-conduction testing on one ear only. Thus, the code 92553 (for pure-tone air- and bone-conduction testing) would be appended as 92553-52 (for reduced services).

A second system, the *Healthcare Common Procedure Coding System*, is maintained by the Centers for Medicare and Medicaid Services. This system uses an alphanumeric code (e.g., V5244) to report diagnoses, disorders, conditions, and symptoms of patients seen for services. The third system is the *International Classification of Diseases, 9th edition, Clinical Modification* (known as ICD-9-CM), which is maintained by the National Center for Health Statistics, Centers for Disease Control and Prevention, and the U.S. Department of Health and Human Services. ICD-9-CM uses a more complicated coding system to report diagnoses, disorders, conditions, and symptoms. For example, the system uses a tabular list organized by three numeric digit codes with third-party payers that expect codes to be carried to a fifth digit to the highest degree of diagnostic certainty. For example, the code for deafness is 389 which is extended to 389.12 for neural hearing loss, if possible. The ICD-9-CM coding system uses supplemental alphanumeric V-codes for recording the purpose of the visit and any circumstances influencing the patient's health status. The system is transitioning to the *International Classification of Diseases, 10th edition, Clinical Modification* (ICD-10-CM) which is to be completed by October 1, 2013.

Adequate reimbursement for auditory rehabilitation by third-party payers requires audiologists and speech-language pathologists to keep up with the latest changes in healthcare policy. One key ingredient for increased reimbursement is an increased emphasis on evidence-based practice (EBP) showing how auditory rehabilitative services and technology improve the lives of patients with hearing loss and balance disorders.

Evidence-Based Practice

Evidence-based practice (EBP) is the combining of clinician expertise, patient values and preferences, and the best available evidence in clinical decision-making (ASHA, 2004c). Chapter 5 discusses the application of EBP to auditory rehabilitation. Too often, scientific evidence and clinical practice are not incorporated on a regular basis for service provision. Students may feel that what they learn in their classes and clinical practica is separate from the concepts they learn in research methods courses. However, as indicated in its definition, EBP requires the interface of clinical expertise, patient values and preferences, and scientific evidence into clinical decision-making. In other words, clinicians should consider whether or not scientific evidence supports what they are doing in the clinic using the following five-step process (Cox, 2005):

- Formulating a clinical research question
- Searching for the evidence
- Evaluating the evidence
- Integrating scientific evidence, clinical expertise, and patient values and preferences for clinical decision-making
- Evaluating the process

EBP should be thought of as a clinical rather than a research skill. Some have felt that EBP de-emphasizes the role of clinicians or desires of patients. However, nothing could be further from the truth! In fact, it takes skillful clinicians to place scientific evidence within the context of what they know works from their professional experience in reverence to and with consultation with patients in finding solutions to problems. However, EBP is a major change in the way that our professions have provided clinical services. Therefore, a change to EBP requires major direction and support from our professional organizations.

In recent years, ASHA has made EBP a focus-based initiative. In addition, ASHA has published a position statement, *Evidence-Based Practice in Communication Disorders* (ASHA, 2005c), and a technical report, *Evidence-Based Practice in Communication Disorders: An Introduction (Technical Report)* (ASHA, 2004c), on the topic. The technical report highlights six steps for the professions to make for EBP. The first step is to provide educational opportunities for clinicians in order to increase their knowledge of and implementation of EBP. Both AAA and ASHA have held conferences on the topic, and ASHA's website has special pages devoted to tutorials and development of its EBP Compendium discussed in Chapter 5. A second step is to assist university programs by teaching faculty how to infuse EBP into their curricula in training the next generation of professionals. However, communication sciences and disorders professionals and students do not learn how to do EBP through content information alone. Students need to have concrete examples of how EBP is related to what they are currently learning and doing in the classroom. In addition to an entire chapter on EBP, readers will notice sections in this textbook called "What does the evidence show?" relating current research findings directly to key concepts. Professors and supervisors need to make EBP an integral part of clinical practice and professional training. Therefore, a third step toward EBP is to showcase exemplary uses of EBP by researchers and clinicians on the websites and at annual conventions. Both AAA and ASHA have EBP materials and tools available on their websites for professionals and students. Similarly, over the past several years, both professional organizations have emphasized EBP in educational offerings at their professional meetings.

A fourth step is to ensure that various stakeholders (e.g., editors, reviewers, and authors) associated with AAA and ASHA journals that publish our research is familiar with the latest recommendations regarding the quality of scientific investigations. Using EBP is of little value if the overall quality of research studies in the professions is flawed. Both AAA and ASHA have provided information on their website with links to resources about standards for conducting and reporting diagnostic and interventional studies. They also have incorporated

EBP into the development of clinical practice guidelines. Editors', reviewers', and authors' familiarity with best practices in the dissemination of diagnostic and interventional research increases the applicability of content from ASHA's journals into EBP. Chapter 5 goes over the basics of sound research design and how to evaluate the rigor of studies in auditory rehabilitation. A fifth step is to encourage audiologists and speech-language pathologists to realize that the systematic review of evidence requires a lot of time, resources, training, and impartiality. A special type of study, a systematic review, often takes 2 or more years and involves the commitment of several team members. **Systematic reviews** are highly structured research methodologies that seek to assess the available scientific evidence pertaining to a well-asked question. Systematic reviews employ secondary measurement methods in that rather than collecting data, they analyze the data that has been collected and analyzed by other investigators. Until recently, systematic reviews were a relatively new concept to audiologists and speech-language pathologists. However, more and more systematic reviews are being published in our journals. We will talk more about systematic reviews in Chapter 5 on EBP in auditory rehabilitation. Finally, the sixth step was for ASHA to be an independent, broadly representative task force composed of researchers, clinicians, members, related professionals, and consumers to focus on EBP.

In addition to ASHA's efforts regarding EBP, AAA has made significant steps toward EBP. For example, a Task Force on the Health-related Quality of Life Benefits of Amplification was established, which conducted a systematic review of the health-related quality-of-life benefits derived from the use of hearing aids (Chisolm et al., 2007). They found that good evidence exists that the use of amplification enhances the health-related quality of life for adults with sensorineural hearing loss. The information will be useful to healthcare providers who make recommendations to their adult patients considering the use of hearing aids. Moreover, AAA established the Task Force for Guidelines for the Audiologic Management of Adult Hearing Impairment and developed the first set of clinical practice guidelines based on scientific findings complete with level of evidence, grading, and declaration of either *effectiveness* or *efficacy* for each clinical recommendation (Valente et al., 2006). We will discuss levels of evidence, grading, and the meaning of effectiveness and efficaciousness in Chapter 5 in addition to this new clinical practice guideline in Chapter 6.

Ethics in Auditory Rehabilitation

Audiology and speech-language pathology are professions whose members should uphold and maintain high ethical standards by complying with codes of conduct (Freeman, 2006; Loh, 2000). When audiologists and speech-language pathologists join professional organizations such as AAA and ASHA, they agree to abide by their respective codes of ethics. Violations of these principles may be reported to the Ethical Practices Committee of AAA, for example. AAA has an **ethical practice board** that investigates and adjudicates members who have reportedly violated the academy's code of ethics. Substantiated violations of the code of ethics may result in reprimand of the offending professional. The codes of ethics for both AAA (www.audiology.org) and ASHA (www.asha.org) are available on their websites; readers are advised to obtain copies of these documents. There are many principles common to both documents, and many have direct relevance to auditory rehabilitation. A few principles from the AAA Code of Ethics will be used to illustrate these points.

- Principle 1 states, "Members shall provide professional services and conduct research with honesty and compassion, and shall respect the dignity, worth, and rights of those served."

As discussed in the last chapter, audiologists and speech-language pathologists should not discriminate against patients based on cultural or linguistic backgrounds or their ability to pay. Judging someone without reason is prejudice; discrimination occurs when prejudice results in differential treatment of people.

- Principle 2 states, "Members shall maintain high standards of professional competence in rendering services."

Earlier in the chapter we discussed how the skill of respecting professional boundaries established in scope of practice documents is necessary for cross-professional competence. It is a violation of the AAA Code of Ethics to provide services outside one's scope of practice. In Chapter 2, we discussed the need for audiologists and speech-language pathologists to recognize when nonprofessional counseling is not enough for patients and their families and that their issues may require referral to appropriate mental health professionals. In addition, professionals need to acknowledge when their knowledge and skills are inadequate and/or outdated in a particular area of practice, necessitating a referral to a more qualified colleague. Intraprofessional and interprofessional documents emphasize that professionals should have expertise in particular areas of practice to best suit the needs of patients. **Intraprofessional documents** are those that are generated by professional organizations (e.g., ASHA or AAA) to guide their members (e.g., audiologists and speech-language pathologists). **Interprofessional documents** are those that are generated by a group of individuals who represent different professional organizations, usually different professions, on multidisciplinary issues. One such document, the Joint Committee on Infant Hearing Year 2007 Position Statement, states that young children identified in early hearing detection and intervention programs and their families should be seen by professionals with expertise appropriate for this area of practice. It was advised that otolaryngologists serving these children should have experience with pediatric hearing loss. Moreover, all professionals, including educators of the deaf, audiologists, and speech-language pathologists providing early intervention services for infants with hearing losses and their families, should have expertise in hearing loss.

To keep up-to-date, professionals are bound by the code of ethics to participate in **continuing education**, or formal acquisition of knowledge and skills beyond those obtained in professional training programs. State licensure boards, ASHA, and ABA require specific numbers of continuing education credits for professionals to maintain their credentials. Audiologists and speech-language pathologists have many options for continuing education activities in a variety of venues, including face-to-face meetings, online courses, and self-study. Technological advances in auditory rehabilitation, particularly in the areas of hearing aids and cochlear implants, require that professionals stay on the cutting edge to provide adequate services.

Other relevant parts of the AAA Code of Ethics include the following:

- Principle 4 states, "Members shall provide only services and products that are in the best interest of those served."
- Principle 5 states, "Members shall provide accurate information about the nature and management of communicative disorders and about the services and products offered."

Above all, audiologists and speech-language pathologists should hold the well-being of the patients they serve as paramount. Communication sciences and disorders professionals should avoid any situations that present a **conflict of interest**, which are characterized by the following descriptions (Kukula, 2006, pp. 133–134):

- when personal interests and the professional duties of a person are at odds
- when the potential for personal gain is in conflict with professional decision making
- when a result of incentives such as cash or trips entices or creates the appearance of enticing professionals to act in their own personal interest

Situations providing conflicts of interest can arise from a variety of sources. Hearing aid manufacturers have been known to discount the wholesale price of hearing aids to audiologists or to buying groups that dispense a large quantity of devices (Hawkins, Larkin, & Tedeschi, 2006). Could a temptation of a discount for selling lots of hearing aids cloud an audiologist's judgment in trying to sell more hearing instruments to patients who may not need them? Could an audiologist be tempted to exaggerate the expected benefits of hearing aids, or a particular brand of hearing aids, in order to make a sale? Maybe, maybe not! Audiologists need to look deep inside themselves for the answer. In such circumstances, it is advisable for audiologists to avoid even the *appearance* of any conflicts of interest that may arise from their relationships with hearing aid manufacturers, including business development plans and reward banks; loans for audiologic equipment; continuing education events at exotic locations; and cash rebates, cruises, vacation packages, and/or convention parties and dinners (Hawkins et al., 2006). AAA has published *Ethical Practice Guidelines on Financial Incentives from Hearing Instrument Manufacturers* that present the following basic principles of conduct (AAA, 2004b):

1. When potential for conflict of interest exists, the interests of the patient must come before those of the audiologist.
2. Commercial interest in any product or service recommended must be disclosed to the patient.
3. Travel expenses, registration fees, or compensation for time to attend meetings, conferences, or seminars should not be accepted directly or indirectly from a manufacturer.
4. Free equipment or discounts for equipment, institutional support, or any form of remuneration from a vendor for research purposes should be fully disclosed and the results of research must be adequately reported.

The AAA guidelines also include a common question-and-answer section clarifying specific issues for audiologists.

Abel and Hahn (2006) stated that audiologists should do what they can to prevent healthcare fraud. To do so requires knowledge of two federal laws: (1) Stark Law, and (2) Anti-kickback Statute. The **Stark Law** (42 U.S.C. 1395nn) is civil law that prohibits physician "self-referral" in that physicians cannot refer patients to entities in which they or their family members have financial holdings (for additional information, see www.cms.hhs.gov). Although audiologists and speech-language pathologists are not physicians, they should pattern their professional dealings according to the same high standards and avoid conflicts of interest by not referring patients to other healthcare professionals with whom they have financial interests. Another law, the **Federal Anti-kickback Statute** (42 U.S.C. 1320a-7b) prohibits healthcare professionals from receiving payments for referrals to providers for services reimbursable through federal programs such as Medicaid or Medicare (Abel & Hahn, 2006; Kukula, 2006).

In summary, we have discussed only a few ethical issues in the provision of auditory rehabilitation services to patients with hearing loss and their families. Audiologists and speech-language pathologists are obligated to uphold the codes of ethics of their professional organizations in order to protect their respective professions and their patients.

SUMMARY

One intention of this chapter has been to provide readers with an understanding of the complementary roles of audiologists and speech-language pathologists in providing auditory rehabilitation. Because hearing loss can affect many aspects of a person's life, auditory rehabilitation often requires not only that audiologists and speech-language pathologists be technically skilled, but also adept at working with others as part of a team. This chapter discussed the importance of developing cross-professional competence in providing services to patients with hearing loss and their families. In addition, this chapter has presented the knowledge and skills recommended for audiologists and speech-language pathologists to have in the provision of auditory rehabilitative services (ASHA, 2001). In conclusion, comtemporary issues of reimbursement, EBP, and the impact of ethics on auditory rehabilitation were examined.

LEARNING ACTIVITIES

- Interview an audiologist or speech-language pathologist who participates on a team that provides auditory rehabilitation. How is the team approach beneficial for patients? What are the most difficult aspects of team management?
- If you are a student member of AAA or ASHA, go to their websites, search for professional documents that pertain to auditory rehabilitation that interest you or that are discussed in this textbook, download them on your computer, or print them out for the development of your own resource notebook.

CHAPTER five

Evidence-Based Practice in Auditory Rehabilitation

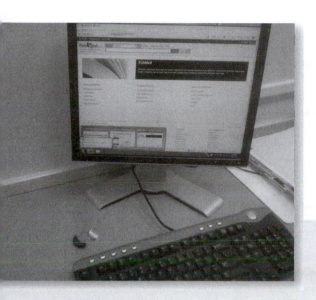

LEARNING *objectives*

After reading this chapter, you should be able to:

1. Define and understand the process of evidence-based practice (EBP).
2. Use tools and resources for EBP.
3. Understand the importance of EBP in auditory rehabilitation.

"Wow, that class was so boring!" remarked Kendra, a first-year doctor of audiology student.

"Yeah, I worked on my clinical report. I feel sorry for Dr. Taylor. Most of us use his class to work on other assignments!" admitted Summer, Kendra's classmate.

"Why do they make us take a research methods class anyhow?" wondered Kendra. "I decided to get my Au.D., not Ph.D., so I wouldn't have to study research methods. I want to do clinical work with patients."

"Me, too," Summer agreed. "After all, what does research have to do with clinical work anyway?"

Like Kendra and Summer, many communication sciences and disorders students wonder about the relevance of research to clinical practice. The number of students pursuing doctor of philosophy degrees (Ph.D.) in speech and hearing sciences has decreased somewhat in recent years. Is research relevant to clinical practice in audiology and speech-language pathology? Is research relevant to auditory rehabilitation? No one would disagree about the importance of research to medicine, especially in using the best diagnostic methods and treatment protocols for cancer. After all, clinical oncology deals with treating patients who have cancer, a potentially fatal disease. How does a physician decide which treatment option has the greatest likelihood for success, does not compromise quality of life, and is the safest?

Oncologists, like other physicians, practice *evidence-based medicine*, which can be defined as the "conscientious, explicit, and judicious use of current best evidence in making sound decisions about the care of individual patients" (Sackett, Rosenberg, Gray, Haynes, & Richardson, 1996). The key term in this definition is **best evidence**. "Best" is excelling all others; "evidence" is that which furnishes proof. Therefore, the best evidence may be defined as scientific proof that exceeds all others. As with EBM, clinical decisions in auditory rehabilitation should be based on the best scientific evidence or that which has the least amount of **bias**, or the influence that factors unrelated to the treatment have on patient outcomes. Bias may come from a motivated researcher who developed a new treatment or from a patient who is convinced that a new medicine will cure his or her illness. Biomedical research studies are ranked according to **levels of evidence** or hierarchies-based on the consistency of results and degree of experimental control to minimize bias. In other words, studies that show consistent results across investigations that have minimized sources of bias are at the highest levels of evidence. For example, systematic reviews of randomized, controlled clinical trials are at the highest level of evidence.

Systematic reviews involve asking research questions; searching, evaluating, and analyzing results of several studies together through special statistical procedures called **meta-analysis**; and making overall conclusions regarding the consistency of findings for a particular treatment. **Double-blinded prospective randomized, controlled clinical trials** (DBPRCTs) are single experimental studies that minimize bias through random assignment of patients to treatment and control groups and concealment of this information to participants and researchers. Therefore, systematic reviews that combine the results of all high-quality DBPRCTs about the effectiveness of a particular treatment satisfy requirements for the highest level of evidence. We will expand on this concept later in the chapter.

However, scientific evidence is only one piece of the puzzle in clinical decision-making. Clinical acumen in auditory rehabilitation is another important factor and requires experienced audiologists or speech-language pathologists. Clinical expertise is the sum total of a practitioner's knowledge, skills, and experience. It is the art of clinical practice that cannot be learned from reading a book, but instead is honed through years of learning about, diagnosing, and managing hearing loss. Still another piece of the puzzle is the patient, his or her family, and their unique set of characteristics. As defined in Chapter 4, evidence-based practice (EBP) is integrating high-quality research evidence, practitioner expertise, and patient preferences and values into the process of making clinical decisions (ASHA, 2004c, 2005c).

Evidence-based practice has signified a paradigm shift for auditory rehabilitation, as it has for all areas of practice in communication sciences and disorders. How is this approach different from the way most audiologists and speech-language pathologists have been trained and now practice? In the past, students learned of normal human communication processes and disorders, observed treatment procedures, and subsequently implemented those techniques in clinical practicum. However, Cox (2004) stated that in EBP, first priority is given to the results of original research that actually measures treatment success on patients in the real world. If a treatment has not shown evidence of real-world effectiveness, clinicians must accept uncertainty of the value of the intervention (Cox, 2004). Let's see how EBP is important for the decisions to be made by the Smiths and the Washingtons.

Casebook Reflection

Quality of Life and Hearing Aids – Part 1

Irene and Charles Smith were sitting at the breakfast table reading the paper. Charles, 70, is professor emeritus in the biology department at their local university. He was just diagnosed as having a moderate-to-severe sensorineural hearing loss. Charles grew up respecting the value of a dollar.

"Don't forget your appointment at the Speech and Hearing Clinic today, dear," reminded Irene. "Today, you need to consider the latest technology and decide whether or not to get hearing aids. I am not going to nag you anymore. It is your decision. That is why I'm staying home."

"I know, I know. The hearing aids will help me hear better, but I want to know if they are going to improve our communication," Charles said. "I am tired of arguing with you and the children. I don't want to be embarrassed in public. I am not sure if hearing aids will improve my overall quality of life."

"You be nice to those sweet young ladies at the clinic, you hear?" warned Irene. "You were quite demanding with that student, Kendra, during your evaluation."

"Oh, I'll be good, dear. Don't you worry," said Charles, who didn't feel that Irene sensed his degree of frustration.

Dr. Weil and Kendra knew that Charles was concerned whether the hearing aids would improve his quality of life.

Casebook Reflection

Cochlear Implants for Joshua – Part 1

"Honey, come to bed. You've been glued to the computer since you put Josh to bed. What's so interesting?" asked Leon, wondering what was keeping his wife.

"Wow, it's 11:30!" exclaimed Debbie. "Where has the time gone?"

Debbie and Leon Washington are parents of Joshua, a 13-month-old with a profound sensorineural hearing loss who was fit with hearing aids when he was just a few weeks old. His parents have been heavily involved in his aural habilitation sessions. Unfortunately, Joshua has not been making the progress that he should with his hearing aids. The Washingtons were referred by Dr. Trenoth to the cochlear implant center for an evaluation. The cochlear implant team believed that Joshua was an excellent candidate for bilateral cochlear implants placed simultaneously, during a single surgery. Long before Joshua's cochlear implant evaluation, Debbie had read about cochlear implants and had assumed that one of Joshua's ears would be implanted during the surgery, with the other ear possibly receiving an implant in the future. Simultaneous implantation seemed to Debbie like a lot for a single surgery.

"I'm concerned about Joshua undergoing a bilateral cochlear implantation during a single surgery. I'd like to talk to Dr. Trenoth," Debbie said as she logged off her computer.

"Call her in the morning and let's make an appointment," Leon suggested.

Dr. Trenoth, the audiologist who diagnosed Joshua's hearing loss, had become a trusted professional to the Washingtons. She had recommended, in conjunction with the Washingtons' pediatrician, that Joshua have an evaluation for a cochlear implant at the local hospital.

"I'll do that," Debbie said.

The next morning Debbie called Dr. Trenoth's office. "Hello, Becky, this is Debbie Washington. How are you?"

"I'm fine, and you?" replied Becky.

"Great! Is Dr. Trenoth in?" Debbie asked.

"Yes, I believe she is between appointments. Hold on," said Becky.

"Dr. Trenoth. It's Debbie Washington on line 2."

"Thanks, Becky," said Dr. Trenoth. "Mrs. Washington, how are you and Joshua?"

"Just fine! Joshua is growing like a weed. I was wondering if my husband and I can talk to you about Joshua's cochlear implantation evaluation and recommendation," Debbie explained.

"Yes, just set it up with Becky. See you soon," Dr. Trenoth.

"Thank you, very much. You have done so much for Joshua, and we value your opinion," Debbie explained.

"It's my pleasure. I'll send you through to Becky. Hold on," Dr. Trenoth said.

The Washingtons' and the Smiths' audiologists must use EBP to facilitate the process of making clinical decisions concerning these patients and their families. The purpose of this chapter is to familiarize students with EBP and its relevance to auditory rehabilitation.

FOUNDATIONS FOR EVIDENCE-BASED PRACTICE IN AUDITORY REHABILITATION

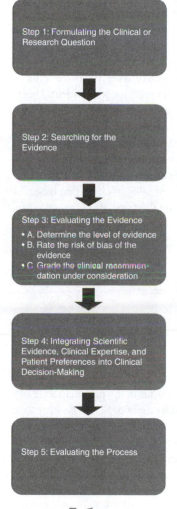

figure *5.1*——————

Five-step process for evidence-based practice.

Source: Based on "Evidence-Based Practice in Provision of Amplification," by R. M. Cox, 2005, *Journal of the American Academy of Audiology, 16,* pp. 419–438.

How do we apply EBP to auditory rehabilitation? We already read about Kendra, Dr. Weil, and Charles and his questions about the quality-of-life benefits of hearing aids. In our other scenario, Debbie Washington had some concerns about the recommendation for bilateral simultaneous cochlear implantation for her son, Joshua. Dr. Elizabeth Trenoth, Joshua's audiologist, was consulted about the Washingtons' questions. In both scenarios, hearing health-care providers must apply EBP procedures in order to make the best recommendations to their patients. Practicing clinicians go through a five-step process for EBM and EBP (Sackett, Straus, Richardson, Rosenberg, & Haynes, 2005). Figure 5.1 shows the five-step process for EBP.

Step 1: Formulating the Clinical or Research Question

The first step is to develop or frame a clinical or research question to be answered in EBP. Typically, clinicians must develop a clinical or research question involving a decision to be made with and about patients and their families surrounding treatments for hearing loss and balance disorders. A helpful procedure is to use the acronym PICO, which stands for **P**opulation, **I**ntervention, **C**omparison (Intervention), and **O**utcome in framing the research question (Cox, 2005). The PICO framework includes spaces for clinicians to write critical elements of a clinical scenario according to the following parameter descriptors:

Population

Intervention

Comparison (Intervention)

Outcome

The PICO rubric may be used with several types of EBP questions encountered in auditory rehabilitation. The most common type of question for auditory rehabilitation is an **intervention question** that focuses on the relative *efficacy, effectiveness,* or *efficiency* of two or more treatments for a specific patient or population. Briefly, **efficacy** is the degree to which intervention results in positive outcomes in ideal settings such as a laboratory (ASHA, 2004c, 2005c). **Effectiveness** is the extent to which treatments provide positive patient outcomes in real-world settings (ASHA, 2004c, 2005c). Finally, **efficiency** is the extent to which one treatment provides relatively better outcomes than other treatments. Scientific evidence helps the clinician decide which treatments are best for patients to consider. It is important to sort out which treatments show promise in laboratory settings, but may not be feasible in the real world. Likewise, EBP assists in selecting the best treatment between two appropriate options for a particular patient.

Auditory rehabilitation may also involve **diagnostic questions** that seek to compare the relative efficacy, effectiveness, or efficiency of two assessment tools. Typically, the accuracy of a new assessment tool is compared against a **gold standard**, which is considered to be the most valid and reliable measure that diagnoses a disease or disorder (e.g., audiogram is the gold standard of measure for hearing loss). Customarily, most students think of diagnostic audiology as involving assessment, whereas rehabilitative audiology focuses on intervention. However, in a later chapter, we will discuss the importance of assessment as part of the rehabilitation process.

Auditory rehabilitation may also involve **etiologic questions** that investigate the relative risk of certain exposures (e.g., noise) for developing a certain disease or disorder (e.g., noise-induced hearing loss). As discussed in Chapter 3, auditory rehabilitation also involves the prevention of hearing loss, so etiologic questions are also relevant.

Examples of other EBP questions for auditory rehabilitation include *patient safety* and *cost-effectiveness* questions. **Patient-safety questions** evaluate the relative risks versus benefits of clinical procedures for specific patients or populations. Some treatments for sensorineural hearing loss involve weighing the benefits of surgically implanted devices (e.g., cochlear implants or bone-anchored hearing aids) versus traditional hearing aids. In one of our Casebook Reflections, Debbie Washington was wondering about the relative safety of a simultaneous bilateral cochlear implantation versus implantation of just one ear. **Cost-effectiveness questions** compare the relative costs versus benefits of clinical procedures. Patients and their families may consider the relative benefits versus the cost of two or more hearing aids prior to purchase. As described earlier, completion of the PICO rubric requires defining the population, intervention, alternative treatment (comparison intervention), and outcome.

Population	
Intervention	
Alternative Treatment	
Outcome	

Population

Defining the population begins with determining salient characteristics of the patient that are relevant to the clinical outcome. The case history provides critical information such as type, degree, and configuration of hearing loss in addition to etiology and age of onset. Other important factors may be previous auditory rehabilitation, including use of hearing aids and any formal communication training. In some situations, patients' cultural, ethnic, and linguistic backgrounds may be important defining characteristics for a clinical population. However, it is important not to be so specific that it is difficult to find relevant evidence. On the other hand, the population should not be so generic that it precludes direct application of recovered evidence to the patient.

In our scenario, Charles is concerned about whether getting hearing aids is going to improve his quality of life. Dr. Weil and Kendra, the doctoral student clinician, will use EBP to help with his decision whether or not to pursue amplification. The possible characteristics for defining the population include the following:

- Age: Adult
- Hearing loss
  - Type: Sensorineural
  - Degree: Moderate to severe
  - Configuration: Sloping
  - Age of onset: Acquired
- Use of hearing aids: No prior experience

Recall that in defining the population for EBP, it is important not to be too specific, which may limit the amount of evidence. Therefore, the defining population for Charles's scenario is adults with sensorineural hearing loss. Similarly, the possible patient characteristics to consider for Joshua include the following:

- Age: 13 months
- Hearing loss
  - Type: Sensorineural
  - Degree: Profound
  - Configuration: Flat
  - Age of onset: Congenital
- Use of hearing aids: Trial period shows inadequate progress

The defining population for Joshua's scenario is an infant with congenital profound sensorineural hearing loss who is not making adequate progress with hearing aids.

Intervention and Alternative Treatment

Determining the intervention and the alternative treatment requires considering the values and preferences of the patient and his or her family in addition to what is logistically available. In some cases, the intervention, hearing aids, may be compared against an alternative treatment of no treatment or postponing amplification, as in the case of Charles. It is important to note that the intervention and alternative treatment boxes on the PICO rubric are different for different types of questions. For etiologic questions, the intervention may be the exposures or characteristics that may put patients at risk for developing hearing loss, whereas the alternative treatment is absence of the risk factor. For patient safety questions, the intervention under consideration may be somewhat invasive compared with a noninvasive alternative. For cost-effectiveness questions, the intervention may be a product or procedure that may be a little more costly than an alternative treatment, but may have the potential of garnering better outcomes. In our other scenario, the interventions under consideration are simultaneous bilateral cochlear implantation versus a unilateral placement of a device during a single surgery.

Outcome

Designating the outcome(s) has to do with what is to be accomplished after treatment and is intimately tied to the values and preferences of patients and their families. In addition, the results of the audiologic and auditory rehabilitation evaluation assist in the determination of appropriate clinical outcomes. For example, the *Client Oriented Scale of Improvement* (Dillon, James, & Ginis, 1997) is a **self-assessment scale** that the audiologist uses to assist the patient to complete during the auditory rehabilitation evaluation. Using the instrument, the patient nominates and prioritizes up to five difficult communication situations to target for improvement. Nominated situations may be tasks such as understanding a spouse in a noisy restaurant, talking on the telephone with grandchildren, or hearing the caller at the bingo hall. Situations such as understanding a spouse in a noisy restaurant can be translated into outcomes that are often dependent variables in experimental studies, such as speech recognition performance in noise. Recognizing key dependent variables assists in search and retrieval of relevant evidence for use in clinical decision-making.

It is important to consider what outcomes are important for our clinical scenarios. For Charles, the outcome is quality of life which, in fact, is measured by several self-assessment scales. For Joshua, the outcome is safety and the degree of benefit received from simultaneous bilateral cochlear implantation. Debbie, Joshua's mother, was essentially concerned about the invasiveness of the surgery relative to the benefits derived from the procedure. Possible outcomes for safety include any complications from the procedure reported in the literature. Outcomes for benefit from cochlear implants for a 13-month-old should focus on speech and language development. See the PICO framework for both scenarios in Table 5.1.

The next step for our scenarios is to frame a focused question using the PICO rubric. Why is the wording of the question so important? The wording focuses the clinican's search of the literature and saves time (Cox, 2004, 2005). Charles was concerned about whether or not getting hearing aids would improve his quality of life. Appendix 5.1 is a worksheet for formulation of clinical research questions using the PICO rubric. An appropriate question for Charles's scenario is, "What are the quality-of-life benefits for adults with acquired sensorineural hearing loss who get hearing aids as opposed to not pursuing amplification?" The clinical research question for Joshua's scenario is a little more complicated, involving two clinical research questions. Recall that Debbie Washington was concerned about the cochlear implant team's recommendation about a simultaneous bilateral cochlear implantation instead

table *5.1*   PICO Rubric for Framing Research Questions for the Two Clinical Scenarios

Charles Smith

Parameter	Descriptors
Population	Adults with acquired sensorineural hearing loss
Intervention	Hearing aids
Comparison (Intervention)	No hearing aids
Outcome	Quality of life

Joshua Washington

Parameter	Descriptors
Population	13-month-olds with a congenital profound sensorineural hearing loss showing inadequate progress with hearing aids
Intervention	Simultaneous bilateral cochlear implantation
Comparison (Intervention)	Unilateral cochlear implantation
Outcome	Complications

Parameter	Descriptors
Population	13-month-old with a congenital profound sensorineural hearing loss showing inadequate progress with hearing aids
Intervention	Simultaneous bilateral cochlear implantation
Comparison (Intervention)	Unilateral cochlear implantation
Outcome	Speech and language development

of just one ear. She wondered about the risk of the procedure in comparison with the benefit of doing one ear only. So, the first question is, "What are the complications of doing a simultaneous bilateral cochlear implantation versus just a single ear?" And the second question is, "What are the relative speech and language benefits of simultaneous bilateral cochlear implantation versus placement of a single implant in a 13-month-old with profound hearing loss?"

Step 2: Searching for the Evidence

The second step involves collecting evidence to answer the question. The task can be quite daunting unless the clinician knows how to conduct effective and efficient searches. The task requires **information literacy**, or the knowledge and skills for effectively and efficiently finding relevant high-quality evidence for clinical decision-making. Most students already have the two resources needed for EBP, a personal computer with Internet capability and access to a comprehensive university library. Next, a search strategy must be designed to retrieve the highest quality information in the shortest amount of time. Recall that high-quality information is that with the least amount of experimental bias and the highest levels of evidence. Therefore, search strategies access the sources most likely to obtain systematic reviews and DBPRCTs first. Finding relevant evidence requires knowledge about databases and effective and efficient search strategies.

Generic and Discipline-Specific Sources of Evidence

Sources of evidence in communication sciences and disorders may be **domestic**, originating in the United States, or **international**, coming from foreign countries. Sources may be **generic** or **discipline specific**. Generic sources of information are used across healthcare disciplines; discipline-specific sources are accessed primarily by audiologists and speech-language pathologists. Table 5.2 shows some major sources and their classifications into these two dichotomies.

table *5.2*   Classifications of Sources of Evidence by Origin and Scope

Source	Origin	Scope
Cochrane Library	International	Generic
Campbell Collaboration	International	Generic
PubMed	Domestic	Generic
Cumulative Index of Nursing and Allied Health Literature	Domestic	Generic
American Speech-Language-Hearing Association Evidence-Based Practice Compendium	Domestic	Discipline specific
Communication Sciences and Disorders DOME (ComDisDome)	Domestic	Discipline specific

Source: Information from *Understanding Research and Evidence-Based Practice in Communication Disorders: A Primer for Students and Practitioners,* by W. O Haynes and C. E. Johnson, 2009, Upper Saddle River, NJ: Pearson.

The **Cochrane Library** (www.cochranelibrary.com), a generic database, is published by Wiley on behalf of the **Cochrane Collaboration** (www.cochrane.org), an international organization devoted to assisting users in making informed healthcare decisions via systematic reviews. The Cochrane Library contains several databases permitting searching for a variety of evidence:

- Cochrane Database of Systematic Reviews provides access to sources that assess the effects of interventions for prevention, treatment, and rehabilitation. The database provides the full texts of rigorous systematic reviews conducted and prepared by the Cochrane Collaboration.
- Database of Abstracts of Reviews of Effects (DARE) summarizes and critiques systematic reviews that have been done by groups other than the Cochrane Collaboration.
- Cochrane Central Register of Controlled Clinical Trials (Central for short) includes specifics (e.g., title, publication information, abstract) or actual publications about clinical trials from other databases and resources.
- The Cochrane Methodology Register provides publications (e.g., journal articles, books, and conference proceedings) that summarize the methods used when conducting clinical trials.
- Health Assessment Database offers information on health technology assessments from all over the world.
- The National Health Service Economic Evaluation Database assists in the decision-making process by providing economic evaluations and assessing their quality, strengths, and recommendations.

Another source for retrieving systematic reviews is the **Campbell Collaboration**, also known as C-2 (www.campbellcollaboration.org), which is an independent nonprofit organization that provides evidence-based information for making decisions regarding social, behavioral, and educational sciences. The C-2 works closely with the Cochrane Collaboration.

PubMed, another generic resource, is a free and accessible online database of biomedical journal citations and abstracts through the United States National Library of Medicine (NLM). PubMed indexes approximately 5,000 journals using the NLM's controlled vocabulary or Medical Subject Headings (MeSH), which consist of hierarchically arranged sets of terms and descriptors that facilitate the search for evidence, from the general to the specific or vice versa (NLM, 2010a, 2010b, 2010c). The largest part of PubMed is the Medical Literature Analysis and Retrieval System Online (Medline) that has over 16 million references to biomedical journal articles (NLM, 2010a). Another generic source of evidence is the Cumulative Index of Nursing and Allied Health Literature (CINAHL), which contains items (e.g., published articles, books, conferences proceedings, and dissertations) referenced since 1982. Although CINAHL does not provide access to the full text of journal articles, citations provide the title, authors' names, and journal citation (e.g., volume number, issue, and page numbers).

The website of the American Speech-Language-Hearing Association (ASHA) (www.asha.org) is an example of discipline-specific source of evidence. Members of ASHA and the National Student Speech-Language-Hearing Association (NSSLHA) have full-text access to articles in the following journals: *American Journal of Audiology, American Journal of Speech-Language Pathology, Contemporary Issues in Communication Sciences and Disorders*, and the *Journal of Speech-Language-Hearing Research*. Available ASHA practice policy documents include clinical practice guidelines, position statements, preferred practice patterns, and technical reports. Users may refine the results of their searches by source (e.g., ASHA website, ASHA journals, *ASHA Leader*, convention materials, *Perspectives* [special interest division newsletters]), ASHA practice policy (e.g., technical reports, practice guidelines, position statements), year, type of information (e.g., web page, PowerPoint, Word document), and topic. The Evidence-Based Practice Compendium (EBC) (www.asha .org/members/ebp/compendium), accessed through the ASHA website, contains guidelines and systematic reviews that are accessible via links organized by topic headings. ASHA's Center for Evidence-Based Practice in Communication Disorders (N-CEP) developed the EBC in the summer of 2005 to promote practice policies that minimize bias.

The Communication Sciences and Disorders DOME (ComDisDome) has been a popular discipline-specific database for audiologists, speech-language pathologists, and students-in-training for almost a decade. Originally, the ComDisDome retrieved information from PubMed, select non-PubMed journals (e.g., *Linguistics and Language Behavior Abstracts*, *Seminars in Hearing*), select grants from the National Institutes of Health and the National Science Foundation, dissertations from ProQuest, books from multiple publishers, profiles of scholars, and related websites. In 2007, the ComDisDome was purchased by CSA Illumina, which provides access to over 100 databases in the natural sciences, social sciences, arts/humanities, and technologies. The change in ownership resulted in loss of some key features (e.g., dictionary and websites).

Macro Versus Micro Search Strategies

Retrieving relevant, high-quality evidence requires the use of strategic **macro search strategies** and **micro search strategies**. Macro search strategies are the order of databases used; micro strategies are the specific techniques for searching within a database. Recall that the aim is to recover the highest-quality evidence possible first. Therefore, Figure 5.2 shows a macro search strategy first seeking systematic reviews with meta-analysis in the Cochrane Database of Systematic Reviews (Cochrane Reviews), the Database of Abstracts of Reviews of Effects (DARE) within the Cochrane Library, and the Campbell Collaboration. Helpful sources of studies based on scientific evidence are shown in Table 5.3, and sources that critically appraise specific interventional methods are shown in Table 5.4.

Ascending down the hierarchy includes searching ClinicalTrials.gov (www.clinicaltrials .gov) and PubMed for randomized, controlled clinical trials. Readers are advised to take the tutorials on how to effectively access each database, increasing the likelihood of efficient recovery of relevant high-quality evidence. Searching databases requires the input of **search strings** or words and phrases that have the greatest likelihood of retrieving relevant articles for a particular EBP question. The best place to obtain terms for search strings is from the contents in the PICO framework. We will come back to this point after discussing importance of documenting the search and retrieval process.

Search and retrieval processes should be documented so that clinicians remember what they have done; in addition, notes from the search and retrieval process provide a hard copy record for the patient and family, other professionals involved in a case, or for those doing research. According to the Cochrane Collaboration's *Cochrane Handbook for Systematic Reviews of Interventions, Version 5.0.2* (Cochrane Collaboration, 2009), adequate documentation of a search includes the following information:

- Title of the database
- Date of search
- Years covered by the search

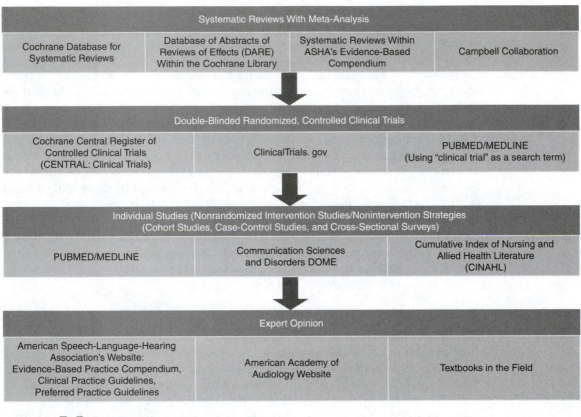

Systematic Reviews With Meta-Analysis			
Cochrane Database for Systematic Reviews	Database of Abstracts of Reviews of Effects (DARE) Within the Cochrane Library	Systematic Reviews Within ASHA's Evidence-Based Compendium	Campbell Collaboration

Double-Blinded Randomized, Controlled Clinical Trials		
Cochrane Central Register of Controlled Clinical Trials (CENTRAL: Clinical Trials)	ClinicalTrials. gov	PUBMED/MEDLINE (Using "clinical trial" as a search term)

Individual Studies (Nonrandomized Intervention Studies/Nonintervention Strategies (Cohort Studies, Case-Control Studies, and Cross-Sectional Surveys)		
PUBMED/MEDLINE	Communication Sciences and Disorders DOME	Cumulative Index of Nursing and Allied Health Literature (CINAHL)

Expert Opinion		
American Speech-Language-Hearing Association's Website: Evidence-Based Practice Compendium, Clinical Practice Guidelines, Preferred Practice Guidelines	American Academy of Audiology Website	Textbooks in the Field

figure *5.2* ————————————————————————————————

Macro search strategy for evidenced-based practice.

Source: Haynes and Johnson, *Understanding Research and Evidence-Based Practice in Communication Disorders: A Primer for Students and Practitioners,* Figure 13.1 "Macro Search Strategy for Evidence in Communication Sciences and Disorders," © 2009. Adapted by permission of Pearson Education, Inc.

- Complete strategy of the search
- Short summary of search strategy
- The absence of any language restrictions

Appendix 5.2 is a worksheet for searching for the evidence. The title of the database, date, and years covered by a search are critical pieces of information because new articles are published every day, and a record of what has been searched saves time from having to duplicate previous efforts and indicates when an update is necessary. It is also important to state any language restrictions for the inclusion of articles. Some clinicians prefer to consider evidence only from articles in English due to limited time and/or resources available for EBP.

Step 3: Evaluating the Evidence

The third step involves formal evaluation or critical appraisal of the evidence that consists of three steps: (1) determine the level of evidence, (2) rate the risk of bias in individual studies, and (3) grade the clinical recommendation under consideration.

table 5.3 Types of Information and Sources Useful in Searching for Scientific Evidence

Type of Information	Database
Systematic Reviews	• Cochrane Collaboration: www.cochrane.org/reviews/clibintro.htm
	• Campbell Collaboration: www.campbellcollaboration.org/
	• What Works Clearinghouse (U.S. Department of Education): www.ies.ed.gov/ncee/wwc/
	• Health Information Resources: www.library.nhs.uk/default.aspx
Research Articles	• Communication Sciences and Disorders Dome: www.comdisdome.com
	• Cumulative Index to Nursing and Allied Health Literature: www.ebscohost.com/cinahl/
	• National Library of Medicine: www.nlm.nih.gov
	• PubMed: www.pubmed.gov

Source: Information from *Steps in the Process of Evidence-Based Practice: Step 2: Finding the Evidence,* by the American Speech-Language-Hearing Association, 2009, retrieved from www.asha.org/members/ebp/finding.htm.

table 5.4 Sources for Critically Appraising Specific Types of Interventional Research

Resource	Application
CONSORT Statement: www.consort-statement.org	• Checklist for assessing reports of intervention studies
STARD Statement: www.stard-statement.org	• Checklist for assessing reports of diagnostic studies
Transparent Reporting of Evaluations with Non-randomized Designs: www.trend-statement.org	• Criteria for assessing quasi-experimental designs
SIGN-50: A Guideline Developer's Handbook: www.sign.ac.uk/guidelines/fulltext/50	Checklists for assessing:
	• Systematic reviews and meta-analyses
	• Randomized controlled clinical trials
	• Cohort studies
	• Case-control studies
	• Diagnostic studies
	• Economic evaluations

Source: Information from *Steps in the Process of Evidence-Based Practice: Step 2: Finding the Evidence,* by the American Speech-Language-Hearing Association, 2009, retrieved from www.asha.org/members/ebp/finding.htm.

table 5.5 Quality of Evidence by Levels

Level	Description
I	Systematic Reviews and Meta-Analyses of Double-Blinded, Prospective, Randomized, Controlled Clinical Trials
II	Double-Blinded, Prospective, Randomized, Controlled Clinical Trials
III	Nonrandomized Intervention Studies
IV	Nonintervention Studies: Cohort Studies, Case-Control Studies, and Cross-Sectional Surveys
V	Case Reports
VI	Expert Opinion of Respected Authorities

Source: Journal of the American Academy of Audiology by AMERICAN ACADEMY OF AUDIOLOGY. Copyright 2005. Reproduced with permission of AMERICAN ACADEMY OF AUDIOLOGY in the format Textbook via Copyright Clearance Center.

Step 3a: Determine the Level of Evidence

How does an audiologist, speech-language pathologist, or patient judge the merit of scientific evidence provided by research studies? The first step is to determine the level of evidence of a particular study. As stated earlier, levels of evidence are hierarchies of rigor used in evaluating research methodology. There is not just one hierarchy, but many, depending on the medical discipline and the type of study.

Table 5.5 depicts six levels, Classes I through VI, of evidence defined by Cox (2004). Class I is the most rigorous and Class VI is the least rigorous. However, the hierarchy of rigor does not necessarily imply a pecking order of utility to the professions. Each level has its place of importance. Before discussing the characteristics of research at each of the six levels of evidence, some general terminology will be defined.

Using our clinical scenarios we can illustrate the results of the search process. Dr. Weil's and Dr. Trenoth's macro search strategies were to search Cochrane Library and ClinicalTrials .gov first to recover systematic reviews and randomized, controlled topics pertinent to their clinical questions. Dr. Weil used search strings such as "hearing aids and quality of life" and "amplification and quality of life." Clinical Trials.gov provided information on completed clinical trials with links to abstracts in PubMed of the resulting scientific articles. Using the same search strings in PubMed yielded additional articles, including a recent systematic review on the topic. Dr. Weil obtained the following systematic review:

Authors/Date	Title	Journal Citation	Level of Evidence and Grading for Risk of Bias
Chisolm, T. H., Johnson, C. E., Danhauer, J. L., et al. (2007)	A systematic review of health-related quality of life and hearing aids: Final report of the American Academy of Audiology Task Force on the Health-Related Quality of Life Benefit of Amplification in Adults	*Journal of the American Academy of Audiology, 18,* 151–183.	?

Similarly, Dr. Trenoth found three articles to assist in her appointment with the Washingtons. The search yielded three recent articles directly related to the safety and potential benefit of a simultaneous bilateral cochlear implantation for Joshua.

Authors/Date	Title	Journal Citation	Level of Evidence and Grading for Risk of Bias
Ramsden, J. D., Papaioannou, V., Gordon, K. A., James, A. L., & Papsin, B. C. (2009)	Parental and program's decision making in pediatric simultaneous bilateral cochlear implantation: Who says no and why?	*International Journal of Pediatric Otolaryngology, 73,* 1325–1328	?
Basura, G. J., Eapen, R., & Buchman, C. A. (2009)	Bilateral cochlear implantation: Current concepts, indications, and results	*Laryngoscope, 119,* 2935-2401	?
Ramsden, J. D., Papsin, B. C., Leung, R., James, A., & Gordon, K. A. (2009)	Bilateral simultaneous cochlear implantation in children: Our first 50 cases	*Laryngoscope, 119,* 2444-2448	?

Some important terms for levels of evidence include dependent variable, independent variable, treatment/intervention, and placebo. In an experiment, there are two types of variables, independent and dependent variables. **Independent variables** are manipulated by the experimenter who is trying to test a hypothesis. For example, a researcher may want to test a hypothesis that vibrotactile cues (i.e., vibrations on the skin from an aid that changes acoustic energy into mechanical vibrations) may aid patients having profound hearing impairment with speechreading. The researcher may test a group of deaf adults with and without the use of the vibrotactile device and then compare the number of sentences recognized correctly in the two conditions. The independent variable is the use of the vibrotactile device. The **dependent variable** is the one that is measured or, in this example, the number of sentences correctly recognized.

Two other important terms are *treatment/intervention* and *placebo*. **Treatments/ interventions** refer to applications or procedures that health professionals administer to lessen the effects of, or cure, a disease or a disorder. In many medical studies, participants with particular diseases or disorders are assigned unknowingly to one of two groups. One group will receive the treatment/intervention being investigated while the other group receives a standard treatment or placebo. **Placebos** are inactive (e.g., sugar pill)/conventional medications or procedures that are administered in the exact same way as the experimental treatment and serve as a comparison. For example, a researcher investigating the effectiveness of a drug in reducing tinnitus may administer the experimental drug to one group of participants and an identical placebo to another group of patients for comparison in the reduction of symptoms.

Appendices 5.3 through 5.5 contain worksheets for the quality assessment of systematic reviews, clinical trials/quasi-experimental studies, and clinical practice guidelines, respectively. Appendices 5.3 and 5.4 require classification of studies or other retrieved sources of information according to their level of evidence. The following section describes the types of research found at each of the levels of evidence.

Class I: Well-designed Systematic Reviews With Meta-Analysis of More Than One Double-Blinded, Randomized, Controlled Clinical Trial.   Research may involve either **primary measurement methods** or **secondary measurement methods**. Primary measurement methods involve investigators collecting and analyzing their own data for a single experiment. For example, primary measurement methods include having participants in a study fill out questionnaires, permit real-ear probe-tube microphone measurements, and so on. Secondary measurement methods involve experimenters or clinicians considering or analyzing data collected in one or more studies conducted by other investigators. For example, some researchers use data already reported in published articles in answering research questions. Clinicians and researchers use secondary measurement methods when they conduct a systematic review of the evidence assessing the effectiveness of a particular diagnostic procedure or treatment of hearing impairment. This definition serves our purposes for auditory rehabilitation, but readers should acknowledge that although the procedures are the same across disciplines, the topics, of course, are not. Systematic reviews can be a qualitative review of the evidence, or quantitative, involving a *meta-analysis*, or the use of special statistical procedures that combine the results of more than one investigation in order to measure the magnitude of a treatment effect. In communication sciences and disorders, some investigations do not have enough participants (subjects) to demonstrate a significant effect of one treatment over another. Systematic reviews with meta-analyses permit the combining of the results of several studies together to increase the magnitude of the effect of the study. A special metric called an *effect size* determines the degree of impact of significant findings and will be discussed later on. Systematic reviews with meta-analyses are needed to validate research because causality between treatment and positive patient outcomes cannot be established on the basis of a single investigation.

Systematic reviews with meta-analyses are done for at least five reasons (McKibbon, Easy, & Marks, 1999).

- First, systematic reviews get to the "bottom line" of all studies involving a particular treatment or intervention. Robey and Dalebout (1998) completed a meta-analysis of a few studies investigating the reduction of self-perceived hearing handicap measured by several self-assessment scales such as the *Hearing Handicap Inventory for the Elderly* (HHIE) (Ventry & Weinstein, 1982) and/or the *Hearing Performance Inventory* (HPI) (Giolas, Owens, Lamb, & Schubert, 1979). They found that hearing aid treatment is effective when indexed as a reduction of patient-perceived hearing difficulty (Robey & Dalebout, 1998).

- Second, systematic reviews are also undertaken to estimate precisely the amount of benefit derived from a treatment or intervention. In their study, Robey and Dalebout (1998) averaged the amount of benefit across investigations to come up with an "effect size," or how much reduction in self-perceived hearing handicap can be expected based on a review of all studies.

- Third, systematic reviews are completed to increase the number of patients in clinically relevant subgroups. The results of many promising studies having low numbers of participants may be combined in a systematic review with meta-analysis to make a powerful statement regarding the effectiveness of a particular treatment.

- Fourth, a systematic review helps resolve discrepancies among the findings of studies. It is not uncommon for some studies to find treatment A more effective than treatment B, and some studies to find the reverse (i.e., treatment B more effective than treatment A), and yet other studies to find the treatments of equal value. In this case, a systematic review can help sort out conflicting results.
- Fifth, a systematic review can help plan future studies. A systematic review guides researchers in designing studies that investigate issues most relevant for a particular intervention, while overcoming pitfalls encountered in previous investigations.

Completion of a systematic review requires five steps that are very similar to the steps we are following in EBP (McKibbon et al., 1999). The first step sets the stage for the review and formulation of experimental questions about the treatment or interventions, populations, settings, outcomes, duration, and inclusion, and exclusion criteria for the studies (McKibbon et al., 1999). For example, 50 million Americans suffer from tinnitus, or the sensation of hearing ringing, buzzing, hissing, chirping, or other sounds either intermittently or constantly, for which there are numerous treatments. Dobie (1999) did a systematic review to answer the question whether there were any well-established treatments, promising developments, and opportunities for improvement in treating tinnitus in adults. The experimenter planned that only DBPRCTs published from 1964 to 1998 would be included in the review.

The second step of a systematic review is to identify, select, and critique studies for inclusion in the study. The search and retrieval process for a systematic review should be nearly identical to that for EBP. In addition to those covered earlier in the chapter, a variety of search methodologies such as the following are applied to databases available in the library and on the Internet along with personal-contact sources (McKibbon et al., 1999):

- Searching general and specific bibliographies
- Using specific index terminology
- **Hand-searching** specific journals, conference proceedings, and meeting abstracts (Hand-searching is searching for articles, conference proceedings, and other materials not referenced in common databases.)
- Contacting authors, other experts in the field, professional organizations (e.g., American Academy of Audiology and the American Speech-Language-Hearing Association), government departments (e.g., Centers for Disease Control and Prevention), and product manufacturers
- Scanning bibliographies of new studies, review articles, book chapters, clinical practice guidelines, theses, and dissertations

For example, Dobie (1999) searched the literature using Medline and Old Medline and hand-searched his notes to include observations found in his own personal files. From this process, 69 DBPRCTs were included in his systematic review that evaluated tocainide and other related drugs (i.e., carbamazepine, benzodiazepines, tricyclic antidepressants), 16 miscellaneous drugs, psychotherapy, electrical/magnetic stimulation, acupuncture, masking, biofeedback, hypnosis, and other miscellaneous nondrug treatments. In addition, he assessed the DBPRCTs for quality.

The third step of a systematic review with meta-analysis is the extraction of data from the studies and their placement into a table for organization into groupings according to the similarity of dependent variables for statistical analysis, and a plan to present the findings in a published form such as an article (McKibbon et al., 1999). Researchers often complete this step two or more times for determining reliability, and seek help from colleagues in double-checking their work. For example, Dobie (1999) compared the studies' specific criteria for DBPRCTs regarding the quality of study design, performance, and analysis.

The fourth step of the systematic review with meta-analysis is to analyze the data using special statistical procedures (McKibbon et al., 1999). During this step, researchers determine whether the data within the studies are similar enough with regard to active participants (e.g., patients), types of treatments, dependent variables, and so on so that an overall statistical analysis can be completed to weigh the preponderance of evidence either for or against a particular treatment. For example, Dobie (1999) inspected the data from the studies for "positive" results in reducing tinnitus and examined them for clinical relevance. From this analysis, he determined that no treatment can be considered well-established in terms of providing replicable long-term reduction of tinnitus that cannot be explained by a placebo effect alone.

The fifth and final step of a systematic review is presentation of the results with a goal of publication in a scholarly journal (McKibbon et al., 1999). All articles for systematic reviews have similar types of tables presenting the data and results from the statistical analyses. These articles also include the following sections: an introduction, methods section, results, discussion, and conclusions. For example, from his systematic review, Dobie (1999) prepared an article that was published in *The Laryngoscope*, a scholarly journal. He concluded that nonspecific support and counseling in addition to tricyclic antidepressants may offer some help to patients with severe tinnitus. Furthermore, he stated that benzodiazepines, newer antidepressants, and electrical stimulation warrant further investigation. Future studies on tinnitus therapy should increase the number of participants, use more clinically relevant dependent variables, and follow-up of patients regarding their outcomes for longer periods of time than the studies included in the review. In conclusion, systematic reviews with meta-analyses are at the highest level of evidence when they combine the results of more than one study, particularly when those studies are DBPRCTs, the gold standard for experimental research.

Class II: Double-Blinded, Prospective Randomized, Controlled Clinical Trials.   Earlier in the chapter, it was mentioned that certain clinical trials that are double-blinded, prospective, and randomized are at a high level of evidence. Readers can best understand DBPRCTs by defining each of the words. **Double-blinding (DB)** means that neither the experimenter nor the participant has knowledge of administration of the treatment/intervention or placebo. *Prospective randomized (PR)* describes studies in which patients are: (1) enrolled as participants prior to conduction of the experiment, (2) randomly assigned to groups receiving either the treatment or a placebo, (3) measured after some period of time, and (4) compared for any statistically significant differences attributable to the treatment or intervention. A major advantage of DBPRCTs is that they are double-blinded, as stated earlier, in that neither the experimenter nor the participant knows whether the treatment or placebo is being administered, eliminating both experimenter and participant bias. Earlier, we defined *bias*, but there are different types of bias. **Experimenter bias** is anything that the experimenter does that has measurable influence on the dependent variable that is not attributable to the independent variable. For example, a researcher may expect more speech recognition errors in noise when scoring a test if they know a participant is wearing a lower-technology hearing aid or a higher-technology device. **Participant bias** is anything that a participant does that has a measurable influence on the dependent variable that is not attributable to the independent variable. For example, participants may rate a more costly digital hearing aid as providing higher quality sound than a more inexpensive analog hearing instrument with the reasoning that if something costs more, it has to be better.

Bentler, Niebuhr, Johnson, and Flamme (2003) investigated whether the label attached to hearing aids would bias outcome measures toward newer high-technology hearing aids. **Outcome measures** are data collected to determine the benefit of treatment. Bentler et al. (2005) matched two groups of participants for age, gender, previous hearing aid experience, and degree/configuration of hearing loss. One group of participants wore two digital hearing aids for one month each. The other group wore the same hearing aid, but was told that they were wearing a digital hearing aid for one period and a "conventional hearing aid" (lower-technology) during the other month. Outcomes measurement consisting of behavioral speech-perception tasks and self-report measures were made at the beginning and end of each trial month. Bentler et al. (2005) found that labeling the hearing aid biased the results in that the hearing aids were rated higher when labeled as digital rather than conventional. The results of this study indicated the need for "double blinding," investigating the effectiveness of the high-technology digital hearing aids as compared with more conventional hearing aids.

Another advantage of DBPRCTs is that participants are randomly assigned to either a control group or treatment group. **Random assignment** implies that each participant has a 50-50 chance of being assigned to receive the experimental or placebo treatment. Random assignment reduces **sampling bias**, or the measurable influence that assignment of participants to treatment or control groups has that is directly not attributable to the independent variable. In other words, assignment of participants must be based on chance alone in order to ensure that any treatment effects measured on the dependent variable are due to the manipulation of the independent variable rather than to inherent differences between the treatment and control groups.

Although considered to be the gold standard for scientific evidence, DBPRCTs present several disadvantages that should be considered prior to their use in experimental implementation. First, DBPRCTs are very difficult to design, execute, and complete. The largest hearing aid clinical trial required collaboration between the Department of Veteran Affairs (DVA), the largest healthcare system in the United States, and the National Institute on Deafness and Other Communication Disorders of the National Institutes of Health (NIDCD-NIH) in order to recruit hundreds of participants meeting specific criteria for a large-scale clinical trial (Beck, 1999; Bratt, 1999; Larson et al., 2000).

Second, DBPRCTs describe outcomes for treatment variables in highly-controlled situations, not those found in the "real world." Outcomes of the DVA-NIDCD hearing aid clinical trial limit generalization to clinical scenarios found specifically within the experimental protocol, not to all patients across service delivery sites.

Third, clinical trials research may pose some ethical dilemmas for researchers, clinicians, and their patients because DBPRCTs require random assignment of participants to treatment and control groups. Random assignment means that half will receive the new treatment and half will receive the placebo or conventional treatment. Is it ethical that some patients are prevented from receiving an experimental treatment that might provide better hearing aid circuitry or, in a more extreme case, a new drug that may shrink or kill their tumors and save their lives?

Fourth, clinical trials research requires a great deal of time in validating treatment regimens, delaying their availability to the public. For example, current estimates state that about 43,000 people are diagnosed with pancreatic cancer each year; about 36,800 will die from the disease during the same time period (National Cancer Institute, 2010). Pancreatic cancer is particularly lethal in that the condition often goes undiagnosed until the later stages of the disease process. In October 2001, scientists at Johns Hopkins University initiated a Phase II clinical trial assessing the effectiveness of a pancreatic cancer vaccine for patients who have had their tumors resected (i.e., removed via surgery) and have no clinical evidence of metastases (i.e., spreading of cancer outside of the pancreas). Unfortunately, only 10% of patients with pancreatic cancer meet these criteria and are eligible to be vaccinated, possibly preventing the recurrence of the disease after surgery. Several more phases of the clinical trial are underway prior to its widespread use of the vaccine on patients who are dying now. Similarly, the DVA-NIDCD hearing aid clinical trial was able to demonstrate that wide-dynamic-range compression was better than compression and peak-clipping analog hearing aids. Although the clinical trial provided important evidence regarding relative outcomes for various circuits in analog hearing aids, the industry had been developing high-technology digital circuitry, and progress would not wait for validation by the scientific community via DBPRCTs.

Fifth, optimal experimental circumstances necessary for clinical trials research may have limited external validity in the real-world clinical practice involving all types of patients across a wide variety of afflictions, behaviors, and service delivery sites (Johnson & Danhauer, 2002a). Indeed, DBPRCTs are needed to demonstrate benefit, improved quality of life, and a reduction of healthcare costs prior to auditory rehabilitation services and products being included in third-party reimbursements. Unfortunately, due to the logistical problems discussed here, DBPRCTs are not too common in communication sciences and disorders.

Class III: Nonrandomized Intervention Studies.   **Nonrandomized intervention studies**, also called **quasi-experimental studies**, use designs that lack characteristics of DBPRCTs such as randomization of assignment of participants into treatment and control groups. These types of studies are the most common in communication sciences and disorders because they are more conducive to the realities of a busy speech and hearing clinic. For example, audiologists and speech-language pathologists often do not have the resources or capabilities to randomly assign patients to treatment and control groups. Therefore, quasi-experimental research designs involve grouping of participants by convenience (Cox, 2005). An audiologist may want to assess any differences in hearing aid satisfaction between new hearing aid wearers who attended group auditory rehabilitation versus those who opted out. Grouping participants by convenience, the audiologist assigns those attending the sessions into the treatment group and those not attending into the control group. Cox (2005) warns that a potential weakness of this design is that the experimenter cannot be sure that the groups are equivalent at baseline or at the beginning of the study and should be matched for critical variables such as age, gender, degree of hearing loss, and so on to strengthen the study. In our example, the audiologist must realize that the treatment and control groups may not be equivalent because those patients who elected to attend these sessions may have been more enthusiastic about auditory rehabilitation or differed in some fundamental way from those who did not.

Class IV: Nonintervention Studies: Cohort Studies, Case-Control Studies, and Cross-Sectional Surveys.   Class IV level of evidence involves nonintervention studies including case-control studies, cohort studies, and cross-sectional surveys, and can be prospective or retrospective (Cox, 2005). **Prospective studies** are those that recruit participants prior to the collection of data. The previous example involved a prospective study in which new hearing aid wearers were assigned into two groups, one whose members attended a hearing aid orientation group and one whose members did not, prior to collecting data regarding the number of postfitting problems, visits to walk-in clinics, and other measures of satisfaction, etc. In **retrospective studies**, data are collected after some sort of event or occurrence. For example, in **case-control studies**, participants are recruited after they have developed some type of pathology (e.g., noise-induced hearing loss [NIHL]) along with a disease-free control group; are measured on some type of predictor variable (e.g., something hypothesized to cause or contribute to developing the condition such as listening to loud music); and then statistically compared for significant difference on (a) predictor variable(s) suggesting possible cause(s) or associative variable(s) for developing NIHL.

Cohort studies can be either prospective or retrospective. **Prospective cohort studies** are those in which participants are recruited in the present, before an outbreak of a disease or disorder to assess who does and does not develop a particular condition in the future (Frattali, 1998). Prospective cohort studies have two purposes: (1) to determine the incidence of certain outcomes over time (i.e., descriptive), and (2) to analyze associations between and/or among risk factors and those outcomes (Cummings, Newman, & Hulley, 2007). **Incidence** is the number of new cases of a disease or disorder that develop over a specified period of time per the number of individuals at risk (Newman, Browner, Cummings, & Hulley, 2007). **Associations** are connections made between risk factors and certain diseases. A prospective cohort study could be used to determine if a significantly higher proportion of a sample of babies who had chronic otitis media (COM) during the first two years of life subsequently develop auditory processing disorders (APD) in the future as compared with individuals who did not have COM. If a significantly higher proportion of individuals with COM during the first few years of life develop APD than those who did not have COM, an association can be made between the presence of COM during the first years of life and the development of APD. Another type of cohort study is a **retrospective cohort study**, which identifies a sample of individuals who already have a disorder and then measures predictor variables (Cummings et al., 2007). Using the previous example, a retrospective cohort design would involve assembling two groups of participants, one with and one without APD, in the present and then determining significant differences between the groups regarding the presence of COM during the first two years of their lives.

Prevalence studies, or **cross-sectional studies**, determine the number of individuals that have a particular disorder or disease at one point in time per the number of people at risk (Newman et al., 2007). **Prevalence** is the number of persons per some number of the population that have some sort of condition. For example, approximately 1 baby per 1,000 born has Down syndrome. In prevalence studies, the investigator makes all of his or her measurements on a single occasion (Newman et al., 2007). The purpose of the study is to describe variables and their distribution patterns (Newman et al., 2007). Prevalence studies have three steps: (1) selecting a sample from the population with a disease or disorder; (2) selecting a disease-free, control sample from the population; and (3) then measuring both the predictor and outcome variables (Newman et al., 2007). Using the same example, a researcher could use a prevalence study to investigate the presence of COM during the first two years of life (e.g., predictor variable) and the development of APD (e.g., outcome variable) by recruiting 1,000 individuals from the population, asking about the presence of COM during the first two years of life via case history, testing for APD, and determining if the prevalence of APD is higher in participants having an early history of COM than those without it.

Class V: Case Studies or Reports.   **Case studies** or reports study specific individuals in detail and compare the results to historical controls or what has been typically expected. Case-study research is used when other experimental designs are impossible, and have advantages in the following applications (McReynolds & Thompson, 1986; Schiavetti, Metz, & Orlikoff, 2010):

- Investigating rare clinical occurrences
- Aiding in the development of clinical insights

- Examining exceptions to accepted rules
- Describing/identifying potential variables for evaluation in experimental studies

A major disadvantage of case-study designs is that little or no generalization of results can be expected from a small number of participants (Schiavetti et al., 2010). Case-study designs frequently employ A-only or B-only single-participant designs. The A-only designs are diary or longitudinal studies of participants that involve copious description of the patients' experiences. For example, Yellin and Johnson (2000) describe the progression of symptoms and diagnosis of Susac syndrome in a 43-year-old woman. Patients with Susac syndrome present initially with only one of a clinical triad of symptoms: (1) encephalopathy, (2) branch retinal artery occlusions, and (3) sensorineural hearing loss (Susac, 1994). However, over the course of the disease, additional symptoms may appear and fluctuate (Yellin & Johnson, 2000). Susac syndrome is seen almost exclusively in women in the 20- to 40-year age range and is frequently misdiagnosed as multiple sclerosis (Yellin & Johnson, 2000). Surprisingly, the symptoms extend only over a one- to two-year period of time and then go into remission (Yellin & Johnson, 2000). The case study served to investigate a rare clinical occurrence and aided in the development of insight into the clinical manifestations of Susac syndrome. Alternatively, using a B-only or treatment-only design, Spencer, Tye-Murray, Kelsay, and Teagle (1998) conducted a four-year case study on a young child who had made good progress after receiving treatment with a cochlear implant, despite the presence of family issues (e.g., possible unreliable reports of child's progress, limited parental interaction with the child, etc.) and school-related issues (e.g., questionable educational programming and support services) before implantation. The case study demonstrated an exception to traditional expectations of poor prognosis postimplantation for children whose families do not meet all patient selection criteria for cochlear prostheses.

Class VI: Expert Opinion.   **Expert clinical opinion** involves the knowledge and skills of recognized leaders in the field who have established themselves through clinical work and/or scholarly activity. Professional organizations such as ASHA and AAA rely on expert clinical opinion for many pursuits such as appointing editors for their journals (e.g., *Journal of the American Academy of Audiology*; *Journal of Speech, Language, and Hearing Research; American Journal of Audiology*), selecting review panels for submissions of presentation to annual conventions, and developing clinical practice standards. Standards of clinical practice are documents published by ASHA and AAA regarding guidelines for service provision. **Clinical practice standards** are an explicitly and systematically defined set of required procedures and practices based on scientific evidence and/or expert opinion that have been designed to yield specific, well-defined outcomes (AAA, 2009b). The AAA and ASHA websites provide access to these types of documents on auditory rehabilitation. Although these documents are based on scientific evidence, it has not been until recently that our professions have recognized the need for developers to rigorously search, retrieve, and critically review all relevant research prior to guideline development. However, until EBP becomes routine in the development of clinical practice standards, any resulting documents (e.g., clinical practice guidelines, position statements, preferred practice patterns, and technical reports) may only be considered expert opinion.

Consensus means reaching agreement regarding important issues facing the professions. For example, the American Academy of Audiology published a position statement regarding the academy's view of Auditory Integration Training (AIT) developed by Guy Berard, which has been touted as an effective treatment protocol for patients who have dyslexia, learning disabilities, pervasive developmental delays, and so on (AAA, 1993). Specifically, AIT is completed in 10 hours over a 10-day period by listening to filtered, electronically modulated music. However, no results of Class I or II levels of evidence investigations on AIT have been published in peer-reviewed journals. Therefore, the academy document stated that AIT is purely investigational at this time and that the status of the technique must be explained to consumers (AAA, 1993).

Step 3b: Rate the Risk of Bias of the Evidence

The quality assessment of the evidence may be accomplished using Appendices 5.3 through 5.5 and ultimately results in determination of the risk of bias. Critically appraising systematic reviews is different than for DBPRCTs/quasi-experimental studies, and therefore requires different worksheets. Readers are advised to have Appendices 5.3 to 5.5 nearby to refer to when reviewing this section.

Appendix 5.3 is a worksheet for evaluating systematic reviews. Although systematic reviews of DBPRCTs are at Class I level of evidence, these types of investigations are rare in communication sciences and disorders. It is important to note that the level of evidence of a systematic review is that of the majority of included studies. For example, if a systematic review includes nonrandomized intervention studies (quasi-experimental studies), it should be classified as being at Class III level of evidence. Systematic reviews should have a strong rationale and be based on a clearly focused clinical or research question. The search strategy should be transparent and clearly documented such that it could be replicated by others. The reviews should have been conducted by an adequately trained team with members having had opportunities to make independent decisions during the search and quality assessment phases of the study. Provisions for settling any disagreements should be clearly described, preserving the objectivity in decision-making. The exclusion/inclusion criteria for studies must be specific and strictly adhered to so that all available evidence is appropriately considered for inclusion. The included studies must be adequately documented (e.g., patient demographics, interventions, and results) and assessed for quality on specific criteria, which will be discussed later on in the chapter (e.g., level of evidence, power analysis, use of a control group, power analyses, inclusion/exclusion criteria, adequate sampling, random assignment, double-blinding, appropriate statistics, and adequacy of conclusions). Some systematic reviews may include a meta-analysis, or a statistical procedure that combines the results of individual studies to assess overall effectiveness of treatment, for example.

At the end of the worksheet are questions about the overall quality of the systematic review. It is important to determine the relevance of the systematic review to the clinical or research question. Direct relevance means that the population, intervention, comparative treatment, and some or all of the outcome measures are the same as those contained in the PICO rubric used for framing the question. A study is indirectly related if one or more of those variables is different, such as a similar but related population or outcome measure. When two or more of the variables do not match, then the study has very little utility for a specific EBP question. Clinicians should also determine if the conclusions were appropriate based on the strength of the results or treatment effects found. Lastly, the worksheet requires a rating for the degree of overall bias to determine if the methodology minimized risks of bias. These items are graded with either a "+ +," "+," or "−" according to the criteria summarized by Cox (2005, p. 231).

Rating	Interpetation of Rating
+ +	Very low risk of bias. Any weaknesses that are present are very unlikely to alter the conclusions of the study.
+	Low risk of bias. Identified weaknesses or omitted information probably would not alter the conclusions of the study.
−	High risk of bias. Identified weaknesses or omitted information are very likely to alter conclusions of the study.

Source: Journal of the American Academy of Audiology by AMERICAN ACADEMY OF AUDIOLOGY. Copyright 2005. Reproduced with permission of AMERICAN ACADEMY OF AUDIOLOGY in the format Textbook via Copyright Clearance Center.

As indicated in the preceding chart, a rating of + +, +, or − indicates lowest to highest risks of bias, respectively.

Appendix 5.4 is a worksheet for evaluating clinical trials and quasi-experimental studies that should be based on a strong rationale and a focused research question. The worksheet has been adapted from documents called the Consolidated Statement for Report Trials (CONSORT) (Schulz, Altman, Moher, and the CONSORT Group, 2010), a critical appraisal sheet from the Center for Evidence-Based Medicine (CEBM, 2006), and a form available from the *Scottish Intercollegiate Guidelines Network (SIGN) Guideline Developer's Handbook*, referred to as SIGN-50 (Scottish Intercollegiate Guidelines Network, 2008). These documents were developed by leading authorities in EBP. The **CONSORT Statement** is a document designed to improve the quality of reporting of clinical trials particularly in medicine. The aim of the **Center for Evidence-Based Medicine** (CEBM), based in England, is "to promote evidence-based healthcare and provide support and resources to anyone who wants to make use of them" (www.cebm.net). The **Scottish Intercollegiate Guidelines Network** is a group devoted to improving the quality and consistency of healthcare for the citizens of Scotland.

Review of the article begins with recording the complete bibliographic citation for the study and level of evidence. The inclusion/exclusion criteria for participants should be stated and the sample should adequately represent the population from which it was drawn. **Inadequate sampling** and **subject self-selection bias** decrease the overall rigor of a study. Inadequate sampling occurs if the participants in a sample do not represent the population of patients from which results are to be generalized. Frequently, studies do not adequately account for factors such as cultural diversity, gender, and socioeconomic status when sampling from a population. Subject self-selection bias may occur when patients who volunteer for an experiment differ in some way from those who opt not to, possibly affecting results. For instance, patients who see a flier posted in the waiting room and enroll as a participant in a study may be more motivated than would those persons not responding to the ad, possibly inflating the effectiveness of a particular treatment.

Another weakness is the recruitment of too few or too many participants in a sample. Frequently, investigators mistakenly believe that 10 or 12 participants constitute an adequate sample size. Alternatively, some researchers believe that the more participants recruited for a study, the better. On the one hand, too few participants may not have enough statistical power to provide meaningful results. **Statistical power** is the degree with which a significant difference between group(s) or condition(s) may be found if, in fact, it exists. Recruiting too many participants, on the other hand, is overkill and may waste precious resources. Therefore, researchers should conduct a statistical procedure called a **power analysis,** which determines appropriate sample sizes for adequate statistical power in a particular experimental design.

The important point is that a power analysis was completed to determine the appropriate number of participants in a study. The details of conducting power analyses are beyond the scope of this textbook; see Haynes and Johnson (2009).

Participants should be randomly assigned to treatment and control groups. Both researchers and participants should be blinded to the randomization process and treatment allocation (e.g., assignments to treatment and control groups). If possible, studies should always have a control group that should be equivalent on baseline at the beginning of the study, to the greatest extent possible, to those receiving the treatment. It is important for the study to have a high degree of **internal validity**, or the degree of certainty that any measurable treatment effects on the dependent variable were due to the independent variable and not to other factors (Haynes & Johnson, 2009). Internal validity is established through a strong methodological control in an experiment such as the training of research assistants, multiple observations, reliability assessments, and so on. The outcome measures (i.e., dependent variables) must be reliable, valid, and administered appropriately with participants.

Other weaknesses are failure to mention or have procedures to account for participants who did not complete the experimental protocol, also known as **dropouts**. Frequently, experimenters do not report the number of persons recruited for the study and include only the data from those participants who completed the experimental protocol. These practices may bias results because those who completed the study may differ in fundamental ways from those who did not, thereby affecting outcomes. Therefore, investigators should report the number and reasons why participants did not complete the study. Moreover, the data from those dropouts should be included in a special statistical procedure called an **intention-to-treat analysis**. This procedure compares the results of patients in groups to which they were originally assigned, requiring obtaining their data regardless of whether or not they completed the experimental protocol (Hollis & Campbell, 1999). Obtaining follow-up data from patients who failed to complete a study may be difficult and time consuming, but improves the validity of the study. Any adverse effects or logistical problems should be reported, particularly those resulting in the loss of participants.

Another weakness to assess for is the use of **surrogate endpoints** as evidence for the effectiveness of auditory rehabilitation. Surrogate endpoints are outcomes (i.e., dependent variables) that do not reflect the long-term status. For example, many studies assessing the effectiveness of amplification concentrate on improved speech recognition in noise measured in clinical settings that may or may not have relevance to real-life listening conditions, a long-term effect on patients' quality of life. More recently, researchers have focused on the impact of auditory rehabilitation on patients' health-related quality of life (Abrams, Chisolm, & McArdle, 2005), which provides indications on the effectiveness of treatment in day-to-day life and for longer periods of time.

One issue in auditory rehabilitation research is how soon outcomes should be measured after hearing aid fitting. Should it be one month, three months, or six months postfitting? What role does **acclimatization**, or the accommodations that the brain must make due to the changes of acoustic information coming from the periphery due to amplification, play in the timing of outcome measurement? How do outcomes change over time? These are important questions because they may impact the measurement of effectiveness of auditory rehabilitation. Therefore, researchers should account for surrogate (e.g., short-term) versus long-term effectiveness of intervention.

Another important question is whether statistically significant differences found on outcomes among treatment options are clinically significant. Studies should employ a metric, or **effect sizes** with corresponding **confidence intervals**, to determine if statistically significant

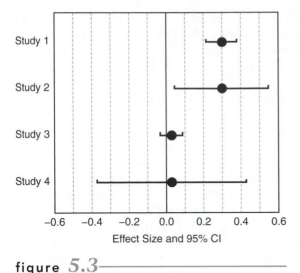

figure 5.3——————————————

Forest plots.

Source: Journal of the American Academy of Audiology by AMERICAN ACADEMY OF AUDIOLOGY. Copyright 2005. Reproduced with permission of AMERICAN ACADEMY OF AUDIOLOGY in the format Textbook via Copyright Clearance Center.

differences are clinically significant. Cox (2005, p. 432) defined effect size as a "metric that expresses the magnitude of a result, such as the differences in mean scores for two different hearing aids, within the context of the individual variation in scores." Effect sizes are frequently accompanied by confidence intervals that are specified by a percentage. A commonly used confidence interval is 95%, which represents a range of where the results may fall 95 times out of every 100 times the study was replicated (Cox, 2005). Effect sizes are meaningful in that 0.2 is a small effect size, 0.5 is a medium effect size, and 0.8 and greater is a large effect size. Confidence intervals are important for deriving meaning from findings in that they should not cross the zero line. Zero for an effect size means that a treatment does not have any significant effect. If a 95% confidence interval does cross the zero line, then clinicians cannot be 95% sure ($p < 0.05$) that a treatment does have an effect. Figure 5.3 shows **forest plots**, or graphs of effect sizes and corresponding confidence intervals, from four studies. For example, forest plots for studies 1 and 2 show moderate effect sizes of 0.3 and corresponding confidence intervals, meaning that this is where results are expected to fall 95 of every 100 times the study is conducted. The effect sizes for studies 3 and 4 are close to zero with confidence intervals that cross the zero line, indicating that the independent variable or treatment did not have any effect.

Specifics of computation of these values are beyond the scope of this textbook; see Cox (2005) and Haynes and Johnson (2009) for additional explanations. However, readers should know that effect sizes provide some indication of the real-world effects or impact of statistically significant differences found between or among groups of participants receiving different interventions. For example, if one group of children receiving one type of training had a statistically significantly higher mean speech perception performance than another group of children who received an alternative treatment, that difference does not necessarily translate into treatment effects. Effect sizes from individual studies may be combined to determine the overall clinical significance of a particular intervention in a systematic review. Effect sizes and confidence intervals are also good for grading clinical recommendations based on scientific evidence. As with the evaluation of systematic reviews, the overall assessment of the clinical trial/quasi-experimental study requires rating the relevance of the study to the clinical or research question, adequacy of the conclusions, and the risk of bias in the study.

Appendix 5.5 contains a worksheet for evaluating **clinical practice guidelines** (CPGs). Field and Lohr (1990) defined CPGs as "systematically developed statements to assist practitioner and patient decisions about appropriate health care for specific circumstances." CPGs are common in medicine and in allied-health professions such as audiology and speech-language pathology. In other chapters, we have defined and discussed professional documents such as scopes of practice, preferred practice patterns, position statements, and practice guidelines developed by the American Speech-Language-Hearing Association and the American Academy of Audiology that clinicians use to drive service delivery. There is a major fundamental difference between CPGs in medicine versus CPGs in communication sciences and disorders professions. Medical CPGs are almost always evidence-based with graded clinical recommendations; most in communication sciences and disorders are not. The medical community and governmental agencies have developed specific criteria for high-quality CPGs.

Several governmental agencies and professional organizations have participated in developing evidence-based CPGs. For example, the **Agency for Healthcare Research and Quality** (AHRQ), part of the Department of Health and Human Services concerned with health services research, supports research to improve the quality, safety, efficiency, and effectiveness of healthcare (AHRQ, 2010). The AHRQ partnered with the American Medical Association to develop the National Guidelines Clearinghouse that houses and provides resources about evidence-based CPGs. One important document is the **Conference on Guidelines Standardization Statement** (COGS) that consists of 18 characteristics of evidence-based CPGs (Shiffman et al., 2003). The document was the result of a 2002 meeting of 23 experts held in New Haven, Connecticut, to discuss the difficulties of and possible solutions for the lack of cohesiveness of CPGs both within and across medical disciplines. An international group of experts developed a similar evaluative tool, **Appraisal of Guidelines for Research and Evaluation Instrument** (AGREE), which is applicable in the assessment of any CPG (AGREE, 2001).

CPGs using a systematic process requiring a rigorous use of evidence-based review of clinical recommendations have begun to be used in the area of audiology and speech-language pathology. For instance, AAA developed the **Clinical Practice Guidelines Development Process** (AAA, 2006b), which describes an evidence-based procedure for the development of CPGs that is fairly compatible with the rigor of the COGS and AGREE instruments. The **Guidelines for the Audiologic Management of Adult Hearing Impairment** is one of the first CPGs developed using a process similar to the new process. The guidelines and their application are thoroughly discussed in Chapter 6. In time, more and more CPGs will be evidence-based. In addition, the American Speech-Language-Hearing Association will make all of these evidence-based CPGs available in the Evidence-Based Practice Compendium available online to all ASHA and NSSLHA members.

CPGs should involve a clearly focused area of clinical practice for audiologists, speech-language pathologists, or both in treating a clearly defined patient population in a particular area of practice. The group developing the document should be composed of recognized leaders in the field with full disclosure of conflicts of interest regarding the development of the CPG. A thorough search for and critical assessment of relevant evidence should drive the development of any clinical recommendations. The search should be transparent and well-documented so that it may be replicated by others. Specific criteria should be used to determine the risk of bias in the experimental studies. Rubrics for rating the risk of bias of evidence should be described so that any clinical recommendations and associated grades may be used appropriately for EBP. Final drafts of the CPG should be available for peer review and should currently be up-to-date. Finally, the overall assessment of CPGs should include its relevance to the clinical or research question, whether recommendations were evidence-based, and the overall risk of bias.

Step 3c: Grade the Clinical Recommendation Under Consideration

Appendix 5.6 is a worksheet to use in grading clinical recommendations based on the summary of articles, their level of evidence, and risk of bias. Please note that the results of this process should be classified according to how relevant the evidence is to the clinical or research question for a particular patient. Therefore, the clinical or research question should be written at the top of the form to keep focused. Let's use this worksheet and apply it to the clinical scenarios. Dr. Weil was fortunate to find a systematic review on the health-related quality-of-life benefits of hearing aids. Although published in 2007, the systematic review was rigorous and included a meta-analysis. The 16 studies that met the criteria for inclusion consisted of randomized controlled clinical trials, quasi-experimental studies, and nonexperimental prepost designed studies, which are Classes II, III, and IV levels of evidence, respectively. Recall that systematic reviews have a level of evidence consisting of those of the included studies. Therefore, the levels of evidence for this systematic review ranged from II to IV. Because the retrieval of studies and their systematic review were conducted using rigorous standards, the risk of bias was very low, warranting a grade of "+ +."

Reference	Level of Evidence	Risk of Bias
Chisolm, T. H., Johnson, C. E., Danhauer, J. L., et al. (2007). A systematic review of health-related quality of life and hearing aids: Final report of the American Academy of Audiology Task Force on the Health-Related Quality of Life Benefit of Amplification in Adults. *Journal of the American Academy of Audiology, 18,* 151–183.	II–IV	+ +

Dr. Trenoth found three articles to assist her with the Washingtons' concerns regarding the safety and relative benefits of simultaneous bilateral cochlear implantation over unilateral placement. In rapidly developing areas of auditory rehabilitation, it is not uncommon to have limited articles available to assist with clinical decision-making. It may be some time before large studies report the achievements of children who undergo these procedures. Two of the retrieved studies were case series or noninterventional studies of the Class IV level of evidence and the third was expert opinion, or Class VI, level of evidence. The results of the two case-series studies have a risk of bias because the results are from a single cochlear implant program warranting a grade of "+."

Reference	Level of Evidence	Risk of Bias
Ramsden, J. D., Papaioannou, V., Gordon, K. A., James, A. L., & Papsin, B. C. (2009). Parental and program's decision making in paediatric simultaneous bilateral cochlear implantation: Who says no and why? *International Journal of Pediatric Otolaryngology, 73,* 1325–1328.	IV	+
Basura, G. J., Eapen, R., & Buchman, C. A. (2009). Bilateral cochlear implantation: Current concepts, indications, and results. *Laryngoscope, 119,* 2395–2401.	VI	N/A
Ramsden, J. D., Papsin, B. C., Leung, R., James, A., & Gordon, K. A. (2009). Bilateral simultaneous cochlear implantation in children: Our first 50 cases. *Laryngoscope, 119,* 2444–2448.	IV	+

Cox (2005) developed a grading paradigm that appears in the following chart:

Grade	Criteria for Grade Assignment
A	Level I or Level II studies with consistent conclusions
B	Consistent Level III or IV studies or extrapolated evidence (generalized to a situation in which it is not truly relevant) from Level I or II studies
C	Level V studies or extrapolated evidence from Level III or IV studies
D	Level VI evidence or inconsistent or inconclusive studies of any level or any studies that have a high risk of bias

Source: Journal of the American Academy of Audiology by AMERICAN ACADEMY OF AUDIOLOGY. Copyright 2005. Reproduced with permission of AMERICAN ACADEMY OF AUDIOLOGY in the format Textbook via Copyright Clearance Center.

Evidence receives a grade of "A" when it presents with consistent results at Level I (i.e., systematic review with meta-analysis of well-designed clinical studies) or II (i.e., double-blinded randomized controlled clinical trials). A grade of "B" requires consistent results at Level III (i.e., nonrandomized intervention or quasi-experimental studies) or IV (i.e., non-intervention studies, cohort studies, case-control studies, or cross-sectional surveys) of evidence that directly relate to the research question. In addition, this grade is also assigned from Level I or II evidence that may be generalized from studies that do not exactly pertain to the research question. Such studies may involve the treatments and outcomes relating to the clinical question, but may differ in the population under consideration. Findings from these studies can be applied to the clinical question only through extrapolation. A grade of "C" requires evidence at Level V (i.e., case studies) or from Levels III or IV that do not directly pertain to all aspects of the clinical question. And finally, a grade of "D" corresponds to Level VI (i.e., expert opinion) or for any other evidence with inconsistent results. Obviously, the higher the grade, the stronger is the clinical recommendation.

Dr. Weil and Kendra reviewed the systematic review and found that Chisolm et al. (2007) assigned a grade of "B" to the clinical recommendation that hearing aids improve the health-related quality-of-life benefits for adults with sensorineural hearing losses. Alternatively, Dr. Trenoth decided not to grade the evidence for the clinical recommendation of the safety and relative benefits in speech and language development from simultaneous bilateral cochlear implantation compared to unilateral or sequential procedures. As Ramsden et al. (2009) found, decisions on this topic are highly individualistic and complex, requiring input from multiple stakeholders. Dr. Trenoth's plan was to be a sounding board for the Washingtons regarding their decision. She decided to explain that often, few studies are found on the cutting edge of technology. She planned to provide the Washingtons with the evidence she found and how it related to their situation.

Step 4: Integrating Scientific Evidence, Clinical Expertise, and Patient Preferences Into Clinical Decision-Making

The next step in evidence-based practice is integrating scientific evidence, clinical expertise, and patient factors into decision-making (see Appendix 5.7). We have just discussed the search and appraisal of scientific evidence. We will now focus on combining this with **clinical expertise** (i.e., knowledge, skills, and experiences of the practitioner in addition to recommendations from CPGs) while considering patient and family values and preferences. How do clinicians accomplish this? How do clinicians measure patients' and their families' values and preferences? How can their needs be matched to appropriate treatment options? How can attainment of goals be normalized to commonly used outcome measures for benchmarking? In incorporating all three elements of EBP, clinicians must be careful to consider the evidence, their own experiences, and the clinical guideline recommendations within the context of the patient and family's values and preferences prior to discussing options.

Dr. Weil had given the systematic review on the quality-of-life benefits of hearing aids to Kendra and told her to review it before her presession planning meeting for Charles's hearing aid evaluation. Kendra told Dr. Weil that she was familiar with that type of study because it had been covered in her research methods course. Kendra now wished she had paid a little more attention in class. She carefully studied her notes and textbook prior to her preplanning meeting.

Casebook Reflection

Quality of Life and Hearing Aids – Part 2

Kendra was nervous about the upcoming hearing aid evaluation with Charles Smith. Kendra had done the audiologic evaluation and enjoyed working with him, but she felt a little uneasy about his inquisitive nature.

"Kendra, are you ready for Dr. Smith?" asked Dr. Weil, Kendra's clinical instructor, poking her head into the consultation room.

"Yes, Dr. Weil," stated Kendra in an apprehensive voice.

"What's wrong, Kendra?" asked Dr. Weil.

"I guess I'm just nervous. Dr. Smith asks so many questions. I feel like he's trying to put me on the spot," offered Kendra. "I hope I can answer his questions."

"I don't think he's trying to put you on the spot. He's a scientist and I think it's his nature to do so," explained Dr. Weil. "If you can answer Dr. Smith's questions, you'll be able to handle any patient. I'm not sure that even I can answer all of his questions to his satisfaction. Relax and I'll jump in if I sense you need help."

"Thanks," Kendra said with a feeling of relief. At that moment, the phone rang and the receptionist told Kendra that Dr. Smith had arrived.

"Showtime!" remarked Dr. Weil, walking with Kendra to the waiting room.

"Dr. Smith, it's good to see you again. I'll be your audiologist today. Kendra is a doctor of audiology student who was involved in your audiologic evaluation a few weeks ago," explained Dr. Weil. "How are you today?"

"Well, I'm doing just fine. It's good to see you, Dr. Weil, and you also, Kendra," Charles said while shaking each clinician's hand, respectively.

"Thank you," responded Kendra. "We'll be down in room 3 to discuss possible options, answer your questions, and if you decide to pursue amplification, we'll go get some additional measures and take some ear impressions."

"Sounds good to me," Charles said, walking down the hall behind the clinicians.

After everyone was seated at the table, Kendra explained Charles's loss on the Count-the-Dot Audiogram, reviewed the advantages and disadvantages of various styles of hearing aids, and so on. Charles was then asked to nominate three to four situations in which he would like to improve his hearing.

"We'll, I'd like to be able to hear in meetings better, particularly women's voices. I'd also like to be able to hear what my wife is saying when we go out to eat. Most of the restaurants that we go to are really noisy and I can't understand a thing,"

Charles explained. "I'd also like to be able to hear the man call the numbers at bingo. I am pretty sure that the hearing aids will help me hear better, but I just want to know if they will improve my relationships in my family and help with the awkwardness in social situations. I want to know if hearing aids will improve my quality of life."

"Yes, I remembered that this was a big concern for you," remarked Kendra, placing a copy of the article in front of the patient. "Dr. Weil brought this article to my attention. It is a recent systematic review of evidence for the improvement of the health-related quality of life for adults with sensorineural hearing loss after getting hearing aids. We made a copy for you."

"Thank you," said Charles. He then took a few minutes to look at the abstract and at the conclusions of the study. Being a scientist, he understood the implications of the study. He looked over at Dr. Weil and winked and then asked Kendra. "Can you tell me about this systematic review?"

Kendra took a deep breath and provided a good explanation of what a systematic review was, what was done, and the conclusions. She then added, "It is important, though, to realize that the hearing aids won't solve all of your problems. You and members of your family need to work together to improve communication, particularly in difficult listening situations."

Realizing that Kendra was touching on a "hot button issue," Dr. Weil quickly added, "Yes, if you do your part and give these hearing aids a chance, your family members need to meet you halfway by decreasing communication barriers like distance when trying to initiate a conversation. Kendra is right. If you decide to try hearing aids, we strongly suggest that you attend group hearing aid orientation sessions with other couples. You'll find that many couples are experiencing some of the same issues. If at the end of 30 days nothing has changed, you can return the hearing aids and get your money back minus a small fee."

For the first time, Charles felt supported in Dr. Weil's acknowledgement that not all of the frustration he was experiencing was his fault. He no longer felt ashamed and alone with his problem, knowing that other couples had the same

struggles. "Well, show me what options you have available for me. . . ."

Also for the first time, Kendra made the connection between research and clinical work. "I guess we have an ethical responsibility to be up on the latest research findings when making recommendations to our patients," Kendra reasoned. "I was amazed at how presenting evidence to Dr. Weil made such a difference."

"I guess Dr. Smith appreciated our honesty and felt that he had nothing to lose considering he had a 30-day trial period," remarked Dr. Weil. "Do you have any questions about today's case?"

"No, I don't think so," said Kendra. "Thanks, Dr. Weil. I'll have the rough draft of the report in to you by tomorrow." Kendra excused herself from the office and went to work on her report.

A few days later, Kendra and Summer were back in Dr. Taylor's research methods course.

"Wow, what's up with you?" asked Summer, observing Kendra reading the textbook before the class. "Kendra? Did you hear me?"

"What?" answered Kendra.

"Why the sudden interest in research?" asked Summer.

"I had a case the other day. I realized that research has A LOT to do with what we do in the clinic. I figured I would understand Dr. Taylor better if I read the assigned chapters before the lecture," explained Kendra.

"Whatever," Summer said, rolling her eyes.

In the meantime, Dr. Weil had a feeling that Dr. Smith would agree to at least try hearing aids. She realized that his recent retirement, turning 70, and an increase in tension with his family members over his hearing loss had made him feel that he had become old overnight. He knew that hearing aids would help him hear better, but he wanted some evidence that they would improve his quality of life, particularly in his interactions with his family. He also understood that he and his wife could benefit from group hearing aid orientation sessions to talk with other couples facing the same problems.

And for Kendra's part, she was even more motivated now that she understood the importance of the content of Dr. Taylor's research methods class!

Casebook Reflection

Cochlear Implants for Joshua – Part 2

Dr. Trenoth has carefully read the articles retrieved for counseling the Washingtons. She had originally recommended the family to Dr. Keith's cochlear implant program at the hospital. She believed strongly that the recommendation made in the center's report for Joshua to undergo a simultaneous bilateral cochlear implantation was the right thing to do. However, her role was to help the Washingtons make an evidence-based decision they felt was best for their son.

"Hi, Mr. and Mrs. Washington, sorry I'm running a bit behind," apologized Dr. Trenoth, greeting the Washingtons in the waiting room. "Let's go back to my office so we can talk."

"How have you been?" asked Dr. Trenoth.

"Busy, busy, busy," Debbie replied. "Sometimes it seems as if I spend more time in the car than at home. Thanks so much for fitting us in."

"No problem. How is Joshua doing this week?" asked Dr. Trenoth.

"Oh, he is doing very well indeed," remarked Debbie. "You did get the results of the cochlear implant evaluation from the hospital, didn't you?"

"Yes, I did," remarked Dr. Trenoth. "You said on the phone that you are a bit uneasy about the recommendation for simultaneous cochlear implantation. Can you tell me about that?"

"Oh, I was just getting used to the idea of Joshua receiving one cochlear implant and the possibility of receiving one for the other ear later on when he is older. He is just a year old and the idea of implanting both ears during the same surgery took me by surprise. I just wanted to talk to you because you have been so good with Joshua over the past year," Debbie said, squeezing her husband's hand.

"Thank you, Debbie. You two have been through a lot the last year. We audiologists are so happy when parents get as involved as you two have. I know it has been difficult for you to be told that Joshua is not making adequate progress with hearing aids," Dr. Trenoth offered. "In preparation for today's meeting, I've done a bit of research regarding your question of the procedure's safety in relation to the possible benefits for Joshua from receiving two implants at the same time. I found three articles and have made copies for you."

"Thank you," said Debbie, placing the articles on the table.

"Please understand that bilateral simultaneous cochlear implantation in young children is a relatively new development. Therefore, there isn't as much research out as I would have preferred," Dr. Trenoth said. "However, the study by Ramsden and colleagues out of the Hospital for Sick Children in Toronto concedes that not all children are suitable for this procedure. It seems, though, that the cochlear implant team states in the report that Joshua is an excellent candidate for the procedure. However, the study also confirms that even though he is a good candidate, some parents do not want their child to undergo the procedure. So, you are not alone in your concerns."

As Debbie positioned herself in her chair, Dr. Trenoth added, "The second study from the same hospital reported on their first 50 pediatric patients who underwent simultaneous bilateral cochlear implantation in comparison to other children who had sequential implantation. You'll be pleased to know that there were no differences in complications, length of hospital stay per procedure, or use of certain medications. In fact, those undergoing a single simultaneous bilateral implantation had shorter cumulative hospital stays and surgical times than children undergoing two sequential procedures. Of course, the outcomes may be different for our local hospital. I assure you, though, that Dr. Keith's program is the best in the state, and they will provide similar statistics for you. Also, two separate procedures would mean that Joshua would have to undergo the risks of general anesthesia twice, not to mention the additional stress of preparing for two surgeries."

Debbie looked over at Leon and squeezed his hand again and said, "I didn't think about that."

"Yeah, that is a really good point," Leon added. "Dr. Trenoth, if Joshua were your child, what would YOU do?"

A few moments passed while Dr. Trenoth looked down at her desk while formulating her answer.

"That's difficult for me to answer and I don't like making decisions for my patients and their families. However, I know that you and Debbie will make the decision you feel is best for Joshua. Please understand that this is only my personal opinion—but speaking as a parent, I would go through with the simultaneous bilateral cochlear implantation. I believe that the benefits outweigh any risks," explained Dr. Trenoth. "Unfortunately, because this is a rapidly developing area, there isn't much data on the benefits attributable to this decision compared to receiving only one implant and possibly another one in the future. However, providing binaural input to Joshua via cochlear implants as soon as possible will help him take advantage of critical periods of auditory development and make the progress he was not able to with his hearing aids. . . . The article by Basura and colleagues published in 2009 describes some of the benefits of bilateral cochlear implantation. I strongly advise you to ask for the opportunity to talk with parents who have elected for their children to undergo this procedure through the local program. Then make your decision."

"Thank you, Dr. Trenoth," said Debbie in a relieved tone of voice. "I appreciate the time you have taken to speak with us and for your personal opinion. Of course, we will talk with Dr. Keith and ask for the outcomes from their program and for the names of other parents we can talk to."

"It's been my pleasure," Dr. Trenoth said, shaking Leon's and then Debbie's hand. "Please let me know what you've decided."

In the previous example, Dr. Trenoth demonstrated the principles of EBP in her consultation with the Washingtons. She carefully listened to the parents' concerns, searched for scientific evidence, and then carefully read the cochlear implant evaluation report from the expert team at the local hospital to assist the Washingtons with their decision. She wanted the Washingtons to dialogue with Dr. Keith and the cochlear implant team regarding the outcomes from their program for young children who had undergone a simultaneous bilateral cochlear implantation. Dr. Trenoth felt it would be helpful if the Washingtons actually talked to other parents of children who had undergone the procedure.

The fifth and final step of EBP is to evaluate the process.

Step 5: Evaluating the Process

Figure 5.1 shows the EBP process. Let's review it . . . Dr. Weil, Kendra, and Dr. Trenoth progressed through the first four steps of EBP in our clinical scenarios to assist their patients with clinical decision-making. For Charles, it was a decision to try hearing aids; for the Washingtons, it was considering simultaneous bilateral cochlear implantation for their son, Joshua. The first step was to frame the clinical research question(s) using the PICO rubric to help clarify the populations, intervention, alternative treatment, and the outcomes. Both Drs. Weil and Trenoth developed search strings that were submitted to databases using a macro strategy aimed at obtaining the highest level of evidence in the shortest amount of time. The articles obtained were critically appraised and both audiologists used scientific evidence, clinical expertise, and patients' values and preferences for assistance in clinical decision-making.

The final step of evaluating the process may take weeks, months, or years to assess the long-term outcomes of patients' decisions. In the short-term, Dr. Smith adjusted well to the use of amplification. The group hearing aid orientation session helped Charles and Irene learn how to work together in easing any communication breakdowns. Charles was open with his adult children and their families about how he had been feeling and how it affected his relationships with them. Debbie and Leon found Dr. Keith and his cochlear implant team very helpful in answering their questions and in making it possible for them to talk to other parents. Joshua's simultaneous bilateral cochlear implantations was successful, and he is now progressing as expected in achieving speech, language, and auditory milestones through auditory habilitation.

MOVING THE PROFESSIONS TOWARD EVIDENCE-BASED PRACTICE

What must the professions of audiology and speech-language pathology do to move toward EBP? Cox (2005) suggested that the following steps could help professionals support the work required of EBP:

- Create continuing education opportunities for audiologists and speech-language pathologists on EBP skills in critically reviewing research.
- Ensure that researchers do systematic reviews on treatments and publish results that are accessible to clinicians in journals.
- Request that researchers:
  - denote the essential features by including them in the key words indexing.
  - write structured abstracts so that key components of a study are quickly reviewed and categorized regarding the level of evidence (e.g., statement of the question, research design).
- Insist on higher levels of evidence on research concerning auditory rehabilitation.
- Train tomorrow's audiologists and speech-language pathologists to appreciate and use the principles of EBP.

Undergraduate students in communication sciences and disorders programs usually do not study research methodology until enrolled in graduate or professional degree programs. However, they can lay the foundation for EBP by following several suggestions. First, students can question the validity or truth of the information regarding auditory rehabilitation. Students must distinguish between peer-reviewed and non-peer-reviewed publications. **Peer-reviewed publications** are those that are reviewed by experts in the field and must meet certain criteria for publication. Some examples of peer-reviewed journals in the field include the *American Journal of Audiology*, *Ear and Hearing*, the *Journal of the American Academy of Audiology*, the *Journal of Speech, Language, and Hearing Research*, and so on. Non-peer-reviewed journals have articles that do not have to be reviewed, and include *The Hearing Journal*, *The Hearing Review*, and so on. Both peer- and non-peer-reviewed publications have their place in the professions. Second, students should consider the hierarchy of scientific rigor according to levels of evidence when reading research findings in professional publications and use correct terminology when stating conclusions. For example, the terms *efficacy* and *efficacy research* imply answering questions about the process of intervention requiring assessment under ideal or laboratory conditions more often at the Class I or II or experimental level of evidence. The terms *effectiveness* or *treatment effectiveness* address whether treatments work in the real world, usually at the Class III level or quasi-experimental level of evidence. Only Class I and II or experimental research can imply a cause-and-effect relationship between variables. Third, students should use an evidence-based approach in the classroom and in clinical practicum by asking questions and stimulating discussions regarding treatment approaches in communication sciences and disorders. For example, students should *not* be afraid to ask their clinical supervisors about the scientific evidence supporting the effectiveness of speechreading therapy with elderly hearing aid wearers. Readers should adopt an evidence-based mindset in their study of communication sciences and disorders. After all, today's students are tomorrow's researchers and clinicians.

SUMMARY

This chapter discussed the importance of evidence-based practice in audiologic/auditory rehabilitation. The term *levels of evidence* was defined as a hierarchy of rigor used in evaluating research methodology. Examples of different methodologies were provided for each level. The process of evidence-based auditory rehabilitation was developed through the use of two scenarios. Students were encouraged to use an evidence-based mindset in their studies of communication sciences and disorders.

LEARNING ACTIVITIES

Present a controversial topic to the class, based on something related to the subject of this chapter. Then divide the class into two teams to research and debate opposing viewpoints of this topic.

- Complete a systematic review of a particular treatment used to lessen the effects of hearing loss.
- Observe clinical practicum and determine if audiologists are using an evidence-based approach with their patients.
- Go through a few professional journals and classify the types of studies according to their level of evidence.

APPENDIX 5.1

Worksheet for Formulating Clinical or Research Questions

Clinician's Name: _____

Date: _____

Step 1: Formulating the Clinical or Research Question

INSTRUCTIONS: *Please use the rubric below to define the patient population, intervention, comparison treatment, and outcomes to formulate the clinical research question.*

Population	
Intervention	
Alternative Treatment	
Outcomes	

_____

_____

_____

_____

Source: Based on *Understanding Research and Evidence-Based Practice in Communication Disorders: A Primer for Students and Practitioners,* by W. O. Haynes and C. E. Johnson, 2009, Upper Saddle River, NJ: Pearson.

APPENDIX 5.2

Worksheet for Searching
for the Evidence

Clinician's Name: _____

Date: _____

Step 2: Searching for the Evidence

INSTRUCTIONS: *Please complete the information about the specific database search and log the authors, name of the study, and journal information of each article in the appropriate spaces below.*

Title of Database: _____

Years Covered by the Search: _____

Language Restrictions: _____

Description of Search (Search Strings): _____

_____

_____

Authors/Date	Title	Journal Citation

NOTES: _____

_____

_____

_____

Source: Based on *Understanding Research and Evidence-Based Practice in Communication Disorders: A Primer for Students and Practitioners,* by W. O. Haynes and C. E. Johnson, 2009, Upper Saddle River, NJ: Pearson.

APPENDIX 5.3

Worksheet for Quality Assessment of Systematic Reviews

Clinician's Name: _____

Date: _____

Step 3A: Assessing the Quality and Rating the Risk of Bias

INSTRUCTIONS: *Please provide the bibliographic reference, level of evidence, assessment of quality indicators, and overall risk of bias for the systematic review.*

Bibliographic Reference: _____

_____

_____

Level of Evidence of Studies Included in the Systematic Review

I   II   III   IV   V   VI

Quality Indicators

1. Was the rationale for conducting the study strong?

   Yes   No   Can't tell

2. Was the research question clearly focused?

   Yes   No   Can't tell

3. Was the search strategy clearly documented, complete, and up-to-date?

   Yes   No   Can't tell

4. Were review team members adequately trained?

   Yes   No   Can't tell

5. Were procedures in place to ensure independent decisions of review team members?

   Yes   No   Can't tell

6. Were impartial methods for settling disagreements among team members in place?

   Yes   No   Can't tell

7. Were inclusion/exclusion criteria for studies clear and adhered to?

   Yes   No   Can't tell

8. Were the included studies adequately described in terms of participants' demographic data, outcome measures, results, and so on?

   Yes   No   Can't tell

9. Were included studies adequately assessed for quality on appropriate factors (e.g., level of evidence, use of a control group, power analysis, inclusion/exclusion criteria, random assignment)?

Yes   No   Can't tell

10. Was a meta-analysis conducted based on reasonable grouping of findings of similar studies?

Yes   No   Can't tell

Overall Assessment of the Study

1. Was the systematic review relevant to the clinical or research question?

Yes   No   Can't tell

2. Were the conclusions adequate based on the results of the systematic review?

Yes   No   Can't tell

3. What is the overall risk of bias in this systematic review?

++	Very low risk of bias. Any weaknesses that are present are very unlikely to alter the conclusions of the study.
+	Low risk of bias. Identified weaknesses or omitted information probably would not alter the conclusions of the study.
−	High risk of bias. Identified weaknesses or omitted information are very likely to alter conclusions of the study.

NOTES: _____

_____

_____

_____

Sources: Based on *Center for Evidenced-Based Medicine,* by the Center for Evidence-Based Medicine, 2010, retrieved from www.cebm.net; *Cochrane Handbook for Systematic Reviews of Interventions, Version 5.0.2,* by the Cochrane Collaboration, 2009, retrieved from www.cochrane-handbook.org/; *Understanding Research and Evidence-Based Practice in Communication Disorders: A Primer for Students and Practitioners,* by W. O. Haynes and C. E. Johnson, 2009, Upper Saddle River, NJ: Pearson.

APPENDIX 5.4

Worksheet for Quality Assessment of Clinical Trials and Quasi-Experimental Studies

Clinician's Name: _____

Date: _____

Step 3A: Assessing the Quality and Rating the Risk of Bias

INSTRUCTIONS: *Please provide the bibliographic reference, level of evidence, assessment of quality indicators, and overall risk of bias for the clinical trial or quasi-experimental study.*

Bibliographic Reference: _____

_____

_____

Level of Evidence of the Study

I   II   III   IV   V   VI

Quality Indicators

1. Was the rationale for conducting the study strong?
   Yes   No   Can't tell

2. Was the research question focused?
   Yes   No   Can't tell

3. Are participant inclusion and exclusion criteria provided?
   Yes   No   Can't tell

4. Does the sample adequately represent the population from which it was drawn?
   Yes   No   Can't tell

5. Were power analyses completed to determine adequate sample size?
   Yes   No   Can't tell

6. Were participants randomly assigned to treatment and control groups?
   Yes   No   Can't tell

7. Were research assistants or those administering tests blinded to treatment allocation?
   Yes   No   Can't tell

8. Were participants blinded to treatment allocation?
   Yes   No   Can't tell

9. Was a control group used?
   Yes   No   Can't tell

10. Were treatment and control groups equal at baseline?
    Yes   No   Can't tell

11. Was treatment allocation the only difference between treatment and control groups?

Yes   No   Can't tell

12. Were outcome measures (e.g., dependent variables) reliable, valid, and normed for appropriate use with the participants in the study?

Yes   No   Can't tell

13. Were methods (e.g., training of research assistants, multiple observations, interobserver reliability) employed to increase the internal validity of the study?

Yes   No   Can't tell

14. Were dropouts discussed?

Yes   No   Can't tell

15. Were dropouts accounted for (e.g., intention-to-treat analysis)?

Yes   No   Can't tell

16. Were any adverse events reported?

Yes   No   Can't tell

17. Were outcome measures merely surrogate endpoints or was some measure of long-term status made?

Yes   No   Can't tell

18. Were effect sizes and confidence intervals computed to provide an indication of significant treatment effects?

Yes   No   Can't tell

Overall Assessment of the Study

1. Was the study relevant to the clinical or research question?

Yes   No   Can't tell

2. Were the conclusions adequate based on the results found in the study?

Yes   No   Can't tell

3. What is the overall risk of bias of this study?

+ +	Very low risk of bias. Any weaknesses that are present are very unlikely to alter the conclusions of the study.
+	Low risk of bias. Identified weaknesses or omitted information probably would not alter the conclusions of the study.
–	High risk of bias. Identified weaknesses or omitted information are very likely to alter conclusions of the study.

NOTES: _____

_____

_____

_____

Sources: Based on *Center for Evidenced-Based Medicine*, by the Center for Evidence-Based Medicine, 2010, retrieved from www.cebm.net; *Understanding Research and Evidence-Based Practice in Communication Disorders: A Primer for Students and Practitioners,* by W. O. Haynes and C. E. Johnson, 2009, Upper Saddle River, NJ: Pearson; *SIGN-50: A Guideline Developer's Handbook*, by Scottish Intercollegiate Guidelines Network, 2008, Edinburgh, Scotland: Author.

APPENDIX 5.5

Worksheet for Quality Assessment
of Clinical Practice Guidelines (CPGs)

Clinician's Name: _____

Date: _____

Step 3A: Assessing the Quality and Rating the Risk of Bias

INSTRUCTIONS: *Please provide the reference for the CPG, sponsoring professional organization, and date of publication.*

CPG Reference: _____

Sponsoring Professional Organization: _____

Date of Publication: _____

Quality Indicators

1. Does the CPG involve a clearly focused area of clinical practice?
   Yes   No   Can't tell

2. Is the CPG specified for a specific communication disorder professional?
   Audiologist   Speech-Language Pathologist   Both

3. Is the CPG for use with a specific patient population?
   Yes   No   Can't tell
   Specify: _____

4. Are the authors of the CPG recognized leaders in the field?
   Yes   No   Can't tell

5. Are there any potential conflicts of interest with authors?
   Yes   No   Can't tell

6. Was there a thorough and transparent search of the evidence concerning this topic?
   Yes   No   Can't tell

7. Was the evidence critically assessed for level of evidence and risk of bias?
   Yes   No   Can't tell

8. Were specific criteria mentioned for rating the risk of bias and for grading of clinical recommendations?
   Yes   No   Can't tell

9. Was a draft of the CPG available for peer review?
   Yes   No   Can't tell

10. Is the CPG up-to-date?
    Yes   No   Can't tell

Overall Assessment

1. Was the CPG relevant to the clinical or research question?

   Yes   No   Can't tell

2. Were the clinical recommendations adequate based on the evidence?

   Yes   No   Can't tell

3. What is the overall risk of bias in this CPG?

++	Very low risk of bias. Any weaknesses that are present are very unlikely to alter the conclusions of the study.
+	Low risk of bias. Identified weaknesses or omitted information probably would not alter the conclusions of the study.
–	High risk of bias. Identified weaknesses or omitted information are very likely to alter conclusions of the study.

NOTES: _____

_____

_____

_____

Sources: Based on *AGREE Collaboration, 2007,* retrieved July 15, 2007 from www.agreecollaboration.org; "Evidence-Based Practice in Provision of Amplification," by R. M. Cox, 2005, *Journal of the American Academy of Audiology, 16,* pp. 419–438; *Understanding Research and Evidence-Based Practice in Communication Disorders: A Primer for Students and Practitioners,* by W. O. Haynes and C. E. Johnson, 2009, Upper Saddle River, NJ: Pearson; "Standardized Reporting of Clinical Practice Guidelines: A Proposal from the Conference of Guidelines Standardization," by R. N. Shiffman, P. Shekelle, J. M. Overhage, J. Slutsky, J. Grimshaw, and A. M. Deshpande, 2003, *Annals of Internal Medicine, 139*, pp. 493–498.

APPENDIX 5.6

Worksheet for Grading the Clinical Recommendation

Clinician's Name: _____

Date: _____

Step 3C: Grading the Clinical Recommendation

INSTRUCTIONS: *Please write the clinical research question, then provide information about key sources of evidence according to their relevance.*

Clinical or Research Question: _____

_____

_____

Directly Relevant Evidence

Reference	Level of Evidence	Risk of Bias
		++ + −
		++ + −
		++ + −
		++ + −
		++ + −

Indirectly Relevant Evidence

Reference	Level of Evidence	Risk of Bias
		++ + −
		++ + −
		++ + −
		++ + −
		++ + −

Clinical Recommendation: _____

_____

_____

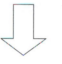

Grade	Criteria for Grade Assignment
A	Level I or Level II studies with consistent conclusions
B	Consistent Level III or IV studies or extrapolated evidence (generalized to a situation in which it is not truly relevant) from Level I or II studies
C	Level V studies or extrapolated evidence from Level III or IV studies
D	Level VI evidence or inconsistent or inconclusive studies of any level or any studies that have a high risk of bias

NOTES: _____

_____

_____

_____

APPENDIX 5.7

Worksheet Integrating Scientific Evidence, Clinical Expertise, and Patient Factors Into Clinical Decision-Making

Clinician's Name: _____

Date: _____

Step 4: Integrating Scientific Evidence, Clinical Expertise, and Patient Preferences into Clinical Decision-Making

INSTRUCTIONS: *Please write down the clinical or research questions and use the following areas to note critical points that will impact clinical decision-making.*

Clinical or Research Question: _____

_____

_____

Scientific Evidence
Clinical Expertise
Patient Factors

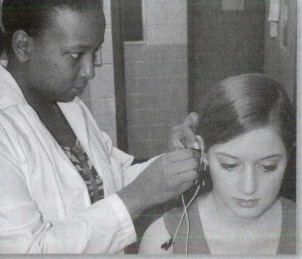

CHAPTER six

An Introduction to Amplification

LEARNING *objectives*

After reading this chapter, you should be able to:

1. Trace the history of hearing aids.
2. Explain the characteristics, advantages, and disadvantages of contemporary styles of hearing aids.
3. Compare and contrast:
   - Analog, digitally programmable, and completely digital hearing aids
   - CROS, BICROS, and transcranial CROS
   - Bone-conduction and bone-anchored hearing aids
   - Piezoelectric and electromagnetic implantable hearing aids
4. List and explain the tools that audiologists need to dispense hearing aids.
5. Understand the principles of and parameters for an electroacoustic analysis of hearing aids.
6. Describe the process in the management of hearing impairment through amplification.

adly, only 20% of the estimated 30 million Americans with hearing loss have
selected to seek help through amplification. Hearing aids are not just a present-day
phenomenon; use of these devices dates back to the 16th century. In this chapter,
the history of hearing aid technology is reviewed. Hearing aids have made considerable
advancements in the last 50 years, are available in different sizes/styles, and offer amplification capabilities for varying degrees of hearing loss. Hearing aid manufacturers'
product lines are now digital rather than analog technology and provide patients with
the latest advancements in signal processing. Hearing aid styles, the advantages/
disadvantages of each, and how these devices work are covered in this chapter. Different types of hearing aids other than those that amplify acoustic energy only will also be
covered including bone-conduction hearing aids, bone-anchored hearing aids, and
implantable hearing aids.

Earlier, we discussed the impact of hearing impairment on the health-related quality of life (HRQoL) for patients of all ages. Dr. James Jerger, one of the founding fa-
thers of audiology, called hearing aids the "cornerstone" of auditory rehabilitation
(Jerger, 2007). A recent systematic review with meta-analysis concluded that hearing
aids reduced the social and emotional impact of hearing loss on adults with sensorineural hearing loss (Chisolm et al., 2007). Hopefully, the results of this study will
encourage primary care physicians (PCPs) to refer patients with sensorineural hearing
losses to audiologists for diagnostic assessment leading to the selection, evaluation,
and fitting of hearing aids.

Evidence-based practice (EBP), a major theme in this textbook, has been applied in
the development of new clinical practice guidelines (CPGs). In the previous chapter,
Field and Lohr (1990) defined CPGs as "systematically developed statements to assist
practitioner and patient decisions about appropriate healthcare for specific circumstances." The American Academy of Audiology's *Guidelines for the Audiologic
Management of Adult Hearing Impairment* (Valente, Abrams, et al., 2006) is one of the
first CPGs complete with level of evidence and graded recommendations for specific
procedures. This chapter follows the guidelines for a process-driven approach to amplification that is best understood when applied to patients as they go through the hearing
healthcare continuum. We will explore the management of hearing loss in an elderly
patient through the use of hearing aids.

HISTORY OF HEARING AIDS

As early as the 16th century, Giovanni Battista Porta described the first hearing aids as being made of wood and shaped like animal ears (American Academy of Otolaryngology—
Head and Neck Surgery Time Line, 2006). In the 1800s, other nonelectric hearing aids
such as speaking tubes and ear trumpets were used. These early, nonelectric hearing
aids amplified sound on the basis of **resonance**, or the tendency for objects to vibrate
when energy at its natural frequency is applied, resulting in amplification. Ear trumpets were made of silver or tortoise shell with some models having special features of
collapsibility for portability, selective amplification of different pitches, and/or concealment in other objects (e.g., canes) (Kenneth Burger Hearing Aid Museum [KBHAM],

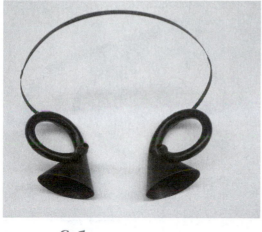

figure *6.1*—————————————

Aurolese phone made by F. C. Rein Company.

Source: Becker Medical Library, Washington University School of Medicine. Used with permission.

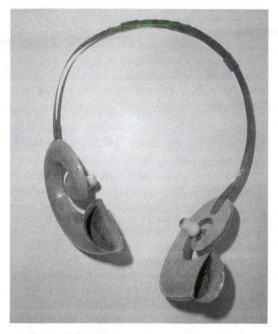

figure *6.2*—————————————

A more decorative Aurolese phone made by F. C. Rein Company.

Source: Becker Medical Library, Washington University School of Medicine. Used with permission.

2009). After the development of ear trumpets, the industry sought to hide the use of these devices in any way possible. Combining the element of disguise with functionality for people with mild-to-moderate hearing loss was almost an art form (Washington University School of Medicine, Bernard Becker Medical Library [WUSM-BBML], 2009). In fact, acoustic headbands were the earliest known attempts at concealing hearing aids (WUSM-BBML, 2009). These devices, such as the Aurolese Phones made by F. C. Rein Company, functioned much like cupping hands to the ears and consisted of irregularly shaped ovoids, barrels, or convoluted shells that fit over or under the ear (KBHAM, 2009; WUSM-BBML, 2009). Two such headbands, made by the F. C. Rein Company, are shown in Figures 6.1 and 6.2.

Figure 6.3 is an ad from the F. C. Rein catalog that showed how its Invisible Aurolese Phones could be hidden in scarves and hats (WUSM-BBML, 2009). Other types of nonelectric hearing aids were concealed in acoustic fans made of thin metal that could be held behind users' ears to direct and amplify sound (WUSM-BBML, 2009). Figure 6.4 shows another example of a water canteen receptor with a shoulder strap that collects sound and funnels it into a tube that goes into users' ears (WUSM-BBML, 2009).

During the early 1900s, hearing aid technology transitioned from nonelectric to electric instruments through the use of batteries. The first electric hearing instruments, in 1902, were carbon hearing aids, available in large models that had to be placed on tables (KBHAM, 2009; WUSM-BBML, 2009). These early wearable models used large 3- or 6-volt batteries and were popular through the 1940s (KBHAM, 2009; WUSM-BBML, 2009). Figure 6.5 shows a wearable carbon hearing aid that was suitable *only* for people with up to moderate hearing losses.

The next generation of electric hearing instruments was more efficient in amplifying electrical signals. Vacuum tube hearing aids had greater acoustic gain and could benefit patients with more severe hearing losses (WUSM-BBML, 2009). These hearing aids were first available in 1921 but did not become practical until the early 1930s (KBHAM, 2009). The first vacuum tube hearing aids were very large and were not easily transported. Figure 6.6 shows the Precision Electric Company table hearing aid, which is camouflaged as a radio, available in 1941 (WUSM-BBML, 2009).

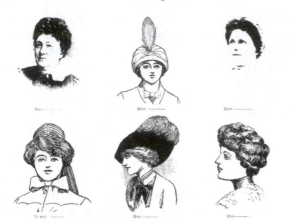

INVISIBLE "AUROLESE" PHONES IN ACTUAL USE.

figure *6.3*

An ad from the F. C. Rein catalog showing how hearing devices could be hidden in scarves and hats.

Source: Becker Medical Library, Washington University School of Medicine. Used with permission.

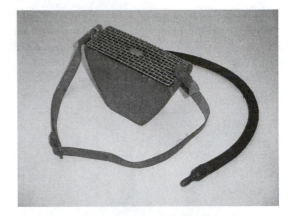

figure *6.4*

Water canteen receptor hearing aid.

Source: Becker Medical Library, Washington University School of Medicine. Used with permission.

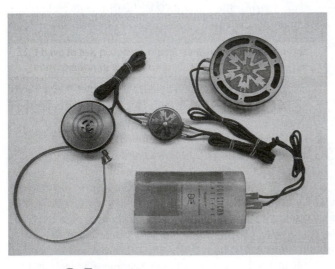

figure *6.5*

A wearable carbon hearing aid.

Source: Becker Medical Library, Washington University School of Medicine. Used with permission.

Wearable vacuum tube hearing aids were not available until 1934, and required two large batteries, weighing as much as 2 1/2 pounds (KBHAM, 2009). One A battery was needed to warm the filament in the vacuum tube, and a second one, a B battery, was needed to amplify the sound (WUSM-BBML, 2009). The batteries had to be worn in a holder under the clothes or in pockets with straps that connected to the hearing aid unit (WUSM-BBML, 2009). Figure 6.7 shows an Aurex Corporation wearable vacuum tube hearing aid. In 1947, improvements in technology enabled miniaturization of batteries such that they could be housed inside the hearing aid unit (WUSM-BBML, 2009).

Transistor hearing aids became available in 1952 and completely replaced vacuum tube hearing aids by the end of 1953 (KBHAM, 2005). These devices required the use of only one battery, resulting in the reduction of the size of body-worn units and the development of styles such as eyeglass and behind-the-ear hearing aids (KBHAM, 2005). The first eyeglass hearing aids were available in the United

States in 1954, and by the end of the decade these devices accounted for about half of the market share (WUSM-BBML, 2009). Figure 6.8 shows the Sonotone Model 400 eyeglass hearing aid circa 1957.

Behind-the-ear hearing instruments were first introduced in the late 1950s and soon overtook eyeglass hearing aids in popularity (WUSM-BBML, 2009). In the 1960s, in-the-ear styles of hearing aids became available, first in stock or noncustom devices, then in custom models that partially filled the concha (e.g., half shell). They also became available in models that filled the external portion of the ear canal (e.g., in-the-canal). Along with the miniaturization of hearing aid styles the circuitry inside these devices progressed from analog, to analog-digital (i.e., hybrid), and then to completely digital technology, which is discussed later on in the chapter. In the 1990s, completely-in-the-canal styles, which fit around the first bend of the ear canal, became popular due to their invisibility. Today, the latest style of hearing aids is the open-ear fitting, which is a small behind-the-ear device.

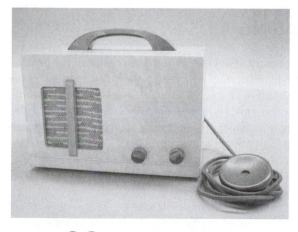

figure *6.6*

A Precision Electric Company table hearing aid.

Source: Becker Medical Library, Washington University School of Medicine. Used with permission.

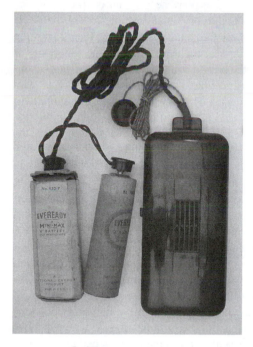

figure *6.7*

An Aurex Corporation wearable vacuum tube hearing aid.

Source: Becker Medical Library, Washington University School of Medicine. Used with permission.

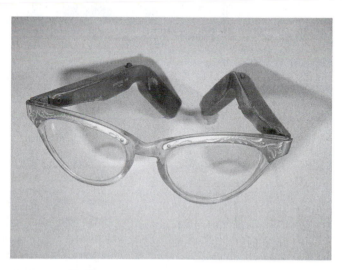

figure *6.8*

A Sonotone Model 400 eyeglass hearing aid from around 1957.

Source: Becker Medical Library, Washington University School of Medicine. Used with permission.

CONTEMPORARY STYLES OF HEARING AIDS

Although this section is called "Contemporary Styles of Hearing Aids," some of the devices are much less common than others. Style of hearing aid refers to the type of casing that a hearing instrument has and how it is coupled or attached to the ear. Styles of hearing instruments can be categorized into two general groups: (1) those requiring earmolds to couple the hearing aid to patients' ears, and (2) those in which the electronic components are housed within the earpiece. An **earmold** is a specially fit or custom-made device that couples hearing aids to patients' ears. *Couple to the ear* means how the hearing aid attaches to the ear.

Hearing Aids Requiring Earmolds

The three styles of hearing aids requiring the use of earmolds are (1) body, (2) eyeglass, and (3) behind-the-ear hearing aids. The **body hearing aid** acquired its name because it is worn on the body (e.g., in a pocket) with the receiver situated at the patient's ear, coupled by means of a snapring earmold. The receiver is attached to the hearing aid by means of a cord. Figures 6.9 and 6.10 show a body hearing aid and a diagram of its parts, respectively.

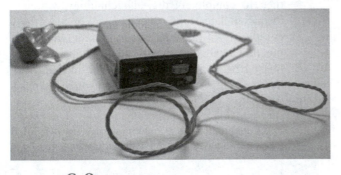

figure 6.9

A body hearing aid.

The body hearing aid is appropriate for slight-to-profound hearing losses, but it is most frequently used with patients with the most severe hearing losses. The advantages of the body hearing aid include high gain or amplification, large controls for patients with manual dexterity problems (e.g., arthritis), reduced likelihood of feedback due to the distance between the microphone and the receiver, durability, and limited susceptibility to moisture problems. **Feedback** is a whistling sound that has come out of the hearing aid receiver that is picked up again by the microphone. In other words, feedback is the reamplification of previously amplified sound and is very annoying to patients. Some of the disadvantages of body hearing aids include poor cosmetic appeal and the location of the microphone when worn on the body of the patient. Patients report hearing the clothing noise when they move and experience "body baffle" or the enhancement of low-frequency sounds. The body hearing aid accounts for so few devices sold that they are not included in annual industry surveys of instruments sold (Kirkwood, 2009).

The **eyeglass hearing aid** has its electronic components housed in the temple of the glasses and is coupled to the ear by means of an earmold using tubing. Eyeglass hearing aids are appropriate for slight to profound hearing losses. Figure 6.11 shows an eyeglass hearing aid.

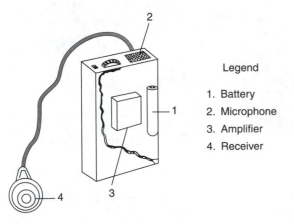

Legend

1. Battery
2. Microphone
3. Amplifier
4. Receiver

figure 6.10

A diagram of a body hearing aid and its parts.

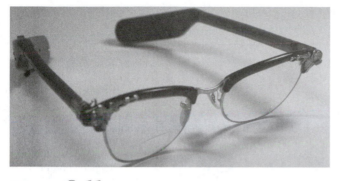

figure *6.11*

An eyeglass hearing aid.

Eyeglass hearing aids share some of the advantages of body hearing aids such as durability and limited susceptibility to moisture damage. Some patients prefer the convenience of having their hearing aids built into their glasses. However, some patients feel that it is a disadvantage because they cannot use hearing aids without having to wear glasses. Similarly, patients may have to do without glasses when their hearing aids are sent to the manufacturer for repair. Another disadvantage of eyeglass hearing aids is their poor cosmetic appeal. The eyeglass style also is not reported in annual industry surveys of hearing aids sold (Kirkwood, 2009).

The third style of hearing aid requiring an earmold is the **behind-the-ear (BTE)**, or postauricular, hearing aid. The behind-the-ear hearing aid is coupled to the ear via an earmold, and its electrical components are housed in a plastic case positioned behind the pinna. The BTE is appropriate for slight-to-profound hearing losses. The BTE comes in different size cases appropriate for use by infants to adults. Figures 6.12, 6.13, and 6.14 show

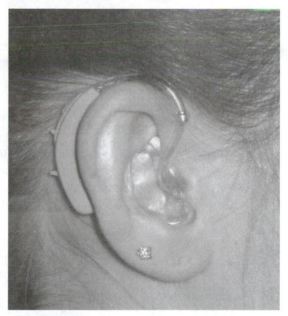

figure *6.13*

A behind-the-ear hearing aid as worn.

Source: Reprinted with permission from "The 'Hearing Aid Effect' 2005: A Rigorous Test of the Visibility of New Hearing Aid Styles," by C. E. Johnson, J. L. Danhauer, R. B. Gaven, S. R. Karns, A. C. Reith, & I. P. Lopez, *American Journal of Audiology, 14,* 169–175. Copyright 2005 by American Speech-Language-Hearing Association.

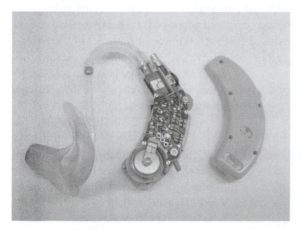

figure *6.12*

A behind-the-ear hearing aid.

Source: Becker Medical Library, Washington University School of Medicine. Used with permission.

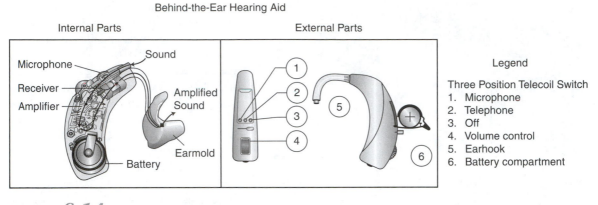

figure *6.14*

A diagram of a behind-the-ear hearing aid and its parts.

a behind-the-ear hearing aid, how it looks when it is worn, and a diagram of its parts, respectively.

The BTE shares some of the same advantages as the two previously discussed styles in that it is durable and less susceptible to moisture damage than in-the-ear hearing aids. Another advantage of the BTE is the space that is available for circuitry and additional accessories. For example, BTEs can be equipped with **direct-audio input (DAI)**, a series of electrical contacts, that allows a signal from one device to enter into to the hearing aid by means of a cord and plug. The BTE is the style of choice for children under 13 years of age, a durable instrument that can accommodate a growing ear by simply replacing the earmold. On the other hand, BTEs provide the most "burden" or hassle for the elderly because the aids have two separate parts, an earmold and a hearing aid to keep up with and manage (May, Upfold, & Battaglia, 1990). Another disadvantage of BTEs is the lack of cosmetic appeal. BTE styles of hearing aids have accounted for approximately 63% of the market share of hearing aids sold in recent years (Kirkwood, 2009). This style has shown a recent surge in popularity because of the availability of open-ear devices that are also considered a type of BTE hearing aid.

Earmolds are available in various styles, depending on the acoustic needs of the patient. Earmolds vary in degree of occlusion, from skeleton to full-shell earmolds, as shown in Figure 6.15. Some skeleton earmolds other than the type shown on the left, do not occlude the ear canal at all.

Earmolds can be modified to alter the acoustic outputs of hearing aids, ensuring a better fit for patients' hearing losses and listening preferences. For example, **acoustic dampers** can be placed in the tubing of an earmold or earhook (e.g., tone hook) of a BTE hearing aid with a net result of smoothing out any acoustical peaks in the output of the hearing aid that may be painful to patients. An **earhook** or **tone hook** is part of a BTE hearing aid that rests on top of the pinna, securing the device in place on the ear.

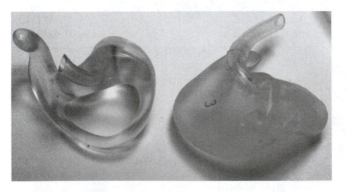

figure *6.15*

A skeleton (left) and shell (right) earmolds.

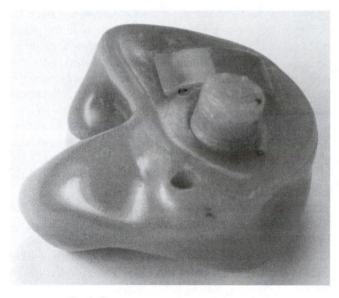

Similarly, many earmolds have **vents**, tunnels connecting the outside environment to the inside of the ear canal, which can taper the amount of low-frequency amplification through the use of little plugs with holes of different diameters. To reduce the amount of low frequencies, plugs with holes with larger diameters are used in the vent, rather than those with openings of smaller diameters. In addition, use of a **libby horn**, in which the diameter of the tubing gets larger from the earhook to its connection to the earmold, can increase the amount of high-frequency amplification. These modifications are typically considered when earmolds are ordered and utilized during the fine-tuning stages of hearing aid fittings.

figure *6.16*

An in-the-ear hearing aid.

In-the-Ear Hearing Aids

Another major category is **in-the-ear (ITE) hearing aids**, which include those styles in which the electronic components are housed completely within a custom-made shell or earpiece. The **classic ITE hearing aid** fills the concha portion of the pinna. The ITE, however, is also available in a half-shell model that does not completely fill in the concha. The ITE is appropriate for slight-to-severe hearing losses. Figure 6.16 shows a classic in-the-ear hearing aid, and Figure 6.17 provides a diagram of its parts. Figure 6.18 shows how full (left) and half-shell (right) in-the-ear hearing aids look when worn.

Some of the advantages of ITEs are their cosmetic appeal and simplicity in manipulation for the elderly, especially when ordered with notches for easy insertion and removal and a raised volume control wheel for easy adjustment. Another advantage of the ITE style of hearing aid over previously described models is the natural location of the microphone. For

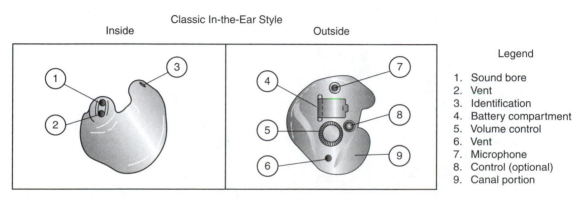

figure *6.17*

A diagram of an in-the-ear hearing aid and its parts.

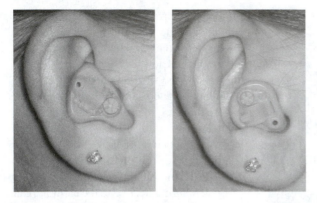

figure *6.18*

A full- (left) and half-shell (right) in-the-ear hearing aids as worn.

Source: Reprinted with permission from "The 'Hearing Aid Effect' 2005: A Rigorous Test of the Visibility of New Hearing Aid Styles," by C. E. Johnson, J. L. Danhauer, R. B. Gaven, S. R. Karns, A. C. Reith, & I. P. Lopez, *American Journal of Audiology, 14,* 169–175. Copyright 2005 by American Speech-Language-Hearing Association.

example, the microphones for the eyeglass and BTE hearing aids are near the ear, but not in the pinna. Some disadvantages of ITEs are their fragility as compared with the previously described styles and their susceptibility to moisture damage because the electronics are built into the earpiece. In addition, the close proximity of the receiver to the microphone increases the likelihood of feedback. Recently, the following market share values have been obtained for ITEs: (1) 6.5% for half-shell, (2) 13.1% for full-shell, and (3) 0.7% for other styles (Kirkwood, 2009).

The **in-the-canal (ITC)** style of hearing aid also fits into the external ear canal, leaving most, if not all, of the concha unaffected. The natural resonance of the concha amplifies sounds at 4000 to 5000 Hz, about 4 to 5 dB (Ballachandra, 1997). The ITC hearing aid is appropriate for up to moderate hearing losses. Figures 6.19, 6.20, and 6.21 show a photograph of an in-the-canal (ITC) hearing aid, a diagram of its parts, and how it looks when it is worn, respectively.

Advantages of ITC hearing aids are cosmetic appeal, the natural microphone placement in the external auditory meatus, and that many patients are able to use the phone naturally. Like the ITE hearing aid, some of the disadvantages are its fragility and susceptibility to moisture damage. The close proximity of the microphone and receiver increases the likelihood for feedback, plus the limited fitting range reduces the applicability of this style to many patients. Moreover, its small controls and batteries make it difficult to manipulate for patients with manual dexterity problems. Similarly, the

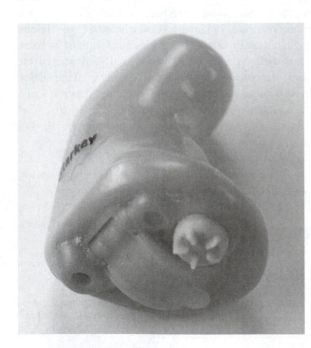

figure *6.19*

An in-the-canal hearing aid.

In-the-Canal Style

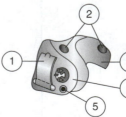

Legend

1. Battery compartment
2. Vent
3. Canal portion
4. Volume control
5. Microphone

figure *6.20*

A diagram of an in-the-canal hearing aid and its parts.

small size of the device limits the amount of circuitry that can fit inside the casing. For 2009, ITC hearing aids accounted for 8.5% of the market share of all devices sold (Kirkwood, 2009).

One of the most unobtrusive styles of hearing aid is the **completely in-the-canal (CIC)** model. The style is also known as a deep-canal fitting because the hearing aid is lodged out of sight, around the first bend of the ear canal, frequently requiring use of an extraction string for removal. Because of their location, CICs do not have external controls such as on/off switches or volume control wheels. The CIC hearing aid is appropriate for up to moderate losses in the lower frequencies and up to severe losses in the higher frequencies. The hearing aid's placement in the external auditory canal places it very close to the tympanic membrane. This interaction of the aid with the physical properties of the ear enables additional gain in the higher frequencies. Figure 6.22 shows a completely-in-the-canal (CIC) hearing aid.

One of the greatest advantages of CIC hearing aids is cosmetic appeal, often invisible to the candid observer. Other advantages include comfort, normal telephone use, and reduction of feedback, wind noise, and the occlusion effect. Because CICs are placed beyond the cartilaginous portion of the external ear, patients do not experience that "plugged up" sensation resulting from the **occlusion effect**. This phenomenon occurs when patient-generated sounds (e.g., vocalizations) vibrate the mandible, which in turn does the same thing to the cartilaginous walls of the outer ear canal, which increases the sound pressure level of low-frequency energy in an occluded ear (MacKenzie, Mueller, Ricketts, & Konkle, 2004). In a 2009 article, Kirkwood reported that CICs accounted for 7.8% of the market share for hearing aids sold.

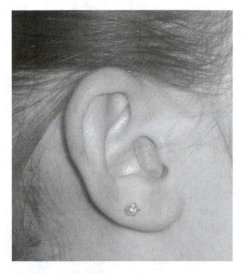

figure *6.21*

An in-the-canal hearing aid as worn.

Source: Reprinted with permission from "The 'Hearing Aid Effect' 2005: A Rigorous Test of the Visibility of New Hearing Aid Styles," by C. E. Johnson, J. L. Danhauer, R. B. Gaven, S. R. Karns, A. C. Reith, & I. P. Lopez, *American Journal of Audiology, 14,* 169–175. Copyright 2005 by American Speech-Language-Hearing Association.

Open-Ear Fittings

Open-ear fitting hearing aids are a relatively new style of a hearing instrument. Most open-ear hearing aids consist of three parts: (1) a sound processor, (2) a thin plastic tube, and (3) a soft plastic tip or dome. The sound processor fits in the small pocket behind the pinna. The thin tube and the dome come in different lengths and sizes, respectively, and are individually fit to each patient. The physical size of the speaker and dome minimizes the components that are placed into the ear canal, enabling patients with smaller ear canals to benefit from this style. The previously described hearing aid styles require either custom-made earmolds (i.e., body, eyeglass, or BTE hearing aids) or hearing aids (i.e., ITE, ITC, or CIC hearing aids) in which an ear impression is made and sent to an

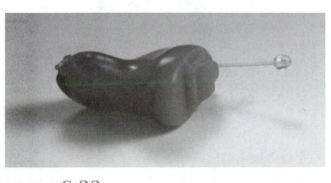

figure *6.22*

A completely-in-the-canal hearing aid.

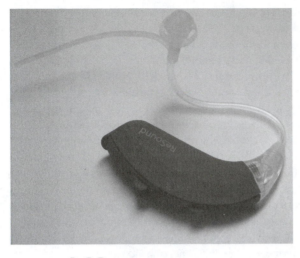

figure *6.23*

An open-ear hearing aid.

earmold or hearing aid manufacturer, respectively, adding an extra week or two to the rehabilitation process. With open-ear fittings, audiologists are able to fit patients during the initial counseling session by simply selecting the appropriate tube and dome. Open-ear fittings are appropriate for slight-to-moderate, and in some cases severe hearing losses; one is shown in Figure 6.23. The degree of noticeability varies based on viewing angle. Figure 6.24 shows the open-ear hearing aid when worn as viewed from 90-degree (left) and 135-degree (right) angles.

Other advantages of the open-ear fitting hearing aids include comfort, superior cosmetic appeal, improved sound quality, and reduction of feedback and the occlusion effect. Similar to the CIC style, the dome attached to the tubing is placed deep into the ear canal, decreasing the volume between the tip and the tympanic membrane and increasing the gain in the higher frequencies. Open-ear fittings account for over 40% of the market share in recent years and are the major reason for the surge in popularity of BTE hearing aids (Kirkwood, 2009; Mueller, 2006).

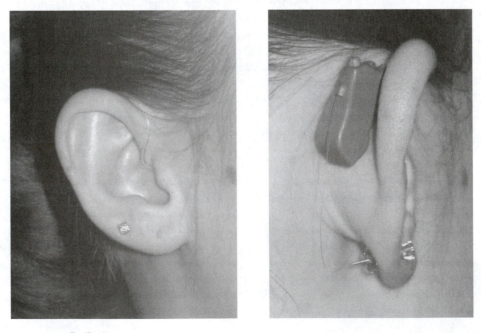

figure *6.24*

An open-ear hearing aid as worn from 90- (left) and a 135- (right) degree angles.

Source: Reprinted with permission from "The 'Hearing Aid Effect' 2005: A Rigorous Test of the Visibility of New Hearing Aid Styles," by C. E. Johnson, J. L. Danhauer, R. B. Gaven, S. R. Karns, A. C. Reith, & I. P. Lopez, *American Journal of Audiology*, 14, 169–175. Copyright 2005 by American Speech-Language-Hearing Association.

CLASSIFICATION OF HEARING AIDS

In the next section, we discuss how hearing aids may be classified based on their type of circuitry and applicability for specific patient needs.

Analog, Digitally Programmable, and Completely Digital Hearing Aids

Analog hearing aids are based on a technology in which sound pressure is turned into an analogous waveform represented by variations in electrical voltage for processing (Dillon, 2001). Since the invention of the telephone, use of analog technology has been pervasive in everyday life. However, within the past 10 to 15 years, analog technology has been replaced by digital technology. Audiocassettes, videotapes, and analog cell phones have been replaced by compact discs, digital video discs, and digital cell phones, respectively. Today, digital hearing aids have all but replaced analog hearing aids. Currently, hearing aids can be classified as analog, digitally programmable analog, or digital.

The basic functioning of analog hearing aids can be described using a **block diagram** that shows how energy flows through the components of an electronic device. Figure 6.25 shows a block diagram of an analog hearing aid. The **microphone** is an input transducer that changes sound pressure into variations in electrical voltage. A **transducer** is anything that changes one form of energy to another and is classified by the transformation that takes place. A microphone is an acoustic-electric transducer. We will discuss microphones in more detail a bit later. The electric voltage is amplified and then turned back into sound pressure by the **receiver**. The receiver is an electric-to-acoustic output transducer. The net result of the entire process is an increase in the sound pressure level of the signal going into the patient's ear. In the past, analog hearing aids were adjusted using a screwdriver on small gauges called potentiometers, or trimpots, that adjusted various aspects of hearing aid function. These potentiometers were labeled to relate to each different electroacoustic parameter under control (e.g., OSPL90, or output saturation sound pressure level 90), a pneumonic device for what was being changed (e.g., "H" for high frequency), or for the audiometric configuration of the patient (Dillon, 2001).

Digitally programmable analog or **hybrid hearing aids** transform sound pressure into electrical voltage for processing by digitally controlled circuits manipulated externally by the audiologist using a computer or by the user via a remote control (Dillon, 2001). The advantages of digitally programmable hearing aids are greater flexibility in adjustment of electroacoustic parameters; the option of using a remote control (e.g., instead of a volume control wheel), fewer mechanical parts (decreasing the likelihood of malfunction), ease in setting for electroacoustic parameters for quicker fits, opportunities for paired-comparison listening by patients for fine-tuning, and decreased manufacturing costs. Figure 6.26 shows a block diagram of a digitally programmable analog hearing aid in which the controller circuit adjusts the signal via a programmer unit.

Digital hearing aids change sound pressure to electrical voltages that are converted to a binary number by the analog-to-digital (A/D) converter, which in turn is processed by a computer chip, then sent to the digital-to-analog (D/A) converter that changes the

figure *6.25*

A block diagram of a hearing aid.

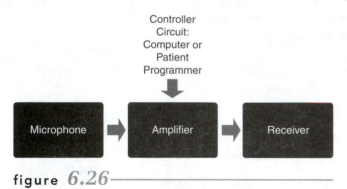

Controller
Circuit:
Computer or
Patient
Programmer

Microphone → Amplifier → Receiver

figure *6.26*

A diagram of a digitally programmable analog hearing aid.

binary number code back into electrical voltage that is changed and delivered by the receiver to the patient's ear as shown in Figure 6.27.

Some of the advantages of digital hearing aids include better sound quality, feedback reduction, noise reduction, and speech enhancement through complex signal processing.

Hearing Aids for Specific Patient Needs

The majority of sensorineural hearing losses are bilateral and fairly symmetrical, or the same, in both ears. Most degrees and configuration of hearing loss may be amplified using the circuitry in today's digital hearing aids. However, some patients may have unique needs that require hearing aids with features such as special circuitry, variable routing of the signal, or differential transformation of energy. Additionally, some patients may need hearing aids that are surgically implantable. For example, some patients with relatively good hearing in the low frequencies but severe impairment in the higher frequency regions may benefit from special circuitry. Other patients who have normal or "near" normal hearing sensitivity in one ear with the other being unaidable may benefit from a hearing aid arrangement that picks up sound on the nonfunctional side and sends it to the good one. Ears may be unaidable for a variety of reasons, including a lack of adequate sensitivity, limited prior stimulation, or congenital malformation. It is important to note that just because two patients have very similar audiograms, they will not necessarily select the same type of hearing aids. Other factors, including prior history of amplification, communication needs, and personal preferences weigh into the amplification decisions patients make along with their audiologists. The following section focuses on some hearing aid options for patients with specific needs.

Hearing Aids for Patients With Severe High-Frequency Hearing Loss

Proportional frequency compression hearing aids are an option for patients who have hearing losses greater than 60 dB HL in the higher frequencies. The circuitry actually moves critical "high-frequency" speech information into the lower frequency regions where patients have better hearing sensitivity (Davis, 2001). The reason these patients can benefit from this type of processing is that when traditional circuitry amplifies sound in the higher frequencies, it can cause distortion, having a detrimental effect on speech recognition for some users (Ching, Dillon, & Byrne, 1998; Davis, 2001; Hogan & Turner, 1998). Turner and Hurtig (1999) examined proportional frequency compression as a strategy for enhancing the speech recognition of patients with high-frequency hearing loss. They found

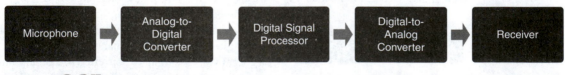

Microphone → Analog-to-Digital Converter → Digital Signal Processor → Digital-to-Analog Converter → Receiver

figure *6.27*

A block diagram of a digital hearing aid.

that although high-frequency amplification is still the most effective strategy for these patients, proportional frequency compression should be considered for some individuals.

Hearing Aids for Unilateral or Asymmetrical Sensorineural Hearing Losses With an Unaidable Ear

CROS, BICROS, and transcranial CROS hearing aids are for patients who have one ear that is normal or a hearing loss that is aidable and another ear that is unaidable or nonfunctional. Basically, these options are for patients that have one ear that does not work. The acronym CROS stands for **contralateral routing of the signal**; the hearing aid arrangement is shown in Figure 6.28.

Patients with unilateral hearing losses, normal or "near normal" in one ear and a nonfunctional or unaidable ear in the other, are candidates for a CROS fitting. In these situations, amplifying the poorer ear is rarely done due to the large disparity in functionality between the two ears, particularly if the poorer ear has never been fit with a hearing aid. In these cases, **auditory deprivation** may occur which is when auditory pathways lose functionality due to a lack of stimulation. Placing a hearing aid on an ear with auditory deprivation may cause interference with the better ear. Recall that patients with unilateral hearing losses do not receive the benefits

Unaidable Ear
Directional
microphone
and FM
transmitter

1. Acoustic energy is picked up by a directional microphone and turned into electrical energy

2. The FM transmitter changes the electrical energy into radio waves

3. FM signal sent to receiver

Normal or
Near-Normal
Ear
"Open"
earmold, mild
amplifier, and
FM receiver

5. Receiver changes electric energy into acoustic energy for delivery to patient's ear via an earmold

4. The FM signal is picked up by the receiver that changes it into electrical energy that is slightly amplified

figure *6.28*

A diagram of how a contralateral routing of the signal (CROS) hearing aid arrangement works.

of binaural hearing, or hearing with two ears. The inability to **localize**, the "**head shadow effect**," and difficulty understanding speech in noisy situations are just some of the frustrations experienced by patients with unilateral hearing losses. Localization is the ability to tell from what direction sound is coming and is based on both the time of arrival and intensity differences in the two ears. The two ears work together for sound localization. Generally, sound is perceived to come from the side of the head that it arrives at first and is perceived to be the loudest. Therefore, patients with unilateral losses have variable localization skills. The head shadow effect occurs when high-frequency sound is presented at the deaf ear and bounces off the head which creates an acoustic shadow and attenuates energy arriving at the opposite ear. The size of the head relative to the wavelength of the sound determines which sounds are diffracted or can bend around and be heard by the other ear. Sounds whose wavelengths are larger than the diameter of the head will be diffracted. Alternatively, those sounds with smaller wavelengths are the ones that cannot bend around and be heard by the better ear. The head shadow creates as much as a 15 dB reduction of sounds with frequencies greater than about 1500 Hz. The head shadow effect can be problematic for patients with significant unilateral losses when someone talks at the poorer ear. Many important high-frequency cues for adequate speech recognition performance are inaudible to these patients when soft speech is presented to the poor ear. Additionally, patients with unilateral losses experience difficulty in noisy situations, particularly when the noise source is present at the better side and someone is speaking to them at their poorer ear. Generally, patients do not experience significant improvement in localization abilities when using CROS hearing aids, but do demonstrate some improvement in speech recognition in noise (Baguley, Bird, Humphriss, & Prevost, 2006).

The CROS hearing aid arrangement is available in BTE or ITE styles. Generally, these models consist of a microphone pick-up on the poorer side that sends the signal to the receiver on the good ear by either hardwire or FM radio waves as described in Figure 6.28. For FM transmission, the microphone on the poorer ear contains an FM transmitter that broadcasts the signal to the receiver on the better ear. The signal is then delivered to the better ear. The hearing aid on the better ear does not contain a microphone because sound on that side goes directly in and is heard by the good ear. Therefore, the earmold on the good ear should be a non-occluding or open mold.

Table 6.1 shows models, arrangements, and characteristics of CROS hearing aids as they have developed over time. Initially, the transmitter and receiver of CROS hearing aids were connected by means of a wire. Later models included the use of wireless, programmable, and digital technologies.

CROS fittings have received variable reports of benefit from patients. Valente et al., (1995) stated that the original CROS hearing aids provided minimal amounts of amplification between 800 and 1500 Hz and significant gain above 1500 Hz in the better ear. Early studies found that the CROS fitting was more successful for patients who had some degree of loss above 1500 Hz in the better ear (e.g., Courtois, Johansen, Larsen, & Beilin, 1988; Punch, 1988; Valente et al., 1995) than for patients who had hearing within normal limits in the better ear.

Another option for patients with normal hearing in the better ear is the **transcranial CROS**, which involves fitting a high-gain output ITE or BTE to the unaidable ear such that sound from that side is amplified and then transferred to the cochlea of the better or normal ear via bone conduction through the cranium (Valente, Potts, et al., 1995). Some advantages reported by users of the transcranial CROS include (1) more "natural" sound than the traditional CROS, (2) improved localization, and (3) improved listening in noise when the source of the noise is on the poor side (e.g., McSpaden, 1990). Therefore, the transcranial CROS may be an option for patients who are

table *6.1* Models, Arrangements, and Characteristics of CROS Hearing Aids

Models of CROS	Arrangement	Characteristics
Wired Analog	• Microphone placed over unaidable ear to pick up sound from that side • The output of the microphone is wired to an amplifier with a volume control wheel via a headband	• An earmold in the better ear channels the sound into the better ear • No amplification below 800 Hz, marginal gain from 800 to 1500 Hz, and slight to mild gain above 1500 Hz

Wired Programmable with Directional Microphone	• Microphone placed over unaidable ear to pick up sound from that side
	• The output of the microphone is wired to an amplifier
	• Remote control designates:
	  • Omni- versus directional microphone
	  • Telecoil
	  • Volume control wheel
		• An earmold in the better ear channels the sound into the better ear

Wireless Analog	• Wireless behind-the-ear hearing aid to in-the-ear or behind-the-ear	• Uses amplitude-modulated carrier frequency • Distance between transmitter and receiver is about 6 1/2 inches • For each inch increase in distance, gain decreases by 3 to 4 dB • No amplification below 800 Hz, marginal gain from 800 to 1500 Hz, and slight to mild gain above 1500 Hz
Wireless Digital	• Wireless behind-the-ear hearing aid to in-the-ear or behind-the-ear • Wireless in-the-ear to in-the-ear	• Contains multichannel digital signal processing • Can shape amount of gain for those users with pure-tone thresholds of 20 dB HL in the better ear

Source: Information from *Fitting Options for Patients with Single Sided Deafness*, by M. Valente, M. Valente, and K. Mispagel, 2006, retrieved from www.audiologyonline.com/articles/article_detail.asp?article_id=1629.

not satisfied with traditional CROS arrangements. However, audiologists should follow suggested fitting and verification procedures (Valente et al., 1995). Furthermore, Valente, Valente, & Mispagel, (2006) believe that this hearing aid arrangement is truly **quasi-transcranial** rather than transcranial because the mode of signal transmission to the better ear is actually via bone conduction and air conduction.

The acronym **BICROS** stands for **bilateral contralateral routing of the signal** and is shown in Figure 6.29. The BICROS hearing aid arrangement is for patients who have asymmetrical losses with the better ear having a significant but aidable loss and the poorer one being nonfunctional. Patients with this type of loss experience the same disadvantages as those with unilateral hearing losses. The BICROS arrangement is similar to the CROS, and

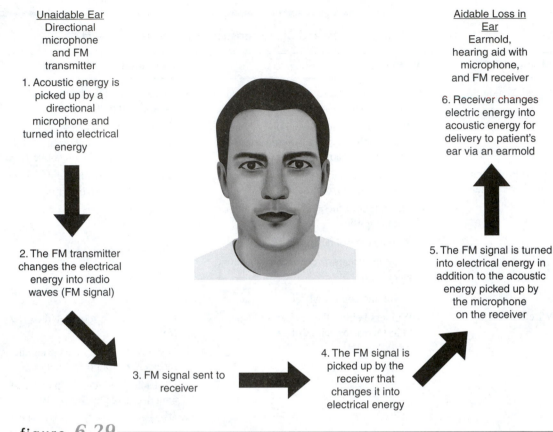

Unaidable Ear
Directional microphone and FM transmitter

1. Acoustic energy is picked up by a directional microphone and turned into electrical energy

2. The FM transmitter changes the electrical energy into radio waves (FM signal)

3. FM signal sent to receiver

4. The FM signal is picked up by the receiver that changes it into electrical energy

5. The FM signal is turned into electrical energy in addition to the acoustic energy picked up by the microphone on the receiver

6. Receiver changes electric energy into acoustic energy for delivery to patient's ear via an earmold

Aidable Loss in Ear
Earmold, hearing aid with microphone, and FM receiver

figure *6.29*

A diagram of how the bilateral contralateral routing of the signal (BICROS) hearing aid arrangement works.

in fact, the components on the poorer ear are exactly the same, consisting of a microphone pick-up and FM transmitter. However, the device aid on the better side is not only an FM receiver, but also a hearing aid with a microphone to amplify sounds for the better ear that also has a significant hearing loss. Therefore, the appropriate earmold is whatever is suitable for the degree of loss.

Hearing Aids for Patients Who Cannot Use Air-Conduction Hearing Aids: Bone-Conduction Hearing Aids and Bone-Anchored Hearing Aids

Most patients with hearing loss can benefit from traditional **air-conduction hearing aids** (ACHAs) that have output transducers that convert the amplified signal from electric to acoustic energy that goes through the outer, middle, and then inner ears. However, patients with some auditory disorders (e.g., chronic otitis media with continuously draining ears, congenital atresia, congenital or acquired middle ear malformations, otosclerosis, sequelae of skull-base surgery, ossicular-chain discontinuity or fixation, or unilateral deafness) may not benefit maximally from ACHAs. Moreover, in some patients the use of ACHAs exacerbates their chronic external otitis or outer ear infection. In patients with **congenital aural atresia** combined with **microtia** or **anotia**, the fitting of ACHAs may be impractical or of little or no benefit if the atresia is complete. Congenital aural atresia is the absence or failure of the development of the external auditory canal apparent at birth. Microtia is deformity of the pinna, which is usually smaller than normal. Anotia is absence of a pinna. Some patients with otosclerosis may want to avoid surgery (e.g., stapedotomy) to improve their hearing sensitivity. **Otosclerosis** is a disease in which a bony growth forms on the stapes footplate. The stapes is the smallest and most medial bone of the ossicular chain, and its footplate is attached to the oval window by means of the annular ligament. For some of these patients, conventional **bone-conduction hearing aids** (BCHAs) may help. Conventional BCHAs utilize a vibrator that is pressed firmly against the skin of the skull via a steel spring coupled to a band that may cause discomfort, pressure sores, and headaches (Bance, Abel, Papsin, Wade, & Vendramini, 2002).

Bone-anchored hearing aids (BAHAs) may provide benefits for these individuals who cannot tolerate wearing the band and transducer of the BCHA. The Food and Drug Administration (FDA) approved the BAHA in 2002. It was first developed by Entific Medical Systems and is now offered through Cochlear Corporation. Patient selection criteria vary according to the type of loss: patients with conductive hearing losses should have more than an average air-bone gap of 30 dB at 500, 1000, and 2000 Hz. Generally, the greater the air-bone gap, the greater should be the amount of benefit in comparison to traditional hearing aids.

Patients with mixed hearing losses should benefit if they also have average air-bone gaps of 30 dB at 500, 1000, and 2000 Hz in addition to mild-to-moderate sensorineural hearing losses. BAHAs may be of benefit for patients having **single-sided deafness**, or a normal ear on one side and a deaf or nonfunctional ear on the other. These patients should have average audiometric thresholds of less than or equal to 20 dB HL at 500, 1000, 2000, and 3000 Hz in the better ear.

The BAHA System is an osseointegrated bone-conduction implant shown in Figures 6.30 and 6.31 that combines a sound processor with a small titanium fixture implanted behind the ear that allows energy conduction through the bone rather than via the middle ear—a process known as direct bone conduction.

The BAHA surgery is minor, during which a small titanium implant is placed in the skull, more specifically, in the mastoid area behind the ear where it adheres to surrounding tissue through a process called **osseointegration** (Cochlear, 2009). It takes about three months for the implant to osseointegrate with the mastoid bone before the BAHA device can be snapped into the abutment (Valente, Valente, & Mispagel, 2006). For patients with chronically draining ears, the BAHA allows infection (itching, pain, and unpleasant discharge) to heal. In the United States, the BAHA is approved for patients who are at least 5 years old. Younger children may still benefit from the BAHA via use of a soft band that goes around the head, securing the device in place at the appropriate location. Several studies have demonstrated that the BAHA is safe and reliable, and provides better audiometric outcomes than BCHAs and, to a lesser extent, ACHAs (Browning & Gatehouse, 1994; Håkansson, Carlsson, Tjellström, & Lidén, 1994). Some studies found patients reported positive impressions about their

1. Sound processor

2. Titanium skin penetrating abutment

3. Titanium fixture/implant

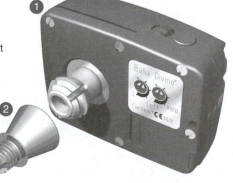

figure *6.30*

A bone-anchored hearing aid (BAHA).

Source: Picture provided courtesy of Cochlear™ Americas, © 2005 Cochlear Americas. Reprinted with permission.

1. Sound processor

2. Titanium skin penetrating abutment

3. Titanium fixture/implant

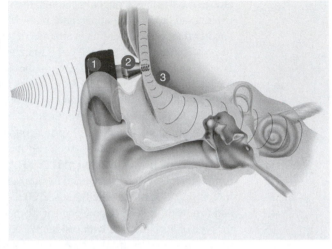

figure *6.31*

The bone-anchored hearing aid as implanted in the head.

Source: Picture provided courtesy of Cochlear™ Americas, © 2005 Cochlear Americas. Reprinted with permission.

listening performances with BAHAs in different situations (Mylanus, Snik, & Cremers, 1995). BAHA hearing aids have been shown to improve the HRQoL benefits of patients who did not achieve acceptable outcomes from ACHAs or BCHAs (Hol et al., 2004). A recent systematic review with meta-analysis found patients with acquired single-sided deafness did not have improved localization abilities with either CROS hearing aids or BAHAs, but did show improvement in speech recognition in noise with the BAHA providing more favorable results than the CROS hearing aids (Baguley et al., 2006). As previously stated, BAHAs are currently manufactured by Cochlear Corporation, which has made several developments in circuitry resulting in a programmable sound processor designed specifically for bone conduction.

Middle-Ear Implantable Hearing Aids

Middle-ear implantable hearing aids are for patients with mild-to-severe sensorineural hearing losses who cannot wear or who are dissatisfied with traditional hearing instruments. These devices have all or most of their parts implanted into the middle ear and are of two basic types: (1) **piezoelectric** and (2) **electromagnetic devices**. Piezoelectric devices send electrical current through components containing piezoelectric crystals that result in vibration (Shohet, 2010). Basically, Shohet (2010) described the following four steps required for the Envoy Esteem piezoelectric implantable middle ear device to work:

- The tympanic membrane actually works as a microphone or transducer for the system that vibrates in response to sound energy.
- A sensor containing a piezoelectric crystal on the incus transduces the vibrations into electrical current that is sent to the sound processor implanted in the mastoid bone.
- The sound processor amplifies, filters, and sends the current to the driver on the stapes in the form of vibration with increased amplitude.
- The increased vibration of the stapes delivers amplified energy to the inner ear via the oval window.

Several piezoelectric devices are available. Chen et al. (2004) conducted a small clinical trial to investigate the safety and patient outcomes of a piezoelectric implantable middle ear device. The results showed that five of seven patients with functioning devices experienced improved performance in speech recognition over traditional hearing aids, but obtained similar results in functional gain and speech reception thresholds. **Functional gain** is the difference in unaided and aided thresholds for warbled tones presented through loudspeakers in an audiometric test booth.

The Vibrant Soundbridge, an electromagnetic device, is only partially implanted, necessitating an externally worn component that looks like a BTE aid and contains an electromagnetic coil (Shohet, 2010). The surgically implanted device is a receiver called a vibrating ossicular prostheses (VORP) containing a floating mass transducer consisting of a coil on the long process of the incus that surrounds a magnet that drives the stapes (Shohet, 2010). Briefly, the microphone on the externally worn processor changes acoustic energy into electric energy which, in turn, is changed into electromagnetic energy that is sent out through a coil across the skin. The signal in the form of electromagnetic energy is received by the VORP, which sets the stapes footplate into vibration.

Patients have reported positive outcomes for the device. A retrospective study of the first 125 patients who received the device from 1997 to 2001 in France found that the large majority were "satisfied" or "very satisfied" with their devices, but their ratings did not correlate with objective performance measures of how well they did with them (Sterkers et al., 2003). Moreover, another retrospective chart review of 20 patients who had their implants for at least two years concluded that the limited benefits of implants as compared with risks for surgery should preclude their use with patients except for those who cannot use traditional amplification (e.g., chronic external otitis) (Schmuziger, Schimmann, àWengen, Patscheke, & Probst, 2006).

Now that we have provided a general introduction to hearing aids, we will describe the tools and equipment needed for audiologists to select, evaluate, and fit them.

THE AUDIOLOGIST'S TOOLS

Audiologists have a variety of tools and equipment that assist in the selection, evaluation, and fitting of hearing aids. Some of these tools are used in the diagnostic evaluation that provides the data for determining patients' needs for auditory rehabilitation. For example, the audiometer, test booth, various transducers (e.g., circumaural and insert earphones, loudspeakers, bone oscillators), and sources of input (e.g., microphone and CD player) are used in assessing patients' degree of hearing impairment and ultimately their candidacy for hearing aids and hearing assistive technology (HAT). In addition, audiologists frequently use commercially available assessment tools such as the Hearing in Noise Test (HINT) (Nilsson, Soli, & Sullivan, 1994) to quantify differences in speech recognition performance in noise from the unaided to the aided condition.

Other tools are specifically for the evaluation and fitting of hearing aids such as hearing aid analyzers and real-ear probe-microphone measurement systems, often found within the same unit. A **hearing aid analyzer** is a device that is used to determine if a hearing aid is functioning according to the manufacturer's specifications. A picture of a hearing aid analyzer and output of the results of an electroacoustic analysis is shown in Figure 6.32.

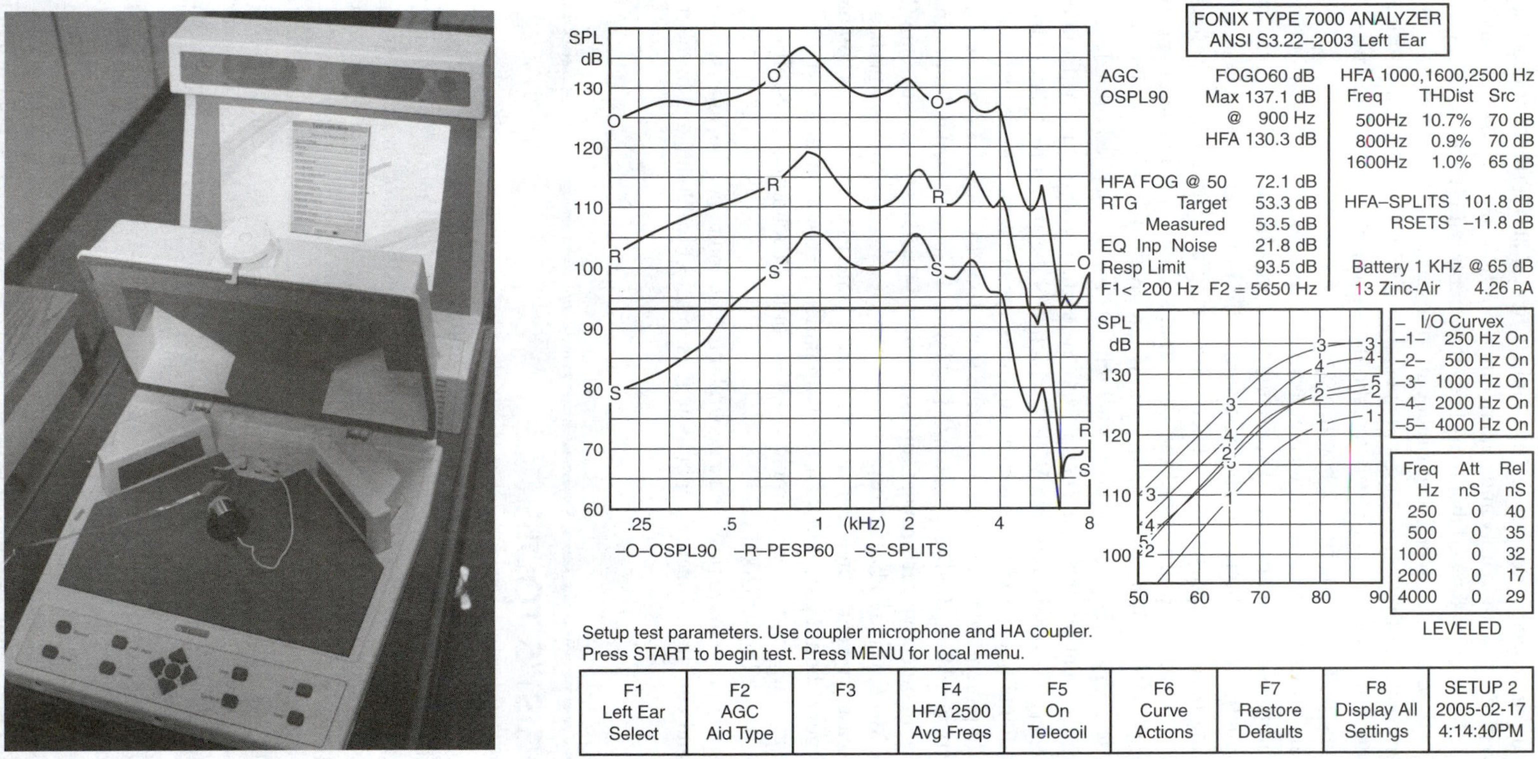

figure 6.32

A hearing aid analyzer and output of the results of the electroacoustic analysis.

Sources: Electroacoustic analysis from *FONIX: ANSI '03 Workbook*, 2005, Frye Electronics, Tigard, OR. Used with permission.

In short, the hearing aid is attached to a **2-cc coupler**, which is a hollow, hard-walled chamber that simulates a human ear for the purposes of standardized assessments of hearing instrument functioning. The hearing aid analyzer sends sound stimuli of known acoustic properties into the hearing instrument via the microphone and then analyzes its output from the receiver. The output is presented on the screen and printed out for comparison to the manufacturer's specification on specific parameters which is covered a little later.

The **real-ear probe-tube microphone measurement system** measures what the hearing aid is doing *inside* the patient's ear. Why is that important? Why does an audiologist need these measurements in addition to the information provided by the hearing aid analyzer? The 2-cc coupler used by the hearing aid analyzer does not represent the human ear, which is unique to each patient in terms of its size and shape. Therefore, the output of a hearing aid measured in a patient's ear differs from that when it is coupled to a 2-cc coupler. The volume of the 2-cc coupler is typically greater than that of the human ear canal, particularly when the ear has a hearing aid or earmold attached to it. The output of a hearing aid measured in a 2-cc coupler may underestimate the actual sound pressure level in the ear canal, especially if the patient is a child. Children's ear canals are even smaller in volume than those of adults. The sound pressure level of a sound increases when measured in a smaller cavity (e.g., ear canal) than when in a larger one (2-cc coupler). Therefore, the gain and output of a hearing aid should be verified via real-ear probe-tube microphone measurement to ensure it is appropriate for the patient. Table 6.2 contains some measures obtained during real-ear probe-tube microphone measurement, as shown in Figure 6.33.

Another tool of an audiologist is networking of computers that integrate patient files, manufacturers' software programs, and equipment. In addition, the computer network may include connections between and among several computers in a clinical office. The Hearing Instrument Manufacturers' Software Association (HIMSA, www.himsa.com) has developed

table *6.2*   Common Measures for Real-Ear Probe-Tube Microphone Measurements (Expressed in SPL or gain as a function of frequency with measurements made with the probe-tube microphone at a specified distance from the tympanic membrane for a calibrated sound field)

Parameter	Measurement Condition or Method of Calculation	Purpose
Real-ear unaided response (REUR)	Unoccluded ear	To determine resonance of external ear
Real-ear occluded response (REOR)	Hearing aid in place and shut-off	To measure the response with the hearing aid off and in place
Real-ear aided response (REAR)	Hearing aid in place and turned on	To measure the response with the hearing aid on
Real-ear insertion response (REIR)	Difference between REAR-REUR	To see the net SPL or gain provided by the hearing aid Real-ear insertion gain at each frequency can be obtained
Real-ear saturation response (RESR)	Hearing aid in place and turned on with a loud input sound	To measures the response with the hearing aid at maximum output

Source: Information from *Probe Microphone Measurements: Hearing Aid Selection and Measurement*, by H. G. Mueller, D. B. Hawkins, and J. L. Northern, 1992, San Diego, CA: Singular.

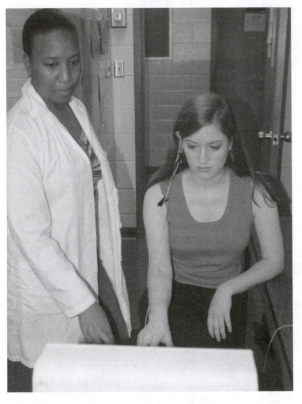

figure *6.33*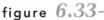

A patient undergoing real-ear probe-tube microphone measurement.

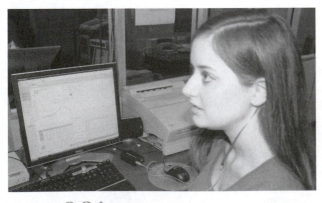

figure *6.34*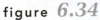

A patient whose hearing aid is hooked up to the NOAH software.

the NOAH software, which provides a unified system for performing patient-related tasks. The NOAH software system has an "integration framework" with the participation of over 90 hearing care companies permitting audiologic measurement (e.g., audiometry, real-ear probe-tube microphone measurement, immittance, electrophysiology, otoacoustic emissions, and video-otoscopy), hearing aid fitting (e.g., NOAHFit and/or HIMSA member modules), and office automation (e.g., demographics, scheduling, accounting, and/or marketing) (HIMSA, 2009). For example, an audiologist can create a patient record; perform an audiologic evaluation; use important data for hearing aid selection, fitting, and evaluation; and then append critical information into the database. Figure 6.34 shows a patient whose hearing aid is hooked up to the NOAH software system during a hearing aid fitting appointment.

Finally, audiologists also have tools for making ear impressions and modifying earmolds and/or hearing aids. As mentioned earlier, earmolds and in-the-ear styles of hearing aids require the making of ear impressions of patients' ears. This procedure must be done carefully to ensure safety of the patient and an accurate impression of the ear(s). The first step is to carefully view the patient's outer ear using an **otoscope**, which is an illuminated, magnifying scope. Otoscopes vary in price and sophistication, but ideally audiologists should have both handheld models and **video otoscopes**. (Handheld otoscopes are handy to have in each audiologic examination and consult room.) Video otoscopes are equipped with an illuminating light and camera contained within a probe placed at the outer opening of the ear canal. Patients' outer ear canals and tympanic membranes are visible on a video screen. Photographs of the results can be taken and archived in patients' folders. Video otoscopes are particularly useful in becoming familiar with the topography of patients' ear canals necessary for insertion of an otoblock—a small sponge—that serves as a barrier between the impression material and the tympanic membrane. The audiologist prepares the material (e.g., silicone) and carefully inserts the material via a syringe or gun into patients' ears. It takes several minutes for the material to harden prior

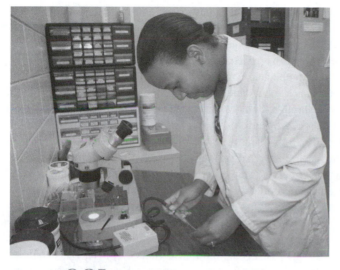

figure *6.35*

An audiologist at work in her hearing aid laboratory.

to the removal of the ear impression and re-inspection of the ear canal to verify that no debris is remaining. Ear canal impressions are sent either to hearing aid manufacturers to serve as the molds for in-the-ear hearing aids or to a company that produces earmolds.

Audiologists also usually have a small room or workbench that serves as a hearing aid laboratory for modifying and/or making minor repairs on earmolds and/or hearing instruments. Typically, the work area has a magnifying lamp; a drill; a sander; a stocked cabinet of different parts for earmolds (e.g., tubing, vents, dampers) and hearing aids (e.g., wax guards, battery doors); and supplies (e.g., earmold impression material, otoblocks, batteries). Patients often present to walk-in clinics with problems with their hearing aids, many of which can be fixed without having to be sent back to the manufacturer. For example, earmold tubing can be replaced, cerumen (i.e., earwax) can be removed from the receiver of an ITE hearing aid, and battery doors can be replaced on most styles of hearing aids. Sometimes, hearing aids need to be sanded and buffed on those areas causing sores in patients' ears. Figure 6.35 shows an audiologist's hearing aid laboratory.

HEARING AID ELECTROACOUSTICS

Hearing aids have not only increased in sophistication in style, but in circuitry as well. In fact, some of the changes in hearing aid style were due to technological advances in the power supplies and electrical components of hearing instruments. This section is about **electroacoustics**, which is the process of how acoustic energy enters a hearing aid, is changed to electrical energy, is processed, and then changed back to acoustic energy for delivery to patients' ears. We will discuss electroacoustics in very simple terms to provide the necessary conceptual framework for the understanding of the technical aspects of hearing aids.

First, all hearing aids, regardless of their sophistication, have the same basic parts. Note how the analog, digitally programmable analog, and digital hearing aids described previously all had microphones, amplifiers, and receivers. The primary purpose of hearing aids is to amplify sound for people who have hearing loss, and more specifically to make soft speech audible. The amount of amplification is determined by the gain, or the number of decibels that is added to the signal by the hearing aid. For example, if a 65 dB SPL signal goes into the microphone (i.e., input) and 95 dB SPL comes out of the hearing aid (i.e., output), then the amount of gain provided is 30 dB. Gain can also be defined by a simple equation of gain = output − input.

As mentioned in the previous section, audiologists use hearing aid analyzers for **electroacoustic analyses**, which determine if hearing instruments are functioning according to manufacturer's specifications. The process is based on the premise that if a known acoustic stimulus of a certain frequency and sound pressure level enters the microphone and the output from the receiver is measured, the hearing aid analyzer can assess the functioning of the device. The American National Standards Institute (ANSI), in standard S3.22.2003, has specified the parameters to be included in an electroacoustic analysis and their **tolerance values**, or how accurately a hearing aid must perform on each measure to be considered to be in line with the manufacturer's specifications. (An updated ANSI standard, ANSI S 3.22 (2009), has been published and has been recognized as a valid standard by the Food and Drug Administration (FDA), but the FDA has not gone through the necessary legal proceedings to make it the labeling standard for the United States.) Appendix 6.1 has a listing and description of some of these electroacoustic parameters. The S3.22 hearing aid standard has defined the performance for hearing aids since 1977 and has been revised periodically to keep up with the changes in technology (Frye, 2005). With today's hearing aids, audiologists may require information from the manufacturer to set hearing aids appropriately for testing. For example, sometimes different programs are used by manufacturers to assess different parameters. ANSI 3.22.2003 guidelines also provide guidance as to how electroacoustic analyses are to be performed.

The first step in an electroacoustic analysis is determining if the hearing aid analyzer and environment meet specifications (ANSI S3.22.2003, Sections 4.1, 5.1). For example, the hearing aid analyzer's manual will specify if the equipment has appropriate sound sources, frequency accuracy, coupler types, and so on. Moreover, the test environment must have an appropriate ambient temperature, humidity, and atmospheric pressure, which are generally satisfied except under extreme conditions.

Another important consideration is the type of hearing aid being tested. We have discussed different styles and circuits within hearing aids, but they can differ in other ways, too, which may determine how to perform an electroacoustic analysis. ANSI S3.22.2003 recognizes four types of hearing aids:

- **Linear hearing aids** have a direct and predictable output as a function of input level of the signal and gain of the device. For example, Figure 6.36 shows that the input level in dB SPL on the horizontal axis, the output level in dB SPL on the vertical axis. If we use the equation gain = output − input, we can determine that the gain of the hearing aid is 40 dB (e.g., at 1000 Hz: output of 100 dB SPL − input of 60 = 40 dB of gain). As the input increases, so does the output in a predictable fashion, creating a straight line on the graph that could theoretically go on forever. Eventually, however, the hearing aid will reach its saturation point, creating distortion and limiting output via a process called **peak clipping**. When linear hearing aids reach their maximum output limit, successive increases in input do not result in complementary increases in the output of the signal whose amplitude is trimmed.

- **Automatic gain control (AGC) hearing aids** automatically control the gain based on the level of the signal being amplified (ANSI S3.22.2003, Section 3.16; Frye, 2005). AGC hearing aids are for patients who have recruitment or an abnormal growth in the sensation of loudness. These hearing aids seek to minimize the range of output levels compared with

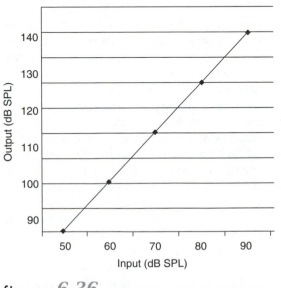

figure *6.36*

An input-output function of a hearing aid.

the range of levels found in the input signal (Frye, 2005). In other words, circuits in these hearing aids compress the wide range of input levels found in everyday sounds that go into the hearing aid into a smaller range in the output signal that ultimately goes into patients' ears. Therefore, these types of hearing aids are called **compression hearing aids**. There are several types of compression, but two common types are **input** and **output compression**. Input compression, or dynamic range compression, reduces the gain of the hearing aid based on the input level in order to match the range of sound pressure levels that are both audible yet comfortable for patients (Frye, 2005). Alternatively, output compression, or output-limiting, compresses or reduces gain in order to limit the maximum output so that it is not uncomfortable to patients (Frye, 2005).

- **Directional hearing aids** have microphones that change their output as a function of the direction from which sound waves arrive at the input of a hearing aid (Frye, 2005).
- **Special purpose hearing aids** amplify at pitch regions outside of that which would be considered conventional, also known as low-frequency– or high-frequency– emphasis hearing aids.

Other preparations prior to performing an electroacoustic analysis are setting the instrument controls and selecting the appropriate coupler. Table 6.3 shows common hearing aid parameters to be tested, their input stimuli, what is analyzed, and tolerance values. For example, the first parameters assessed in an electroacoustic analysis are the **output saturation sound pressure level-90 (OSPL90) curve**, **high-frequency average OSPL90**, and the **maximum OSPL90**. The ANSI standards state that for these parameters, the input to the hearing aid, generated by the hearing aid analyzer, is a pure tone that sweeps from at least 200 to 5000 Hz at a sound pressure level (SPL) of 90 dB. The hearing aid is set such that it produces its maximum output both internally and externally. For example, audiologists have ways of adjusting the hearing aid for different output levels and these methods differ based on whether the device is analog or digital. Recall that analog hearing aids have **potentiometers** that are manipulated by screwdrivers, and typically have volume control wheels (VCWs). Digital and digitally programmable hearing aids are most often adjusted via computer with a click of the mouse. The hearing aid analyzer graphs the OSPL90 curve in sound pressure level as a function of frequency. According to ANSI S3.22 (2003), the maximum OSPL90 is the highest point on the OSPL90 curve and must be no higher than 3 dB of the manufacturer's specifications. High-frequency average OSPL90 is also obtained from the same graph; it is the average output taken at 1000, 1600, and 2500 Hz and must be within ± 4 dB of the manufacturer's specifications.

Other important parameters include the **full-on gain curve**, **high-frequency full-on average gain,** and **reference test gain**. The input to the hearing aid for measurement of these parameters is either a 50 or 60 dB SPL tone that sweeps from at least 200 to 5000 Hz. For full-on gain, the input level is 50 or 60 dB SPL. The hearing aid is set for maximum output, set to full-on. The hearing aid analyzer graphs the full-on gain curve as the *gain* of the hearing aid as a function of frequency. The decibel values on the vertical axis are much smaller on the gain graph than on the OSPL90 graph because the input is subtracted from output (i.e., gain = output − input) to obtain this measure across the frequency range. High frequency full-on average gain is the average gain taken at 1000, 1600, and 2500 Hz and must be within 5 dB of manufacturer's specifications.

A similar parameter for AGC hearing aids is the **reference test gain**, which is a measurement with the gain or volume control set at a specific level or at which a 60 dB SPL input yields an output that is 17 dB below the HFA OSPL90. The reason this is done is to try to simulate a gain level used by most hearing aid wearers for everyday purposes

table *6.3*   Input Stimuli, Output, and Tolerance Values for Output and Gain Parameters in Electroacoustic Analyses of Hearing Aids

Hearing Aid Parameter	Hearing Aid Setting	Input Stimuli	Output	Tolerance (Re: Manufacturer's Specifications)
Saturation Sound Pressure Level 90 (OSPL90) Measures	Set for the highest output and the broadest frequency response	A 90 dB SPL pure-tone that sweeps the frequencies from at least 200 to 5000 Hz		
OSPL90 Curve			Output of the hearing aid as a function of frequency	
High-Frequency Average OSPL90			Average output taken at 1000, 1600, and 2500 Hz on the OSPL90 curve	Within ± 4 dB
Maximum OSPL90			Maximum output on the OSPL90 curve	No more than 3 dB higher
Full-on Gain Measures	Set for the highest output and the broadest frequency response	A 50 or 60 dB SPL pure-tone that sweeps the frequencies from at least 200 to 5000 Hz		
Full-on Gain Curve			Gain of the hearing aid as a function of frequency	
High-Frequency Full-on Average Gain			Average gain taken at 1000, 1600, and 2500 Hz	Within ± 5 dB
Reference Test Gain Measure	Set with the gain control or volume wheel so that the output is 17 dB below the High-Frequency Average OSPL90	A 60 dB SPL pure-tone that sweeps the frequencies from at least 200 to 5000 Hz		N/A

Source: Information from *Standards for Specification of Hearing Aid Characteristics, S3.22-2003,* by the American National Standards Institute, 2003, New York: Author.

of communication. Frye (2005) explained that the average level of conversational speech is 65 dB SPL at 1 meter from the speaker and may vary by as much as +12 to −18 dB. Therefore, the maximum level of conversational speech is 77 dB SPL. (i.e., 65 dB SPL + 12 dB = 77 dB SPL). So, setting the reference test gain such that the output is 17 dB below the HFA OSPL90 ensures that the range of amplified conversational speech falls at or below the hearing aid saturation level (Frye, 2005). ANSI S3.22 (2003) does not have tolerance values for reference test gain.

We reviewed three parameters that are assessed during an electroacoustic analysis. Other parameters and the reasons for their inclusion in an electroacoustic analysis include the following:

- **Frequency response curve/frequency range (f1 and f2):** Assesses whether the hearing aid is amplifying a range of frequencies specified by the manufacturer.
- **Percent total harmonic distortion:** Determines if the hearing aid is adding extra energy at frequencies that are whole-number multiples of input stimuli, which could compromise the quality of the output signal, particularly if it is speech.
- **Equivalent input noise (EIN) level:** Evaluates if the hearing aid is producing noise on its own.
- **Battery current drain:** Tests if the hearing aid is drawing an appropriate amount of power from the battery.

Furthermore, some parameters are assessed depending on whether a hearing aid is a linear versus an AGC hearing aid or compression device. For example, AGC hearing aids have additional parameters that assess the functioning of their compression circuits: (1) **input/output function**, (2) **attack time**, and (3) **release time**. To obtain an input/output function, the hearing aid is set to reference test gain position; the input stimulus is a pure tone of a single frequency that rapidly increases in 5 dB steps from 55 to 90 dB SPL, simulating the onset of a loud sound. An input/output function is plotted with the dB SPL of the input to the hearing aid on the horizontal axis and that for the output on the vertical axis. Recall that the function of the compression circuit is to limit the output of the hearing aid so that it will not be painful to the listener. The input/output function shows where the compression starts to limit the output at specified levels based on patients' loudness discomfort levels. Moreover, attack time is the length of time, in milliseconds, that it takes for the compression circuit to activate after onset of a loud sound. It is important for the compression circuit to be fast acting so that it activates quickly enough to ensure that sounds going into patients' ears are not too loud. Alternatively, the release time is the length of time, in milliseconds, that it takes for a compression circuit to deactivate after a decrease in sound level. When intense sounds are no longer entering the hearing aid, compression circuits need to deactivate to not further influence signal processing. A detailed discussion of all of these parameters is beyond the scope of this textbook; readers are referred to Kates (2008) and Ricketts, Bentler, and Mueller (2008). Now that we've discussed some of the basic electroacoustic aspects of hearing aids, we will go through the process of managing hearing loss through amplification.

AUDIOLOGIC MANAGEMENT OF ADULT HEARING IMPAIRMENT THROUGH AMPLIFICATION

The selection, evaluation, and fitting of hearing aids have been described as involving both science and art. The scientific aspect of the process may appear to be all of the measurements made with sophisticated equipment. The art of hearing aid fitting is understanding and meeting patients' communications needs through appropriate amplification and auditory rehabilitation. Numerous clinical practice guidelines (CPGs) have been written on the topic, but until recently EBP has not been incorporated into these documents. Let's consider an evidence-based CPG discussed in the following What Does the Evidence Show?

What Does the Evidence Show?

In the chapter on professional issues in auditory rehabilitation, we defined **clinical practice guidelines** as a systematically defined set of recommended procedures based on scientific evidence and/or expert opinion that have been designed to yield specific, well-defined outcomes. Unfortunately, in communication sciences and disorders, CPGs have been based more on expert opinion than on scientific evidence. In the creation of these documents, a group of experts in a particular clinical area convene and recommend a set of best practices. In addition, as we learned in the last chapter, expert opinion is at a low level of evidence; to achieve a higher level of evidence, EBP requires integrating expert opinion, patient preferences, *and* scientific evidence for clinical decision-making.

Toward this ideal in 2003, the American Academy of Audiology assembled a Task Force for Developing Guidelines for the Audiologic Management of Adult Hearing Impairment with the following individuals: Michael Valente (chairperson), Harvey Abrams, Darcy Benson, Theresa Chisolm, Dave Citron, Dennis Hampton, Angela Loavenbruck, Todd Ricketts, Helena Solodar, and Robert Sweetow. Their specific goal was to provide a set of statements, recommendations, and strategies for best practices in the provision of comprehensive treatment to adults with hearing loss.

For one of the first times, EBP principles were incorporated into the development of CPGs in Audiology. Members of the task force were assigned to specific areas of the guidelines to review and assess available scientific evidence supporting clinical procedures. In addition, members rated the level of evidence for each clinical procedure using the same classification system introduced in the last chapter (e.g., Cox, 2005):

- Level I: Systematic reviews and meta-analysis of randomized controlled trials (RCT) or other high-quality studies
- Level II: Well-designed RCTs
- Level III: Nonrandomized treatment studies
- Level IV: Cohort studies, case-control studies, cross-sectional surveys, and uncontrolled experiments
- Level V: Case reports
- Level VI: Expert opinions

Then, members of the task force assigned a Grade of Recommendation based on the level of evidence and consistency of findings using the rubric also introduced in the last chapter (e.g., Cox, 2005):

- A: Level I or II with consistent conclusions
- B: Levels III or IV studies or extrapolated evidence (generalized to a situation where it is not fully relevant) from Level I or II studies
- C: Level V studies extrapolated from Level III or IV studies
- D: Level VI evidence or inconsistent or inconclusive of any level or any studies that have a high risk of bias

A final step involved labeling the evidence as Effective (EV) or Efficacious (EF). Valente, Abrams, et al. (2006) explained that the label of EV is evidence measured in the "real world," while EF evidence was measured under ideal laboratory conditions. At the end of each section of the guidelines are charts providing this information for each recommendation, facilitating EBP for clinicians.

We will use the CPG as a framework for discussing the following continuum of hearing healthcare in selection, evaluation, and fitting of amplification.

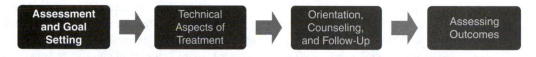

Assessment and Goal Setting

The first stage of the process contains three steps:

- Auditory assessment and diagnosis
- Self-perception of communication needs, performance, and selection of goals for treatment
- Nonauditory needs assessment

Auditory Assessment and Diagnosis

According to the guidelines, the purpose of this stage of the process is to diagnose the type and degree of hearing loss and determine if patients are candidates for hearing aids. The outcomes for auditory assessment and diagnosis are the following (Valente, Abrams, et al., 2006):

- Diagnosis, type, and extent of hearing loss
- Determination and need for medical referral to a licensed physician
- Provision of audiometric results and treatment options through appropriate patient and family/caregiver counseling
- Determination of candidacy for amplification and counseling and patient's attitude toward the treatment plan
- Determination of lifestyle through needs assessment techniques
- Determination of need for medical clearance as determined by the guidelines established by the FDA

Audiologic evaluation determines whether the hearing loss is conductive, sensorineural, or mixed. Any type of hearing loss that can be treated medically should receive a referral to a licensed physician. Provision of audiometric results and treatment options through appropriate patient and family/caregiver counseling sets the tone for the auditory rehabilitation process. Audiologists should use **informational counseling** to explain audiometric findings and treatment options. Recall that informational counseling was discussed in Chapter 2 and is intended to provide the knowledge and understanding about patients' hearing losses and the steps needed for management (Margolis, 2004). It has been found that patients remember only about 50% of information provided by healthcare providers (Shapiro, Boggs, Melamed, & Graham-Pole, 1992) with 40% to 80% of the information immediately forgotten (Margolis). Margolis explained how patient factors, mode of presentation, and clinician characteristics can affect the retention of information. For example, patients who have suspicions or previous knowledge of, or are experienced with hearing loss should retain more information than others who are not. Moreover, audiologists, who calmly use clear language with simple sentence structure and present the information according to the method of explicit categorization, may facilitate patients' retention of information. Recall that the **method of explicit categorization** is presenting information to patients in specific, rank-ordered categories of recommendations, diagnosis, test results, and then prognosis. In addition, it is helpful to supplement verbal facts with written, graphical, and/or pictorial information to help patients understand and retain information about their hearing loss and treatment options.

Another important step is to determine candidacy for amplification that is initially made on the results from the audiologic evaluation. Generally, there are no hard and fast rules for candidacy based on audiometric results. In fact, many audiologists agree that if patients' pure-tone thresholds are between 20 and 25 dB HL, then hearing aids would probably not be of much benefit (Mueller, Johnson, & Carter, 2007). However, as thresholds get appreciably worse, particularly at 2000 Hz and higher, the likelihood of significant benefit from amplification increases (Mueller et al., 2007). Additionally, plotting audiometric thresholds on Mueller and Killion's Audibility Index or Count-the-Dot Audiogram, discussed in Chapter 1 (see Figure 1.10), can be useful in both determining candidacy and for counseling the patient.

Recall that the Audibility Index or Count-the-Dot Audiogram by Mueller and Killion (1990), modified later by Lundeen, consists of 100 dots representing the percent of audible speech energy available for soft speech. Notice that the dots are plotted on a regular audiogram so that audiologists can superimpose patients' pure-tone air-conduction thresholds, connect them with straight lines, and then determine the audibility index by counting the number of dots that are found *below* the audiometric thresholds (toward the bottom of the audiogram). Mueller et al. (2007) stated that patients who have an audibility index below 85% are candidates for amplification if they are experiencing communication difficulties and are motivated to try hearing aids. Although someone may be a candidate for a hearing aid based on his or her audiometric profile, a patient may not accept that he or she has a problem. The Count-the-Dot Audiogram can be used to counsel patients regarding the audibility of speech when considering their degree of hearing loss.

Prospective hearing aid wearers should then be counseled regarding appropriate expectations of the benefits derived from the use of amplification. Table 6.4 shows some realistic expectations to share with patients about their audiologist, hearing aids, and themselves (Allen, 2002; Kochkin, 2006; Weinstein, 2000). For example, patients need to have an idea about the role of the audiologist, the provision of a 30-day trial period, and the necessity of attending follow-up appointments. State laws ensure that patients have at least a 30-day trial period with their hearing aids before deciding on their purchase. Moreover, audiologists communicate closely with patients during this time regarding any difficulties and see them for follow-up appointments so that adjustments can be made on their hearing aids. Most importantly, however, patients need to know that hearing aids do not restore hearing to normal and that they must be patient when adjusting to amplification. Laying the groundwork with appropriate expectations may increase the likelihood for patient satisfaction.

The FDA oversees and regulates the manufacture and sale of hearing aids. The FDA has established guidelines which state that patients must be referred to a physician if they have any of the following conditions:

- Deformity of the ear that was present at birth or caused by some type of trauma
- Active drainage from the ear during the previous 90 days
- Sudden or rapidly progressive hearing loss during the previous 90 days
- Sudden or long-term dizziness
- Sudden or recent unilateral hearing loss during the previous 90 days

- Air-bone gaps equal to or greater than 15 dB HL at 500, 1000, and 2000 Hz
- Significant cerumen (i.e., earwax) buildup or foreign body in the ear canal
- Ear pain or discomfort

table *6.4* Realistic Expectations for Patients About Their Audiologists, Hearing Aids, and Themselves

Expect your audiologist to:
- Be knowledgeable, courteous, and accommodating
- Suggest a referral to a physician to rule out any medical conditions
- Assess your hearing difficulties in several environments
- Define individual goals for you
- Offer a 30-day trial period
- Provide an initial orientation session on how to handle and care for your hearing aids
- Schedule multiple follow-up appointments
- Evaluate the benefits of your hearing aids

Expect your hearing aids to:
- Cost more than you expected
- Fit comfortably
- Allow you to hear:
  - Soft speech audibly
  - Conversational speech comfortably
  - Loud speech without discomfort
- Not filter out noise completely
- Provide some protection from loud sounds
- Deliver sounds that at first may seem different (e.g., your own voice and footsteps)
- Require repairs from time to time
- Whistle or feedback if the earmold or hearing aid are not seated properly

Expect yourself to:
- Require presentation of the same information about and practice of new skills with your hearing aids more than once prior to feeling comfortable with the situation
- Require a period of adjustment with your hearing aids
- Experience some difficulty in noisy situations
- Buy batteries
- Benefit from an orientation group for new hearing aid wearers
- Purchase hearing aids about every 5 years
- Enjoy better hearing!

Sources: Information from *Hearing Aids: Reasonable Expectations for the Consumer*, by R. Allen, 2002, retrieved from www.audiologyonline.com/articles/article_detail.asp?article_id=347; *Hearing Solutions—Expectations—A Key to Success*, by S. Kochkin, 2006, retrieved from www.betterhearing.org/hearing_solutions/expectations.cfm; *Geriatric Audiology*, by B. E. Weinstein, 2000, New York: Thieme Publishers.

Audiologists must obtain a written statement from the patient that is signed by a licensed physician. Additionally, the statement must be signed and dated within the previous six months, confirming that the patient's ears have been evaluated, and that he or she is cleared to pursue amplification. However, patients who are 18 years of age and older can sign a waiver of the medical evaluation. Audiologists should not encourage signing of the waiver as it is in the best interest of the patient to have medical clearance from a physician.

In the following Casebook Reflections, we will follow Bill and Dottie Roberts through the management of Bill's hearing loss through the fitting of hearing aids and auditory rehabilitation. Bill Roberts, a 65-year-old retired carpenter has been accompanied by his wife Dottie to his audiologic evaluation conducted by Yan Chew, Au.D. The clinical scenario exemplifies clinical recommendations from the guidelines that are listed at the end of each Casebook Reflection along with the grade based on available evidence.

Casebook Reflection

Bill and Dottie Roberts: Auditory Assessment and Diagnosis

Dr. Yan Chew just completed an audiologic evaluation of Bill Roberts, a 65-year-old retired carpenter, who came to the appointment with his wife, Dottie. A few years ago, the Roberts had taken an early retirement and moved to a golfing community in Florida. Dr. Chew had been recommended to the Roberts by their family physician. Dottie had noticed that Bill's hearing had become worse during the last year, making communication difficult in some situations at home and during some of their activities. Bill knew that he had some hearing loss from exposure to artillery fire in the Vietnam War and machinery at his job.

Dr. Chew: "Mr. Roberts, we are all done with testing. I'd like to explain the results of my evaluation with you."

Bill: "Can you get Dottie, my wife, out of the waiting room? I'd like for her to be part of this."

Dr. Chew: "Bernice, can you please ask Mrs. Roberts to come back to the consultation room? Thanks!"

Dr. Chew: "I have some news that you were expecting. I think you're an excellent candidate for binaural hearing aids. Mr. Roberts, you have a moderate-to-severe sensorineural hearing loss as shown on the audiogram with the red symbols representing the results for your right ear and blue ones for your left ear. . . . I have also plotted the audiometric results on this Count-the-Dot

Audiogram. Do you notice the gray area at the top of the page with the dots?"

Bill: "Yes, I do."

Dottie: "Yes. . . ."

Dr. Chew: "The gray area represents where conversational speech has its energy. There are 100 dots, with each one representing one percentage point of speech energy. If all of your audiometric thresholds were within the normal range, you would have 100% of the energy of conversational speech that would be audible for you. However, notice that you have only 27% audibility for the right ear and 24% audibility for the left ear."

Bill: "What exactly does that mean?"

Dr. Chew: "It means that with your hearing loss, you can only hear about 25% of the energy of conversational speech. Do you notice how there are more dots in the higher frequencies than in the lower frequencies?"

Dottie and Bill: "Yes. . . ."

Dr. Chew: "The greater density of the dots in the higher frequencies represents the fact that critical energy for speech intelligibility is located above 1000 Hz, where you have the greatest amount of hearing loss. You are missing all of the dots in the higher frequencies in quiet situations. In noisy situations, audibility is worse because the noise covers over the energy that you do hear."

Bill: "Yes, you're right. Will hearing aids help me?"

Dottie reached over and held Bill's hand.

Dr. Chew: "Yes, they will, but it is important to note that hearing aids do not restore your hearing to normal, although their circuitry has improved in recent years through digital technology. We also recommend that you get hearing aids for both ears for the following reasons. . . ."

Bill, Dottie, and Dr. Chew discussed the importance of binaural amplification. Deep down, Bill was getting up the courage to discuss how the hearing aids might look. Being bald, he knew that there was no chance of any hair concealing his hearing aids.

Bill: "Dr. Chew, what styles of hearing aids could I use?"

Dr. Chew: "I'll go get them so you can see what is available."

Dr. Chew could tell from Bill's voice that he was really concerned about hearing aid cosmetics. Due to his level of anxiety, Dr. Chew felt that Bill should complete the *Expected Consequences of Hearing Aid Ownership* (Cox & Alexander, 2000) to determine his level of expectations of hearing aid use. Dr. Chew wanted to be prepared to address any of Bill's concerns.

Dr. Chew modeled and explained the characteristics, advantages, and disadvantages of the BTE, ITE, ITC, and CIC in his right ear. Simultaneously, he wore an open-ear fitting in his left ear.

Dr. Chew: "I have one more style of hearing aid that I need to tell you about, which I have been wearing in my left ear since we started talking."

Bill: "I can't see it!"

Dottie: "Me either!"

Dr. Chew: "Do you see this little wire?"

Bill: "Well, now that you mention it, yes!"

Dr. Chew took the open-ear hearing aid out of his ear and explained its characteristics, advantages, and disadvantages. Bill and Dottie were really excited about this style of hearing aid. Dr. Chew sensed a really positive attitude toward auditory rehabilitation and amplification from this couple who were ready to begin seeking amplification immediately.

Because Bill was referred from his primary care physician, he elected to sign a medical waiver so he could pursue amplification. Dr. Chew discussed the rest of the process with the Roberts.

Clinical Recommendations

- Patients should complete self-assessment tools prior to hearing aid fitting to identify communication needs, present level of functioning, and goals.

  GRADE: B

- Self-assessment tools should address user expectations of hearing aid use.

  GRADE: B

Self-Perception of Communication Needs, Performance, and Selection of Goals for Treatment

If auditory rehabilitation is to be successful, the goals must be patient specific. There are self-assessment instruments available that assist the audiologist and patient in documenting communication needs. In that way, management plans can be tailored to meet patient-specific goals. Some audiologists have deemed measurement tools used during this phase of the rehabilitation process as "income" measures because patients' perceptions at this point in treatment establish a baseline of functioning against which postfitting performance will be compared (Johnson & Danhauer, 2002a).

Several self-report instruments are available for use in measuring functioning across the domains of the World Health Organization International Classification of Functioning,

Disability, and Health (2001) (described in Chapter 1 and integrated into the auditory rehabilitation model) and are defined as follows:

- **Impairment** is a loss or abnormality of a bodily structure or of a physiological or psychological function.
- **Activity limitation** is an inability to carry out activities of daily living (ADL) involving hearing, speech understanding, and communication.
- **Participation restriction** is an inability to communicate with specific partners in specific situations.

Assessing impairment, as in hearing impairment, is completed during the audiologic evaluation and includes measures such as the audiogram and the **Audibility Index**, which is the amount of speech information audible to the listener. The goals in the impairment domain include increasing patients' ability to detect sounds through the use of amplification. As described previously, the Audibility Index can be calculated from the patient's audiometric results superimposed on the Count-the-Dot Audiogram and can be used as an income measure for the impairment domain against which postfitting measures can be made. However, increased audibility post–hearing aid fitting does not necessarily translate into better communication or interpersonal interactions (Abrams, 2000). Therefore, income measures must be made for the activity limitation and participation restriction domains through self-assessment instruments.

Fortunately, there are several self-assessment scales or instruments available that tap into the activity limitation domain. These measures deal primarily with the patient's ability to hear for the purposes of carrying out everyday activities. Two such instruments include the *Client Oriented Scale of Improvement* (COSI) (Dillon et al., 1997) (see Appendix 6.2) and the *Abbreviated Profile of Hearing Aid Benefit* (APHAB) (Cox & Alexander, 1995) (see Appendix 6.3). Use of the COSI is conducted in two phases: (1) Phase I: Identification of Specific Listening Situations, and (2) Phase II: Assessment of Improvement and Final Listening Ability. During Phase I, audiologists ask the patient to identify up to five *specific* listening situations in which he or she would like to hear well. The operative word is "specific" in that goals such as "I want to hear better in restaurants" are not precise enough. However, a goal such as "I would like to hear my wife better when we are sitting and eating at the Red Lobster on a Saturday night" is specific enough. The situations are recorded onto the COSI form. Patients should be encouraged to prioritize the situations by placing a number by each on the COSI form. In addition, each listening situation should be classified into one of the 16 listening categories listed on the COSI form. For Phase II, completed after the hearing aid trial period, audiologists ask patients to rate the degree of change in hearing ability for each situation by selecting one of the following choices: "worse," "no difference," "slightly better," "better," or "much better." In addition, the patient is instructed to rate his or her final speech understanding in each of the situations. The COSI assists audiologists in forming partnerships with patients by selecting goals for rehabilitation that are unique for each hearing aid wearer.

The APHAB is a 24-item self-assessment inventory in which patients report the amount of difficulty they are having with communication or sources of noise in everyday situations. The 24 items are equally divided among four subscales: (1) Ease of Communication (EC), (2) Reverberation (RV), (3) Background Noise (BN), and (4) Aversiveness (AV). The first three subscales ask about speech understanding in everyday listening situations. The fourth subscale asks hearing aid wearers about their reactions to environmental sounds. As an example, patients respond to statements such as "When I am in a crowded grocery store, talking with the cashier, I can follow the conversation" by selecting from an array of choices ranging from "A = Always (99%)" to "G = Never (1%)." The APHAB takes about 10 minutes to complete; hearing aid benefit is calculated by comparing patients' ratings in the unaided mode to when they wear hearing aids.

Similarly, there are several self-report scales that tap into the participation restriction domain. The most commonly used tools in this domain are the *Hearing Handicap Inventory for the Elderly* (HHIE) (Ventry & Weinstein, 1982), (see Appendix 6.4) and the *Hearing Handicap Inventory for Adults* (HHIA) (Newman, Weinstein, Jacobson, & Hug, 1991). The HHIE is to be used with independent adults aged 65 years and older; the HHIA is to be used with adults under 65 years of age. Briefly, the HHIE is a 25-item assessment tool that measures the social and emotional consequences of hearing loss of noninstitutionalized elderly persons (Ventry & Weinstein, 1982). The Social Scale includes 13 of the 25 items that measure the perceived effects of hearing loss in social situations (Huch & Hosford-Dunn, 2000). The Emotional Scale consists of 12 of the 25 items and measures patients' attitudes and emotional reactions toward hearing loss (Huch & Hosford-Dunn, 2000). An example of an item is "Does a hearing problem cause you to feel embarrassed when meeting new people?" to which patients select either "yes" (4 points), "sometimes" (2 points), or "no" (0 points). Scoring entails adding up the points based on patients' responses to determine three scores: total score, subtotal social score, and subtotal emotional score. Total scores range from 0 (i.e., no hearing handicap) to 100 (i.e., maximum hearing handicap). Total scores from 0 to 16 indicate no handicap, 17 to 42 signals mild-to-moderate difficulties, and scores of 43 or more indicate significant problems (Ventry & Weinstein, 1982). The HHIA is also a 25-item self-assessment scale that measures the same domain as the HHIE. The HHIA is almost the same as the HHIE except for changes in one emotional and two social questions to make the scale appropriate for use with adults under 65 years of age who may be still employed (Newman et al., 1991).

Other types of baseline measures include patients' expectations of amplification and health-related quality of life. One self-report scale that measures patients' expectations of hearing aids prior to the fitting is the *Expected Consequences of Hearing Aid Ownership* (ECHO) (Cox & Alexander, 2000) (see Appendix 6.5). The ECHO measures and provides a global score and scores on four subscales: (1) Positive Effect, (2) Service and Cost, (3) Negative Features, and (4) Personal Image. The ECHO is effective for identifying unrealistic expectations prior to hearing aid fitting so that appropriate issues can be addressed through counseling. **Health-related quality of life** (HRQoL) is an individual's physical, mental, and social well-being that may be reduced by untreated sensorineural hearing loss (Abrams, Chisolm, & McArdle, 2005). HRQoL is frequently measured using self-assessment scales and can be used across healthcare conditions to compare the relative benefits or interventions for various diseases. One instrument for measuring HRQoL includes the *Medical Outcomes Survey—Short Form 36* (SF-36) (Ware & Sherbourne, 1992). The SF-36 has been used in numerous investigations assessing the effectiveness of amplification in enhancing generic HRQoL. The SF-36 does not seem to be sensitive enough to measure the consequences of or the effectiveness of interventions for hearing impairment (Abrams et al., 2005; Bess, 2000). Fortunately, another generic HRQoL measure, the *World Health Organization's Disability Assessment Schedule* (WHO-DAS II) (World Health Organization, 1999), appears to have sections that measure the consequences of hearing loss (Abrams et al., 2005). Briefly, it is a 36-item questionnaire that measures six domains: (1) communication, (2) self-mobility, (3) self-care, (4) interpersonal, (5) life activities, and (6) participation in society.

The purpose of obtaining income measures is to assist patients in setting some goals for their auditory rehabilitation programs. Valente, Abrams, et al. (2006) stated that goals can either be **cognitive** or they can be **affective**. Cognitive goals are objective statements of the ability to hear during certain activities, such as "to be able to hear my grandchildren on the telephone" or "to be able to hear the doorbell when I'm in my bedroom." Affective goals include the psychosocial implications of hearing loss, such as "I don't want to feel embarrassed anymore because of not hearing," or "I don't want to feel isolated because of my hearing loss." Setting goals establishes a partnership between patient and audiologist in addition to making both accountable to the process.

Casebook Reflection

Bill and Dottie Roberts: Self-Perception of Communication Needs, Performance, and Selection of Goals for Treatment

Dr. Chew: "What I'd like to discuss is the specific communication problems that you are having. In particular, I'd like for you and Dottie to select some specific goals to focus on for treatment. I have some tools that will assist us with this. The first is the Client-Oriented Scale of Improvement in which I'd like you to nominate and prioritize at least four situations in which you'd like to hear well. Be specific on what you want to hear and where. Does that make sense?"

Bill and Dottie: "Yes, it does!"

With Dr. Chew's help, the Roberts came up with five goals (from most important to least important):

1. Understand Dottie when seated and eating at their favorite restaurant even when it is noisy.
2. Understand friends when seated at Bill's weekly Kiwanis lunches.
3. Hear the speaker at his weekly Kiwanis meetings.
4. Understand his grandchildren on his cell phone without having the speaker on full volume.
5. Hear the television without having the volume up so high that it is offensive to others.

Dr. Chew also could sense that Bill's hearing impairment had an impact on his psychosocial well-being and requested his completion of the Hearing Handicap Inventory for the Elderly to document any social and emotional impact of his hearing loss. In addition, Dr. Chew wanted Bill and Dottie to state some affective goals.

Dr. Chew: "Bill, could you tell me about how your hearing loss has impacted your interactions with others?"

Bill was caught off guard by this question and he was not comfortable talking about his feelings. "Well. . . ."

Dottie: "I don't want to speak for Bill, but it has been a source of frustration for us," Dottie said, gently touching her husband's hand.

Bill: "Yes, it has. Also, I feel anxious before going to my weekly Kiwanis meetings for fear of seeming 'out of it' when I lose track of the conversation. . . . I also feel that my grandchildren feel sorry for me."

Dr. Chew: "Yes, your descriptions of your feelings are consistent with your results on the HHIE. So, you would like to reduce feelings of frustration, anxiety, and pity from others associated with your hearing loss?"

Bill: "Yes, I would."

Clinical Recommendations

- Each patient should complete self-assessment instruments prior to hearing aid fitting to identify communication needs, functions, and goals.

  GRADE: B

- Goals should be patient specific and have cognitive and affective components.

  GRADE: B

- Self-assessment scales may determine readiness for pursuing amplification.

  GRADES: B AND C

- A variety of tools should be used to assess patient readiness for amplification.

  GRADE: B

Nonauditory Needs Assessment

In other chapters, we have discussed the importance of how multiple areas of patients' lives can affect the rehabilitation process. For example, in Chapter 12 involving elderly adults, we mention that Lesner and Kricos (1995) advocated a "holistic" approach to auditory rehabilitation involving assessing multiple areas of patients' lives that are impacted by hearing loss: physical status, psychological status, sociological status, and communication status.

Valente, Abrams, et al. (2006) suggested that audiologists ask about or even screen for general health, manual dexterity and finger sensitivity, near vision, support systems, motivation, and prior experience with amplification. For example, case history forms usually inquire about patients' health histories. Kricos (2006a) suggested that the *Purdue Nine-Hole Peg Board Test* (Mathiowetz & Weber, 1985; Tiffin & Asher, 1948) be used to screen patients' degree of manual dexterity in addition to more informal evaluations, including just asking the patient to pick up a hearing aid, adjust the controls, and lift the device to ear level. Similarly, Kricos also suggested the use of the *Semmes-Weinstein Monofilaments test* (Bell-Krotoski & Tomancik, 1987; Weinstein, 1993) to assess patients' finger sensitivity. Knowledge of patients' limitations in these areas can assist with hearing aid selection.

Casebook Reflection

Bill and Dottie Roberts: Nonauditory Needs Assessment

Dr. Chew was not really concerned about nonauditory factors impacting Bill's use of amplification and his treatment plan. After all, Bill was a vibrant 65-year-old who was active, fit, and in overall good health without any chronic health conditions or any signs of cognitive decline. Dr. Chew did ask about his manual dexterity, finger sensitivity, and the last time Bill had a visual examination. He noted that Bill squinted quite a bit and held things at arm's length to see them better. Dr. Chew had discovered that Bill hadn't had his eyes examined in five years. Therefore, Dr. Chew recommended that Bill see his ophthalmologist for an examination and get an updated prescription for his glasses.

Clinical Recommendations

- Nonauditory needs of patients should be considered because they may impact prognosis.
  GRADE: B

- Patients should be asked about or even screened on general health, manual dexterity, vision, support systems, and so on.
  GRADE: B

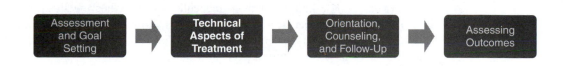

Assessment and Goal Setting → Technical Aspects of Treatment → Orientation, Counseling, and Follow-Up → Assessing Outcomes

Technical Aspects of Treatment

Technical aspects of treatment include (1) hearing aid selection (i.e., style, external/internal features, and monaural versus binaural fittings), (2) quality control, (3) fitting and verification (i.e., physical fit, occlusion effect, selection of assessment signal, gain verification, output verification, aided sound-field verification, and verification of special features), and (4) hearing aid assistive technology.

Hearing Aid Selection

Valente, Abrams, et al. (2006) stated that the goal of this part of the fitting process is to select the appropriate amplification system and HAT for the patient based on auditory and nonauditory needs. The hearing aid selection process involves some decisions made by the audiologist alone and others by the patient in consultation with his or her hearing healthcare provider. For example, selection of hearing aid style involves a decision made by the patient based on recommendations from the audiologist. However, some selections, particularly those about what is happening inside the hearing aid, such as gain processing and frequency shaping, involve the audiologist alone. Selection involves style, external features, internal features, type of fitting (e.g., monaural versus binaural), and special applications.

Hearing Aid Style.   One of the first and greatest concerns for patients is the selection of hearing aid style. Characteristics, advantages, and disadvantages of the various styles of hearing aids along with general patient factors to consider were discussed earlier in the chapter. To assist patients with this decision, each audiologist should have a complete set of custom "dummy" hearing aids made that represent all possible styles. Audiologists simply have to have ear impressions made for an earmold for a BTE style, a full-shell ITE, a half-shell ITE, an ITC, a mini-ITC, and a deep-fitting CIC. Most hearing aid manufacturers will provide "dummy" aids for free or a nominal charge. Custom-made "dummy" hearing aids enable audiologists to contrast styles of well-fitting hearing instruments in addition to providing close inspection and manipulation of the devices. Dr. Chew used this technique in counseling Bill Roberts on different styles of hearing aids.

Selection of hearing aid style is based on both auditory and nonauditory factors. Degree of hearing loss often precludes the use of some hearing aid styles for some patients. Patients with a severe hearing loss may have to settle for an ITE hearing aid rather than an ITC hearing aid. Similarly, characteristics of patients' outer ear canals may preclude the use of CIC hearing aids if canals are too short, narrow, or curvy. Elderly patients with manual dexterity problems may do better with ITE hearing aids than BTE, ITC, or CIC hearing instruments. In addition to patient characteristics, the degree of occlusion can play a major role in the selection of hearing aid style.

Occlusion is the degree to which an earmold or hearing aid blocks the ear canal. The occlusion effect occurs when an object completely fills the outer portion of the ear such that sound in the external auditory canal is projected back toward the tympanic membrane, increasing the sensation of loudness of patients' voices; often a complaint of new hearing aid wearers (Ross, 2004). Smaller, more cosmetically appealing hearing aids provide less occlusion than larger, bulkier hearing aids. Moreover, some hearing aids and earmolds are more occluding than others. Selection of an appropriate hearing aid and/or earmold also has to take into account the technical aspects of occlusion.

Valente, Abrams, et al. (2006) explained that signal processing in conventional hearing instruments with increased gain may produce unwanted feedback unless there is considerable separation between the microphone and receiver, possibly necessitating a larger style, particularly if there is no **digital feedback suppression scheme**, which is an internal feature in a hearing aid that eliminates feedback before it is noticeable to the patient. Valente, Abrams, et al. (2006) also suggested that, although uncomfortable or impossible with some ear canals, extending the shell of the hearing aid to the bony portion of the ear canal or use of a digital feedback reduction may reduce the problem.

External Features of Hearing Aids. Volume control wheels adjust the loudness of sound coming out of the hearing aid. Customarily, patients turn the volume wheel down so they will not experience any discomfort from loud sounds. Conversely, patients turn up the volume of their hearing aids to hear soft sounds. However, with many of the compression systems used in today's hearing aids that make soft sounds audible, conversational speech comfortable, and loud stimuli tolerable, many hearing aids do not need a volume control wheel. Elderly patients may find these aids without volume control wheels more manageable. For example, Dillon (2001) suggested ordering wide dynamic range compression and no volume control wheels for manageability. Additionally, he suggested ordering an automatic control in addition to a manual one that can be locked, if needed.

A **telecoil** (sometimes called a t-coil) is an induction coil (i.e., metal rod surrounded by many turns of a copper wire) that produces a voltage that can be amplified by the hearing aid when in close proximity to an alternating magnetic field, such as from a telephone, that flows through it (Dillon, 2001). The alternating magnetic field can originate from a telephone receiver, a neckloop attached to an FM receiver, and so on. Neckloops and FM receivers are discussed in more detail in the next chapter. Telecoils are most frequently found in ITE and BTE hearing aids. On older hearing aids, a switch designates whether the microphone or telecoil is accessed by using a toggle switch labeled M for *microphone*, T for *telecoil*, and O for *off*. Some hearing aids have an M-MT-T switch in which the MT stands for *microphone-telephone*, enabling the use of the microphone and telecoil simultaneously. More technologically advanced hearing aids access the telecoil via a program. Telecoils are essential for patients with severe-to-profound hearing loss, but patients with slight-to-mild hearing impairment may be able to use the telephone without their hearing aids, affected greatly by the style of hearing aid. Moreover, telecoils are appropriate for patients with all degrees of hearing loss who use inductive coupling for HAT. Another way of coupling hearing aids is through the use of **direct audio input (DAI)**, which electrically connects an external signal source to the input of a hearing aid, bypassing the microphone, as discussed in the next chapter. The DAI on the hearing aid consists of electrical contacts that patients can attach to a plug or audio shoe. The electrical signal that goes into the hearing aid can come from a handheld microphone, FM receiver, and so on (Dillon, 2001).

Microphones can be **directional** or **omnidirectional**. Directional microphones pick up sounds from the front of the hearing aid wearer; omnidirectional microphones transduce sounds from all around the listener. Directional microphones have been popular for more than 50 years, declining in popularity during the 1980s and 1990s and then making a comeback recently due to the development of the listener-control-of-microphone mode based on environmental conditions (Bentler, 2005). Directional microphones help for speech recognition in difficult listening situations (e.g., trying to have a conversation in a noisy restaurant by zeroing in on the speaker in front and attenuating noise from the back). Adaptive directional microphones automatically switch between modes based on listening conditions and have shown some advantages over listener-controlled devices, particularly when noise is coming from the side of the hearing aid wearer (Ricketts & Henry, 2002).

Internal Features of Hearing Aids. **Gain processing** is how hearing aid circuitry amplifies sounds in certain frequency regions. One of the advantages of digital signal processing is the flexibility with which processing schemes increase the audibility of sounds while minimizing discomfort to the patient through manipulation of compression (e.g., input specific band dependence, greater number of channels, and kneepoints) (Ricketts, 2005). For the past 50 years, prescription of gain was accomplished via **prescriptive methods**, which are formulas that determine the amount of gain based on patients' audiometric thresholds and other measures. One approach is the National Acoustics Laboratory NL1 (NAL-NL1: Byrne, Dillon, Ching, Katsch, & Keidser, 2001) that aims to make the output comfortable; gain is based on patients' audiometric thresholds. NAL-NL1 is most frequently used with adults, but is also used for children (Ching, Scollie, Dillon, & Seewald, 2010; Scollie, Ching, Seewald, Dillon, Britton et al., 2010). Another method, the Desired Sensation Level (Scollie, Seewald, Cornelisse, Moodie, et al., 2005), is used most often with children and ensures that conversational speech is audible while avoiding loudness discomfort. The selection, evaluation, and fitting of hearing aids on children are discussed at the end of this chapter. Many of the popular prescriptive methods are included within the software that comes with real-ear probe-tube microphone measurement systems. The amount of gain at each frequency may be customized to meet the unique needs of each patient. **Frequency shaping** is differentially amplifying sound from certain frequency regions or "sculpting" the frequency response of a hearing aid to accommodate various configurations of hearing loss via the use of more than one channel or frequency band. If a patient's audiometric thresholds vary greatly across the frequency range (e.g., 50 dB HL at 250 Hz, 70 dB HL at 500 Hz, 40 dB HL at 1000 Hz, 30 dB HL at 2000 Hz, 60 dB HL at 4000 Hz, and 80 dB HL at 8000 Hz), the gain in the individual frequency bands can be adjusted to provide the precise amount of amplification. It is important to know that multiple channels or frequency bands in hearing aids can be used for purposes other than frequency shaping. For example, hearing aid channels or bands can be used to ensure that sounds remain comfortable to the patient. Valente, Abrams, et al. (2006) stated that hearing aids typically use four to eight separate bands.

Earlier in this chapter, various hearing aid parameters used in electroacoustic analyses of hearing aids were explained. One parameter was **output** and **output sound pressure level-90 (OSPL90)**. Recall that the output of the hearing aid is simply the sound pressure level coming out of the receiver. OSPL90 is the output of the receiver measured in a 2-cc coupler with the input to the microphone being a tone, sweeping from low to high frequencies, at 90 dB SPL with the hearing aid settings set for maximum output capabilities. The microphone attached to the 2-cc coupler records the output of the hearing aid (OSPL90) on a graph that has sound pressure level on the vertical axis and frequency on the horizontal axis. Recall that hearing aid test systems obtain information from the graph such as peak OSPL90, high-frequency average OSPL90, and the OSPL90 curve.

These data are important in hearing aid selection because the audiologist wants to select and adjust hearing aids so that the OSPL90 curve does not reach patients' **loudness discomfort levels (LDLs)**. Loudness discomfort levels are levels of sound that are judged to be uncomfortable by the patient. There are several methods for obtaining patients' LDLs. Customarily, patients listen to frequency-specific narrow bands of noise and are asked to indicate levels that are uncomfortable by raising their hands, pressing a button, or pointing to words such as "uncomfortably loud" on a loudness scale. Patients with sensorineural hearing loss frequently have **recruitment**, which is the abnormal growth in the sensation of loudness of sounds. For most listeners with normal hearing there is a large decibel range—known as **dynamic range**—between thresholds (e.g., 10 dB HL) and sounds that are uncomfortably loud (e.g., 90 dB HL). Patients with recruitment have a restricted dynamic range (e.g., threshold at 2000 Hz of 50 dB HL and at LDL of 80 dB HL), making it difficult for hearing aids to make sounds loud enough to be audible, but not uncomfortable.

Loudness discomfort measures also have been included as part of published hearing aid fitting protocols spanning the past 50 years (Mueller & Bentler, 2005). There are two: (1) obtaining *unaided* LDL measurements through earphones (i.e., prefitting measure), and (2) measuring *aided* loudness discomfort (Mueller & Bentler, 2005). These prefitting measures are used for setting the OSPL90 of the hearing aid in addition to certain aspects of compression systems to ensure patients' listening comfort. Many of the hearing aid manufacturers use these data in their software fitting programs to determine what an instrument will do. Aided loudness discomfort measures do not seek to determine patients' LDLs, but determine if loud sounds picked up by hearing aids are too loud for the patient. If so, then they are adjusted.

Hawkins and Schum (1991) published a face-to-face debate on the topic of appropriate uses of LDL measurements. David Hawkins felt that patients' unaided LDLs are worth measuring if three conditions could be met. First, the patient must be able to make loudness judgments. In other words, the patient is reliably able to classify sounds of different hearing levels according to his or her perceived loudness. Second, the instructions must be clear to the patient as to categories of loudness to be used, such as uncomfortably loud; loud, but ok; comfortable, but slightly loud; comfortable; comfortable, but slightly soft; soft; and very soft. Third, the LDL values must be expressed in useful values, such as SPL in a 2-cc coupler, so that comparisons to the OSPL90 data from hearing aids are possible. Audiologists frequently measure patients' LDLs in dB HL using an audiometer. However, measurements of hearing aid output are made in SPL. Audiologists must convert HL to SPL. Alternatively, Hawkins advised measuring LDLs through an insert earphone with a probe-tube microphone to measure the SPL in the ear canal at the point of loudness discomfort. Donald Schum, on the other hand, felt that obtaining patient LDLs prior to hearing aid selection may not be the most efficient use of audiologists' time. Because hearing aids can be adjusted for patients with significant recruitment, Schum does not make *a priori* measurements of patients' LDLs for hearing aid selection. Schum believes that it is more important to spend time counseling patients about issues with loudness. His procedure measured patients' responses to loud sounds with the hearing aids on and then making any necessary adjustments. He advised patients to be particularly sensitive to loudness issues during the trial period.

In summary, obtaining patients' LDLs has a long history in hearing aid fitting and is routinely used by many audiologists. However, is there any scientific evidence to show that these practices result in positive patient outcomes? In Chapter 5, we discussed the importance of EBP in auditory rehabilitation. The following What Does the Evidence Show? discusses the available evidence regarding the effectiveness of measuring patients' LDLs before or after the fitting of hearing aids.

What Does the Evidence Show?

Mueller and Bentler (2005) conducted a systematic review of the evidence pertaining to the use of obtaining unaided and aided LDL measurements. They explained that because unaided and aided measures of discomfort were made at different times during the hearing aid fitting process, evidence for both methods should be evaluated separately. Their experimental question was, "Are the clinical measurements of LDL for adult patients predictive of aided acceptance and satisfaction of loudness for high inputs in the real world?" In other words, do patients' LDLs predict their acceptance and satisfaction of how they hear loud sounds through their hearing aids when worn in the real world? Using relevant search strings, Mueller and Bentler (2005) searched PubMed, Medline, CINAHL, and EMBASE databases for articles to include in their systematic review (see Chapter 5). Included articles had to have been published from 1980 to 2005; use a randomized control clinical trial, or quasi-experimental, or nonintervention descriptive research design; use adult participants with sensorineural hearing loss; involve either unaided or aided LDL measures; and use self-report of loudness acceptance with hearing aids used in the real world. The search strategy resulted in 187 articles from which 173 were eliminated, with 14 articles remaining for further consideration. Of those, 11 were further eliminated in a second-round review, resulting in 3 articles for inclusion in the systematic review. The articles included only unaided LDL measurements that were at level 4 of evidence. No studies obtaining aided LDLs were included. The results of this systematic review indicated some evidence supporting unaided LDLs, but it was not worthy of a strong recommendation that doing so results in aided acceptance and satisfaction of loudness in the real world. Further, it shows how some measurements that audiologists routinely make in hearing aid evaluations are not strongly supported by scientific evidence.

Memories or **programs** are different settings on the hearing aid that listeners may use for various listening situations. Each memory or program changes the internal functioning of the hearing aid to suit patients' needs in certain listening situations. For example, patients, along with their audiologists, may prioritize communications situations in which they need help such as in understanding a dinner companion in a noisy restaurant. Separate programs may be needed for listening on the telephone, for example.

Hearing aid manufacturers have developed digital noise reduction (DNR) algorithms that acoustically analyze sound coming into the hearing aid and change the gain and output to minimize the amplification of noise (Bentler & Chiou, 2006). How does a hearing aid do this? Although there are several methods of DNR, the most common is the detection of the difference in amplitude or intensity modulation between speech and noise. Because syllables vary in duration from 75 to 150 milliseconds, speech has 4 to 6 modulations per second (Mueller & Ricketts, 2005). During syllable production, amplitude increases and between syllables, it decreases creating modulation. In a quiet environment, DNR is not activated because the hearing aid is able to recognize the amplitude modulation of speech. Alternatively, constant noise, such as that encountered at a party, has a fairly consistent amplitude over time. Therefore, when the steady state amplitude of noise is detected, the hearing aid reduces the gain in certain frequency regions to reduce its masking effects on speech (Ricketts, 2005).

Another complaint of new hearing aid wearers, particularly those who wear high-powered instruments, is feedback. Hearing aid manufacturers have developed digital feedback suppression schemes that monitor for the presence of feedback and then eliminate it through cancellation systems or notch filtering (Ricketts, 2005). Older styles of hearing aids with analog circuitry required that patients turn down their volume control wheels to reduce feedback. Digital feedback suppression schemes eliminate the problem before it becomes noticeable to patients.

Monaural Versus Binaural Fittings. One decision to be made is whether patients should receive amplification to one ear (i.e., monaural) or two (i.e., binaural). It is widely accepted that binaural amplification is the fitting strategy of choice for patients with bilateral

table *6.5*   Reasons Why People Should Wear Two Hearing Aids

1. Better understanding of speech
2. Better understanding in group and even noisy situations
3. Better ability to tell the direction of sound
4. Better sound quality
5. Smoother tone quality
6. Wider hearing range
7. Better sound identification
8. Keeps both ears active resulting in less hearing loss deterioration
9. Hearing is less tiring and listening more pleasant
10. Feeling of balanced hearing
11. Reduced feedback and whistling
12. Tinnitus masking
13. Consumer preference
14. Customer satisfaction

Source: Reprinted with permission from "The Consumer Handbook on Hearing Loss & Hearing Aids—A Bridge to Healing." Auricle Ink Publishers, 2009, pp. 96–98. Developed further at: The Gellar Hearing Institute www.betterhearing.org.

sensorineural hearing loss. Simply stated, two ears are better than one. Kochkin (2000) provided a handout (see Table 6.5) that states reasons why someone with a bilateral hearing loss should consider binaural amplification. Refer to Kochkin (2000) for an excellent discussion of the psychoacoustic and acoustic evidence for the binaural advantage.

Some patients, however, should be considered for monaural fittings. A typical scenario for these patients is that they are experienced hearing aid users who were originally fit with monaural amplification. Patients with these profiles may have experienced auditory deprivation, defined earlier as some loss of integrity of the sensory system due to a lack of external auditory stimulation (Kochkin, 2000). In other words, failing to amplify an ear with a significant hearing loss for an extended period of time may result in a lack of the necessary stimulation of the auditory pathways for maintaining speech recognition skills. For example, Silman, Gelfand, and Silverman (1984) compared the pure-tone thresholds, speech-recognition thresholds, and speech-recognition scores of the right and left ears of participants in one of two groups: (1) those with binaural amplification and (2) those with monaural fittings. Present performances were compared with those measured four to five years before being fit with hearing aids. The results indicated that there were no significant differences over time for pure-tone thresholds or speech-recognition thresholds between the ears for both groups of hearing aid users. However, the group of patients with monaural hearing aid fittings showed a significant decrease in speech recognition performance in the unaided ear, demonstrating the possible effects of auditory deprivation. These patients may prefer to continue with monaural fittings because aiding a previously unaided ear may not be desirable for some.

Let's look in on Bill and Dottie and see what progress has been made in terms of hearing aid selection.

Bill and Dottie Roberts: Hearing Aid Selection

The Roberts, in consultation with Dr. Chew, already had made several decisions regarding hearing aid selection during the counseling session. For example, they had decided on binaural open-ear digital hearing aids. Regarding external features, the open-ear model that Bill was considering did not have a volume control wheel, but a switch to select different programs for setting the loudness in different listening situations and when using the telecoil. Bill and Dottie were also excited about the adaptive directional microphones that automatically focus on amplifying speech energy based on location of the speaker. Moreover, regarding internal features, Bill's hearing aids would have digital noise reduction and a feedback suppression scheme.

Dr. Chew, though, needed to obtain some additional measurements to select certain parameters related to gain processing using a prescriptive method. Dottie remained in the consultation room as the others went back to the audiometric suite.

Dr. Chew: "Bill, I need to obtain some additional measurements in the audiometric booth. I'm going to be playing some noise to you through the insert earphones to determine your loudness discomfort levels for low-, medium, and high-frequency sounds. I'd like you to use the following chart by pointing to the words that indicate your perceptions of the loudness of the noise."

The chart showed the following seven categories of loudness (Cox, 1995):

- Uncomfortably loud
- Loud but OK
- Comfortable but slightly loud
- Comfortable
- Comfortable but slightly soft
- Soft
- Very soft

The testing resulted in identification of dB HL levels for narrow bands of noise centered at 500,

1000, 1500, and 3000 Hz that Bill had labeled as "Loud but OK" and "uncomfortably loud." These data along with the audiometric thresholds enable Dr. Chew to use settings for gain, OSPL90, and compression circuitry. For example, the audiometric thresholds are used to predict the amount of gain needed from a hearing aid: "Loud but OK" indicates levels that are acceptably loud, and "uncomfortably loud" indicates LDLs. That is, the OSPL90 of the hearing aid should not exceed the LDL measurements. This information will be input into NOAH and used during the hearing aid fitting process.

Clinical Recommendations

- The style of hearing aid should be selected based on factors such as gain/output, ear canal size, cosmetics, and so on.
  GRADES: B AND C

- Binaural amplification is recommended for most patients.
  GRADE: B

- Direct-audio-input and telecoil circuitry should be considered when appropriate.
  GRADES: Telecoil: C

- Gain characteristics provided by the hearing aid should be based on prescriptive methods.
  GRADE: B

- Output and OSPL90 should be based on measures of threshold of discomfort.
  GRADE: B

- Multiple memories may be helpful when specific signal processing is needed in select environments.
  GRADE: A

- Digital noise reduction may make the quality of sound better and provide more comfort for patients.
  GRADE: D

- Switchable directional/omnidirectional microphones are recommended for patients who report difficulty understanding speech in noise.
  GRADE: B

- Output and OSPL90 should be based on measures of threshold of discomfort.
  GRADE: B

Quality Control

Valente, Abrams, et al. (2006) stated that the primary purpose of quality control is to ensure that selected hearing aids meet standards prior to hearing aid verification and fitting on patients. Quality control includes executing a visual and listening check of hearing aids and earmolds, if applicable, in addition to an electroacoustic analysis to verify functioning according to the manufacturer's specifications. Audiologists should not assume that hearing aids arriving from the manufacturer are functioning properly. For example, a hearing aid may be dropped during shipment and may not work at all. Valente, Abrams, et al. (2006) stated verification should also include substantiation of earmold/shell style, appropriate venting, color, as well as mechanical and hearing aid processing features.

Casebook Reflection

Bill and Dottie Roberts: Quality Control

Dr. Chew had already performed a visual/listening check of the hearing aid and performed electroacoustic analysis and determined that both instruments were functioning according to the manufacturer's specifications.

Clinical Recommendations

- An electroacoustic analysis should be done on new hearing aids.
  GRADE: D

Fitting and Verification of Hearing Aids

Valente, Abrams, et al.'s (2006) objective for fitting and verification of hearing aids consists of a process that results in an optimal fitting for the patient and establishes a baseline of performance against which future adjustments will be compared. The fitting and verification process includes consideration of (1) physical fit, (2) occlusion effect, (3) selection of assessment signal, (4) gain verification, (5) output verification, (6) aided sound-field threshold, and (7) verification of special features.

Valente, Abrams, et al. (2006) recommended that audiologists check the physical fit of the hearing aids according to the following criteria: (1) ease of insertion and removal, (2) patient comfort during both static and dynamic jaw movement, (3) appropriateness of microphone angles, and (4) no audible feedback. Patients should be easily able to insert and remove hearing aids without difficulty, and they should not have to struggle or strain to insert or remove their hearing aids. Likewise, the earmolds or hearing aids should be comfortable when in the ear, with or without jaw movement. Finally, proper earmold and hearing aid fitting should not result in audible feedback. Unfortunately, these problems may not be evident during the initial fitting and may present during follow-up appointments.

Audiologists should also assess for the occlusion effect both through subjective patient report and objective physical measurement. Patients' subjective complaints may include that their own voices sound loud or funny (Staab, Dennis, Schweitzer, & Weber, 2004). In addition, the occlusion effect can be objectively measured using real-ear probe-microphone measurements or through using the Occlusion Effect Meter ER-33, manufactured by Etymotic Research, by comparing the open-ear unoccluded response during patient vocalization to the occluded (e.g., with an earmold or hearing aid in place) responses (MacKenzie et al., 2004). The occlusion effect is the difference in dB SPL between the "unaided," or unoccluded, ear and "aided," or occluded, response for each ear (MacKenzie et al., 2004). The larger the difference in SPL, the greater is the occlusion effect. The occlusion effect can be minimized through the use of venting. Audiologists should use both subjective and objective data in determining the most appropriate vent size for the patient. Other styles of hearing aids, such as deep-canal fitting CICs, may eliminate the occlusion effect.

With many of today's hearing aids, the manufacturers' software on NOAH (e.g., NOAHFit) can program patients' hearing aids based on their audiometric thresholds and LDL measurements. The hearing aids are connected to the computer system and programmed automatically. Many manufacturers have fitting programs that allow patients to get accustomed to their new hearing aids via **first-fit programming**. As the patient gets used to his or her hearing aids, these settings are gradually changed to achieve maximum audibility of speech without loudness discomfort. For the most part, first-fit programming is based on well-known prescriptive fitting methods. Nevertheless, many audiologists like to verify fittings using real-ear probe-tube microphone measurements to ensure that targets have been reached.

Considerable debate has been devoted to what type of test signal should be used in verifying gain and output of hearing aids via real-ear probe-tube microphone measurements. One question under consideration is, "Should a speechlike stimulus be used or a nonspeech stimulus in verifying gain and output?" Another issue is how gain and output should be adjusted and verified. Let's see what the evidence shows.

What Does the Evidence Show?

Mueller and Bentler (2005) conducted a systematic review of the evidence supporting the use of prescriptive methods for selecting and verifying hearing aid parameters. Specifically, the experimental question was "Are there real-world outcome measures from adult patients who show a preference for the gain prescribed by a specific prescriptive fitting procedure?" In other words, what types of outcomes are obtained from patients whose gain targets are described by different prescriptive methods? Mueller used relevant search strings in research databases (i.e., PubMed, Medline, CINAHL, and EMBASE) to retrieve titles of studies to possibly include in the systematic review. The included studies had to have been published between 1985 and 2005; employ a randomized control, randomized crossover, a quasi-experimental, or noninterventional descriptive research design; employ adult participants with hearing impairment; use real-ear probe-tube microphone measurements for verification of attainment of prescribed targets; use consistent technology through the course of the investigation; have participants use hearing aids in the real world; and provide data from outcome measures pertaining to use of gain, self-report of prescriptive gain preference, or real-world benefit (Mueller & Bentler, 2005). Mueller's search and retrieval process uncovered 136 initial articles for review of which 94 articles were eliminated, leaving 42 articles to consider for inclusion in the systematic review. Ultimately, 11 articles were included in the systematic review. Mueller concluded that the evidence supported use of a speechlike stimulus in the verification of gain and that use of first-fit programming by manufacturers is acceptable, providing it prescribes gain similarly to the NAL-RP/NL1 prescriptive method verified via real-ear probe-microphone measurement of real-ear insertion gain (REIG) or real-ear aided response (REAR). The evidence also supported adjustment of gain/compression parameters to within 2 to 3 dB or as much as 5 dB of targets at key frequencies for adult patients with mild to moderately severe sensorineural hearing loss (Mueller & Bentler, 2005).

Other types of verification include aided sound-field thresholds and assessment of special features. In the past, obtaining aided sound-field thresholds, or functional gain, was one of few hearing aid fitting verification measures. Briefly, patients were placed in a sound field, and thresholds were obtained for warbled tones transduced through loudspeakers. The difference between unaided and aided thresholds was the functional gain of the hearing aids. The evidence is not strong for using functional gain as a valid verification measure due to the lack of standardization of the test environment, for example (Valente, Abrams, et al., 2006). Verification of special features of hearing aids is important, particularly for patients with specific needs. For example, the functionality of adaptive directional microphones may be accomplished by determining how much improvement in signal-to-noise ratio (S/N) is provided to patients, resulting in 50% correct recognition of sentences using the HINT Test (Nilsson et al., 1994).

Casebook Reflection

Bill and Dottie Roberts: Fitting and Verification of Hearing Aids

Dr. Chew set Bill's open-ear hearing aids using the manufacturer's first-fit program. He then fit the hearing aids to Bill's ears using appropriately sized speaker links and domes. He verified the physical fit of the hearing aids with Bill. He then provided Bill with a mirror.

Dr. Chew: "How do they look and how do they feel?"
Bill: "They look great!"
Dottie: "Yes, they do!"
Dr. Chew: "How do they sound?"
Bill: "They sound pretty good, but maybe a little loud."
Dr. Chew: "Are they uncomfortably loud?"
Bill: "No, just loud. . . ."
Dottie: "Well, you haven't been hearing much!"
Bill: "Guess not!"
Dr. Chew: "We need to do some verification measurements, and it may take 10 to 20 minutes. It is

called real-ear probe-tube microphone measures, which will verify that the hearing aids are hitting their targets and that they won't be too loud. We need to insert a probe into your ear and would like you to remain very still. Let me turn the hearing aids off and take them out of your ears. Once we set up for real ear, I will put the hearing aids back in and will be asking you a few questions throughout the process."

Dottie watched with excitement as Dr. Chew performed real-ear measurements on her husband while periodically asking him some questions. He tried to explain what he was doing to Dottie at the same time, but she got glassy-eyed from hearing more details than she found interesting. At the end of testing, Dr. Chew had verified that the manufacturer's first-fit program hit targets for gain based on a reputable prescriptive method (i.e., NAL-RP/NL1) and provided output that did not exceed Bill's LDLs.

Clinical Recommendations

- Gain characteristics provided by the hearing aid should be based on prescriptive methods.

  GRADE: B

- Speech or speechlike signals should be used in hearing aid verification, particularly when the outputs are based on speech input.

  GRADE: B

- Appropriateness of the physical fit of hearing aids should be verified.

  GRADE: C

- Verification of prescribed gain via real-ear probe-tube microphone measurements should be co-validated using a validated prescriptive method.

  GRADE: B

- Output verification using real-ear measurement techniques should determine if levels exceed patients' thresholds of discomfort.

  GRADE: B

Hearing Assistive Technology (HAT)

For some patients, hearing aids are not enough to meet all of their communication needs. Valente, Abrams, et al. (2006) reviewed the following four areas of communication needs mentioned by Compton (1999):

- Live face-to-face communication (e.g., playing bridge, listening to a sermon, talking with friends at a cocktail party)
- Broadcast and other electronic media (e.g., watching television, listening to the radio, watching a DVD)
- Telephone conversation (e.g., talking to family members on the telephone)
- Awareness of alerting signals (e.g., hearing the phone ring, knocks at the door, or alarm clock) and environmental stimuli (e.g., hearing the dog barking, an automobile horn, a baby crying)

The selection, evaluation, and fitting of HAT are discussed in Chapter 7. Generally, the patients' goals for amplification are reviewed, and HAT is a consideration if some objectives may not be met through the use of hearing aids alone.

Casebook Reflection

Bill and Dottie Roberts: Hearing Assistive Technology

One of Bill's goals was to hear better on his cell phone without having to turn the volume all the way up and turning the speaker on. Dr. Chew knew that was a problem that couldn't be fixed by hearing aids alone. So, he inquired about the make and model of his cell phone and then contacted a local cell phone store selling accessories. He asked if there was a neckloop that could be used with that make and model of cell phone. The manager said yes and ordered one to be sent to Dr. Chew's practice, which he would provide at a few dollars above cost to account for time spent in fitting the HAT.

Clinical Recommendations

- Hearing assistive technology should be considered for patients' communication needs not met through the use of hearing aids alone.

  GRADES: B AND C

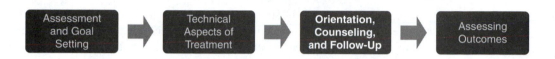

Orientation, Counseling, and Follow-Up

The primary objective of orientation, counseling, and follow-up is to facilitate patients' and their families' acquisition of benefits derived from the use of amplification (Valente, Abrams, et al., 2006). Specifics for patients of different ages and their families are covered in Chapter 12, discussing auditory rehabilitation across the life span.

Hearing Aid Orientation

The hearing aid orientation period begins during the hearing aid delivery and may extend throughout the trial period. The hearing aid delivery should include the patient and one other family member and/or significant other. The hearing aid orientation consists of the audiologist conveying device-related and patient-related information that should be presented orally and in writing (Valente, Abrams, et al., 2006).

Device-Related Information.   Device-related information should include a description of hearing aid features (e.g., use of multiple programs, telephone-coil operation, directional microphones, direct-audio input; insertion/removal of the hearing aid; battery use [including sizes used, how to change, disposal, purchase options, and so on]; care and cleaning; comfort; feedback; telephone use; and warranty protection [Valente, Abrams, et al., 2006]).

Insertion and removal of hearing aids can be a challenge for patients and their family members. Orientation for this skill must be explained, demonstrated, and practiced by the patient and/or family member. Patients should be reminded that their hearing aids should be off or at low volume during insertion and removal to avoid feedback. Audiologists should require that the patient independently complete this task at least once before leaving the appointment. Some patients, particularly those who are elderly, may not be able to complete this task without assistance and therefore must rely on significant others. Patients should be reminded to practice insertion and removal over a soft surface (e.g., sitting on a bed or standing over a soft carpet) in case they drop their hearing aid. Initially, patients should use a mirror to check to see that their hearing aid is inserted properly.

Patients should be told that hearing aid batteries come in different sizes that are indicated by number and a standardized color coding scheme. Common hearing aid battery sizes range from very small to large: 5 (red tab), 10 (or 230) (yellow tab), 312 (brown tab), 13 (orange tab), and 675 (blue tab), respectively (Rayovac, 2006). Patients should expect their hearing aid batteries to last approximately 5 to 7 days, based on the number of hours of use per day and the type of hearing aid. Patients should be told that removal of the colored tab on the hearing aid activates the battery, and its placement back on the battery will not deactivate it. Therefore, patients should be absolutely sure that the battery needs replacing prior to activating another one. Explanation of how to change a battery should include *both* audiologist and patient demonstration of this task, particularly the new elderly hearing aid wearer with arthritis. Therefore, special tabbing by battery manufacturers should be used for ease in changing. Two strategies are helpful in knowing when to replace a battery. One is for the patient to purchase an inexpensive battery tester. Another strategy is for the patient to keep a battery calendar by placing its tab on the day of activation. Patients can get an idea of how long to expect their batteries to last based on their individual needs. If the batteries need to be changed more frequently than usual, hearing aids may be malfunctioning. Batteries should be stored in a cool, dry place. Patients and their family members should be advised on options for purchase. For example, many audiologists operate battery clubs offering discounts for batteries bought by the case, as patients can expect a shelf life of at least three years. Hearing aids and batteries should be kept safely away from children and pets. Patients should be given the number of the National Button Battery Ingestion Hotline, which is (202) 625-3333. If a hearing aid battery is swallowed, a trip should be made to the emergency room at the nearest hospital for X-rays to determine the location of the battery to see if it is lodged in a particular area needing surgery for removal or if it will pass out of the body naturally.

Proper care and cleaning of hearing aids can extend their lives and are important components of the orientation. First, patients need to be instructed on how to clean their hearing aids and earmolds. Each night the hearing aid and earmold should be wiped off with a soft and dry cloth to remove excess moisture, earwax, and body oils. Excess moisture can be minimized using a forced-air bulb, and earwax can be removed with wax loops and soft brushes. Care should be taken using these tools on in-the-ear hearing aids (e.g., classic ITE, ITC, and CIC) so that damage is not done to the receiver. Special devices, called earwax guards, prevent cerumen impaction from damaging hearing aids. It should also be emphasized that moisture can cause damage, and hearing aids should be inserted only into ears that are dry, particularly after showering.

At night, hearing aids should be kept with their battery doors open in a dehumidifier to draw out excess moisture. Dehumidifiers can be elaborate or simple. For example, Dry 'N Store is an elaborate electrical unit with a drawer for placement of hearing aids for an eight-hour cycle that includes exposure to an ultraviolet light to kill bacteria, circulating warm/dry air to release moisture and loosen extra earwax, and a desiccant brick to absorb excess moisture. A picture of this device is shown in Figure 6.37.

Dri-Aid Kits are simple dehumidifiers in which hearing aids are placed nightly with battery doors open so that a desiccant can absorb any moisture from the devices. Figure 6.38 shows a Dri-Aid Kit (top), which consists of a metal canister containing **silica gel**, a desiccant material, that pulls moisture out of the hearing aid that is placed into the bag at night. The Super Dri-Aid Kit (bottom) works on the same principle except that the dessicant material is located under a sponge upon which hearing aids with battery doors open are placed at night with the cap sealed on the jar.

Last, hearing aids should not be exposed to conditions of extreme heat or humidity such as placement on heaters,

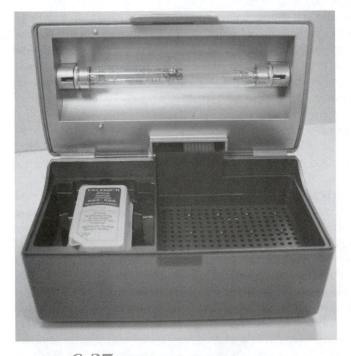

figure *6.37*

A Dry 'N Store hearing aid dehumidifier and cleaner.

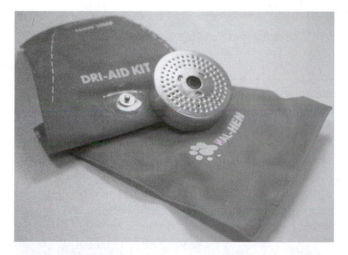

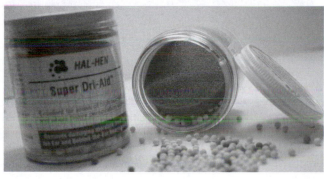

figure *6.38*

Dri-Aid kits.

radiators, or on the dashboards of cars on hot days. Likewise, hearing aids should not be worn in situations of extreme humidity such as in a steam bath.

Patients should be given a troubleshooting guide similar to the one shown in Table 6.6 that provides possible problems, things to check for, and solutions. Patients should be encouraged to solve simple problems before calling their audiologists.

In brief, four common problems and their possible solutions are shown as follows:

- **If the hearing aid produces no sound**–Patients should check/correct for closure of the battery compartment, battery positioning, voltage, and contact corrosion; switches in the "on" position and volume control wheel setting; and/or the existence of earwax in the receiver/earmold bore or moisture in the tubing.

- **If the sound is weak or intermittent**–Patients should check/correct for battery voltage, contact corrosion, and/or existence of earwax in the receiver or earmold bore.

- **If the hearing aid feedbacks or whistles**–Patients should check/correct for proper fit of the earmold/hearing aid, too high of a volume, or existence of a crack in the tubing or hearing aid case. If all else fails, patients should make an appointment with an audiologist or physician who can check for impacted cerumen.

- **If the hearing aid produces poor sound quality**–Patients should check/correct for battery voltage, contact corrosion, or moisture in the tubing or the earmold.

Patients should expect that their hearing aids should be physically comfortable and not give feedback. Patients should return to the audiologist if the hearing aids or earmolds cause the development of sore spots in their ears. Blisters and tender spots indicate a need for modification in the audiologist's laboratory. Similarly, feedback, or whistling, is another problem needing attention to ensure that amplified sound from the receiver is not picked up by the microphone. Modifications include isolating the receiver from the microphone, replacing or modifying the earmold or hearing aid casing, removing excessive cerumen in the external ear canal, and so on. Patients should be instructed to contact their audiologist if they are experiencing excessive feedback.

Audiologists should explain, demonstrate, and require patient mastery of telephone use with hearing aids during the hearing aid delivery. Patients who use ITC and CIC hearing aids can use the telephone naturally by simply placing the telephone receiver up to their ear as usual. However, some BTE hearing aids have microphone-telephone-off

table *6.6*   Hearing Aid Problems: Things to Check for and Possible Solutions

Problem	Check	Solution
No sound	• Closure of the battery compartment door	• Secure the door
	• Battery	
	• Positioning	• Position the battery correctly
	• Voltage	• Change the battery
	• Contacts for corrosion	• Clean the battery contacts
	• Switches	
	• On-off	• Turn the hearing aid on
	• Volume control wheel	• Turn the volume wheel up
	• For wax	• Use wax pick or soft brush
	• In the earmold bore	
	• Receiver	
	• For moisture in the tubing	• Use forced-air bulb to blow moisture out of the tubing
Sound is weak and/or intermittent	• Battery	
	• Voltage	• Change the battery
	• Contacts for corrosion	• Clean the battery contacts
	• For wax	• Use wax pick or soft brush
	• In the earmold bore	
	• Receiver	
Feedback or whistling	• Fit of earmold or hearing aid	• Position earmold or hearing aid properly to avoid sound leakage
	• Volume	• Turn down the volume
	• Cracks in the hearing aid/or tubing	• Contact your audiologist
	• Excessive wax in the ear canal	• Contact your audiologist or physician
Poor sound quality or scratchiness	• Moisture in the tubing	• Use forced-air bulb to blow moisture out of the tubing
	• Battery	
	• Voltage	• Change the battery
	• Contacts for corrosion	• Clean the battery contacts

Sources: Information from "A Troubleshooting Guide for Your Hearing Aid Patients and Families," by R. L. Martin, 1999, *The Hearing Journal, 53*(2), p. 66; *Troubleshooting Your Hearing Aid*, by M. Ross, 2006, retrieved from http://www.healthyhearing.com/articles/7835_troubleshooting_your_hearing_aid.htm.

(MTO) switches, and many ITEs have telecoil switches that must be used to access the telecoil and volume control wheels. For BTEs, the telephone receiver should be placed near the hearing aid, not the patient's ear, and some experimentation may be needed to achieve optimal positioning for maximum signal viability. For ITEs, the telephone receiver should be held near the hearing aid. For BTEs without telecoils, the telephone receiver should be placed in close proximity to the microphone. For ITEs without t-coils, the telephone receiver should be in close proximity to the hearing aid. However, if feedback occurs, a phone pad or WhistleStop accessory (i.e., a cylinder of plastic snapped onto the telephone receiver should be used for isolation and funneling of sound to the microphone without feedback) on the telephone receiver. Elderly patients may need extensive practice in mastering telephone use with their hearing aids.

Patients should be told about the details of their hearing aid warranty. Patients may not know what they need to know. Critical information includes warranty expiration, additional coverage after initial expiration, what is covered and what is not, loss and damage, and shipping costs (Meier, 2006). Different hearing aid manufacturers have different warranties, but most are for one year and some are for two years. Patients can purchase extended warranties from the manufacturer, their audiologists, or insurance companies (Meier, 2006). Most warranties cover all internal parts of a hearing aid and any manufacturer defects in the casing or shell, but may not cover shipping costs for repair (Meier, 2006).

Patient-Related Information.   Patient-related information includes wearing schedule (i.e., goals/expectations and adjusting to amplification), environmental issues (e.g., family, social, school, and work settings), improved hearing aid listening strategies, speechreading, monaural/binaural hearing aid use, and postfitting care (Valente, Abrams, et al., 2006). Patients should slowly adjust to amplification by initially wearing their hearing aids a few hours a day in quiet environments, then gradually increasing their use to longer periods of time in a variety of situations. Patients must have realistic expectations regarding the benefits derived from the use of amplification and be patient with the process. Review of the nomination and prioritization of problem listening situations on the COSI establishes patients' focus, accountability, and active participation in the adjustment process. Audiologists should underscore that hearing aids alone cannot solve all communication problems. Patients need coaching on improved listening and communication strategies involving significant others. Table 6.7 shows tips for spouses and significant others and for new hearing aid wearers, respectively (Wayner & Abrahamson, 2001). For example, spouses or significant others should be considerate in communicating by making sure that their loved one has their full attention before speaking. Furthermore, they should not try to communicate in the kitchen with the dishwasher on. Likewise, new hearing aid users need to be effective communicators by providing feedback to speakers, paying attention, observing the talker, and so on.

Coaching on environmental issues is critical for new hearing aid users to achieve maximum benefit from amplification. Specific instruction should be tailored to the particular features on patients' hearing aids. New hearing aid wearers with programs for specific environments (e.g., use of directional microphones in restaurants) need to be reminded of the existence of those programs and when and how to use them. Specific assignments involving these situations could be incorporated into their adjustment schedules, ensuring the application of new knowledge and skills with their hearing aids. Moreover, patients need consciousness-raising in seeking the best location in certain environments and being assertive about their communication needs. For example, new hearing aid wearers should know how to find and ask to be seated in the area providing the best communication environment. Details of these strategies are provided in Chapter 12.

New hearing aid wearers should be instructed on the information provided by visual aspects of communication through **speechreading**, which is a process by which listeners put

table *6.7* New Hearing Aid Wearers: Communication Tips for Spouses and Significant Others

- *Get the listener's attention* before you speak.
- *Do not shout* because talking louder does not help.
- *Slow down a bit* to aid listeners' reception of information.
- *Get closer* to reduce the urge to shout and improve listeners' understanding.
- *Speak clearly* by finishing all of the speech sounds of one word before beginning the next, but do not overexaggerate pronunciation.
- *Rephrase your message* when listeners do not understand the first time by using different words to express the same idea.
- *State the topic* of conversation at the start and whenever the topic changes.
- *Use gestures* to augment your message.
- *Minimize the effects of noise* either by turning things off (e.g., fan) or moving to a quiet area.
- *Confirm comprehension* of information by politely double-checking listeners' receipt of important details (e.g., times and places).
- *Be visible* by making sure that listeners can see your face.
- *Simplify the message* by eliminating useless details.

Source: Information from *Learning to Hear Again: An Audiologic Rehabilitation Curriculum,* Second Edition, by D. S. Wayner and J. E. Abrahamson, 2001, Lantham, NY Hear Again.

together information from a variety of sources to derive meaning. The sources of information include lipreading; facial expressions; gesture, posture, and movement; situational cues; the topic of conversation; rules of the language; news of the day; motivation to understand; and residual hearing (Cherry & Rubenstein, 1988). Patients need to be told that speechreading is not just **lipreading**, which is watching the speaker and deriving meaning from recognition of the visible aspects of articulation. Patients should be advised that confusion often occurs because some sounds look the same on the mouth. For example, /p/, /b/, and /m/ all look the same on the mouth and are all in the same *viseme group*, which are sounds grouped together that look the same on the mouth. The phonemes /f/ and /v/ form another viseme group. It should be explained that ambiguous lipreading cues can cause confusion, but can be overcome using other elements of speechreading. For example, a new hearing aid user's audiovisual perception of a sentence may have been, "The pan gave a speech at the banquet," but because of their knowledge of language, he or she knows that the correct message was, "The man gave a speech at the banquet."

New hearing aid wearers with binaural fittings should be advised to use both hearing aids in order to adjust properly to amplification. They may need to be reminded about the benefits derived from the use of binaural amplification covered earlier in this chapter. During the hearing aid delivery, audiologists should emphasize the importance of adherence to follow-up appointments and attendance at a hearing aid orientation group.

Counseling and Follow-Up

As will be discussed in Chapter 12, group hearing aid orientation classes have been shown to result in the reduction of self-perceived hearing handicap, improved quality of life, improvement in specific communication situations, and reduction in the return-for-credits

table *6.8* Topics to Be Covered in Refresher Courses for New and Experienced Hearing Aid Wearers

- Basic anatomy and physiology of the hearing process
- Understanding the audiogram
- Problems associated with understanding speech in noise
- Appropriate and inappropriate hearing and listening behaviors
- Listening and repair strategies
- Controlling the environment
- Assertiveness
- Realistic expectations
- Stress management
- Basic speechreading
- Hearing assistive technology
- Helpful hints for communicating with spouse
- Helpful hints for spouse communicating with patient
- Hearing aid use and care
- Community resources

(Abrams, Chisolm, & McArdle, 2002; Abrams, Hnath-Chisolm, Guerreiro, & Ritterman, 1992; Beyer & Northern, 2000; Chisolm, Abrams, & McArdle, 2004; Valente, Abrams, et al., 2006). Typically, these groups involve new hearing aid wearers, spouses, and/or significant others and focus on ways to minimize the deleterious effects of hearing loss on communication through the use of amplification. Moreover, they may be suitable as a "refresher course" for experienced hearing aid users (Valente, Abrams, et al., 2006). Table 6.8 shows topics to be covered in these sessions. Counseling can also be accomplished in individual sessions and sometimes may be needed for patients having complications.

Casebook Reflection

Bill and Dottie Roberts: Hearing Aid Orientation, Counseling, and Follow-Up

It had been a long afternoon, but Dottie had not seen Bill so motivated about getting hearing aids. It was mid-afternoon, and Dr. Chew suggested that Bill and Dottie take a break to have some coffee and donuts and then join him in the consultation room.

Dr. Chew: "Well, it is has been a long day. Now, I will tell you about the care, use, and maintenance of your new hearing aids. We're going to go over a lot of information. However, everything I'm going to tell you is written down in this information packet. Be sure to ask me any time that you have a question. We will begin with insertion and removal of your hearing aids. I will first demonstrate with an exact duplicate of your hearing aid. Make sure that the hearing aid is off so it does not squeal when you put it in. Put the part that fits into your ear first, then gently drape the speaker loop around the top of your ear and rest the device in the pocket behind your ear. OK, you try it."

Dr. Chew proceeded to cover all of the device-related information (e.g., use of multiple programs, telephone coil operation, directional microphones, direct-audio input, insertion/removal of the hearing aid, battery use [including sizes used, how to change, disposal, purchase options, and so on], care and cleaning, comfort, feedback, telephone use, and warranty protection). He also reviewed Bill's goals for amplification so that they would be on the same page.

Dr. Chew: "Don't wear your hearing aids when driving home. Start wearing them at home first for a few hours a day, then gradually increasing to all day and in all situations. Let me know if you have any questions, discomfort, or difficulty in operating your remote control. . . . I want to see you here in a week at 3:00 p.m. for a follow-up appointment and then at 3:30 p.m. for the first meeting of the Hearing Aid Counseling group. . . . Let me remind you that it is going to take some time to get used to hearing sounds that you haven't heard in a while, including how speech may sound different. This process is called acclimatization."

Bill: "Thank you, Doctor."

Dottie: "Yes, thank you."

Bill and Dottie returned the following week for a follow-up appointment and attended the group counseling sessions. Bill needed several adjustments to his programs and had some difficulties operating the remote control. At first, Bill had been reticent about joining other couples to talk about his hearing loss. However, once other participants opened up about how they felt, Bill didn't feel so alone. He found suggestions from others helpful and felt that Dottie benefited from the input of other spouses of new hearing aid wearers. In addition, she was able to open up about her feelings of frustration about which she would never have confronted her husband.

Clinical Recommendations

- Important information about hearing aid use and maintenance should be presented to patients and at least one significant other during hearing aid orientation.
  GRADES: B and C

- Postfitting counseling and follow-up should be provided to new and experienced hearing aid wearers.
  GRADES: A and B

- Hearing aid orientation and counseling should include patients' significant others.
  GRADE: B

- Hearing aid orientation and counseling may be provided on a one-on-one basis or in group situations.
  GRADE: B

- The hearing aid orientation counseling should cover a variety of topics.
  GRADES: A and B

- Patients and their family members need to be counseled that getting used to amplification may take a while.
  GRADE: B

Assessment and Goal Setting → Technical Aspects of Treatment → Orientation, Counseling, and Follow-Up → **Assessing Outcomes**

Assessing Outcomes

Outcome measurement is the last step in the process. The objective of this segment of the process is to validate the hearing aid fitting by measuring the effects on patients' impairment, activity limitations, participation restrictions, and quality of life (Valente, Abrams, et al., 2006). Moreover, other important outcome measures have to do with hearing aid satisfaction. Measuring outcomes takes place after the patient has acclimatized to amplification and should include revisiting some of the income measures used during the assessment and goal-setting stage. Measurements made at this time are now outcome measures. For example, it is now time for the audiologists, patients, and their families to evaluate the situations nominated and prioritized on the COSI to determine progress regarding activity limitations. Similarly, patients may fill out the HHIA and HHIE so that comparisons can be made to pretreatment results.

Some outcome measures are completed only at the end of the auditory rehabilitation process. For example, one particularly useful outcome measure is the *International Outcome Inventory for Hearing Aids* (IOI-HA) (Cox & Alexander, 2002), which can be found in Appendix 6.6. The IOI-HA has seven items for measuring the outcomes of hearing aid treatment. The IOI-HA has been found to be psychometrically fit and has two statistically sound domains: (1) benefit and (2) residual problems (Cox & Alexander, 2002). Furthermore, it has been found that the two outcome items on the COSI correlate well with patients' scores on the benefit domain, but not the residual problem domains on the IOI-HA (Stephens, 2002). The IOI-HA has been translated into several languages promoting international agreement for use of outcome measures (Cox, Stephens, & Kramer, 2002). Appendix 6.7 shows commonly used outcome measures in audiology as a function of domain. In addition, audiologists should informally ask patients and their family members whether their affective goals have been achieved through amplification.

Casebook Reflection

Bill and Dottie Roberts: Outcome Measures

Bill and Dottie had a final follow-up appointment with Dr. Chew to review the results of the outcome measures that were completed during the last group counseling session. Recall that Bill had nominated and prioritized four specific situations on the COSI, completed the HHIE, and talked about some personal affective goals for amplification. For all situations nominated on the COSI, he rated his degree of change as either "Better" or "Much Better," and his ability to hear in all situations with his hearing aids as either "Most of the Time" (i.e., 75%) or "Almost Always" (i.e.,

95%). Bill also completed the HHIE again, which was scored and showed a significant reduction on the social and emotional impact of hearing loss. Dr. Chew also had Bill complete the IOI-HA during this last follow-up meeting, which followed with a discussion of the results.

Dr. Chew: "Bill and Dottie, it is great to see you once again. I've reviewed the results of the outcome measures, the COSI, the HHIE, and the IOI-HA. It seems that the hearing aids and auditory rehabilitation have met all of your needs and reduced the negative impact of hearing loss on your psychosocial well-being. Also, the results on the IOI-HA are consistent with the other measures, which indicate that you're satisfied with your hearing aids."

Bill: "Yes, I am so pleased with the results. I should have done this earlier!"

Dr. Chew: "You had mentioned some affective goals. Do you still feel anxious or frustrated?"

Bill: "Well, old feelings take some time to change. I still feel anxious before my Kiwanis meetings, but feel empowered by the new strategies I've learned and the assistance provided by my hearing aids. Also, I don't feel pitied anymore by my grandchildren."

Dottie: "Also, the hearing aids and the group counseling situation improved our communication. I don't feel frustrated anymore. Thank you so much, Dr. Chew."

Dr. Chew: "Oh, my pleasure. I wish all of my patients could have as much success as you've had. I'll see you in one year for a hearing reevaluation and hearing aid check."

HEARING AID SELECTION AND FITTING IN CHILDREN

We conclude this chapter by discussing hearing aid selection, evaluation, and fitting on children. Children and their parents go through similar stages as those outlined earlier in this chapter for adults that consist of (Beauchaine, 2001):

- Making ear impressions for earmolds
- Making preliminary measurements
- Determining gain and output using a prescriptive approach
- Selecting the hearing aids
- Verifying the progress toward the target
- Validating the fitting and following up with parents

At the time of diagnosis of hearing loss, audiologists frequently follow the parents' lead in when to begin the intervention process, which commences with the making of earmold impressions. As discussed in Chapter 9, some parents may want to make earmold impressions during the diagnostic evaluation; some may prefer to wait until their next appointment to allow time to adjust to the diagnosis of hearing loss in their child. It is important that the earmolds are made of a soft, flexible material such as vinyl and that they fit securely and comfortably without feedback (Cunningham, 2007).

The second step in the process is measuring **real-ear–to-coupler difference (RECD)**. Earlier in the chapter it was mentioned that real-ear probe-tube microphone measures were necessary to measure what hearing aids are doing inside the patients' ear canals. However, real-ear measurements require the cooperation of the patient, needing them to hold still while delicate measurements are made with a real-ear probe-tube microphone positioned in the ear canal. Young children rarely have the patience to cooperate for extended periods of time. The RECD is the difference between sound pressure level as a function of frequency measured at a specific point in the ear canal to that when measured in a 2-cc coupler. Measuring the RECD requires the cooperation of young children, but for shorter durations than real-ear probe-tube microphone measurements. The materials needed for this procedure are a hearing aid analyzer/real-ear probe-tube microphone measurement system, a child's custom earmold or insert earphone, and comply wrap or other sticky material. The comply wrap is used to connect the child's earmold or insert earphone to the probe-microphone tip. The audiologist must ensure that the real-ear probe-tube microphone measurement system is calibrated and that the child's audiometric thresholds are entered into the computer. The computer sends an acoustic signal to the 2-cc coupler via the child's earmold or insert earphone; its response (i.e., SPL as a function of frequency) is measured with the probe tip, and presented on the computer screen. Next, the process is repeated, this time with the probe-tip positioned about 11 mm from the opening of the canal and attached to the child's earmold or insert earphone. The same stimulus is presented in the ear canal, the response is measured, and is also shown on the computer screen. The real-ear probe-tube microphone measurement system then computes the RECD. Some children may be too active to obtain RECD measurements. In this case, it may be advisable to use age-appropriate normative data for estimating RECD (Cunningham, 2007). Some experts have advised against using these values because of the wide variability of values across young patients (Cunningham, 2007). Next, the Desired Sensation Level (Scollie et al., 2005) prescriptive method determines the **SPL-O-GRAM**, or output targets for hearing aids, to ensure audibility of the **long-term average speech spectrum (LASS)**. The LASS is the sound pressure level as a function frequency for speech. The **SPL-O-GRAM** assists the audiologist in selecting children's hearing aids that have the electroacoustic characteristics that will make soft speech audible while avoiding loudness discomfort. The hearing aid evaluation should verify that hearing aids, in fact, are accomplishing their goals. RECDs should be measured every few months to account for growth and other factors that change during the first few years of life. As ear canal volume increases, the amount of gain needed to achieve targets diminishes, necessitating a change in hearing aid settings.

Chapter 9 explains important factors in delivering hearing aids to parents in addition to tools for validating fittings. It is important for parents to feel comfortable managing hearing aids and to make the connection between full-time device use and their children's achievement of positive outcomes in speech and language development (Moeller, 2010; Robbins, 2002). Follow-up appointments are critical for answering parents' questions and following children's compliance in wearing hearing aids. Parents' qualitative reports about infants' auditory behaviors and vocalizations assist the audiologist in determining benefits derived from the use of amplification. Consultation with a speech-language pathologist is necessary to determine if children are making adequate progress with hearing aids or if a referral to a cochlear implant center is warranted.

SUMMARY

This chapter has provided an introduction to amplification. The history and the contemporary styles of hearing aids were reviewed. Different types of hearing aids based on circuitry and patients with special needs were also reviewed. Readers were introduced to all of the tools used by audiologists prior to the discussion of the electroacoustic characteristics of these devices. One of the first evidence-based CPGs was discussed and used as a model in a process-driven approach to the selection, evaluation, and fitting of these devices.

LEARNING ACTIVITIES

- Visit the websites mentioned in the first section on the history of hearing aids.
- Make contact with an audiologist and arrange to observe a patient throughout the entire hearing healthcare continuum.
- Borrow one hearing aid of each style and learn how to identify each of the parts.
- Ask an audiologist or a speech-language pathologist to teach you how to complete a visual and listening check of a hearing aid.
- Visit the Internet sites of two to three hearing aid manufacturers. Visit the pages for prospective hearing aid wearers concerning their latest product lines.
- Interview an audiologist regarding his or her use of outcome measures.

APPENDIX 6.1

Parameters for Electroacoustic Analysis of Hearing Aids

Tests for Linear Instruments

Test	Test Conditions
OSPL90 curve	Input level: 90 dB SPL; gain control full-on
OSPL90 max	From OSPL90 curve
OSPL90 (HFA or SPA)	From OSPL90 curve
Full-on gain (HFA or SPA)	Input level: 50 dB SPL; gain control at full-on
Reference-test gain	OSPL90 (HFA or SPA) 77 dB, or full-on gain, whichever is lower
Frequency response curve	Input level: 60 dB SPL; gain, control at reference-test position
Frequency range (f_1 and f_2)	From frequency response curve; draw line at HFA (or SPA) level 20 dB
Percent total harmonic distortion	500 Hz (or half the low SPA freq) @ 70 dB SPL; 800 Hz (or half the mid SPA freq) @ 70 dB SPL; 1600 Hz (or half the high SPA freq) @ 65 dB SPL; gain control at reference-test position; 12 dB-rule applies
Equivalent input noise (EIN) level	Very quiet ambient conditions; input signal off; gain control at reference-test position; subtract HFA gain value found with a 50-dB-SPL input signal from the rms output
Battery current: drain	Input level: 65 dB SPL @ 1000 Hz; gain control at reference-test position
SPLITS curve	Magnetic field of 6 milliamperes divided by number of coils; gain control at reference-test position; hearing aid in telecoil mode
HFA- or SPA-SPLITS	HFA or SPA value found using decibel values on SPLITS curve
Relative Simulated Equivalent Telephone Sensitivity (RSETS)	Subtract HFA (or SPA) found, with aid in normal mode with gain control at reference-test position and input signal of 60 dB SPL from the HFA- or SPL-SPLITS value

Tests for AGC Instruments

Test	Test Conditions
OSPL90 curve	Input level: 90 dB SPL; gain control full-on; compression controls set to minimum
OSPL90 max	From OSPL90 curve
OSPL90 (HFA or SPA)	From OSPL90 curve
Full-on gain (HFA or SPA)	Input level: 50 dB SPL; gain control full-on; compression controls set to minimum
Reference-test gain	OSPL90 (HFA or SPA) 77 dB, or full-on gain, whichever is lower; compression controls set to minimum
Frequency response curve	Input level: 60 dB SPL; gain control at reference-test position; compression controls set to minimum
Frequency range (f_1 and f_2)	From frequency response curve; use line at HFA (or SPA) level 20 dB
Percent total harmonic distortion	500 Hz (or half the low SPA freq) @ 70 dB SPL; 800 Hz (or half the mid SPA freq) @ 70 dB SPL; 1600 Hz (or half the high SPA freq) @ 65 dB SPL; gain control at reference-test position; compression controls set to minimum; 12 dB-rule applies
Input-output (I/O) characteristic	Input frequency of 250, 500, 1000, 2000, or 4000 Hz, or any combination of those frequencies; input level varies from 50 to 90 dB SPL in 5-dB steps; gain control in reference-test position; compression controls set to maximum
Attack time	Input frequency of 250, 500,1000, 2000, or 4000 Hz, or any combination of those frequencies; input level switched abruptly from 55 to 90 dB SPL; compression controls set to maximum
Release time	Input frequency of 250, 500, 1000, 2000, or 4000 Hz, or any combination of those frequencies; input level switched abruptly from 90 to 55 dB SPL; compression controls set to maximum
Equivalent input noise (EIN) level	Very quiet ambient conditions; input signal off; gain control at reference-test position; subtract HFA gain value found with a 50-dB-SPL input signal from the rms output; compression controls set to minimum
Battery current drain	Input level: 65 dB SPL @ 1000 Hz; gain control at reference-test position; compression controls set to minimum
SPLITS curve	Magnetic field of 6 milliamperes divided by number of coils; gain controls at reference-test position; compression controls set to minimum; hearing aid in telecoil mode
HFA- or SPA-SPLITS	HFA or SPA value found using decibel values on SPLITS curve
Relative Simulated Equivalent Telephone Sensitivity (RSETS)	Subtract HFA (or SPA) found with aid in normal mode with gain control at reference-test position and input signal of 60 dB SPL from the HFA- or SPL-SPLITS value

Source: From *FONIX: ANSI '03 Workbook,* by G. Frye, 2005, Frye Electronics, Tigard, OR. Used with permission.

APPENDIX 6.2

NAL Client Oriented Scale of Improvement

Name : _____

Audiologist : _____

Category:　New _____

　　　　　　Return _____

Date : 1. Needs Established _____

　　　　2. Outcome Assessed _____

SPECIFIC NEEDS

Indicate Order of Significance

☐ ──────────────────────────────

☐ ──────────────────────────────

☐ ──────────────────────────────

☐ ──────────────────────────────

☐ ──────────────────────────────

Degree of Change

Worse	No Difference	Slightly Better	Better	Much Better	CATEGORY

Final Ability (with hearing aid)

Person can hear

	Hardly Ever	Occasionally	Half the Time	Most of Time	Almost Always
%	10%	25%	50%	75%	95%

Categories

1. Conversation with 1 or 2 in quiet
2. Conversation with 1 or 2 in noise
3. Conversation with group in quiet
4. Conversation with group in noise
5. Television/Radio @ normal volume
6. Familiar speaker on phone
7. Unfamiliar speaker on phone
8. Hearing phone ring from another room
9. Hear front doorbell or knock
10. Hear traffic
11. Increased social contact
12. Feel embarrassed or stupid
13. Feeling left out
14. Feeling upset or angry
15. Church or meeting
16. Other

Source: From Client Oriented Scale of Improvement, H. Dillon, A. James, and J. Ginis, 1997, National Acoustics Laboratory, 2010, retrieved from www.nal.gov.au/pdf/COSI_Questionnaire.pdf. Reprinted with permission.

217

APPENDIX 6.3
Abbreviated Profile of Hearing Aid Benefit

Name: _____   Date: _____   File No.: _____

INSTRUCTIONS: *Please circle the answers that come closest to your everyday experience. Notice that each choice includes a percentage. You can use this to help you decide on your answer. For example, if the statement is true about 75% of the time, circle C for that item.*

A	Always (99%)
B	Almost always (87%)
C	Generally (75%)
D	Half the time (50%)
E	Occasionally (25%)
F	Seldom (12%)
G	Never (1%)

If you have not experienced the situation we described, try to think of a similar situation that you have been in and respond for that situation. If you have no idea, leave that item blank.

Notice that for some items, an answer of Always (99%) means you have few problems. Other items are written so that an answer of Always (99%) means you have a lot of problems. Here is an example. In item (a), an answer of Always (99%) means that you usually have problems. In item (b), the same answer means that you only have problems once in a while.

EXAMPLE:

		Without Hearing Aids	With Hearing Aids
(a)	When I'm talking with a friend outdoors on a windy day, *I miss a lot of the conversation.*	A B C D E F G	A B C D E F G
(b)	When I am in a meeting with several other people, *I can comprehend speech.*	A B C D E F G	A B C D E F G

Please begin answering the questions on the next page.

A	Always (99%)
B	Almost always (87%)
C	Generally (75%)
D	Half the time (50%)
E	Occasionally (25%)
F	Seldom (12%)
G	Never (1%)

	Without Hearing Aids	**With** Hearing Aids
1. When I am in a crowded grocery store, talking with the cashier, I can follow the conversation.	A B C D E F G	A B C D E F G
2. I miss a lot of information when I'm listening to a lecture.	A B C D E F G	A B C D E F G
3. Unexpected sounds, like a smoke detector or alarm bell, are uncomfortable.	A B C D E F G	A B C D E F G
4. I have difficulty hearing a conversation when I'm with one of my family at home.	A B C D E F G	A B C D E F G
5. I have trouble understanding the dialogue in a movie or at the theater.	A B C D E F G	A B C D E F G
6. When I am listening to the news on the car radio, and family members are talking, I have trouble hearing the news.	A B C D E F G	A B C D E F G
7. When I'm at the dinner table with several people, and am trying to have a conversation with one person, understanding speech is difficult.	A B C D E F G	A B C D E F G
8. Traffic noises are too loud.	A B C D E F G	A B C D E F G
9. When I am talking with someone across a large empty room, I understand the words.	A B C D E F G	A B C D E F G
10. When I am in a small office, interviewing or answering questions, I have difficulty following the conversation.	A B C D E F G	A B C D E F G
11. When I am in a theater watching a movie or play, and the people around me are whispering and rustling paper wrappers, I can still make out the dialogue.	A B C D E F G	A B C D E F G
12. When I am having a quiet conversation with a friend, I have difficulty understanding.	A B C D E F G	A B C D E F G
13. The sounds of running water, such as a toilet or shower, are uncomfortably loud.	A B C D E F G	A B C D E F G
14. When a speaker is addressing a small group, and everyone is listening quietly, I have to strain to understand.	A B C D E F G	A B C D E F G
15. When I'm in a quiet conversation with my doctor in an examination room, it is hard to follow the conversation.	A B C D E F G	A B C D E F G

A	Always (99%)
B	Almost always (87%)
C	Generally (75%)
D	Half the time (50%)
E	Occasionally (25%)
F	Seldom (12%)
G	Never (1%)

	Without Hearing Aids	**With** Hearing Aids
16. I can understand conversations even when several people are talking.	A B C D E F G	A B C D E F G
17. The sounds of construction work are uncomfortably loud.	A B C D E F G	A B C D E F G
18. It's hard for me to understand what is being said at lectures or church services.	A B C D E F G	A B C D E F G
19. I can communicate with others when we are in a crowd.	A B C D E F G	A B C D E F G
20. The sound of a fire engine siren close by is so loud that I need to cover my ears.	A B C D E F G	A B C D E F G
21. I can follow the words of a sermon when listening to a religious service.	A B C D E F G	A B C D E F G
22. The sound of screeching tires is uncomfortably loud.	A B C D E F G	A B C D E F G
23. I have to ask people to repeat themselves in one-on-one conversation in a quiet room.	A B C D E F G	A B C D E F G
24. I have trouble understanding others when an air conditioner or fan is on.	A B C D E F G	A B C D E F G

© University of Memphis, 1994

Comments: _____

_____

_____

_____

Source: From "The Abbreviated Profile of Hearing Aid Benefit," by R. Cox and G. Alexander, 1995, *Ear and Hearing, 16,* pp. 176–183. Reprinted with permission from R. M. Cox, University of Memphis.

APPENDIX 6.4

Hearing Handicap Inventory for the Elderly

Name: _____ Gender: **M F** **Date of Birth:**__/__/__ **Today's Date:** __/__/__

INSTRUCTIONS: *The purpose of this scale is to identify the problems your hearing loss may be causing you. Answer YES, SOMETIMES, or NO for each question. Do not skip a question if you avoid a situation because of your hearing problem. If you use a hearing aid, please answer the way you hear without the aid.*

	Yes (4)	Some-times (2)	No (0)
S-1. Does a hearing problem cause you to use the phone less often than you would like?	_____	_____	_____
E-2. Does a hearing problem cause you to feel embarrassed when meeting new people?	_____	_____	_____
S-3. Does a hearing problem cause you to avoid groups of people?	_____	_____	_____
E-4. Does a hearing problem make you irritable?	_____	_____	_____
E-5. Does a hearing problem cause you to feel frustrated when talking to members of your family?	_____	_____	_____
S-6. Does a hearing problem cause you difficulty when attending a party?	_____	_____	_____
E-7. Does a hearing problem cause you to feel "stupid" or "dumb"?	_____	_____	_____
S-8. Do you have difficulty hearing when someone speaks in a whisper?	_____	_____	_____
E-9. Do you feel handicapped by a hearing problem?	_____	_____	_____
S-10. Does a hearing problem cause you difficulty when visiting friends, relatives, or neighbors?	_____	_____	_____
S-11. Does a hearing problem cause you to attend religious services less often than you would like?	_____	_____	_____
E-12. Does a hearing problem cause you to be nervous?	_____	_____	_____
S-13. Does a hearing problem cause you to visit friends, relatives, or neighbors less often than you would like?	_____	_____	_____
E-14. Does a hearing problem cause you to have arguments with your family members?	_____	_____	_____

	Yes (4)	Some- times (2)	No (0)
S-15. Does a hearing problem cause you difficulty when listening to TV or radio?	_____	_____	_____
S-16. Does a hearing problem cause you to go shopping less often than you would like?	_____	_____	_____
E-17. Does any problem or difficulty with your hearing upset you at all?	_____	_____	_____
E-18. Does a hearing problem cause you to want to be by yourself?	_____	_____	_____
S-19. Does a hearing problem cause you to talk to family members less often than you would like?	_____	_____	_____
E-20. Do you feel that any difficulty with your hearing limits or hampers your personal or social life?	_____	_____	_____
S-21. Does a hearing problem cause you difficulty when in a restaurant with relatives or friends?	_____	_____	_____
S-22. Does a hearing problem cause you to feel depressed?	_____	_____	_____
S-23. Does a hearing problem cause you to listen to TV or radio less often than you would like?	_____	_____	_____
E-24. Does a hearing problem cause you to feel uncomfortable when talking to friends?	_____	_____	_____
E-25. Does a hearing problem cause you to feel left out when you are with a group of people?	_____	_____	_____

FOR CLINICIAN'S USE ONLY: Total Score: _____

Subtotal E questions: _____

Subtotal S questions: _____

Note: "E" = Emotional
       "S" = Social

Source: From "The Hearing Handicap Inventory for the Elderly: A New Tool," by I. Ventry and B. E. Weinstein, 1982, *Ear and Hearing, 3*, pp. 128–134. Reprinted with permission.

APPENDIX 6.5

Expected Consequences of Hearing Aid Ownership (ECHO)

Name: _____ **Gender: M F** **Date of Birth:__/__/__** **Today's Date: __/__/__**

INSTRUCTIONS: *Listed below are statements about hearing aids. Please circle the letter that indicates the extent to which you agree with each statement. Use the list of words on the right to determine your answer.*

A	Not at all
B	A little
C	Somewhat
D	Medium
E	Considerably
F	Greatly
G	Tremendously

How much do you agree with each statement?

1. My hearing aids will help me understand the people I speak with most frequently.	A B C D E F G
2. I will be frustrated when my hearing aids pick up sounds that keep me from hearing what I want to hear.	A B C D E F G
3. Getting hearing aids is in my best interest.	A B C D E F G
4. People will notice my hearing loss more when I wear my hearing aids.	A B C D E F G
5. My hearing aids will reduce the number of times I have to ask people to repeat.	A B C D E F G
6. My hearing aids will be worth the trouble.	A B C D E F G
7. Sometimes I will be bothered by an inability to get enough loudness from my hearing aids without feedback (whistling).	A B C D E F G
8. I will be content with the appearance of my hearing aids.	A B C D E F G
9. Using hearing aids will improve my self-confidence.	A B C D E F G

A	Not at all
B	A little
C	Somewhat
D	Medium
E	Considerably
F	Greatly
G	Tremendously

How much do you agree with each statement?

10. My hearing aids will have a natural sound.	A B C D E F G
11. My hearing aids will be helpful on most telephones without amplifiers or loudspeakers. (If you hear well on the telephone *without* hearing aids, check here ☐)	A B C D E F G
12. The person who provides me with my hearing aids will be competent.	A B C D E F G
13. Wearing my hearing aids will make me seem less capable.	A B C D E F G
14. The cost of my hearing aids will be reasonable.	A B C D E F G
15. My hearing aids will be dependable (need few repairs).	A B C D E F G

Please respond to these additional items.

Lifetime Hearing Aid Experience (includes all old and current hearing aids)	**Daily Hearing Aid Use**	**Degree of Hearing Difficulty** (without wearing a hearing aid)
☐ None ☐ Less than 6 weeks ☐ 6 weeks to 11 months ☐ 1 to 10 years ☐ Over 10 years	☐ None ☐ Less than 1 hour per day ☐ 1 to 4 hours per day ☐ 4 to 8 hours per day ☐ 8 to 16 hours per day	☐ None ☐ Mild ☐ Moderate ☐ Moderately severe ☐ Severe

© **University of Memphis, 1999**

APPENDIX 6.6

International Outcome Inventory for Hearing Aids (IOI-HA)

1. Think about how much you used your present hearing aid(s) over the past two weeks. On an average day, how many hours did you use the hearing aid(s)?

none	less than 1 hour a day	1 to 4 hours a day	4 to 8 hours a day	more than 1 hour a day
☐	☐	☐	☐	☐

2. Think about the situation where you most wanted to hear better, before you got your present hearing aid(s). Over the past two weeks, how much has the hearing aid helped in those situations?

helped not at all	helped slightly	helped moderately	helped quite a lot	helped very much
☐	☐	☐	☐	☐

3. Think again about the situation where you most wanted to hear better. When you use your present hearing aid(s), how much difficulty do you STILL have in that situation?

very much difficulty	quite a lot of difficulty	moderate difficulty	slight difficulty	no difficulty
☐	☐	☐	☐	☐

4. Considering everything, do you think your present hearing aid(s) is worth the trouble?

not at all worth it	slightly worth it	moderately worth it	quite a lot worth it	very much worth it
☐	☐	☐	☐	☐

5. Over the past two weeks, with your present hearing aid(s), how much have your hearing difficulties affected the things you can do?

affected very much	affected quite a lot	affected moderately	affected slightly	affected not at all
☐	☐	☐	☐	☐

6. Over the past two weeks, with your present hearing aid(s), how much do you think other people were bothered by your hearing difficulties?

bothered very much	bothered quite a lot	bothered moderately	bothered slightly	bothered not at all
☐	☐	☐	☐	☐

7. Considering everything, how much has your present hearing aid(s) changed your enjoyment of life?

worse	no change	slightly better	quite a lot better	very much better
☐	☐	☐	☐	☐

8. How much hearing difficulty do you have when you are **<u>not</u>** wearing a hearing aid?

severe	moderately-severe	moderate	mild	none
☐	☐	☐	☐	☐

Norms for the IOI-HA

Item	Individual Clients		Groups of Clients	
	Mild-moderate lower/upper	*Mod-severe lower/upper*	*Mild-moderate mean/SD*	*Mod-severe mean/SD*
1. use	3/5	4/5	3.73/1.17	4.5/.96
2. benefit	3/4	3/4	3.39/.98	3.52/1.08
3. RAL	3/4	2/4	3.4/.95	3.19/1.05
4. satisfac.	2/4	3/5	3.2/1.21	3.84/1.17
5. RPR	3/4	3/4	3.57/1.13	3.38/1.11
6. imp-oth	3/5	2/4	3.79/1.13	3.38/1.1
7. QofLife	3/4	3/4	3.19/.93	3.68/1.02

The category of norms used should depend on the patient's answer to the eighth item of the questionnaire. If they choose "none," "mild," or "moderate," use the "mild/moderate" norms. For the other two options, use the "mod/severe" norms.

The norms for individual clients are the middle 50% of the data. Hearing aids were: single-channel, single-memory, ITE; all bilateral fittings; all compression (any type); standard fitting protocol; purchased between Aug/00 & Jan/01.

IOI-HA Norm Template for Individual Scores

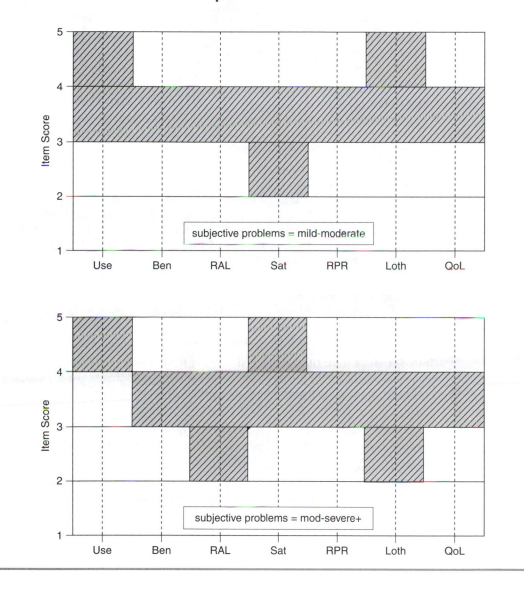

APPENDIX 6.7

Common Outcome Measures as a Function of Domain

- **Impairment**
  - Audibility
  - Functional gain
  - Real-ear probe-microphone measurements
  - Speech recognition measures

- **Activity Limitation**
  - Abbreviated Profile of Hearing Aid Benefit (APHAB)—Cox and Alexander (1995)
  - Client-oriented Scale of Improvement (COSI)—Dillon, James, and Ginis (1997)
  - Hearing Aid Performance Inventory (HAPI)—Walden, Demorest, and Helper (1984)
  - Hearing Performance Inventory–Revised (HPI-R)—Lamb, Owens, and Schubert (1983)
  - Hearing Performance Inventory (HPI)—Giolas, Owens, Lamb, and Schubert (1979)
  - Shortened Hearing Aid Performance Inventory (SHAPI)—Schum (1992)

- **Participation Restriction**
  - Hearing Handicap Inventory for Adults (HHIA)—Newman, Weinstein, Jacobson, and Hug (1990)
  - Hearing Handicap Inventory for the Elderly (HHIE)—Ventry and Weinstein (1982)

- **Both Activity Limitations and Participation Restriction**
  - Communication Profile for the Hearing-Impaired (CPHI)—Demorest and Erdman (1987)
  - Glasgow Hearing Aid Benefit Profile (GHABP)—Gatehouse (1999)

- **Satisfaction**
  - Hearing Satisfaction Survey (HSS)—Kochkin (1997)
  - Satisfaction of Amplification in Daily Life (SADL)—Cox and Alexander (1999)

- **Health-Related Quality of Life**
  - Medical Outcomes Survey Short-Form 36 (MOS SF-36)—Ware and Sherbourne (1992)
  - World Health Organization Disabilities Assessment Schedule–II (WHO-DAS II)—(World Health Organization, 1999)

Source: Based on *Outcome Measures in Audiology: Knowing We've Made a Difference*, by H. B. Abrams, 2000, retrieved from www.audiologyonline.com/articles/article_detail.asp?article_id=236.

CHAPTER seven

Introduction to Hearing Assistive Technology

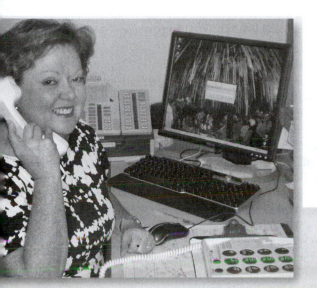

LEARNING *objectives*

After reading this chapter, you should be able to:

1. Define assistive technology, hearing assistive technology (HAT), assistive technology system, and HAT system.
2. List and describe the characteristics of HAT.
3. Discuss how aspects of context can affect the use of HAT.
4. List the major pieces of legislation affecting HAT.
5. Explain the major categories of HAT and describe devices within each category.
6. Envision audiologists' responsibilities in evaluating, selecting, and fitting HAT.
7. Identify and discuss HAT for individuals who are deaf-blind.

Assistive technology is defined as a "broad range of devices, services, strategies, and practices that are conceived and applied to ameliorate the problems faced by individuals who have disabilities" (Cook & Hussey, 2002, p. 5). The Technology Related Assistance Act of 1988 first defined assistive technology as "products, devices or equipment, whether acquired commercially, modified or customized, that are used to maintain, increase or improve the functional capabilities of individuals with disabilities." In considering auditory rehabilitation, we can modify the definition to be specified as **hearing assistive technology (HAT)** or **assistive listening devices (ALDs)**, which include a range of devices, services, strategies, and practices that are conceived and applied to ameliorate the problems faced by individuals who have hearing loss. In discussing HAT, we do not just consider the device that the person uses, but acknowledge the **assistive technology system**, consisting of the device, a human operator of the instrument, and an environment in which a functional activity is to take place (Cook & Hussey, 2002). Audiologists and speech-language pathologists may modify the previous definition of the **HAT system**, consisting of the device, a user of the instrument, and an environment in which listening activity is to take place. Figure 7.1 represents an assistive listening technology system.

In the previous chapter, hearing aids were discussed and described as the cornerstone of auditory rehabilitation (Jerger, 2007). Some patients with hearing loss, however, do not pursue amplification and opt for the use of HAT. Alternatively, some hearing aid wearers may find that the use of hearing aids is not enough and may need to use HAT. The need for HAT is highly variable from patient to patient depending upon his or her degree of loss, communication demands, activities, and interactions with others. Audiologists and speech-language pathologists must realize that HAT systems exist within unique milieus consisting of the setting within social, cultural, and physical contexts. Successful selection, evaluation, and fitting of HAT requires acknowledgement of the multidimensional aspects of *context*, or the who, what, where, when, and why of use. In this chapter, readers will learn the basics of HAT.

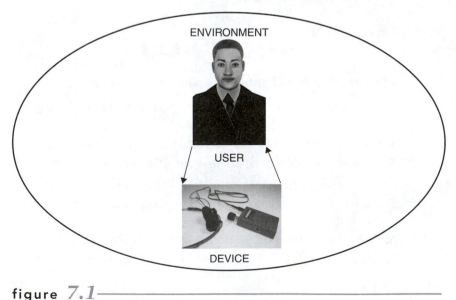

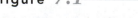

figure *7.1*

An assistive technology system.

CHARACTERISTICS OF HEARING ASSISTIVE TECHNOLOGY

Hearing assistive technology shares the same characteristics as other assistive technologies used by persons with disabilities, which are as follows:

- Assistive versus rehabilitative versus educational technologies
- Low versus high technology
- Hard versus soft technologies
- Appliances versus tools
- Minimal versus maximal technology

First, HAT serves primarily an assistive role rather than an educational or rehabilitative role. In other words, HAT is used to carry out a functional daily activity associated with hearing, such as enabling a person who has a hearing loss to hear the telephone ring or understand what is being said. An example of HAT with an educational or rehabilitative role may be software that teaches those with hearing loss how to speechread.

Second, HAT can range from low to high technology. A low-technology example is a Whistle Stop, consisting of a cylinder of plastic that snaps onto the receiver of a telephone, which decreases the likelihood of feedback from a hearing aid. Alternatively, a high-technology device may consist of a transmitter that sends a clear signal from a speaker via infrared light directly to a receiver coupled to listeners' ears.

Third, appropriate use of HAT requires the use of hard and soft technologies. **Hard technologies** are the actual devices or parts that can be easily purchased by the consumer, assembled, and used (Cook & Hussey, 2002). On the other hand, **soft technologies** are human components such as decision-making strategies and training. Audiologists may develop the acumen for solving communication difficulties by assisting patients in developing unique strategies (i.e., soft technologies) with specific types of devices (i.e., hard technologies) in order to listen to television.

Fourth, HATs may involve **appliances** or **tools**. Appliances are devices that provide benefits to patients irrespective of their individual skill level. Tools, on the other hand, require the development of skills for optimal use (Cook & Hussey, 2002). For example, HAT such as visual and auditory alerting smoke detectors are appliances because they do not require any skill to operate, if properly set. However, a wireless FM transmitter sending a speaker's voice to an FM receiver is considered a tool because training on the importance of strategic microphone placement is required to maximize the signal-to-noise ratio and patient benefit from the equipment.

Fifth, successful use of HAT may range in the use of minimal to maximal technology. **Minimal technology** are those devices that augment patients' listening abilities, whereas **maximal technology** replaces hearing with other senses, such as visual or tactile. For example, minimal technologies to aid in hearing the telephone ring may include increasing the loudness or changing the pitch of the bell. However, maximal technology would replace hearing the phone ring with seeing a lamp flashing.

CONTEXTS FOR ASSISTIVE TECHNOLOGY USE

Four primary contexts to be considered for the use of HAT are illustrated in Figure 7.2.

The first context is the setting, or where the HAT is to be used. Patients may use the HAT device at home, at work, at school, at church, or enjoying leisure time activities.

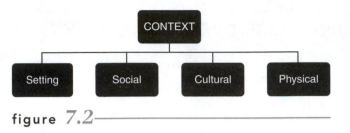

figure *7.2*

Four contexts of assistive technology.

Source: Based on *Assistive Technologies: Principles and Practice* (2nd ed.), by S. M. Cook and S. M. Hussey, 2002, St. Louis, MO: Mosby.

Acknowledgment of the setting is key for successful selection, evaluation, and fitting of HAT. For example, what functional academic activities in a noisy classroom are difficult for the child? Or, for an adult, what day-to-day tasks at work are difficult even when the adult is wearing his or her hearing aids? Or, for an elderly patient, what tasks involving hearing are difficult for this person at home? Other aspects of setting include what federal laws apply regarding patients' rights to have communication access using a HAT device. In other chapters, more detail is provided for specific types of patients (e.g., the elderly) in a variety of settings (e.g., long-term residential care facilities for the elderly).

Communication sciences and disorders professionals must also consider the social context for patients' HAT usage with peers, nonpeers, strangers, or with no one, for example, when listening to music. Most importantly, how do patients feel when using HAT in public? Do they feel self-conscious, embarrassed, or stigmatized? Audiologists need to probe for these feelings, otherwise HAT may never be used by some patients. How will a teacher and classmates react to a child's use of HAT in a classroom? Or, will a 40-year-old businessman's coworkers feel inconvenienced passing a microphone from speaker to speaker during a meeting? How will an elderly woman's spouse feel about her using HAT? The social context is an important determinant of whether patients use or do not use HAT.

Cultural context is important to consider when dispensing HAT to diverse patient populations. Table 7.1 shows the cultural factors that affect use of HAT. It has been found that Caucasians are more likely to use assistive technology than people of color partly due to limited access, lack of awareness, and possible linguistic barriers (Yeager, Kaye, & Reed, 2007). Moreover, Caucasians are more likely to use high technology devices than people of color (Yeager et al., 2007).

Cultural groups vary on their views of how time is used, the balance of work and play, and use of financial resources. Some cultures value leisure time; others may view it as laziness. Therefore, some cultures may feel that purchasing HAT for watching television is a waste of money. Some cultures may view seeking assistance from others as a weakness. Therefore, some cultures may frown upon seeking assistance from hearing healthcare professionals and purchasing HAT. And still other cultures may value physical appearance and may stigmatize those using hearing aids or HAT.

The physical context includes those aspects of the environment that affect communication—noise, reverberation, speaker-to-listener distance, or the lighting in the room. How noisy is the setting? **Noise** is any unwanted sound. Its index of severity is **signal-to-noise ratio** (S/N), defined as the relative level of signal, in decibels (dB), in relation to that of the background noise. The lower the S/N, the more prominent is the masking of the noise in relation to the signal. Signal-to-noise ratios for optimal listening should be at least +15 dB for children (Crandell & Smaldino, 2005). Office spaces, classrooms, and dayrooms in long-term residential care facilities for the elderly are often noisy, making speech recognition difficult for listeners. **Reverberation**, the continuation of acoustic energy due to the reflections of that energy off of the floor, ceiling, and walls of a room after the source of the sound has been terminated, also degrades speech recognition. Reverberation causes elongation of vowel sounds such that they mask or "smear" over the softer

---

table *7.1*   Cultural Factors That Affect Delivery of New Assistive Listening Devices

---

- Use of time
- Balance of work and play
- Sense of personal space
- Values regarding finance
- Roles assumed in the family
- Knowledge of disabilities and sources of information
- Beliefs about causality
- Views of inner workings of the body
- Sources of social support
- Acceptable amount of assistance from others
- Degree of importance attributed to physical appearance
- Degree of importance attributed to independence
- Sense of control over things that happen
- Typical or preferred coping strategies
- Style of expressing emotions

Sources: Information from *Assistive Technologies: Principles and Practice* (2nd ed.), by S. M. Cook and S. M. Hussey, 2002, St. Louis, MO: Mosby; "Cultural Influences on Performance," L. H. Krefting and D. V. Krefting, 1991, in *Occupational Therapy,* by C. Christiansen and C. Baum (Eds.), Thoroughfare, NJ: Slack.

consonants that follow. The index of severity for reverberation is **reverberation time**, which is the time it takes for the sound to decrease 60 dB after the source of the sound has been terminated and should be less than about 0.7 seconds, especially for children (Crandell & Smaldino, 2005). The longer the reverberation time, the greater is the degradation on speech understanding. Larger rooms with hard, reflective surfaces have longer reverberation times than smaller rooms with softer surfaces. In addition, large rooms such as auditoriums, places of worship, or large lecture halls may have large speaker-to-listener distances and poor lighting, possibly limiting the visual cues for speech recognition. Therefore, the setting plays an important role in the need for the use of HAT for individuals with hearing loss. In summary, the selection, evaluation, and delivery of HAT occur in and are affected by the various aspects of context.

MAJOR PIECES OF LEGISLATION AFFECTING THE USE AND FUNDING OF ASSISTIVE TECHNOLOGY

Audiologists and speech-language pathologists may have patients they believe may benefit from the use of HAT but who may not be able to afford it. It is important to know about federal legislation affecting funding and the use of HAT, as illustrated in Figure 7.3.

The Rehabilitation Act of 1973 mandated reasonable accommodations for persons with disabilities, including assistive technology, for employment settings subsidized by federal

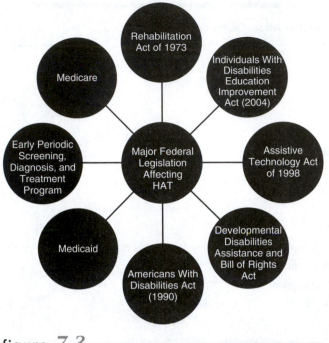

figure *7.3*

Major federal legislation affecting assistive technology.

Source: Based on *Assistive Technologies: Principles and Practice* (2nd ed.), by S. M. Cook and S. M. Hussey, 2002, St. Louis, MO: Mosby.

funding and for higher education. For example, postsecondary institutions of higher learning should have FM systems available for students who are deaf and hard of hearing. For the 0- to 21-year-old population, the Individuals With Disabilities Education Act (IDEA) Amendments of 1997 stipulated the right of every child with a disability to a free and appropriate public education (FAPE) in a least restrictive environment (LRE), which may require the use of HAT. Both the Rehabilitation Act of 1973 and the reauthorized IDEA (2004) are massive laws that mention assistive technology. One significant change from the reauthorization of the IDEA from 1997 to 2004 is the exclusion of implantable technologies such as cochlear implants from the definition of assistive technology. The Assistive Technology Act of 1998 (PL 105-394), which replaced the Technology Related Assistance for Individuals With Disabilities Act of 1988, was the first law specifically addressing assistive technology devices and services. President Clinton signed this piece of legislation into law on November 13, 1998, and it was reauthorized in 2004. It affirms the powerful role of technology in improving the lives of persons with disabilities. In addition, the law defined the responsibility of the federal government to ensure the accessibility of assistive devices to persons with disabilities (Mississippi Project START, 2002).

Several laws and federal programs include mandates of financial assistance in the securing of assistive technology. The Developmental Disabilities Assistance and Bill of Rights Act provides financial assistance to states to provide services and assistive technology to persons with developmental disabilities. The Americans With Disabilities Act (ADA) of 1990 forbids discrimination on the basis of a disability on-the-job, in state and local government, public accommodations, commercial facilities, transportation, and telecommunications. A cornerstone of the ADA is accessibility of people with disabilities to facets of American life through the use of assistive technology.

Medicaid is an income-based program of healthcare that varies by state that includes some assistive technology. Medicaid programs vary based on the age of the group served. For example, the Early Periodic Screening, Diagnosis, and Treatment Program (EPSDTP) mandates services for children (birth to age 21) that may include assistive technology. States must provide these programs for children in order to receive Medicaid money (University of Washington Center for Technology and Disability Studies, 2003). Each state has its own EPSDTP that entitles children to a broad coverage of healthcare services that may include assistive technology. Other Medicaid programs are for people over 18 years of age such as the Community Options Program Entry System (COPES), a community-based program in the state of Washington. COPES offers people over age 18 a choice of receiving institutional-, home-, or community-based services that may include assistive technology (University of Washington Center for Technology and Disability Studies, 2003). And finally, Medicare is a national health insurance program funded by the federal government for people 65 years of age and over and younger people with certain disabilities (University of Washington Center for Technology and Disability Studies, 2003). Medicare may fund assistive technology provided that the following standards and procedures are followed, and HAT is (1) within the scope of its funding, (2) "reasonable and necessary," and that (3) authorization procedures are strictly followed (University of Washington Center for Technology and Disability Studies, 2003).

Audiologists can be instrumental in helping patients navigate through the process of securing funding for HAT, shown in Table 7.2. Audiologists may play a key role in assisting patients' investigations of HAT options to solve their communication problems. Once options have been identified, an assessment should determine the extent of possible benefit received from HAT use within specific contexts, possibly identifying specific funding sources. For example, a student with a severe bilateral sensorineural hearing loss who needs specific HAT for accessibility to nurses' training classes at a junior college may apply to the Division of Vocational Rehabilitation (DVR) for funding. Audiologists can assist the student in clarifying the DVR's eligibility criteria, policies, and procedures. Reports must be meticulously written to support and justify the request for funding from the agency. Appendix 7.1 shows an outline for a justification letter for assistive technology (University of Washington Center for Technology and Disability Studies, 2003). The report should mention the need of HAT support services, which may include user training and programming/configuration, maintenance, and repair (University of Washington Center for Technology and Disability Studies, 2003). For example, funding may be needed for the university speech and hearing clinic to repair the student's HAT. Because not all funding requests are granted, alternative payment arrangements may be explored such as through the university's program for students with disabilities. Securing funding may take time, so

---

table *7.2*   Ten Steps for Securing Funding for Assistive Technology

- Step 1: Investigate options for assistive listening technologies.
- Step 2: Execute assistive listening technology assessment.
- Step 3: Identify funding sources.
- Step 4: Clarify source eligibility criteria, policies, and procedures.
- Step 5: Support and justify the request.
- Step 6: Acknowledge the need for support services.
- Step 7: Explore alternative payment arrangements.
- Step 8: Prepare for delays and persist.
- Step 9: Anticipate an appeal.
- Step 10: Meet deadlines.

Source: Information from *Paying for the Assistive Technology You Need: A Consumer Guide for Funding Sources in Washington State*, by the University of Washington Center for Technology and Disability Studies, 2003, retrieved from http://uwctds.washington.edu/resources/legal/funding%20manual/index.htm.

preparations for delays and persistence in filing appeals may be needed for proposal success. Furthermore, even the best appeals will be denied if deadlines are not strictly met.

BASIC CATEGORIZATIONS OF HEARING ASSISTIVE TECHNOLOGY

Individuals who are deaf and hard of hearing are just like their peers who have normal hearing. Their activities of daily living include communicating on the telephone, answering doorbells, visiting friends and family members, and watching television, which may require the use of HAT. HAT can be classified into three categories: those that help with (1) telephone communication, (2) environmental awareness of sounds, and (3) face-to-face communication and listening to television.

Devices That Assist With Telephone Communication

Hearing Assistive Technology for Landline Phones

Examples of HAT that assist with talking on the telephone range from very simple devices to special telephones. Figures 7.4, 7.5, 7.6, 7.7, and 7.8 show HAT that assists in talking on the telephone.

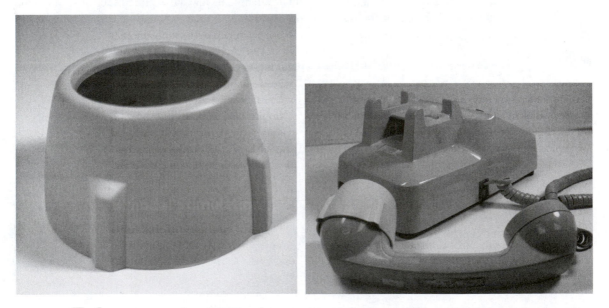

figure *7.4*

The Whistle Stop and its placement on the telephone receiver.

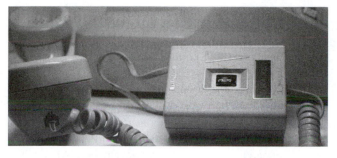

Figure 7.4 on the previous page shows two pictures of the Whistle Stop: by itself (left) and as it is used when the patient snaps it onto the receiver of the telephone (right). The device serves as a funnel for sound and separates the microphone of the hearing aid from the telephone receiver to prevent whistling or feedback. Figure 7.5 shows an in-line amplifier that is inserted between the body and the curly cord of the telephone. The loudness of the telephone can be adjusted by the patient using a volume control wheel. Figure 7.6 is the Clarity phone, which not only is an amplified telephone, but has features for patients with visual problems (e.g., large numbers on keys) and/or manual dexterity problems (e.g., large-button keys). Patients may use the telephone by listening to the amplified sound through the receiver or through the telecoils in their hearing aids. Figure 7.7 shows a portable phone amplifier, which is battery operated and connects to the receiver of the

figure 7.5

The in-line amplifier.

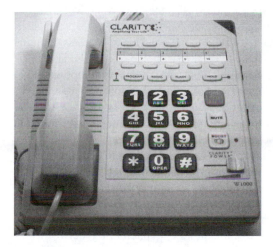

figure 7.6

Clarity phone.

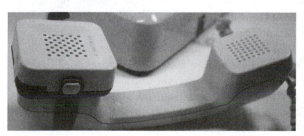

figure 7.7

Portable phone amplifier.

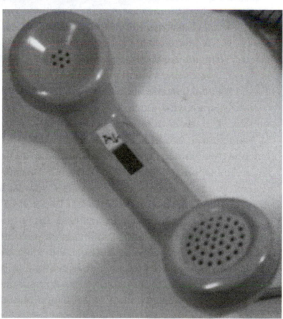

figure 7.8

Replacement handset.

phone. The device may be carried in a pocket or purse. Last, Figure 7.8 displays a replacement handset with a volume wheel for amplifying phone conversation. The user simply switches that handset on his or her regular telephones.

Hearing Assistive Technology for Cell Phones

The telephone is a major source of communication even for people who are deaf or hard of hearing. Almost everyone has a cell phone these days. Cell phones are decreasing in size and increasing in their capabilities to do other tasks such as videorecording and personal computing. Several of the leading cell phone manufacturers have developed HAT to make cell phones accessible to hearing aid wearers. Nokia developed neckloops for use with several models of their cell phones to couple with telecoil-equipped hearing aids. However, earlier on in the hearing aid/cell phone compatibility issue, the Self-Help for the Hard of Hearing (SHHH, now known as the Hearing Loss Association of America) consumer group surveyed its membership and found that they had several preferences regarding use of cell phones (Battat, Berger, Killion, & Kozma-Spytek, 2003). The majority wanted hearing aid compatibility built-in at the design stage of the cell phone precluding the use of HAT such as neckloops. Some hearing aid wearers perceived that neckloops make wireless communication wired and confining. Second, most wanted to have a choice of cell phone options such as styles, features, and prices. Third, hearing aid wearers wanted the option of returning cell phones after a reasonable trial period without penalty. (Most cell phone companies allow only a 10-day trial period with a phone. Hearing aid wearers may need a longer trial period prior to making a decision about purchase.) Fourth, hearing aid wearers wanted cell phone products to have appropriate labeling on their boxes and explanations in the user's manuals regarding cell phone compatibility. Fifth, most wanted audiologists and salespeople to be knowledgeable about finding acceptable cell phone solutions for hearing aid wearers.

Audiologists can assist patients in this endeavor by including an item on the case history form regarding the desire for cell phone use (Johnson, Gavin, & Reith, 2004). Hearing healthcare professionals should seek to understand the interaction between and among major players regarding the hearing aid/cell phone compatibility issue, which includes cell phone manufacturers, cell phone service providers, cell phone retailers, hearing aid manufacturers, and consumer groups. Audiologists should understand why hearing aid wearers have problems using cell phones (Kozma-Spytek, 2003); they should know that consumers want to use cell phones directly with their hearing aids rather than having to use an accessory (e.g., neckloop by Nokia); and they should know that the use of accessories should be only a short-term solution. Audiologists should find out which hearing aids have the greatest immunity to cell phone interference for each manufacturer that is used in their practice.

On August 14, 2003, the Federal Communications Commission (FCC) ruled that wireless phones were no longer exempt from the Hearing Aid Compatibility Act of 1988. Based upon this ruling, the FCC established rules for the hearing aid compatibility of digital wireless phones. Stipulations of this requirement have been slowly phased in over time (for details, see www.fcc.gov/cgb/consumerfacts/hac_wireless.html.) The FCC has mandated that cell phones be rated for the amount of interference to be expected when used with the microphone and/or telecoil of a hearing aid. Scales for both go from 1 to 4 (i.e., 1 = poor, 2 = fair, 3 = good, and 4 = excellent.) Only ratings of 3 or 4 are acceptable for microphones (i.e., M3 or M4) and telecoils (i.e., T3 or T4) for cell phones to be considered hearing aid compatible. Furthermore, patients should be counseled that the majority of salespeople in cell phone retail shops have little or no knowledge about hearing aid/cell phone compatibility issues. Therefore, the patient and the audiologist must work together in requesting extended trial periods for digital cell phones and to eliminate any penalties for switching cell phones. Finding acceptable cell phone solutions is a team effort.

Bluetooth® technology refers to wireless personal area networks (PANs) that provide wireless communication between devices (e.g., mobile phones, laptop computers, digital cameras) via an unsecure short-range radio frequency. For example, when someone synchronizes a personal digital assistant with a personal computer, more than likely it is done via Bluetooth technology. Some manufacturers are using Bluetooth technology to connect hearing aids through a mediating devices such as Phonak's SmartLink. In the near future, hearing aids will directly connect with cell phones via Bluetooth technology.

Devices That Assist With Environmental Awareness of Sounds

Figures 7.9, 7.10, 7.11, and 7.12 show ALDs that are used for environmental awareness of sounds.

Figure 7.9 is the RingMax, which assists patients in hearing the phone ring. The patient can adjust the RingMax for his or her degree and configuration of hearing loss. For example, patients with high-frequency hearing loss can adjust the ring to a lower frequency, increasing the likelihood of

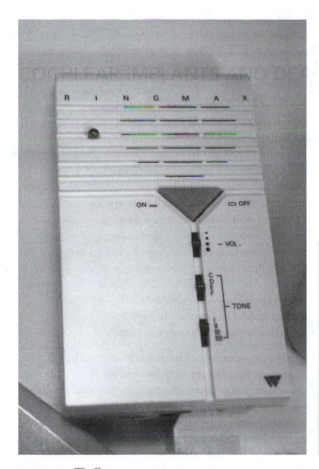

figure *7.9*

The RingMax.

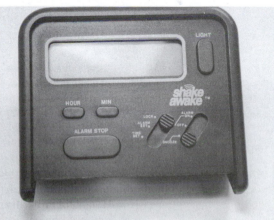

figure *7.10*

The Shake Awake.

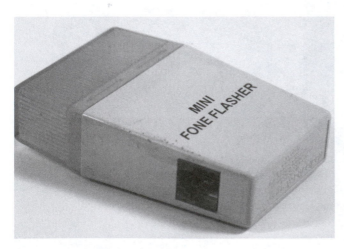

figure *7.11*

Smoke detector that provides both visual and auditory warnings.

figure *7.12*

The Fone Flasher.

detection. In addition, the loudness of ring is adjustable for different degrees of hearing loss. The RingMax requires an external power source. Figure 7.10 shows the Shake Awake, which is a flat, battery-operated alarm clock that vibrates under a pillow, awakening the patient. Figure 7.11 is a picture of a smoke detector that provides both a loud signal and flashing strobe light that alerts patients to the presence of significant smoke. In Figure 7.12 is the Fone Flasher, which connects between the wall jack and the telephone. Its light flashes when the telephone rings, alerting patients to incoming calls.

Devices That Assist With Television Viewing or Interpersonal Communication

Group-amplification systems transmit speakers' voices (either live or via multimedia) to an audience of listeners and are classified by how the signal travels to the listener(s). They consist of a speaker microphone, amplifying unit, and means of transmitting the signal to one or many listeners. It is important to note that even though these devices are referred to as group-amplification systems, frequently they are used on an individual basis, too (e.g., one transmitter to one receiver or one television to one listener). Group-amplification systems can be **wired** or **wireless**.

Wired Systems

Wired systems are also known as **hardwired systems** in which the speaker or sound source like a television is physically tethered to the listener via a wire. Figure 7.13 shows the PockeTalker, a relatively simple and portable hardwired system.

The signal can either be the speaker's voice transduced via a microphone or transmitted from the source (e.g., television) via a jack. The advantage of the hardwired system is that it is relatively inexpensive and

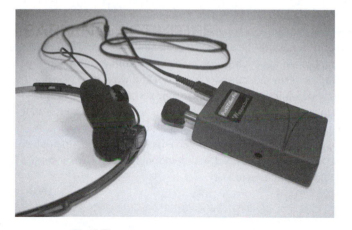

figure *7.13*

The PockeTalker.

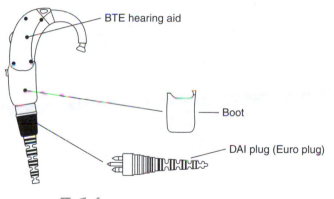

figure *7.14*

Direct-audio input via an audio boot on a hearing aid.

Source: Information from *Comparison of Large Area Wireless Systems*, by C. Compton-Conley, 2006, Washington, D.C.: Gallaudet University, Assistive Device Center.

provides a good signal. The disadvantage is the lack of mobility. Compton (1999) classifies hardwired systems into (1) **hearing aid dependent systems** and (2) **hearing aid independent systems**.

Hearing Aid Dependent Systems. These systems require use of a hearing aid that is coupled or attached to the jack or microphone in one of two ways. Figure 7.14 shows direct-audio input via a boot.

The first coupling method is through **direct-audio input (DAI)** in which the signal, in electrical form, enters the hearing aid through a DAI cord and boot or an audio-shoe attachment. The second coupling method is accessed via the hearing aid telecoil via several different ways. For example, patients can use a **teleloop**, worn around the neck, that changes the signal or electrical energy into electromagnetic energy that is picked up by the telecoil. Patients can also use a **silhouette inductor**, an ear-level device worn behind the ear much like a hearing aid that provides a stable electromagnetic signal to the telecoil. The silhouette is similar in size and shape to a standard behind-the-ear hearing aid, but is only about one-fourth as thick.

Hearing Aid Independent Systems. These systems require the use of a receiver or hardwire amplifier that has an input jack, volume control wheel, and earphone jack. The PockeTalker you saw in Figure 7.13 is an example of a hearing aid independent system.

The output jack can be connected to headphones or earbuds for use by listeners without hearing aids. The hardwired amplifier can also be coupled to hearing aids by the same methods described previously.

Wireless Systems

Wireless systems are those that do not tie the speaker or sound source to the listener with a wire. Just like the hardwired systems, wireless models can be hearing aid dependent or independent. Moreover, new clinical practice guidelines have developed new terminology and refer to some of these systems as "remote microphone" HAT (American Academy of Audiology, 2009). There are three types of wireless systems: (1) **induction loop**, (2) **infrared**, and (3) **frequency modulation (FM) systems**.

Induction Loop Systems.   These systems consist of a microphone, an amplifier, and a large loop that turns the signal into a fluctuating electromagnetic field that is picked up by a telecoil in the listener's hearing aid, whether it is an in-the-ear (ITE) or behind-the-ear (BTE) hearing aid. The input to the amplifier can be the microphone or jack output from a computer, DVD player, or television. Figure 7.15 shows an induction loop system and ways of accessing the signal. The speaker talks into the microphone, which goes to a mixer/amplifier that splits the signal to be presented through a loudspeaker for people with nomal hearing and through an induction loop for people with hearing aids (ITE or BTE) or telecoil receivers.

Sometimes, people either do not have hearing aids or have hearing aids that do not have telecoils. In this case, a telecoil receiver can be used with headphones/earbuds or coupled to patients' hearing aids or cochlear implants via DAI.

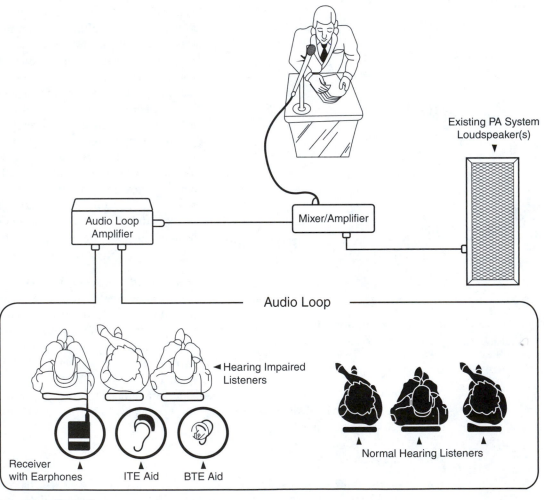

figure *7.15*

An induction loop group amplification system.

Source: This illustration is used with permission by Cynthia Compton-Conley, Ph.D., Gallaudet University, Washington, D.C.

The advantages of the induction loop system are that they provide accessibility to listeners with telecoil-equipped hearing aids, they allow for freedom of movement within the loop, and they are relatively inexpensive. However, induction loop systems have several disadvantages. First, telecoil receivers are required for those without telecoil-equipped hearing aids. Second, induction loop systems are subject to interference from a variety of sources (e.g., 60-cycle hum, fluorescent lights, and other sources of electricity). Third, the electromagnetic field from one induction-loop system can interfere or **spill over** with that from another such as in the case of systems built into the walls of adjacent rooms. For example, a child in one room may hear not only his or her teacher's voice, but the voice of the teacher in the adjacent room. Fourth, in most cases, listeners must often sit within a designated area that contains the induction loop at public events.

The induction loop can be permanent, such as built into the walls of a room, or it can be portable and placed under a mat for special events. A new type of induction loop system, the 3-D loop, overcomes the spillover and inconsistency of signal uniformity that plague traditional built-in systems (Lederman & Hendricks, 2003). The 3-D loop system takes advantage of digital signal processing and consists of four loop wires geometrically arranged in a specific pattern that are sandwiched into a premade flexible mat that can be either 9 × 9 feet or 12 × 12 feet (Lederman & Hendricks, 2003). These mats are placed under a carpet with the possibility of using additional mats to create larger listening areas (Lederman & Hendricks, 2003). Should you wish to contact the manufacturer of 3-D induction-loop systems, you may do so at the following address:

Induction Loop Systems
Oval Window Audio
33 Wildflower Court
Nederland, CO 80466
(303) 447-3607 Phone/TDD/Fax
www.ovalwindowaudio.com

Infrared Systems.   These systems transmit the signal via infrared light rays from a transmitter to a receiver. All listeners must have an infrared receiver. If the listener does not have a hearing aid, he or she can wear headphones or earbuds. Listeners with hearing aids can access the signal via the telecoil or a silhouette or through the use of DAI. Figure 7.16 shows an infrared (IR) receiver and ways of coupling the receiver to the user. For infrared devices, all users must be in direct line of sight so that the transmitter can send the signal from its light-emtting diode to the light-receiving diode on each receiver. Using the under-the-chin receiver, it can be coupled to unaided ears or those with CIC hearing aids. Similarly, body-worn receivers may be coupled to unaided ears or those with CICs. For ITEs and BTEs with telecoils, the signal may be accessed electromagnetically via teleloops (neckloops) or silhouette inductors; BTEs may also connect to infrared body-worn receivers via DAI.

Infrared systems have several advantages. First, the infrared system transmits a high-quality signal to listeners. Second, users are not limited to seating in specific areas as long as transmitting units are positioned in direct lines of light transmission to the receivers. Third, privacy is assured because the infrared signal cannot travel through walls or spill over to adjacent rooms. One disadvantage of the infrared systems is that they are expensive because they require a receiver for each listener. Second, infrared light is degraded by

IR Receiver Coupling Options

1	2	3	4	5
Unaided ear or CIC hearing aid worn with under-the-chin headphone IR receiver	Unaided ear or CIC hearing aid worn with headphones and body worn IR receiver	ITE or BTE hearing aid set to telecoil & worn with neckloop & body worn IR receiver	ITE or BTE hearing aid set to telecoil & worn with silhouette inductor & body worn IR receiver	BTE hearing aid with DAI cord and body worn IR receiver

figure *7.16*

Way of coupling to infrared receivers.

Source: The illustration is used with permission by Cynthia Compton-Conley, Ph.D., Gallaudet University, Washington, DC.

sunlight, precluding its use outside. Third, such things as clothing, children seated on laps, and so on may interfere with signal transmission. Fourth, similar to any light source, the infrared signal may be reflected off of room surfaces. Last, the larger the room, the more light-emitting transmitters are needed to ensure signal integrity.

Frequency Modulation (FM) Systems. These systems consist of a transmitter that sends the signal via radio waves to a receiver. Currently, these are the most popular form of group-amplification system. Compton (1999) stated that the FCC designated two special hearing assistance bands of 72 to 76 MHz and 216 to 217 MHz, the latter offers higher power and transmits over greater distances than the former. Figure 7.17 shows an FM amplification system consisting of a receiver and a transmitter. The receiver is worn on the body.

The speaker talks into the microphone that transduces the acoustic signal into an electric signal, which is in turn sent by radio waves to the receiver. There are a variety of microphones to choose from, which may be particularly critical in classroom situations. The receiver changes the radio waves back into electrical energy, which is amplified, and is then sent to the listeners' ears in a variety of ways. Figure 7.18 shows various coupling options for FM body receivers, which are essentially the same as for the infrared body receivers.

FM systems worn on the body were first available around 1968 and are used today. However, beginning about 1996, ear-level FM receivers became available that may be attached to the bottom of a hearing aid via an audio shoe. Over the years, the ear-level receivers have been reduced in size, one of the many advancements owed to the use of digital technology.

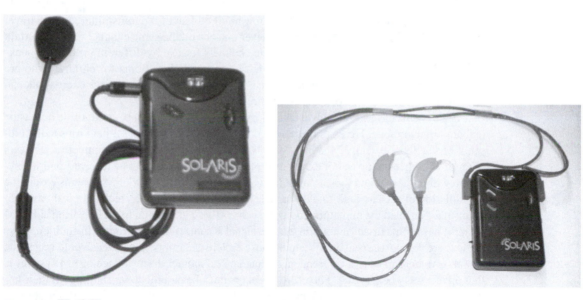

figure *7.17*

An FM amplification system consisting of a transmitter (left) and a receiver (right).

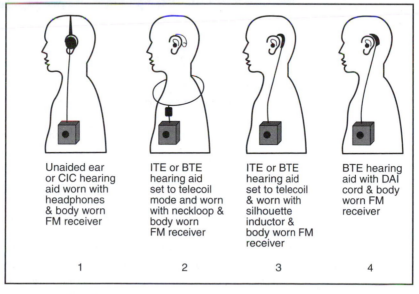

Coupling Options for FM Body-style Receiver

Unaided ear or CIC hearing aid worn with headphones & body worn FM receiver	ITE or BTE hearing aid set to telecoil mode and worn with neckloop & body worn FM receiver	ITE or BTE hearing aid set to telecoil & worn with silhouette inductor & body worn FM receiver	BTE hearing aid with DAI cord & body worn FM receiver
1	2	3	4

figure *7.18*

Ways of coupling to a body-style FM receiver.

Source: This illustration is used with permission by Cynthia Compton-Conley, Ph.D., Gallaudet University, Washington, D.C.

The FM signal is ubiquitous within a few hundred feet of the transmitter and can travel through walls. The transmitter and the receiver must be on the same channel for use. Certain contexts require the availability of multiple channels for use by different groups of speakers and listeners. For example, a school that has several classrooms for children who are deaf and hard of hearing necessitates the use of different channels; otherwise, crosstalk can occur between classrooms or communication groups.

FM systems have several advantages. First, the FM systems can be used inside or outside and are highly mobile. For example, teachers can use the FM system on field trips to the museum or the zoo. Second, FM signals may be broadcast to an unlimited number of receivers without seating restrictions. For example, football fans can check out FM receivers and sit anywhere within the stadium to hear all of the game, play-by-play. Third, FM systems ensure the transmission of a clear, high-quality signal. Fourth, as stated earlier, technological advancements have enabled the miniaturization of receivers that can snap-on to BTE hearing aids. FM systems have some disadvantages in that the signal is subject to interference. In addition, these devices are the most expensive system because each listener must have a receiver to access the signal, and these units require frequent maintenance. Another disadvantage of FM systems is that privacy may be an issue. Therefore, speakers must be careful about shutting off their microphones when they leave the room. Consider the Casebook Reflection that tells the story of Josie Moore, a speech-language pathologist who was just starting a new job at Taft Junior High School in Oklahoma City, Oklahoma. She taught a language group in the afternoon in the self-contained class for students who were either deaf or hard of hearing.

Other types of FM systems include **sound-field amplification systems** that consist of an FM transmitter that sends the speakers's voice to strategically placed loudspeakers in a classroom in order to improve the S/N ratio. We will be discussing the use of these devices in Chapter 10.

Casebook Reflection

Turn That Transmitter Off, Josie!

"Students, students . . . Mrs. Nelson will take over the group for just a few minutes," said Josie. "Thanks, Clarisse, I'll be just a minute. I just can't wait for the bell!"

"No problem! I know how it feels!" replied Clarisse Nelson, the paraprofessional. Clarisse had worked in the self-contained classroom for students with hearing impairment for six years. She had come to realize that these children were just like any other junior high school students—they enjoyed testing the boundaries and could sense fear in a new teacher. She was concerned about Josie Moore, the new speech-language pathologist at the school. Clarisse said, "OK, kids, let's continue. What did you think about the movie *The Outsiders*?"

"The town was like divided," Sue said. "Two groups of kids—the rich kids and the poor kids. The poor kids, I think, were called greasers."

"Yeah, Sue, like you! When was the last time you washed your hair?" Tony asked.

"Very funny, Tony," Sue said. "You should talk!"

As this was occurring in the classroom, Josie ran down the stairs to the teachers' restroom. The new job had been very difficult for her. She felt that the students had been "giving her the business" and testing her limits during the first few weeks of school. She had tried to maintain an authoritarian approach with them, hoping to keep order in the classroom although it was directly in contrast with her easygoing personality. Josie finished in the restroom and flushed the toilet.

Meanwhile, Clarisse was continuing the group discussion about *The Outsiders*. "Yes, Sue, there were two groups of people in the town. The greasers, the poor kids . . .," reviewed Clarisse before the class erupted in laughter. Some of the boys made flushing noises while making a sweeping movement with their hands.

"What's going on?" asked Clarisse.

"Miss Moore must be in the bathroom," Tony said. "We can hear the toilet flush!"

"Oh my, she must have forgotten to turn off the microphone on her transmitter," Clarisse surmised, with a big grin.

Josie wanted to get back and finish the group discussion before the end of the period. She ran up the stairs, down the hall, and entered the classroom to wild cheers and applause. Josie had no idea why she was the center of attention. The class was out of control!

Clarisse pointed to Josie's transmitter and said, "They heard everything. Sorry, I should have reminded you to shut off the microphone."

Josie's face turned a bright red. It was difficult to maintain her no-nonsense, all-business facade. Although embarrassed, she thought it was funny, too. So, she decided to make the most of it by taking a bow and curtsy at her students' applause. At that moment, the students realized that their teacher was human and "cool." It was the break that Josie needed. From that point on, she felt more at ease with her students. In turn, the students felt that their teacher was being "real" with them, and collectively, became more cooperative in the classroom.

OTHER ASSISTIVE TECHNOLOGY FOR THE DEAF AND HARD OF HEARING

Although the following involves mostly the use of vision, other assistive technology involves captioning and video relay services.

Captioned Programming, Closed Captioning, and Real-Time Captioning

As of January 2010, all new programming must be captioned (National Association of the Deaf, 2010b). **Closed captioning** is the process of converting a television program via a decoder or home video's dialogue, sound effects, and narration into words that appear on the screen (National Captioning Institute, 2005). Captioned programming is that which has closed captioning. The Telecommunications Act of 1996 mandated that 15 hours or 75% of the broadcast day for new programming must be captioned. As of January 1, 2006, the requirement was increased to 20 hours or 100% of the broadcast day for new programming that must be captioned. The hours between 2:00 and 6:00 a.m. are not considered part of the mandate. In addition, programs made or originally broadcasted before January 1, 1998, have different requirements. For example, 30% of these programs had to be captioned by January 1, 2003, and 75% of them had to be captioned by January 1, 2008. The Federal Communications Commission (FCC) is the federal agency that ensures that television networks and stations meet these requirements.

The National Captioning Institute (NCI) was established in 1979 and has been the world leader in providing high-quality media accessibility specializing in the following areas (NCI, 2005):

- Local and national news on major broadcast and cable networks
- Primetime and daytime network, cable, and Public Broadcasting Service (PBS) programs

- Children's programming on PBS and cable
- Live sports events
- Public affairs programming, such as C-SPAN and C-SPAN2
- Home video and DVD
- Commercials, infomercials, and music videos
- Local and national government meetings and conferences

The work of the NCI benefits a reported 100 million people, many of whom are deaf or hard of hearing. Other people who benefit from NCI services include those who are learning to read, who speak a foreign language or English as a second language, who are blind or have low vision, or who are otherwise interested in staying informed.

Real-time captioning is using captions that are created and displayed simultaneously for lectures/presentations such as training seminars, corporate meetings, sporting, or other "live" events (Robson, 2008). Captioners can type in excess of 225 words per minute with a high level of accuracy and usually hold credentials through state licensure boards for court reporters or by the National Court Reporters Association (NCRA) (Robson, 2008). Captioners use stenotype machines that are connected to computers with special software that translates stenographic shorthand into caption formats and standard spellings (Robson, 2008).

Telephone Devices for the Deaf

Two ways for the deaf and hard of hearing to communicate by telephone are discussed next. The text telephone has been around for decades, but the video relay services are newer.

Text Telephone

In the past, the deaf have used teletype machines for communication on the telephone. In old movies, teletype machines are often shown sending and receiving the latest news. The term **TTY** is an abbreviation for text telephone or telephone typewriter; it permits the deaf and hard of hearing to communicate by telephone. Figures 7.19 and 7.20 show a picture of a TTY and a graphic explaining how it works, respectively.

The sending teletype has electronic circuitry that changes type into pulses that are sent over the telephone lines to the receiving teletype that receives the pulses and turns them back into type for people to read (Cook & Hussey, 2002). The term TTY is also called a telecommunications device for the deaf or (TDD). The term TTY is used more frequently than TDD.

To use the device, the operator has to put the handset of the telephone into the acoustic cups on the top of the TTY. The operator types a message on the keypad and the letters are turned into electronic pulses that are sent via telephone wire to the recipient who also has a TTY. The TTY receives the electronic pulses, which are changed back into orthographic

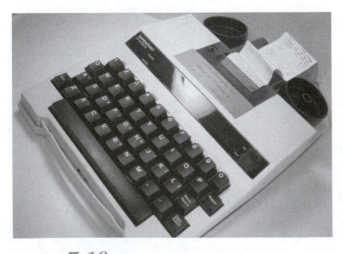

figure *7.19*

A TTY device.

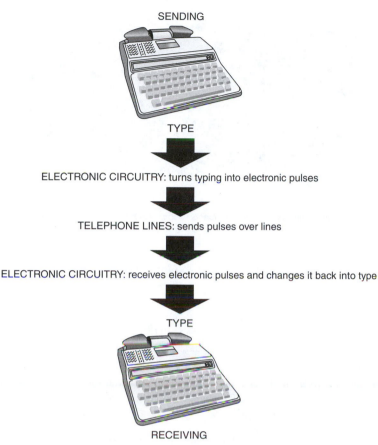

SENDING

TYPE

ELECTRONIC CIRCUITRY: turns typing into electronic pulses

TELEPHONE LINES: sends pulses over lines

ELECTRONIC CIRCUITRY: receives electronic pulses and changes it back into type

TYPE

RECEIVING

figure *7.20*

How the TTY works.

symbols that are displayed on an LED screen for the recipient to read. It is not necessary for a person to have a TTY to send a message to a TTY user. The **Telecommunications Relay Service (TRS)** has special operators available 24 hours a day, seven days a week who can type whatever is said so that it appears on the TTY user's screen. Likewise, that operator can read the response from the TTY user to a person using a regular telephone.

In the past, TTYs could be used only with landline telephones or analog cellular phones and networks. On July 1, 2002, the FCC ruled that TTY users must be able to complete calls with their digital wireless services, provided that they have TTYs and digital wireless handsets that are compatible with one another. To comply with FCC requirements, wireless service providers, handset manufacturers, and TTY manufacturers have made technological changes to their networks and some of their products. Newer TTYs now have symbols identifying them as "compatible with select digital cellular phones." Therefore, users should be able to use their TTY with digital wireless handsets that are designated as compatible with TTYs.

The use of a TTY necessitates that the following rules of etiquette be followed (The Arizona Commission for the Deaf and Hard of Hearing, 2003; Rochester Institute of Technology Libraries, 2003).

- Allow for at least 10 rings before hanging up because it may take TTY users a while to notice the flashing light.
- Introduce yourself when calling because TTY users obviously cannot recognize callers by their voices.
- Use signals such as "ga" for "go ahead" to let the TTY user recognize the end of your message. Similarly, use "sk" for "stop keying" to alert the TTY user of the end of a conversation. To put someone on hold, use "hd," and if it is taking longer than usual, type "hd" again to show that you have not forgotten about them.
- Do not interrupt the TTY user, and let him or her finish the message before typing, otherwise a garbled message will result.
- Print out your TTY conversation to reread after the call to verify its content and then destroy it so that it is not read by an unintended party.

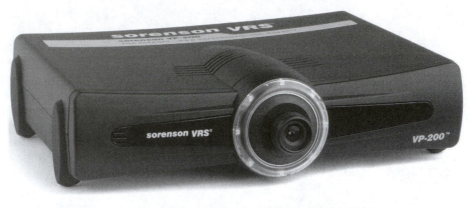

Photo provided courtesy Sorenson Communications.

figure *7.21* ─────────────────────────────

A Sorenson Videophone (VP-200) used to transmit the image of a caller using American Sign Language.

- Type cue signals to denote emotion such as, "HAHAHA," "SMILE," "GRRR," and so on.
- Exercise typical telephone etiquette by explaining why a conversation must be made short and alert the TTY users if anyone else is listening or watching.
- Learn common abbreviations used by TTY users (e.g., abt = about, AM = morning, ans = answer, bec = because, and so on).

Following these and other rules of etiquette can make communication via a TTY a more pleasant experience for all.

Video Relay Services

Users of American Sign Language can now use video relay services to make telephone calls. Sorenson Communications in Salt Lake City, Utah, is an example of one company providing free video relay services to these individuals. Users require a Sorenson Videophone VP-200 (see Figure 7.21), a certified sign-language interpreter, a television, and a high-speed Internet connection to send messages. Figure 7.22 shows how various components of the Sorenson system work together. Users simply have to make a call that goes to an ASL interpreter who serves as a conduit for communication between callers. The caller signs to the interpreter, whom they see on their television screen. The interpreter calls the hearing person on a regular telephone line and relays the conversation between the two individuals (Sorenson Communications, 2010). The interpreter translates the signed message into spoken English for the hearing person. Hearing people can use these services, too, by simply calling the Direct VP Number or the toll-free number: 1 (866) FAST-VRS (1 (866) 327-8877) of the person who is deaf or hard of hearing.

Users of ASL frequently communicate with each other using Skype, the largest voice-communication service over the Internet. Users simply have to have a microphone and video camera connected to their personal computer. The software is free and may be downloaded at www.skype.com. ASL users can sign to each other using the video-transmission capabilities of Skype.

How does Sorenson VRS work?

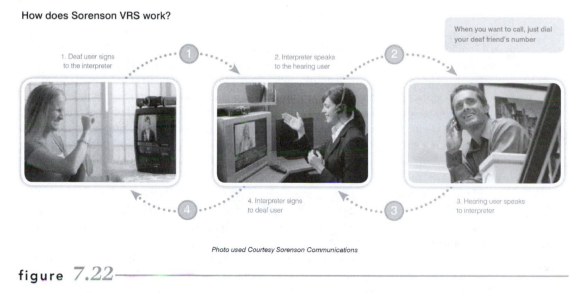

Photo used Courtesy Sorenson Communications

figure 7.22

Sequence of events in using the Sorenson Communications Video Relay Service.

AUDIOLOGISTS' RESPONSIBILITIES IN EVALUATING, SELECTING, AND FITTING HEARING ASSISTIVE TECHNOLOGY

Even though anyone can purchase HAT from a vendor, audiologists should evaluate, select, and fit the devices. HAT can be used by a variety of patients of different ages, varying degrees of hearing losses, including hearing aid and non-hearing aid owners in a variety of settings. In this section of the text, we will discuss and provide specific examples of HAT use across the lifespan within particular attention to the impact of various aspects of context (e.g., setting, social, cultural, and physical). How do you know when someone is a candidate for HAT? The use of HAT is not dependent on age, degree of hearing loss, or whether patients use hearing aids or cochlear implants. Children with the following disorders are candidates for HAT (AAA, 2009d):

- Hearing loss
- Auditory processing deficits
- Learning disabilities
- Auditory neuropathy spectrum disorder
- Language delay/disorder
- Attention deficits
- English as a second language

Parents, classroom teachers, speech-language pathologists, and other professional advisors are instrumental in supporting young children's successful use of HAT. Similarly, there is no upper age restriction for HAT, especially if elderly persons have caretakers to assist with their use. HAT users may have hearing sensitivity that ranges from normal to profound hearing impairment. Similarly, patients may vary in their use of HAT with and without other devices. Some may use only HAT, others may use it with hearing aids and/or cochlear implants.

For pediatric patients, audiologists should consider the acoustic environment, social/emotional considerations, functional status, and available support when determining HAT candidacy (AAA, 2009d). (See Chapters 9 and 10.) With adult patients, audiologists may use self-assessment tools that specifically ask about hearing in different situations with and without hearing aids. For example, Sandridge's (1995) *Listening Questionnaire* asks patients their difficulty in hearing in an automobile, listening to the television or radio, or talking over the telephone, and so on with and without their hearing aids. Patients check "yes," "sometimes," "no," or "not applicable." Audiologists analyze patients' responses to see difficult listening situations that may or may not aided by HAT. In addition, audiologists may look at the listening situations nominated and prioritized by the patient on the *Client Oriented Scale of Improvement* (COSI) (Dillon, James, & Ginis, 1997). In particular, situations rated poorly even after obtaining hearing aids may be improved through the use of a HAT.

So, should patients get hearing aids, HAT, or hearing aids *and* HAT? The previous study showed that for this sample of patients, hearing aids provided more benefit than use of HAT alone. However, each patient is different, and it depends on the individual. For example, for some patients, HAT may be enough. Pruitt (1990) presented a case study in which an elderly woman rejected the use of a hearing aid in favor of HAT. However, some studies have found that patients prefer hearing aids in daily use rather than using HAT (Jerger, Chmiel, Florin, Pirozzolo, & Wilson, 1996). Similarly, 60 veterans—30 with service-related and 30 non–service-related hearing loss—were compared for the amount of improvement in hearing-related quality of life using no assistance, a HAT device, a conventional hearing aid with an omnidirectional microphone, and a programmable hearing aid with a directional microphone (Yueh et al., 2001). Veterans fit with either type of hearing aid showed substantial improvement in hearing-related quality of life over veterans using HAT or no form of assistance. Therefore, research shows hearing aids provided greater improvement with hearing aids over HAT alone. Let's consider two different patients, Jenny and Casey, in the following Casebook Reflections.

Casebook Reflection

HAT Only for Jenny

Jenny Gaylord, a 90-year-old woman, lives in the Golden Sunset Apartments, a residential facility for self-sufficient, low- to middle-income senior citizens. The facility consists of 60 single-bedroom apartments. Residents must be independent and are responsible for their own transportation although the city bus stops in front of the building. Jenny has been a resident of Golden Sunset Apartments for five years. Jenny is rarely home in the evening, as she frequently accepts dinner invitations from her friends and family. Jenny's children, their spouses, and her grandchildren live in the town. Jenny takes great pride in her appearance and independence. She communicates very well in most situations.

Last year, Jenny had an audiologic evaluation performed by a local audiologist as suggested by her primary care physician. Jenny was accompanied by her daughter Trista and was diagnosed with a mild-to-moderate bilateral sensorineural hearing loss. At the time, the audiologist, Dr. Billingsley, suggested, "Mrs. Gaylord, you might benefit from the use of hearing aids."

"Dr. Billingsley, I don't feel that I need them yet. I can hear just fine," said Jenny. "I just have a little difficulty hearing over the telephone, especially when talking to my grandchildren."

"I'm afraid I have to agree with Mom, Dr. Billingsley," Trista said. "Mom really doesn't seem to have difficulty in face-to-face conversations."

"Do you even understand what is being said in a noisy restaurant?" asked Dr. Billingsley.

"Well, yes, I can. However, I have to watch their lips. If I don't understand someone, I'm not afraid to ask the person to repeat what they've said," Jenny said.

"I wish all my patients did that," remarked Dr. Billingsley. "Are you sure you don't want to see the styles of hearing aids and hear about the latest technology that is available?"

"I'm sure," said Jenny. "I just don't think I'm ready for hearing aids yet. Do you have anything that can help me hear over the telephone? I don't like the telephone that I have. Although it cost only $9.95, I can hardly see the buttons and they're difficult for me to press."

"Yes, Mrs. Gaylord. I have an assortment of devices available for use on the phone in our hearing assistive technology center. We say HAT center for short. Your problem may be helped by several HAT devices. I have several to demonstrate for you. First, there is the in-line amplifier. See how it is connected between the body of the phone and the curly cord. It has a wheel that can be used to adjust the volume. Let's try it. I'll call you from the other room. Answer the phone and adjust the volume using the volume wheel," instructed Dr. Billingsley.

"OK," said Jenny looking at her daughter.

"Go ahead, Mom, answer it!" Trista said when the phone rang.

"Hello," Jenny said.

"Can you hear me?" said Dr. Billingsley. "Turn up the volume if necessary."

"Oh, that's wonderful," Jenny said. "I can hear you well!"

"OK, I'm coming back to the HAT center," said Dr. Billingsley. "This is the Clarity phone. It has big numbers for those users with visual or manual dexterity problems. You can have the clarity feature either on or off and can adjust the volume."

"What does the clarity feature do?" Jenny asked.

"It makes the higher frequencies louder," explained Dr. Billingsley. "That will be good for you considering that your hearing loss is mostly in the higher frequencies. Let me go to the other room and call you."

"OK," Jenny said. "Hello?"

"Yes, can you hear me?" asked Dr. Billingsley. "Don't forget to adjust the volume."

"Oh, this is marvelous!" Jenny exclaimed. "I'd like to purchase this telephone! I love the large buttons! The clarity feature allows me to hear the high-pitch sounds!"

Although Jenny opted for purchasing a HAT device only, some patients, such as Casey Scott in the next Casebook Reflection, require both a hearing aid and HAT.

Casebook Reflection

A Hearing Aid and HAT for Casey

Casey Scott, a 65-year-old retired lawyer, enjoys his Lifelong Learners Group at Springfield University. He recently had a significant decrease in hearing sensitivity in both ears from moderately severe to severe-to-profound. His physicians could find no medical reason for the sudden change in his degree of hearing loss. Casey was very frustrated because his old hearing aids did not provide enough gain and he was having difficulty hearing conversations even in quiet environments, on his cell phone, and in a variety of other situations. Casey was particularly distraught because of his inability to hear on his cell phone, dining at restaurants, and hearing speakers at his Lifelong Learners Group, among other once-easy listening situations.

Dr. Cameron, Casey's audiologist, recommended a new hearing aid for Casey that was compatible with Phonak's MLxS FM receiver and SmartLink SX communication device.

"Mr. Scott, in reviewing the situations that you feel provide you with the most difficulty, I am recommending new digital behind-the-ear hearing aids that will be strong enough for you," explained Dr. Cameron. "Also, you have listed several situations in which you can't hear the speaker, especially during your Lifelong Learners classes. What exactly is the problem?"

"In our classes, we have discussions about books we've read. I can't hear speakers that are at a distance from me, even in a quiet room," explained Casey. "They just don't speak loud enough. Also, I have difficulty understanding my wife when we go out to dinner. Her voice is so soft, and most restaurants are quite noisy."

"Well, Mr. Scott, your hearing has gotten significantly worse so that your present hearing aids don't provide much help. However, even if your aids did provide enough amplification for your current degree of loss, distance and noise make understanding speech difficult. When someone's voice travels over a distance, it loses its intensity and is affected by reverberation and noise."

"What difference does reverberation make?" asked Casey.

"Mr. Scott, reverberation is sound reflecting off of the surfaces and objects in a room. The reflection of the sound distorts speech, causing speech sounds to smear, eliminating important cues," explained Dr. Cameron. "Noise covers over the speaker's voice. That is why in addition to new hearing aids, I'm recommending a special FM receiver, the MLxS, that snaps into the bottom of your hearing aids and the SmartLink SX, a compact communication device, which is a microphone with a built-in FM transmitter. I have them here in my hands. See how the MicroLink snaps into the bottom of the hearing aid?"

"Yes," Casey said. "How does this contraption work?"

"The SmartLink SX is a microphone that, as I mentioned, has a built-in FM transmitter. It is placed directly in front of the sound source, which could be a person or a TV set, for instance. There are two different microphones to use, but we will get to that later. The microphone picks up whatever you want to hear and sends the signal via radio waves directly to the FM receivers on your hearing aids, eliminating any effects of reverberation or noise."

"Wow, sounds like exactly what I need!" exclaimed Casey.

"What's convenient is that you can set the microphone on a stand in front of the sound source, or the speaker can clip the SmartLink SX to his pocket so that you can hear your buddy when fishing."

"I can't wait to try it out!" Casey said enthusiastically.

"Another feature of this device is that this has Bluetooth capabilities that can be used with your cell phone."

Several factors should be considered when selecting a HAT for a patient. Audiologists should not just select a device, but form a partnership with the patient. In both cases, the audiologists formed partnerships with Jenny and Casey in selecting their HAT.

Rothstein and Everson (1994) suggested using the following guidelines for selecting HAT for patients. First, look for simple answers; low-technology options are not necessarily inferior to high-technology solutions. Actually, the opposite may be true. Low-technology devices are often less expensive, easier to use, and more reliable than high-technology devices. Second, consider the learning and work style of the user. Audiologists should strongly consider the individual preferences of the patient in selecting appropriate HAT. Which device does the patient seem to prefer? Which device do you feel the patient would use on a long-term basis? For example, Dr. Billingsley allowed Jenny to try several HAT devices that could help her understand better over the telephone before she chose the Clarity phone. Third, consider the long-range implications of patients' hearing impairments. What is the degree of the patient's hearing loss? Will it get worse or fluctuate?

Does the patient use hearing aids or cochlear implants? Which devices can be coupled to the patients' hearing aids or cochlear implants? Will the device have to be replaced if the patient's hearing deteriorates? For Jenny, the Clarity phone should be useable even if her hearing gets worse because it may still be accessed through telecoil-equipped hearing aids. Casey's hearing has already deteriorated, and if it gets even worse, the MicroLink and SmartLink SX should still be useable.

Fourth, look at each piece of equipment. How easy will it be for the patient to assemble, use, and maintain? How long will the device last, be compatible with today's technology, and when will it need to be updated? Will the device be functional for the patient over time? Will the patient have the same communication needs over time? Can the device be easily adapted for a variety of situations and uses? How portable is the device? For example, Casey's device is very compatible with today's technology, will be very functional for use in his activities over time, and in a variety of situations at home and on the go. Other considerations include what other patients and consumers who have purchased the device say about its dependability and durability. If the device malfunctions, can it be easily repaired? Does the manufacturer have technological support available via telephone or the Internet? For example, Dr. Billingsley had good reports from patients who had used the Clarity phone regarding its dependability and durability; rarely were there reports of mechanical difficulties.

Fifth, audiologists should explore as many options as possible with patients prior to the selection of HAT. Much of this work needs to be done prior to deciding to dispense HAT to patients as part of a practice. Audiologists should do preliminary research through contacting different consumer organizations, support groups, and rehabilitation agencies regarding the best manufacturers of HAT. Some agencies have lending libraries or demonstration laboratories with the latest technology. Most professional meetings have exhibits that are attended by leading manufacturers who demonstrate the latest innovations in assistive technology. Audiologists should register for manufacturers' and suppliers' mailing lists to receive the latest catalogs of their product lines. For example, Dr. Billingsley and Dr. Cameron had extensively researched commonly used HAT available from different manufacturers in developing their product lines.

Sixth, audiologists should organize the HAT into categories so that patients can compare products from different manufacturers. If possible, audiologists should secure HAT on consignment for patients to try prior to purchase. Audiologists should be familiar enough with the HAT so that they can easily answer questions about the features and options each offers in addition to the pros and cons of each device. For example, Dr. Billingsley had at least two types of HAT available from different manufacturers for patients to try.

After selection of HAT, audiologists should use the sheet found in Appendix 7.2 (ASHA, 2006b). The report should contain the manufacturer, model, and serial number of the device in addition to an explanation of the rationale for the device, including the results of self-report surveys. In addition, the report should contain a summary of any counseling provided to the patient, including the types of HAT considered and the pros and cons of the selected device(s). The audiologist should also describe any assessments completed with the device. For example, the electroacoustic characteristics of hearing aids may be altered when coupled to HAT. Therefore, reports of electroacoustic analyses and real-ear probe-microphone measurements are essential documentation for HAT that is used when coupled to patients' hearing aids, in addition to their responses to the device and their prognosis for benefit (McPherson, Hickson, & Baumfield, 1992). Audiologists should provide information about orientation and ongoing monitoring.

How should audiologists orient patients to HAT? Compton, Lewis, Palmer, and Thelen (1994) suggested a series of patient outcomes from a HAT orientation (see Appendix 7.3). They suggested that patients should be able to install the device, turn it on and off, change its batteries, and clean and care for it. For example, Dr. Billingsley made sure that Mrs. Gaylord was able to install the Clarity phone, use the clarity feature and volume control, as well as program in frequently used numbers. Patients should be able to select appropriate coupling methods to the ears, and understand the principles of sound-to-source microphone proximity and that the device will work with only one sound source at a time. For example, Dr. Cameron made sure that Casey understood how the Phonak MLxS FM receiver worked with his hearing aids, and that a good signal required that the Phonak SmartLink SX be placed close to the speaker or sound source. Casey was also told that the SmartLink had three microphone modes, the Omni, the Zoom and SuperZoom. The Zoom microphone is used for one-on-one or small-group communication situations. The Super-Zoom microphone is for use in very noisy situations, picking up the signal from the front and attenutating sound from other directions. Compton et al. (1994) suggested that patients should be able to explain to others why they have the device and what it is and does, in addition to its purpose and what a speaker does to be able to use it. Children particularly should develop self-advocacy skills with their use of HAT. If they are comfortable sharing information about these devices, the more others, especially their peers, will understand their purpose. Similarly, Dr. Cameron role-played with Casey so he could practice explaining to other members of the Lifelong Learners Group that the SmartLink SX had to be passed from speaker to speaker for him to be able to participate in class discussions. Audiologists should also brainstorm with patients in inventorying and selecting situations to use the device. For example, besides the Lifelong Learners Group, Dr. Cameron and Casey made a list of other communication situations in which to use the MLxS FM receiver and SmartLink SX. Dr. Cameron showed Casey how to use the devices with his cell phone, his television, and even his geographical positioning system in his car. Patients should demonstrate troubleshooting skills with the device during installation, coupling, and operation. Dr. Cameron demonstrated how to troubleshoot the MLxS FM receiver and SmartLink SX during all phases of its use and then tested Casey's skill and comprehension. In other chapters of the book, we will go into further detail regarding the use of HAT by patients of different ages and in a variety of settings.

ASSISTIVE TECHNOLOGY FOR DEAF–BLIND PERSONS

Dual sensory impairment—having both visual and hearing sensory difficulties—has been discussed in other chapters. People with dual sensory impairment use assistive technology. It is important to realize that both visual and hearing impairment have wide ranges of severity. Some HAT is appropriate for persons with hearing loss and low vision, such as the Walker Clarity phone with its large-numbered keypad. However, for some people with no functional hearing or vision, assistive technology for deaf-blind individuals may be required.

Assistive technology for deaf-blind individuals can involve low or high technology. The first consideration for members of the general public who interact with deaf-blind individuals is to know their preferred method of communication (Deafblindinfo.org, 2010). Some deaf-blind persons use assistance cards that state their needs, preferred method of communication, and type/degree of impairment (Deafblindinfo.org, 2010). Some low-technology communication methods may include the following (Deafblindinfo.org, 2010):

- An Alphabet Glove: a white glove with letters of the alphabet printed in strategic positions so that communication partners can touch the letters to spell words in conveying messages to deaf-blind persons.
- The Brailletalk: a plastic card with a fold-over cover that has raised Braille symbols that co-occur with their corresponding English letters so communication partners can spell words that can be read by deaf-blind persons using Braille.
- Pad and Thick Pen: simply a large pen and a large pad on which large letters can be written that may be read by deaf-blind persons.

Assistive technology for deaf-blind individuals can also involve high-technology devices. A few examples are as follows (Taylor, Booth, & Tindell, 2006):

- Freedom Scientific Face-to-Face Communicator: enables real-time communication between a person with deaf-blindness who types on a special keyboard that sends messages at distances up to 30 feet to Bluetooth® compatible personal computers that display the messages on a screen. The sighted person types responses on the computer keyboard that go in reverse direction to the special keyboard, which displays the message in Braille. Face-to-Face permits saving text files of conversations for archiving, and uses common phrases for easy communication.
- TTY with Braille Display: consists of a regular TTY that is positioned on top of a Braille communicator. Callers who are deaf-blind can make a call by typing their messages on the Braille communicator, which are sent by the TTY as electric pulses over the telephone wires. The caller responds and the message goes in reverse direction and is ultimately shown on the Braille display.
- Captel: a special phone that requires use of a captioning service. Senders type messages on a computer screen in large enough font so that persons who are deaf with limited vision can read it.

SUMMARY

Communication sciences and disorders professionals require an understanding of assistive technology for persons with disabilities, in particular the use of HAT by people who are deaf and hard of hearing. Successful selection, evaluation, and fitting of HAT for patients require knowledge beyond the devices themselves. The chapter has reviewed the use of HAT within various social, cultural, and physical contexts. Readers were exposed to different categories of HAT, including those that help use the telephone, those that help with the awareness of environmental sounds, and those that are used for face-to-face communication and television watching. The accessibility of cell phones was also discussed. Two Casebook Reflections were used to illustrate the selection, evaluation, and fitting process. Last, low- and high-technology assistive devices for individuals who are deaf-blind were presented.

LEARNING ACTIVITIES

- Interview two audiologists who work in two different practice settings (e.g., private practice, hospital setting, and public schools) and ask about how much of their job involves the selection, evaluation, and fitting of HAT.
- Search the Internet and develop a resource notebook for use in a hypothetical clinic with an ample selection of HAT from all three categories, complete with pictures, manufacturer contact information, use, coupling capabilities, and approximate price.

APPENDIX 7.1

Justification Letter
for Assistive Technology (AT)

Date

Addressee:

Re: Consumer's Name

Social Security Number

Policy or Account Number

Dear (name of Medical Consultant, Vocational Rehabilitation Counselor, Personal Care Representative, Special Education Director, etc.):

Paragraph One: Short Introduction

One or two sentences about the device and services requested and why they are needed. Identification of supporting documentation included as enclosures (AT professional evaluation, price quotation from vendor, letters of medical necessity from specialists, brochure, or other information showing device).

Paragraph Two: Information About the Consumer

Personalize the consumer: provide information needed to acquaint the funding source's decision-maker with the situation and requirement for AT. Include the following, as appropriate:

1. Name, age, sex, diagnosis
2. Current housing status (where does consumer live and with whom; availability of, or need for, personal assistance)
3. Current school or employment status
4. Primary care physician, hospital, and clinic affiliation as appropriate
5. Diagnosis, expected clinical course, and prognosis. Be as specific and inclusive as possible. Address changes in condition; height and weight comparisons; planned or completed surgeries; X-ray findings; and other relevant medical diagnostic testing as appropriate.
6. Information regarding functional limitations associated with the diagnosis
7. AT history
8. Current equipment and experiences in using that equipment
9. Cognitive status
10. Describe efforts to obtain funding through other sources

Paragraph Three: Equipment Requested

Describe the equipment needed in detail. A request that simply states "electric wheelchair" or "augmentative communication system" will not be adequate because there are many different varieties of communications systems and power chairs. Address the need for any added components (e.g., cushions, joysticks, positioning belts, mounting devices, etc.). Discuss duration of expected usage of equipment. Describe the consumer's actual experience and success in using the device. Show the functional benefits of the equipment to the consumer; tell the decision-maker what the equipment will allow the consumer to do. You may want to include a picture or video of the consumer using the device.

Explain why other devices were ruled out, especially less expensive devices. Express the need for the device in language that targets the funding source's criteria. For example, language such as: "medical necessity," "achieving a free and appropriate public education," or "overcoming barriers to employment." Describe why the device is not an item of convenience.

Consider addressing the following rationales:

1. Is the device needed to prevent further injury or pain? Is it a cost-effective means of preventing secondary complications or further functional limitations?
2. Is the device needed for effective communication including communication for medical purposes?
3. Is the device needed for safety?
4. What is the impact of the device on the consumer's mental health? How does the consumer's mental health impact medical, educational, vocational status?
5. Will the device reduce dependence upon other services funded by this agency such as nursing care or hospitalization?
6. Is the device a substitute—in effect, a prosthetic or orthotic device—for a lost functional capability such as vision or hearing or mobility?
7. Will the device allow the consumer to resume or improve his employment?
8. Will the device allow the consumer to continue to live at home instead of in a nursing home or hospital?
9. Will it allow the consumer to meet educational goals?

Mention potential for growth-modification and adjustments that will ensure long-term use of the device. Describe the cost of the equipment and why the particular vendor was chosen. For example: good reputation, experience with that vendor, preferred provider with your insurer, only vendor in town.

Paragraph Four: Needed Support Services or Plans for Evaluation

Describe any needed support services such as training, maintenance, and repairs and how these services will be funded, including contributions from any other funding sources.

Paragraph Five: Summary

Identify enclosures if you have not already done so. Identify whom to contact for additional information or questions.

Closure

Thank the agency for its time in reviewing the request. Provide co-signatures of appropriate medical and vocational professionals.

Sample enclosures:

1. Prescription and letter from primary care physician and specialists
2. AT evaluation documents
3. Photographs or videos showing consumer using the requested device
4. Information from vendor on device and costs
5. Brochures or letters describing requested AT device
6. Any required agency forms

Sources: Information from the University of Washington Center for Technology and Disability Studies, retrieved from http://uwctds .washington.edu; the University of Washington Center on Human Development and Disability for the Washington Assistive Technology Act program, retrieved from http://watap.org. Used with permission.

APPENDIX 7.2

Documentation of Hearing Assistive Technology Device Selection Protocol

Rationale for system/device selection:

Counseling provided:

Procedures involved in the assessment of the system/device:

Measures of satisfaction:

Prognosis for benefit:

Plan for monitoring and orientation:

Final disposition/reassessment plan:

Source: From *Preferred Pratice Patterns for the Profession of Audiology [Preferred Practice Pattern],* by the American Speech-Language-Hearing Assocation, 2006, retrieved from www.asha.org/policy. Reprinted with permission.

APPENDIX 7.3

Hearing Assistive Technology Device Fitting and Orientation Checklist

INSTRUCTIONS: *Please assess the following skills after delivery of assistive listening technology.*

Task: Can Patient . . .	Outcome			Comments
Install device?	Yes	No	N/A	
Turn device on and off?	Yes	No	N/A	
Change batteries?	Yes	No	N/A	
Clean and care for device?	Yes	No	N/A	
Select appropriate coupling method?	Yes	No	N/A	
Describe principles of sound source microphone proximity?	Yes	No	N/A	
Explain presence of the device?	Yes	No	N/A	
Explain what the device is?	Yes	No	N/A	
Explain what purpose the device serves?	Yes	No	N/A	
Explain how speakers may use it?	Yes	No	N/A	
List appropriate situations for device use?	Yes	No	N/A	
Troubleshoot installation problems?	Yes	No	N/A	
Troubleshoot coupling problems?	Yes	No	N/A	
Troubleshoot operational problems?	Yes	No	N/A	

Source: Based on *Assistive Technology: Too Legit to Quit,* by C. Compton, D. Lewis, C. Palmer, and M. Thelen, 1994, Pittsburgh, PA: Support Syndicate for Audiology.

CHAPTER eight

An Introduction to Cochlear Implants

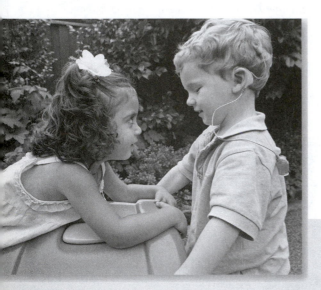

LEARNING *objectives*

After reading this chapter, you should be able to:

1. Describe the basic parts of a cochlear implant and how they work.

2. Navigate websites of the three cochlear implant manufacturers.

3. List pediatric and adult patient selection criteria of two cochlear implant manufacturers.

4. Discuss the preimplant evaluation process and surgery.

5. Articulate postoperative procedures and device orientation.

6. Identify various communication options and therapy programs for those with cochlear implants.

7. Describe pediatric and adult cochlear implant recipients' short- and long-term performance expectations.

8. Define and list some benefits of bimodal stimulation (e.g., hearing aid worn in the ear opposite to the implant), bilateral implantation, and hybrid cochlear implants.

9. Discuss patient candidacy for surgical risks and expected outcomes for auditory brainstem implants.

10. Explain issues that the Deaf community has with cochlear implants.

To the general public, the cochlear implant has been known as the "bionic ear," offering people with severe to profound sensorineural hearing loss an opportunity to hear. At first, only adults with profound sensorineural hearing losses were candidates for cochlear implants. Advancements in technology have resulted in cochlear implantation for children less than a year old. At least 10 years ago, Blanchfield, Feldman, Dunbar, and Gardner (2001) estimated that as many as 738,000 persons in the United States have severe to profound sensorineural hearing loss and may be potential candidates for cochlear implants. Today, that number has grown and the trend is expected to continue in the future.

Some people considering a cochlear implant for themselves or a loved one may believe that those devices will restore hearing to normal. Physicians, audiologists, speech-language pathologists, and other healthcare professionals must be able to provide accurate information to patients and their families that fosters realistic expectations regarding the benefits derived from the use of cochlear implants. Moreover, cochlear implantation requires a strong commitment to auditory rehabilitation to receive maximum benefit from these devices. In this chapter, readers will learn about how cochlear implants work, and follow the experiences of a young girl and her family through the process of receiving a cochlear implant. Considerations for school follow-up, communication options, and examples of therapy programs and materials for children and adults with cochlear implants will be presented. Additionally, other options for patients will be discussed, including bimodal stimulation, bilateral cochlear implants, and hybrid devices. The chapter concludes with an introduction to auditory brainstem implants and a discussion of Deaf culture and cochlear implants.

COCHLEAR IMPLANTS AND THEIR PARTS

Because cochlear implants are surgically implanted, some parts are "inside" components and some are worn externally. Although cochlear implant manufacturers differ in the design and circuitry of their products, most devices have the same basic parts. Figure 8.1 shows and labels the inside parts visible on Cochlear's Freedom Nucleus® cochlear implant. The internal parts of a cochlear implant include the receiver-stimulator, internal receiver, electrode array, and ground. The external parts include a directional microphone, cords, speech processor, and a transmitting coil. Over the years, the speech processors available from different manufacturers have undergone miniaturization. Figures 8.2 and 8.3 show the Nucleus® Freedom baby-worn and behind-the-ear processors. Figure 8.4 shows a child wearing a cochlear implant.

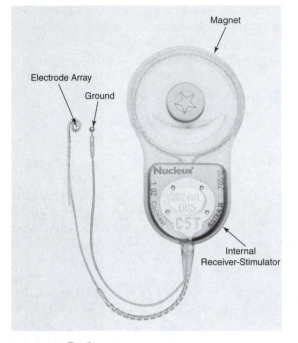

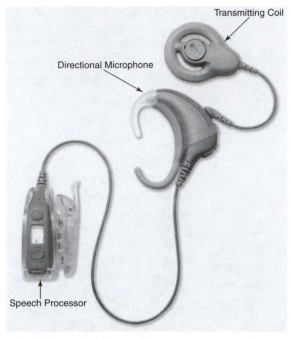

figure *8.1*

Cochlear's™ Freedom Nucleus® cochlear implant.

Source: Picture provided courtesy of Cochlear™ Americas, © 2005, Cochlear Americas.

figure *8.2*

Cochlear™ Nucleus® baby-worn processor.

Source: Picture provided courtesy of Cochlear™ Americas, © 2007, Cochlear Americas.

Figure 8.5 shows how the parts of the cochlear implant work together. Briefly, the directional microphone picks up acoustic energy in front of the patient and changes the signal into electrical energy. The electrical signal is sent to the speech processor that will change it into a digitally coded signal. These processors use special speech coding strategies that determine how loudness, pitch, and timing are processed and sent to nerve fibers. The coded signal is sent via an electromagnetic conductor or FM transmitter to the transmitting coil. The transmitting coil, held in place by a magnet, sends the coded signal across the skin to the internal receiver-stimulator, which changes the coded message into an electrical code. The code is sent to the electrode array that stimulates auditory nerve fibers tuned to a specific frequency. The **electrode array** consists of electrodes that are paired and aligned along a wire that is inserted into the round window (i.e., scala tympani) during surgery. The nerve fibers send this information to the brain. Cochlear implants provide an option for patients who are deaf and hard of hearing who receive little or no benefit from hearing aids. However, not all of these patients are suitable candidates for cochlear implants. We will discuss the criteria for cochlear implant candidacy a bit later on in the chapter.

COCHLEAR IMPLANT MANUFACTURERS

In the United States, there are three cochlear implant manufacturers. They are Cochlear (www.cochlear.com), Advanced Bionics (www.cochlearimplant.com), and Med-El (www.medel.com). All three manufacturers are very competitive with each other in that

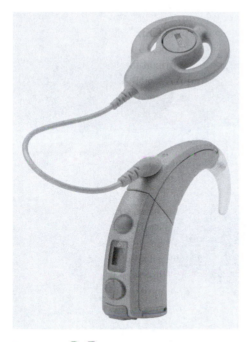

figure *8.3*

Cochlear™ Nucleus® behind-the-ear speech processor.

Source: Picture provided courtesy of Cochlear™ Americas, © 2005, Cochlear Americas.

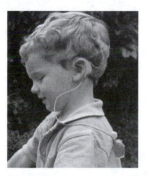

figure *8.4*

A child wearing a cochlear implant.

Source: Picture provided courtesy of Cochlear™ Americas, © 2009, Cochlear Americas.

they produce high-quality products and serviceability. Patients and their families may choose among the three companies, but frequently that choice may be predetermined by the physician performing the surgery or the cochlear implant center that deals specifically with Cochlear. Therefore, if a patient wants an Advanced Bionics cochlear implant, that patient might have to select a cochlear implant center that offers those implants. On each of the manufacturer's websites is a search engine for prospective candidates to find participating cochlear implant centers. Twenty years ago, patients had only a handful of cochlear implant centers to go to, frequently requiring travel to other cities or states. Today, a large urban area may have three or more cochlear implant centers to choose from. However, patients' health insurance companies may limit access to certain cochlear implant centers. Appendix 8.1 provides the contact information for the three cochlear implant manufacturers.

Cochlear implant manufacturers offer a variety of electrode arrays to meet the needs of most patients. Cochlear currently offers the Cochlear™ Nucleus 5® CI 512 cochlear implant which is reportedly 40% thinner than its previous model and 30% thinner than any titanium device on the market. Advanced Bionics' popular cochlear implant is the HiRes® 90K with the HiFocus® Helix or HiFocus® 1J electrodes. Med-El claims to provide the smallest cochlear implant, the Maestro Sonata I100 which is purported to make surgery shorter and less invasive. Manufacturers also offer special electrode arrays for patients who have ossification or bony growths within the cochlea. For example, the Cochlear™ Nucleus® Double Array, an earlier implant, placed 11 electrodes into the first turn of the cochlea and the next 11 electrodes into the second turn (Lenarz, Battmer, Frohne, Büchner, & Parker, 2000).

The type of speech processor used depends on the patients' age and preferences. For example, Advanced Bionics produces body-worn processors for infants and young children, whereas older children and adults may prefer the ear-level speech processors. Some parents may feel inconvenienced dealing with small ear-level devices with their young children. However, parents of infants and toddlers reported ease in manipulating the dials and switches, changing the battery pack, using external sources of input and accessories of ear-level speech processors (Anderson, Schmidt, Buchreiter, & Bisanar, 2004). Furthermore, older children easily transition from body-worn to behind-the-ear (BTE) speech processors (Dodd, Nikolopoulos, Totten, Cope, & O'Donoghue, 2005). Therefore, ear-level devices should be applicable to most patients, even those who are accustomed to body-worn devices. Cochlear™ Nucleus 5® CP 810 Sound Processor is claimed to be the smallest sound processor available today complete with a remote control or assistant. These speech processors have Smart Sound™ 2, which has four possible programs: (1) the Everyday program automatically adjusts in everyday

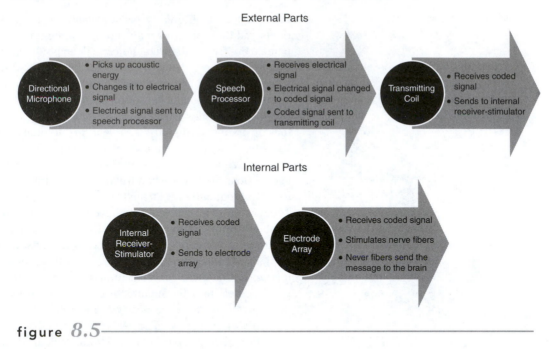

External Parts

Directional Microphone
- Picks up acoustic energy
- Changes it to electrical signal
- Electrical signal sent to speech processor

Speech Processor
- Receives electrical signal
- Electrical signal changed to coded signal
- Coded signal sent to transmitting coil

Transmitting Coil
- Receives coded signal
- Sends to internal receiver-stimulator

Internal Parts

Internal Receiver-Stimulator
- Receives coded signal
- Sends to electrode array

Electrode Array
- Receives coded signal
- Stimulates nerve fibers
- Never fibers send the message to the brain

figure *8.5*

A diagram of how a cochlear implant works.

Casebook Reflection

Getting to Know the Cochlear Implant Manufacturers

Go to each of the cochlear implant manufacturers' websites and compare and contrast what each has to offer. While exploring these webpages, it is immediately apparent that the manufacturers operate on a global basis because accessibility requires selection of a country of origin. Each manufacturer's website has a section tailored to prospective patients and their families that has resources and describes what a cochlear implant is and does, who may benefit, and so on. These individuals may also become members of online communities and post their questions to cochlear implant recipients and their significant others. In addition, each manufacturer provides a detailed description and photographs of each of their products. Furthermore, hearing health professionals are provided with downloadable information on how to best meet the needs of their patients.

---

listening situations; (2) the Focus program is for conversation in noise that emphasizes the speaker directly in front of the listener; (3) the Noise program is for conversations in extremely noisy conditions; and (4) the Music program is used when listening to music. Advanced Bionics' current speech processors are the body-worn Platinum Series and the Auria® Harmony™ BTE models. Similarly, Med-El's BTE-style speech processor is the Maestro OPUS 2 with remote programming. A telecoil and FM battery pack permit wireless connectivity to telephones, public sound systems, MP3 players, and Bluetooth systems.

Regarding accessories, all three manufacturers offer connections for listening through FM receivers, popular personal listening devices (e.g., iPods, MP3 players, Walkmans, and so on), televisions, home stereo systems, personal computers, DVD players, and gaming consoles (e.g., Xbox and Sony Playstations). Earphones are also available for parents and teachers to listen to input to the microphone during visual and listening checks. Most implants can be used with hearing assistive technology (HAT) via a patch cord (e.g., direct-audio input) or via a telecoil through use of a "T" switch on the speech processor (National Public Website on Assistive Technology, 2006). Electrical coupling involves connecting FM receivers via a patch cord to speech processors. Most body-worn speech processors have an audio jack, but ear-level speech processors need special audio covers and/or accessory cables (Thibodeau & Schafer, 2005). Telecoil coupling is accomplished via the t-coil in the speech processor that receives an electromagnetic signal from the body-worn FM receiver via a teleloop (Thibodeau & Schafer, 2005). The Cochlear™ Nucleus 5® System has two ways of accessing the telecoil. The manual telecoil is activated using the switch on the sound processor or remote assistant. AutoPhone™ telecoil automatically detects the electromagnetic energy from the telecoil. Some disadvantages with telecoil coupling are variability of signal viability with t-coil orientation, reduction of low-frequency sounds, and addition of noise to the cochlear implant system (Thibodeau & Schafer, 2005). Research has demonstrated improved speech recognition in noise for children and adults when cochlear implants are electrically coupled with FM systems; this interface does not cause poor signal quality, interference, or system noise (Anderson, Goldstein, Colodzin, & Inglehart, 2005; Schafer & Thibodeau, 2003, 2004; Thibodeau & Schafer). Use of cochlear implants with sound field amplification devices is discussed in Chapter 10.

PATIENT SELECTION CRITERIA AND PREIMPLANT EVALUATION

Cochlear implants are Class III medical devices and, therefore, are regulated by the Food and Drug Administration. Not all patients with hearing loss are candidates for a cochlear implant. Over the past three decades, the criteria for candidacy have expanded to include more patients who may benefit; this trend is expected to continue. For example, it was not until the early 1980s that children were permitted to receive cochlear implants (Moller, 2006). Similarly, the minimum age of implantation was 2 years of age, but now children as young as 12 months and even younger receive cochlear implants.

Determination of who may benefit from a cochlear implant is best accomplished with a multidisciplinary assessment team that includes the following areas of expertise (Schopmeyer, 2001):

- Audiologic evaluation
- Medical examination including otology
- Auditory skills assessment
- Language assessment
- Psychologic assessment

- Educational placement evaluation
- Ophthalmologic evaluation
- Occupational therapy
- Developmental pediatric and neurologic assessments

The purpose of the preimplant evaluation is to provide the patient and his or her family with enough information to make an informed decision about pursuing cochlear implantation. Alternatively, the assessment team collects necessary data to determine patients' eligibility for implantation through a thorough case history and series of examinations. Patient selection criteria and preimplant assessment and patient selection criteria are different for children than for adults. We will first discuss patient selection criteria.

Patient Selection Criteria

As cochlear implants have developed over the past 30 years, the **patient selection criteria** have changed in a variety of ways. Patient selection criteria are requirements that must be met prior to proceeding to implantation. Some of the changes have included who can be implanted, their age, degree of hearing loss, and so on. In 1985 only adults 18 years of age and older with postlingual profound sensorineural hearing loss and no **open-set speech recognition** were candidates for cochlear implants. Open-set speech recognition is a response format in which patients write down or repeat test stimuli instead of selecting a response from a group of options. By 1990, these criteria were expanded to include children 2 years of age and older with either prelingual or postlingual hearing loss. In 1998, children 12 months of age and older could be implanted and adults with either prelingual or postlingual hearing loss could receive cochlear implants. The changed criteria included that adults needed to score less than 42% in speech recognition performance on the *Central Institute for the Deaf Everyday Sentence Test* (CID) (Silverman & Hirsh, 1955). The CID Everyday Sentences consist of 10 lists of 10 everyday sentences (e.g., "Walking's my favorite exercise") (Mendel & Danhauer, 1997). At that time, children had to have a profound sensorineural hearing loss and less than 20% word recognition. It is important to note that patient selection criteria were established by each manufacturer. By 2000, the Cochlear company expanded its criterion for degree of hearing loss to severe to profound sensorineural hearing loss for children age 24 months and older to receive a specific type of implant, a Nucleus® 24 Contour Implant.

Table 8.1 shows current patient selection criteria for two manufacturers, Cochlear and Advanced Bionics, which have similar criteria for adults except that Cochlear requires a moderate-to-profound pre- or postlingual sensorieural hearing loss compared with Advanced Bionics requiring a severe-to-profound postlingual sensorineural hearing loss. Both require 50% or lower on sentence recognition in the ear to be implanted. Adults also must desire to be part of the hearing world and have no medical contraindications. There is no upper age limit for adults, but patients must be healthy enough to undergo the surgery, which requires general anesthesia. Advanced Bionics suggests the following real-life indicators for an adult who is considering cochlear implantation (Advanced Bionics, 2009):

- Difficulty carrying on a conversation on the telephone
- Difficulty understanding speech in group situations or in background noise
- Heavy reliance on lipreading
- Severe activity limitations and participation restrictions

table *8.1*   Adult and Pediatric Patient Selection Criteria of Two Different Cochlear Implant Manufacturers

Adults

Cochlear

- 18 years of age and older
- Moderate-to-profound sensorineural hearing loss, bilaterally
- 50% or less sentence recognition in the ear to be implanted
- 60% or less sentence recognition in the opposite ear or binaurally
- Prelinguistic or postlinguistic onset of moderate-to-profound sensorineural hearing loss
- No medical contraindications
- A desire to be part of the hearing world

Advanced Bionics

- 18 years of age and older
- Severe-to-profound sensorineural hearing loss, bilaterally (>70 dB HL)
- Postlinguistic onset of severe-to-profound sensorinerual hearing loss
- Limited benefit from appropriately fitted hearing aids, scoring 50% or less on a test of open-set sentence recognition (*Hearing in Noise Test* sentences)
- Desire to improve hearing and realistic expectations
- No medical contraindications

Pediatric

Cochlear

25 months to 17 years, 11 months:

- Severe-to-profound sensorineural hearing loss, bilaterally
- Limited benefit from hearing aids or scoring 30% or less on the *Multisyllabic Lexical Neighborhood Test* (Kirk, Pisoni, & Osberger, 1995) in the best aided condition (children 25 months to 4 years, 11 months)
- Limited benefit from hearing aids or scoring 30% or less on the *Lexical Neighborhood Test* (Kirk et al., 1995) (children 5 years to 17 years, 11 months)
- Lack of progress in the development of auditory skills
- No medical contraindications
- High motivation and appropriate expectations from the child, when appropriate, and the family

12 months to 24 months:

- Profound sensorineural hearing loss, bilaterally
- Limited benefit from appropriate binaural hearing aids
- Lack of progress in the development of auditory skills
- No medical contraindications
- High motivation and appropriate family expectations

(*Continued*)

table *8.1*   *(Continued)*

Pediatric

Advanced Bionics

12 months through 17 years, 11 month:

- Profound sensorineural hearing loss, bilaterally (>90 dB HL)
- Hearing aid trial period
  - Six-month trial period for children 24 months to 17 years, 11 months of age
  - Three-month trial period for children 12 months to 23 months of age
- Limited or no benefit from appropriately fit hearing aids
  - Age 3 and younger
    - Failure to reach auditory milestones (e.g., failure to respond to their name or environmental sounds in a quiet environment) measured by the *Infant-Toddler Meaningful Auditory Integration Scale* (Zimmerman-Phillips, Robbins, & Osberger, 2000)
    - Scores of less than 20% on a simple open-set word recognition test such as the *Multisyllabic Lexical Neighborhood Test* (Kirk et al., 1995) administered using live voice at 70 dB SPL
  - Four years of age and older
    - Less than 12% on a difficult open-set word recognition test such as the *Phonetically Balanced Kindergarten Word Lists* (Haskins, 1949) administered using recorded materials at 70 dB SPL
    - Less than 30% on an open-set sentence recognition test such as the *Hearing in Noise Test for Children*
- Motivation to improve hearing
- High motivation and appropriate expectations from the child, when appropriate, and the family

Sources: Information from *Candidacy Criteria,* by Advanced Bionics, 2009, retrieved from www.advancedbionics.com/
For_Professionals/Audiology_Support/Candidacy_Criteria.cfm?langid=1; *Cochlear Implant Candidate Criteria,* by Cochlear
Americas, 2009, retrieved from www.professionals.cochlearamericas.com/sites/default/files/resources/criteria%20card.pdf.

Cochlear and Advanced Bionics have similar patient selection criteria for children. However, there are some differences, too. For example, for those 12 to 24 months of age, Cochlear and Advanced Bionics require bilateral profound sensorineural hearing losses. However, Cochlear permits patients 24 months to 17 years to have severe to profound sensorineural hearing losses, whereas Advanced Bionics prefers to use the same criteria for degree of loss for all children. Another common criterion is that children should receive limited benefit from amplification. Advanced Bionics specifies that patients 24 months to 17 years of age have at least a 6-month trial period with appropriately fit hearing aids, but that time may be reduced to 3 months for infants and toddlers 12 to 24 months of age. Moreover, the hearing aid trial period may be waived if there is evidence of **cochlear ossification** or a build-up of new bone in response to bacterial meningitis that may have caused an infection in the cochlea (El-Kashlan, Ashbaugh, Zwolan, & Telian, 2003). Regarding speech recognition scores, Cochlear requires that children 2 to 4 years of age score 30% or less on the *Multisyllabic Lexical Neighborhood*

Test (MLNT) (Kirk, Pisoni, & Osberger, 1995), and the same for those 5 to 17 years old on the *Lexical Neighborhood Test* (LNT). The test lists consist of vocabulary words that had a high probability of being understood by children with profound sensorineural hearing loss (Kirk, Diefendorf, & Robbins, 1997).

Similarly, Advanced Bionics believes that children failing to reach developmental auditory milestones (e.g., responding to their own name) is an indication for cochlear implantation. Specifically, criteria for children younger than 4 years must achieve 75% consistency on questions 3 and 5 on the *Infant Toddler Meaningful Auditory Integration Scale* (IT-MAIS) (Zimmerman-Phillips, Robbins, & Osberger, 2000). The IT-MAIS is a parent-report tool that asks about children's natural reactions to sound in their environments. Question 3 asks, "Does the child spontaneously respond to his/her name in quiet with auditory cues only (i.e., no visual cues) when not expecting to hear it?" Question 5 asks, "Does the child spontaneously alert to environmental sounds (dogs, toys) in the home without being told or prompted to do so?" Parents' responses are graded on a scale from 0 to 4 (i.e., 0 = Never, 1 = Rarely, 2 = Occasionally, 3 = Frequently, and 4 = Always). Therefore, cochlear implantation is indicated if children do not frequently (i.e., at least 75% of the time) perform these tasks. Similarly, Advanced Bionics also requires that children 2 to 4 years of age achieve 20% or less on the *MLNT* in the child's best aided condition with stimuli presented at 70 dBSPL (50 dBHL) using **modified live voice presentation**. Modified live voice is accomplished when the audiologist presents the speech stimuli via the microphone on the audiometer while modifying the presentation level on a volume meter. Additionally, Advanced Bionics requires that children 4 years of age and older achieve 0 to 12% open-set word recognition on the *Phonetically Balanced Kindergarten Word Lists* (PBK-50) (Haskins, 1949) or 30% or less on open-set sentence recognition on the *Hearing in Noise Test for Children* (HINT-C) (Nilsson, Soli, & Gelnett, 1996; Nilsson, Soli, & Sumida, 1995). The *PBK*-50 lists contain words that have been found to be within the vocabulary of kindergarteners (Kirk et al., 1997). The *HINT-C* was developed as an adaptive procedure to find children's **sentence recognition thresholds** or the lowest signal-to-noise ratio resulting in 50% sentence recognition. **Adaptive procedures** are tests in which the difficulty of the assessment conditions is based on the accuracy of patients' previous responses. Advanced Bionics changed the tests to consist of 13 lists of 10 phonetically balanced sentences each to determine patients' open-set recognition in quiet.

Children and their parents must be motivated for cochlear implantation and be willing to do what is required for auditory habilitation. In addition, older children need to be enrolled in educational programs that foster the development of auditory, speech, and language skills. Most importantly, children and their parents need to have realistic expectations regarding the benefits gleaned from cochlear implantation. If not, extensive counseling may be needed prior to proceeding to candidacy.

Preimplant Evaluation

The preimplant evaluation includes appropriate counseling for patients and their families and evaluations completed by the cochlear implant team. Patients and significant others require a great deal of information regarding cochlear implants in order to make an informed decision. They may have received information from their primary-care physicians, audiologists, and/or speech-language pathologists, but unfortunately some of it may be inaccurate. Recent surveys have shown that the majority of pediatricians who responded serve as medical home providers and do not know current patient selection criteria nor do they feel comfortable counseling families about cochlear implants (e.g., Dorros, Kurtzer-White, Ahlgren, Simon, & Vohr, 2007; Mathews, Johnson, & Danhauer, 2009; Moeller, White, & Shisler, 2006). Therefore, it may be advisable to probe for what is known and ask patients if they have any questions about pursuing cochlear implants. In fact, it does not hurt to repeat what other healthcare professionals may have said about cochlear implants because patients may be unclear about certain aspects of devices or procedures.

Patients and their family members receive a great deal of information during preimplant evaluations. Therefore, informational counseling techniques, covered in Chapter 2, may assist in patients' retention of both general and specific information about cochlear implants. General information includes basics on the anatomy of the ear and hearing loss, patient selection criteria, and appropriate expectations about the use of cochlear implants. Specific information relevant to the cochlear implant includes its parts, surgery, scheduling/procedures for counseling, therapy, overall costs, and processes for insurance approval. The most important aspect of preimplant counseling is to ensure that patients/parents have appropriate short- and long-term expectations of cochlear implants and what it is going to take to be successful. Patients must also have a desire to be part of the hearing world. Children must be enrolled in educational programs that develop auditory, speech, and language skills. Parents/patients should have an opportunity to talk with experienced cochlear implant users and their families. Cochlear implant programs and manufacturers often provide opportunities to talk with cochlear implant recipients and their families through mentoring programs. Recently, cochlear implant manufacturers have established online communities providing opportunities for candidates and their families to communicate with other patients and families who have gone through the process.

The preimplant evaluation involves various members of the cochlear implant team to determine if patients and their families meet all selection criteria. The cochlear implant team may include, but is not limited to, a team coordinator, audiologists, otolaryngologists, otologists, surgeons psychologists, social workers, speech-language pathologists, and teachers of the deaf. The **cochlear implant team coordinator** is the main contact for patients and their families and organizes the preimplant evaluation. The evaluation includes scrutinizing patients' responses on their case histories, audiologic/speech-language evaluations, medical assessments, patients'/parents' expectations, cognitive functioning, and so on. The preimplant evaluation involves assessment by various members of the team. The audiologic evaluation is usually completed first and includes otoscopy, immittance testing (tympanometry and acoustic reflex testing), otoacoustic emissions, auditory brainstem evaluation, including **auditory steady state response** (ASSR) testing, pure-tone air- and bone-conduction testing, speech audiometry, and hearing aid evaluation, as well as an assessment of the amount of benefit. ASSR is an electrophysiological examination that provides an accurate estimation of patients' pure-tone audiograms. The ASSR is particularly useful in assessing patients who cannot provide valid or reliable behavioral responses, such as young children who may need to be sedated for testing.

The physician, typically the otologist, conducts the consultation history and physical. Some possible physical contraindications for implantation include deafness due to lesions in the acoustic nerve or central auditory pathway. **Neurofibromatosis** is a genetic condition that causes tumors to grow on nerves and also causes other problems with skin and bones. There are two types of neurofibromatosis, Type I (NF-1) and Type II (NF-2). NF-1 is more common and is characterized by change in the skin (i.e., café au lait spots) and presence of tumors or bone abnormalities (National Institute of Neurological Disorders and Stroke [NINDS], 2009).

Not as common, NF-2 results in bilateral tumors on nerve VIII precluding viability of nerve fibers to send impulses to the brain and suitability of cochlear implants (NINDS, 2009). Other medical contraindications include external or middle ear infections that may delay implantation. However, pressure equalization tubes in otherwise healthy middle ears are acceptable. Contraindications also may include tympanic membrane perforations, chronic mastoiditis, or cholesteatomas, which must be cleared up before implantation is an option.

The otologist also assesses for cochlear ossification from bacterial meningitis or congenital malformation of the cochlea or temporal bone. Computed-tomography scans (CT scans) and magnetic resonance imaging (MRI) are done on patients' skulls with particular interest paid to the temporal bone and the status of the inner ear. Because the internal parts of the implant go inside the cochlea, it is important to assess for any abnormalities that may limit the usefulness of the device. First, it is important to determine if there are any congenital malformations, such as the Mondini anomaly that frequently presents with a profound sensorineural hearing loss and a flattened cochlea with a single turn. A second abnormality to rule out is **enlarged vestibular aqueduct syndrome** (EVAS). The **vestibular aqueduct** is a small opening in the temporal bone that serves as a passageway for part of the membranous labyrinth, the endolymphatic duct, to travel outside of the inner ear to terminate at the endolymphatic sac at the level of the dura mater. In children with EVAS, the opening in the temporal bone is larger than normal with affected patients having a tendency to present with a progressive sensorineural hearing loss. CT scans and MRIs are also effective in detecting any ossification (build-up of bone) as a result of bacterial meningitis. Presence of other systematic illnesses involving renal problems, bleeding disorders, or risks for anesthesia may present some challenges for the surgeon.

Another useful evaluation is the **promontory stimulation test** in which a needle electrode is inserted through the tympanic membrane and placed on the promontory with a surface electrode placed on the opposite cheek. The promontory is an area on the medial wall of the middle ear cavity. A small electrical current is sent through to the needle electrode and the patient is asked if he or she experiences any sensation from this stimulation. It is a good sign if patients experience sensation because it means that the neurons of the auditory nerve are stimulable and suitable for cochlear implantation. In fact, a relationship has been found between sensations during the test and better speech recognition performance with the cochlear implant (Kuo & Gibson, 2005; Lee, Yoo, Ahn, & Lee, 2007).

In summary, these multidisciplinary teams consider many factors in determining candidacy for cochlear implantation. Some patients are clearly appropriate candidates, some are not, and other cases may need further evaluation. In the following scenarios, evaluate each situation and determine whether you feel the patient in question is or is not an appropriate candidate for a cochlear implant, or if further evaluation is warranted.

What Do You Think, Good Candidate or Not?

Betsy, a 10th-grader at the California School for the Deaf and Blind in Fremont, California, lives in Union City with her hearing parents, Dolores and Frank. Betsy was born with a bilateral profound sensorineural hearing loss that was diagnosed when she was 2 years old. Since then, she has worn behind-the-ear hearing aids. She has received speech and language therapy since early childhood, but has not progressed as her parents had hoped. Children in the mainstream public school made fun of her. Her Individualized Education Plan team felt that the state school for the deaf and blind was a more appropriate placement for her. Although Betsy communicates with her parents via spoken English at home, she uses American Sign Language at school and with her friends. Betsy started dating a fellow student, frequently going to Deaf clubs and socializing with others within the Deaf community. Recently, Betsy's parents have become concerned about their daughter's future. What type of job will she have? Will she be able to support herself? They believed that Betsy's chances for independence would increase if she received a cochlear implant. Betsy gets furious when her parents bring up the subject.

Do you think Betsy is a good candidate for a cochlear implant? Betsy has a bilateral profound prelingual sensorineural hearing loss, receives little or no benefit from hearing aids, and has parents who are motivated and have realistic expectations about cochlear implants. Sounds like she's a great candidate! Right? Think again! Betsy is not a good candidate for a cochlear implant because she has no interest in obtaining the device. Betsy is old enough to decide what is most appropriate for her, feels more part of the Deaf community than the hearing world, and primarily uses American Sign Language. She and her parents should receive counseling to resolve their differences regarding cochlear implantation.

Let's consider another case.

What Do You Think, Good Candidate or Not?

Donna Hoffman, single mother of five children, works a full-time job as a secretary during the day and moonlights as a waitress at a local coffee shop four evenings a week just to make ends meet. She has sole custody of her five children, who range in age from 18 months to 16 years. Fortunately, Bernice, her eldest, is able to care for her siblings on the nights her mother has to work. Donna is exhausted from working 65-hour weeks. Ricky, the 18-month-old, was diagnosed with a bilateral profound sensorineural hearing loss at age 15 months and was immediately fit with behind-the-ear hearing aids. Ricky receives early intervention services through the Alabama Institute for the Deaf and Blind. Unfortunately, Ricky has not made much progress in auditory skill or speech/language development. Tamara Sanchez, Ricky's speech-language pathologist, reports that Ricky has missed more than half of his appointments and when he does attend, he is not wearing his hearing aids. Tamara was surprised by this because Donna appeared so motivated to do anything to help her child succeed. Tamara suspects that Ricky is not wearing his hearing aids at home either. Tamara knows that Donna has her hands full.

Do you think Ricky is a good candidate for a cochlear implant? He seems to have the necessary degree of hearing loss and his mother seems motivated to pursue a cochlear implant and has realistic expectations for her son. Unfortunately, Ricky is *not* a candidate for a cochlear implant, at least not at this time. Why? Because it appears that he has not had an opportunity for consistent use of amplification nor an opportunity to benefit from speech-language therapy. Ricky's mother. Donna, should be reminded that Ricky has not had an adequate opportunity to see if he may benefit from hearing aids, particularly in speech-language therapy. Although Donna probably knows this, her demanding schedule in meeting the basic needs of her family may have precluded following through with Ricky's auditory habilitation. Donna and her family may benefit from a referral to social services so that appropriate resources may be identified to ease some of the family's burden, and Ricky's candidacy should be reconsidered after six months.

Let's try one more scenario.

What Do You Think, Good Candidate or Not?

Isabel Rodriguez, a 6-year-old child who contracted bacterial meningitis, had been in the hospital for weeks. Her parents, Juan and Dolores, were so thankful when their little girl finally came home. It had been a difficult illness that almost claimed Isabel's life. One unfortunate outcome, however, is that Isabel acquired a severe-to-profound bilateral sensorineural hearing loss. Isabel had been a normally developing 6-year-old prior to her illness. Juan and Dolores are very motivated to learn about ways to help their daughter. They know that Isabel's school has excellent support services and programs for children with hearing impairment. Isabel tried binaural behind-the-ear hearing aids, but made little progress in auditory skill development. The audiologist, who diagnosed Isabel's hearing loss and who fit her with hearing aids, has recommended that they consider a cochlear implant.

Is Isabel a good candidate for a cochlear implant? Yes, she is an excellent candidate for a cochlear implant for several reasons. First of all, she acquired her hearing loss at 6 years of age, after she had already developed age-appropriate speech and language skills. Second, her parents are highly motivated for her to do well. Third, she is fortunate to be in a school district that provides excellent special education related services, particularly for students who are hard of hearing. We will check in on Isabel and her family later on in the chapter.

So far we have considered cochlear implant candidacy in three children. What about adults? The following Casebook Reflection tells the story of Stephanie, an undergraduate student at Auburn University in Alabama, who is an excellent candidate for a cochlear implant.

Casebook Reflection

Stephanie's Story: A Sophomore at Auburn University

During the spring of my senior year in high school, I received the highest achievement of my entire life, my acceptance letter to Auburn University. Attending Auburn University had always been a goal of mine, and I achieved it. I was afraid to leave home to go to Auburn for the first time, but my older sister, an Auburn student, told me what to expect. With her guidance, I didn't feel alone, but I had to struggle to do well in my classes. It was really hard for me at first, having a severe-to-profound sensorineural hearing loss and coming from a small, rural high school.

People kept telling me how well I was doing! I surprised many people and never gave up! My experiences have taught me that in everything that a person does, hard work is required; there are no easy ways out in school or in the "real world." I am now working toward my second greatest goal, which is to graduate with my undergraduate degree and begin work toward my doctorate of audiology (Au.D.).

As a small child, I was diagnosed with a profound sensorineural hearing loss in my right ear and a severe sensorineural hearing loss in my left ear. At that time, my audiologist told my parents that I would hear better with hearing aids than I would with a cochlear implant. Every year my audiologist would keep us updated on the advances in cochlear implant technology, but he still felt that I would hear better with hearing aids. However, a year ago my audiologist told us that I may now qualify as a cochlear implant candidate! I want to have a cochlear implant because I am hoping that it will improve my understanding of

speech. I want to be an audiologist to provide hope to people with hearing loss. I know that I will have to work hard to learn to hear better with my new implant, but in my life, I have truly learned that if you set your goal for the moon, at least if you miss, you have still landed on a star. . . .

Stephanie is an excellent candidate for a cochlear implant. Stephanie, her parents, and her audiologist have considered cochlear implantation as an option for many years. Together, they have monitored the technological developments of these devices and expected outcomes. Stephanie is highly motivated and knows that she would have to work hard to adjust and reap the benefits from using a cochlear implant. Once the decision has been made and patients such as Stephanie have been deemed appropriate candidates for cochlear implants, preparing for and undergoing surgery are the next steps.

COCHLEAR IMPLANT SURGERY

Preparations for surgery begin long before the day of the procedure. The patient's primary care physician must provide clearance for surgery requiring general anesthesia (Chang, Ko, Murray, Arnold, & Megerian, 2010). Another hurdle is seeking approval from third-party payers for cochlear implantation. Recall that third-party payer was defined in Chapter 4 as an entity other than the healthcare provider or patient who reimburses for procedures performed, diagnoses made, and certain devices, supplies, and/or other equipment for patients (ASHA, 1996).

Patients and their family members must be counseled regarding the specifics of the surgical procedure. If the patient is a child, then counseling should be aimed at explaining what is going to happen and when and if one or both ears are to be implanted during the procedure. Traditional approaches to implantation have involved selecting the "better" ear, which usually has a larger population of surviving nerves in the **spiral ganglion** to be stimulated by the implant (Megerian & Murray, 2010). The spiral ganglion is a collection of nerves that have fibers that send signals from the cochlea to the brain.

The surgeon carefully selects and orders the most appropriate implant for the patient well in advance of the surgery, in addition to a duplicate device in case something should go wrong. In almost all cases, the surgery takes two to three hours, although some experienced surgeons are able to complete the procedure in half that time, and is performed on an in- or out-patient basis.

In preparation, the scalp around the site for implantation is shaved and cleaned. Intravenous drug lines are inserted into patients' arms to deliver general anesthesia, and masks are placed on their faces to deliver oxygen and anesthetic gases, causing deep sleep. Complications from general anesthesia are rare, and postoperative nausea is decreased with contemporary techniques. Cables, monitors, and patches monitor patients' vital signs and nerve functioning. The function of the facial nerve, cranial nerve VIII, is monitored because of its close proximity to the surgical areas. Although a variety of surgical procedures have been developed, traditional approaches have involved a **mastoidectomy** in addition to a **facial recess approach** in an attempt to preserve key structures (Majdani et al., 2008). A mastoidectomy is partial or complete removal of the mastoid process and bone; a facial recess approach is a way of surgically accessing the middle ear through the mastoid bone through a niche lateral to the facial nerve canal.

The surgeon must perform a **cochleostomy**, which requires drilling a hole into the basal turn of the cochlea to insert the electrode array into the scala tympani. Over the years, surgeons have become more skilled in selecting the best location to drill the hole (Roland, 2008). The location is crucial because the surgeon's aim is to insert the electrode array into the scala tympani with as little trauma as possible, in order to preserve residual hearing (Roland). In addition to the location of the cochleostomy, the softness, flexibility, and delicate nature of the electrode array impact the amount of trauma to the cochlea (Roland). For example, inserting a straight electrode into a curved structure such as the cochlea may damage the outer canal wall or puncture delicate inner ear structures. Further, placing electrodes toward the outer cochlear canal wall may increase the distance from the auditory nerves that are situated toward the center of the cochlea, thereby reducing the accuracy of stimulation of specific neuronal groups (Roland). Newer electrode arrays are soft and flexible and are inserted using a stylette that, when pulled, uncoils the device within the cochlea with minimal trauma and optimal neuronal stimulation (Roland).

Electrophysiological testing within the operating room, or **electric auditory brainstem response** (EABR), confirms the "stimulability" of nerve VIII. EABR is an auditory brainstem response test using an electrical stimulus (Voll, 2005). The integrity of the internal device is tested using a procedure called **telemetry** in which impedances and voltages are measured when current is passed through the system to determine if the electrodes are in compliance with the manufacturer's specifications. Telemetry occurs during and after surgery to determine if there is appropriate impedance and that there are no short circuits. **Impedance** is the opposition to the flow of energy (i.e., electricity). A measure of high impedance means that the circuit is open and the electric signal is flowing. A short circuit means that an electrode or lead wire is in contact with another electrode and modifications must be made. *Telemetry* is a bidirectional communication of data between implants and the programming hardware. *Neural response telemetry* is a noninvasive, objective measure of peripheral nerve function when utilizing a cochlear implant, and also helps to identify problems prior to the patient hook-up. These results, however, do not determine future patient prognosis with the device. Patients and their families are often relieved to find out that the nerve is stimulable. X-rays can also determine if the electrodes have been placed in the densest part of the temporal bone and are oriented in the correct way. When everything has confirmed optimal placement of the electrodes, the cochleostomy is packed with fascia or muscle to seal it up and the surgeon is ready to close.

Some postoperative symptoms include mild pain, vertigo, nausea, and aural numbness, but these are rare. However, tinnitus, or ringing in the ear, is common but transient. Other possible immediate difficulties from the surgery include facial nerve injuries, flap complications, anesthetic complications, reimplantation for device failure, and infections. It is important to note that pain is not limited to just the incision or cochlear implant site, but may occur anywhere on the head, neck, or jaw. The Food and Drug Administration and the Centers for Disease Control and Prevention have found that children and adults with cochlear implants may be more susceptible to developing bacterial meningitis and suggest that these patients are vaccinated according to recommendations for other persons who are at greater risk for this disease (Centers for Disease Control and Prevention, 2010). The surgeon carefully counsels patients and their families prior to surgery about the process and answers their questions. Manufacturers have developed materials to prepare patients and their families for surgery. Cochlear has a play book titled *My Cochlear Implant Story* that has activities to help prepare the child for surgery. Activities include coloring and personalizing the story with pictures of the patient and family members. Let's look in on the Rodriguez family and their surgeon, Dr. Edwards.

Casebook Reflection

Isabel's Presurgery Consultation

"Hi, Mr. and Mrs. Rodriguez. And Isabel, how are you today?" asked Dr. Edwards.

Isabel nodded and smiled.

"The purpose of today's consultation is to explain to you what is going to happen during surgery. I have a play book made by Cochlear that you can go over with Isabel at home."

"Thank you, Dr. Edwards," said Dolores.

"The part of the cochlear implant that we will implant looks just like the one in my hand. It consists of two parts, the body and the electrode array. The body is placed into the bone behind the ear and the electrode array is carefully inserted into the cochlea. As you know, the Cochlear Nucleus 5 is implanted under general anesthesia and the parts are made to last for a lifetime. Isabel is not to have anything to eat or drink after midnight the night before the surgery. You will come to the hospital early in the morning and we will begin the process about 7:00 a.m. Any questions so far?" asked Dr. Edwards.

"No," said Dolores, and Juan agreed.

"In preparation for surgery, a member of the surgical team will shave your daughter's head behind the ear where the implant will be. An incision will be made so that the skin and tissue will be folded back to expose the bone called the mastoid bone. The surgeon will make a small impression in the mastoid bone for the body of the implant. The surgeon must drill through the bone to get to the cochlea to insert the electrode array. Afterward, the incision will be covered, bandages will be placed on Isabel's head, and she will go to the recovery room," explained Dr. Edwards. "Some patients go home the same day, but we'd like to keep Isabel overnight for observation. That's a lot of information. . . . Do you have any questions?"

"No," said Dolores with tears in her eyes, looking at Isabel. "We'll see you bright and early Wednesday morning."

"Thank you, Dr. Edwards, for all that you're doing for Isabel," added Juan.

"It's been a pleasure," said Dr. Edwards, shaking Dolores's, Juan's, and Isabel's hands. "Call me tomorrow if you have any more questions."

"Doctor, I forgot to ask what happens *after* surgery," said Dolores.

"Good question. It will take three to five weeks for the incision to heal. Isabel's hair will grow back, making the implant practically invisible. During that time, we will have her come to the office to check on the healing of the incision. Once healed, Isabel will receive her speech processor and Dr. Boomgartner, our audiologist, will work with Isabel in developing some MAPs, or patterns of electrode stimulation, so that she can hear in a variety of situations. I expect Isabel will do exceptionally well, having developed speech and language before losing her hearing."

"Thanks again, Dr. Edwards," said Dolores. "We'll see you Wednesday!"

WHAT TO EXPECT AFTER SURGERY

After surgery, patients and their families will be scheduled for follow-up appointments. The external parts of the cochlear implant will be delivered and programmed for the patient. Instruction will be provided on the maintenance and use of the device. School personnel must also be contacted regarding the roles that they may serve to ensure patients' success with their cochlear implants.

The "Hook-Up"

As Dr. Edwards told Isabel and her family, three to five weeks are needed for the incision to heal prior to the "**hook-up**," or the initial delivery and fitting of the implant, which usually takes about two hours. During the hook-up, the audiologist provides the newly implanted patient with the external parts of the implant and programs the speech processor. The audiologist performing the programming uses a personal computer with specific software and hardware provided by the manufacturer.

During the initial programming or **mapping** of the cochlear implant, the audiologist determines the type of **speech coding strategy**, the volume setting, the sensitivity setting, program choices, and if any locks on the controls are needed to prevent tampering with the settings (Nussbaum, 2003). Mapping is the setting of the required electrical stimulation by the cochlear implant for the patient to hear soft and comfortably loud sounds. The primary goal of programming is to determine the dynamic range for each electrode such that the signal is comfortable over a wide variety of inputs (Boyd, 2006). The dynamic range is based on the area between the **electrical threshold level** (T-level) and the **maximum comfort level** (C-level). The T-level is the amount of current provided by an electrode that results in the patient being able to just detect the sensation of hearing. T-levels are important in mapping because they tell the audiologist the smallest amplitude of a pulse that is audible to the patients so that soft sounds may be heard. The C-level is the highest current level at which a patient can tolerate a sensation for an extended period of time. The **dynamic range** is the difference in the current level between the T- and C-level for each electrode and is highly variable between electrodes in the same patient and across patients. Therefore, using these terms we can further define **cochlear implant mapping** as the process of setting or adjusting the speech processor based on the dynamic range of each electrode and pair so that soft and comfortably loud sounds may be heard. A patient's MAP is the program for his or her individual speech processor, is often printed out in hard-copy form, and often changes over time.

A variety of speech coding strategies have evolved with cochlear implant technology and are available to meet patients' needs. Cochlear developed the **SPEAK** speech coding strategy, which breaks the signal into many (e.g., 20) bandpass filters, scans for those having the greatest amplitude, and then conveys that information via low pulse rates (e.g., 180 to 300 pulses per second [pps]). SPEAK is based on the principle that frequency regions with the greatest amplitude have the most perceptual salience. Other speech coding strategies use higher pulse rates (e.g., 900 to 2400 pps) that supposedly provide detailed sampling of speech waveforms (Middlebrooks, 2008; Wilson, 1997). The **continuous interleaved stimulation** (CIS) speech coding strategy estimates the envelope of the acoustic wave by coding the amplitude of the signal in six to eight bandpass filters at > 800 pps. Another coding strategy developed by Cochlear, ACE, is a combination of SPEAK and CIS aimed at providing high quality spectral and fast temporal resolution of speech. There are numerous speech coding strategies; researchers have consistently been working on their development in order to improve speech recognition performance of patients with cochlear implants.

The patient's initial MAP is set prior to activation of the microphone that enables the patient to hear with his or her implant. The microphone may be set to different **sensitivity levels**, which determine the softest sounds to be picked up. Patients and their families are also shown how other controls work such as those for volume and user programs. The volume control sets the level of the incoming sound; program switches designate individual listening processing schemes for specific situations. As mentioned earlier, programming is an ongoing process because patients' perceptions with their cochlear implants change over time. Patients typically adapt to their MAPs over time and initial settings may be too weak, requiring adjustment. Fibrous tissue may grow as a reaction to cochlear implantation, which may require greater electrical current for adequate signal strength. Let's check back in with Isabel during her hook-up session.

Casebook Reflection

Isabel's Hook-Up Session

Dolores and Juan Rodriguez had been on pins and needles for the past week, waiting for Isabel's hook-up session. Finally, the day had arrived and the final T- and C-levels had been set. Dr. Boomgartner, the audiologist, activated the microphone.

"Isabel, can you hear me?" asked Dr. Boomgartner, who was at Isabel's side, out of her view.

"Yes!" Isabel said with a wide grin. She looked at her parents and found her mother crying and her dad teary-eyed. So many months and days they had worried about their daughter, first concerned for her life and then about her future after she had acquired a profound sensorineural hearing loss as she fought to survive meningitis.

"Isabel, Isabel, my baby. . . . You can hear me!" exclaimed Dolores.

Isabel couldn't understand what her mother was saying to her, but was aware she was hearing something.

"It will take some time and therapy for Isabel to be able to understand what she is listening to through her cochlear implant. It has been a long process, but this is one of the best moments! I have some instructions for you about the care and use of the device and a diary for you to fill out. We'd like to see you back here next week so that we can review Isabel's progress and adjust her MAP. Your responses in the diary will help us determine if the current settings are loud enough or too loud. We will also be doing some testing that day, too," explained Dr. Boomgartner. "Do you have any questions?"

"No, I don't think so. All of you have been so kind to us. You have done so much for Isabel. Thank you so much!" said Juan, shaking the doctor's hand.

"It's been a pleasure! Please give us a call if you have any questions. We have gone over so much information today. Everything is in the user's manual," reminded Dr. Boomgartner.

During this initial appointment, the audiologist also orients the patient and their family to the device. Care is taken to identify the parts of the implant, how they work, how to put them on, how to wear the headset, and so on. A very important part of the orientation is the care and maintenance of the device. For example, patients and their families should know what type of batteries the speech processor uses, and that spares should by carried in a closed plastic bag so they don't short circuit and/or cause a burn. Patients need to know that rechargeable nickel-cadmium (NiCd) batteries are different than disposable alkaline ones. In addition, patients and their families need to be warned that a discharge of static electricity may damage the electrical components of the cochlear implant system or alter the program in the speech processor. It is recommended that if static electricity is present, cochlear implant users should touch something that should release the charge (e.g., something metal) before any part of the cochlear implant touches someone or something. The static electricity mostly affects the speech processor and does not result in injury to the wearer. Also, like pacemakers for the heart, cochlear implants may activate metal detectors.

Patients' and their family members' questions are also answered during this initial appointment. For example, parents may want to know that their children can go swimming with their implants, provided the microphone headset and speech processor are removed (The Listen-up Web, 2006). In fact, patients can go scuba diving in very deep water without any major effects on cochlear implant functioning (Kompis, Vibert, Senn, Vischer, & Häusler, 2003).

School Follow-Up

Isabel went on to achieve excellent outcomes with her implant. Within a year, she was back performing at grade level with minimal accommodations in the classroom. The cochlear implant center formed an excellent partnership with the school speech-language pathologist, educational audiologist, and Isabel's classroom teacher.

Isabel's parents followed through with four recommendations for parents regarding building successful partnerships with school personnel, as advocated by Zwolan and Sorkin (2006). First, parents should share information with school officials by providing copies of pertinent information such as hard copies of children's MAPs, programming reports, and evaluation results. Similarly, parents should provide copies of relevant school documents to staff at the cochlear implant center. Second, parents should ask teachers to provide feedback on Isabel's progress to cochlear implant center staff and speech-language pathologists. Third, parents should inform teachers about children's appointments at the cochlear implant center in addition to any change in equipment such as an upgrade to a new speech processor. Moreover, teachers may require inservices on troubleshooting the devices. Fourth, parents should encourage communication between the school and cochlear implant center. Children's teachers and/or speech-language pathologists may want to accompany the child to his or her appointments at the cochlear implant center. Alternatively, cochlear implant center staff may even want to visit children's schools to better understand their educational environments. It is important that school officials learn about safety considerations with the cochlear implant. They must be told that the cochlear implant is not waterproof (e.g., can't go swimming or take a shower without removing the external components) and is fragile (e.g., shouldn't be worn while playing rough sports).

Unfortunately, not all children are as fortunate as Isabel, and parents often must self-advocate in selecting an educational setting for their child by asking the following questions (Med-El, 2010):

- What are the school's expectations for a student with a hearing loss?
- What is the school's philosophy with regard to auditory development for a child with a hearing loss?
- If it is a school for the deaf, what opportunities are there for interaction with hearing peers and/or mainstream classrooms?
- How much experience does the school have in educating students with special needs?
- What is the school's policy regarding classroom observations by parents and other team members? Are school personnel willing to work with professionals from a cochlear implant team?
- What is the availability of FM systems to use with the child's cochlear implant? (We will be discussing the use of FM systems in a later chapter.)

In 2003, Sorkin and Zwolan conducted a national survey of school-age cochlear implant users. The most common services used by students with cochlear implants were speech-language pathology services (75%), use of FM systems (65%), and deaf education services (54%) (Sorkin & Zwolan, 2004). In addition, other services utilized by these students included individual or small-group instructional support, use of an interpreter, audiology services, captioning, listening therapy, and acoustical treatment of classrooms (Sorkin & Zwolan, 2004; Zwolan & Sorkin, 2006). Sorkin and Zwolan (2004) also found that 66% of students between 7 to 13 years of age used spoken language with 64% of this group attending public or private mainstream schools.

As more and more children are implanted at 12 months of age and younger, the placement options for children in the public schools will change, along with expectations for their academic achievement. The Individuals with Disabilities Education Improvement Act (IDEA, 2004) is covered in Chapters 9 and 10. The IDEA mandates that children with disabilities are entitled to a free and appropriate public education in the least restrictive environment (LRE). The principle of LRE means that children with disabilities should be educated with their peers in regular education to the greatest extent possible (IDEA, 2004). Mainstreaming is placing children with disabilities into the regular education setting. Mainstreaming is not an all-or-nothing option, but consists of a series of placements along a continuum with complete integration (i.e., 100% into regular education with no support) at one end and complete segregation at the other (i.e., residential school for the deaf).

It is a mistake to believe that placement of the student into regular education is the top priority; decisions concerning mainstreaming should be based on the individual needs of the child (Heavner, 2007). It has been estimated that children who are implanted by 3 years of age are able to be mainstreamed after three or four years of device use (Geers, Nicholas, & Sedey, 2003; Heavner, 2007). Heavner (2007) advised that children with cochlear implants must satisfy the following criteria prior to mainstreaming into regular kindergarten classes:

- A minimum of a 4-year-old language level
- Intelligible speech
- A trend of performance age catching up to chronological age

Further, Heavner (2007) stated that mainstreaming a child is but a first step and that an educational team must be in place for continual success. Table 8.2 provides a checklist of team personnel and their duties for serving on an educational team for children with cochlear implants.

THERAPEUTIC CONSIDERATIONS

In the previous section, we discussed Isabel's journey in receiving a cochlear implant and the teaming with personnel to support her in the school setting. Isabel had a postlingual profound sensorineural hearing loss secondary to bacterial meningitis; her therapeutic considerations will be different from children with congenital and/or prelingual losses. Parents of these children select communication options after considering personal preferences, professionals' recommendations, and children's needs. We will review communication options, therapy programs/materials, and assessment of the auditory progress of patients receiving cochlear implants.

Selection of Communication Options

Parents must consider various communication options for their child. Selection of a communication option should be made only after a careful consideration of the pertinent factors. Table 8.3 shows the various communication options and characteristics, including

table *8.2*   Checklist of Educational Team Members and Their Duties in Serving Students With Cochlear Implants

Speech-Language Pathologists or Auditory/Verbal Therapists
_____ Assess and monitor child's progress
_____ Collaborate between regular education and special education
_____ Provide direct speech and language services
_____ Troubleshoot cochlear implants, hearing aids, and hearing assistive technology
_____ Serve as case manager

Teachers of the Hearing-Impaired (Itinerant Teachers)
_____ Provide one-on-one services
_____ Monitor child's progress in the classroom
_____ Consult with regular classroom teacher
_____ Collaborate with speech-language pathology services to coordinate goals
_____ Provide preteaching to students on concepts prior to their introduction into the regular classroom

Educational Audiologists
_____ Monitor and maintain cochlear implants, hearing aids, and hearing assistive technology
_____ Troubleshoot these devices when found to be malfunctioning
_____ Assist classroom teachers in analyzing room acoustics
_____ Advocate for acoustic modifications and use of FM systems with cochlear implants
_____ Provide inservices on topics related to cochlear implants and recipients' educational needs
_____ Provide direct aural habilitation services

Language Facilitators
_____ Provide preteaching to students on concepts prior to their introduction into the regular classroom
_____ Assist the student with following directions or complex information in noisy environments or events

Classroom Teachers
_____ Meet the acoustic needs of students
_____ Assist students in meeting the demands of the regular curriculum
_____ Make appropriate instructional accommodations
_____ Disseminate class themes and pertinent concepts to the educational team at least one week in advance of their introduction into the classroom curricula
_____ Notify the educational team and family when remedial work is needed

School Psychologists or Counselors
_____ Prepare to deal with social issues of students with cochlear implants who have been mainstreamed
_____ Assess cognitive skills of children with cochlear implants

Cochlear Implant Team
_____ Communicate with students, families, and other members of the educational team
_____ Serve as a resource for other members of the educational team

Parents
_____ Communicate regularly with special and regular education teachers
_____ Discuss class themes and concepts with student
_____ Reinforce curriculum and follow through with students' work at home
_____ Assist with preteaching and remedial work
_____ Facilitate transition of student by instilling confidence and encouraging self-efficacy

Children
_____ Self-advocate for the needs in the classroom
_____ Communicate with the cochlear implant team and other members of the educational team
_____ Communicate concerns to parents and other members of the educational team

Source: Information from "Changing Trends in the Educational Placement for Children with Cochlear Implants," by K. Heavner, 2007, *Advanced Bionics: Loud and Clear, Issue 2,* retrieved from www.advancedbionics.com/UserFiles/File/2-091702%20Loud-Clear-FINAL%20Issue%202%202007.pdf.

table 8.3 Communication Options and Their Characteristics

	Auditory Verbal Unisensory	Oral Auditory-Oral	Cued Speech	Total Communication	American Sign Language/English as a Second Language (ASL/ESL) Bilingual/Bicultural
Definition	A program emphasizing auditory skills. Teaches a child to develop listening skills through one-on-one therapy that focuses attention on use of remaining hearing (with the aid of amplification). Since this method strives to make the most of a child's listening abilities, no manual communication is used and the child is discouraged from relying on visual cues.	Program that teaches a child to make maximum use of his/her remaining hearing through amplification (hearing aids, cochlear implant, FM system). This program also stresses the use of speech reading to aid the child's communication. Use of any form of manual communication (sign language) is not encouraged although natural gestures may be supported.	A visual communication system of eight handshapes (cues) that represent different sounds of speech. These cues are used while talking to make the spoken language clear through vision. This system allows the child to distinguish sounds that look the same on the lips.	Philosophy of using every and all means to communicate with deaf children. The child is exposed to a formal sign-language system (based on English), finger spelling (manual alphabet), natural gestures, speech reading, body language, oral speech, and use of amplification. The idea is to communicate and teach vocabulary and language in any manner that works.	A manual language that is distinct from spoken English (ASL is not based on English grammar/syntax). Extensively used within and among the deaf community. English is taught as a second language.
Primary Goals	To develop speech, primarily through the use of aided hearing alone, and communication skills necessary for integration into the hearing community.	To develop speech and communication skills necessary for integration into the hearing community.	To develop speech and communication skills necessary for integration into the hearing community.	To provide an easy, least restrictive communication method between the deaf child and his/her family, teachers and school-mates. The child's simultaneous use of speech and sign language is encouraged as is use of all other visual and contextual cues.	To be the deaf child's primary language and allow him/her to communicate before learning to speak or even if the child never learns to speak effectively. Since ASL is commonly referred to as "the language of the deaf," it prepares the child for social access to the deaf community.
Language Development (Receptive)	Child learns to speak through the early, consistent and successful use of a personal amplification system (hearing aids, cochlear implant, FM system).	Child learns to speak through a combination of early, consistent, and successful use of amplification and speechreading.	Child learns to speak through the use of amplification, speech reading, and use of "cues" which represent different sounds.	Language (be it spoken or sign or a combination of the two) is developed through exposure to oral speech, a formal sign language system, speech reading, and the use of an amplification system.	Language is developed through use of ASL. English is taught as a second language after the child has mastered ASL.

	(Approach 1)	(Approach 2)	(Approach 3)	(Approach 4)	(Approach 5)
Expressive Language	Spoken and written English.	Spoken and written English.	Spoken English (sometimes with the use of cues) and written English.	Spoken English and/or sign language and finger-spelling and written English.	ASL is the child's primary expressive language in addition to written English.
Hearing	Early, consistent and successful use of amplification (hearing aids, cochlear implant, FM system) is critical to this approach.	Early and consistent use of amplification (hearing aids, cochlear implant, FM system) is critical to this method.	Use of amplification is strongly encouraged to maximize the use of remaining hearing.	Use of a personal amplification system (hearing aids, cochlear implant, FM system) is strongly encouraged to allow the child to make the most of his/her remaining hearing.	Use of amplification is not a requirement for success with ASL.
Family Responsibility	Since the family is primarily responsible for the child's language development, parents are expected to incorporate on-going training into the child's daily routine and play activities. They must provide a language-rich environment, make hearing a meaningful part of all the child's experiences and ensure full-time use of amplification.	Since the family is primarily responsible for the child's language development, parents are expected to incorporate training and practice sessions (learned from therapists) into the child's daily routine and play activities. In addition, the family is responsible for ensuring consistent use of amplification.	Parents are the primary teachers of cued speech to their child. They are expected to cue at all times while they speak; consequently, at least one parent and preferably both must learn to cue fluently for the child to develop age-appropriate speech & language.	At least one, but preferably all family members, should learn the chosen sign language system in order for the child to develop age-appropriate language and communicate fully with his/her family. It should be noted that a parent's acquisition of sign vocabulary and language is a long-term, ongoing process. As the child's expressive sign language broadens and becomes more complex, so too should the parents' in order to provide the child with a stimulating language learning environment. The family is also responsible for encouraging consistent use of amplification.	Child must have access to deaf and/or hearing adults who are fluent in ASL in order to develop this as a primary language. If the parents choose this method they will need to become fluent to communicate with their child fully.
Parent Training	Parents need to be highly involved with child's teacher and/or therapists (speech, auditory-verbal, etc.) in order to learn training methods and carry them over to the home environment.	Parents need to be highly involved with their child's teacher and/or therapists (speech, aural habilitation, etc.) to carry over training activities to the home and create an optimal "oral" learning environment. These training activities would emphasize development of listening, speech reading, and speech skills.	Cued speech can be learned through classes taught by trained teachers or therapists. A significant amount of time must be spent using and practicing cues to become proficient.	Parents must consistently sign while they speak to their child (simultaneous communication). Sign language courses are routinely offered through the community, local colleges, adult education, etc. Additionally, many books and videos are widely available. To become fluent, signing must be used consistently and become a routine part of your communication.	If parents are not deaf, intensive ASL training and education about deaf culture is desired in order for the family to become proficient in the language.

Source: Courtesy of MED-EL and BEGINNINGS.

definitions, primary goals, language development (receptive and expressive), emphasis on hearing, family responsibilities, and parent training.

For parents of children with cochlear implants, the selection of a communication option should be one that has a strong emphasis on the development of auditory/oral communication. In considering the various communication options, the **Auditory/Verbal approach** has the strongest emphasis on auditory/oral communication in that it is a unisensory approach, encouraging the child to develop the use of his or her residual hearing through amplification without relying on visual cues. The clinician minimizes the availability of visual cues during therapy, encouraging the child to use his or her residual hearing with the aid of amplification to understand what is being said. The focus on hearing strengthens that sense, but may be too difficult for some children. The Auditory/Verbal approach is a widely used approach for patients with cochlear implants reporting good results (Goldberg & Flexer, 2001). Considerable parental involvement is required because training must be incorporated into the family's daily routine creating a language-rich environment, making hearing a meaningful part of all of the child's experiences and ensuring the full-time use of amplification. For example, the following View on Intervention describes the types of activities that parents implement in the home using auditory/verbal therapy.

View on Intervention

Auditory/Verbal Therapy at Home: Teaching Tips and Techniques for Parents

Auditory/verbal therapists agree that parental participation is key for a child's success with auditory/verbal therapy. By creating a listening environment and interacting with your child through spoken language, you will help enhance his or her learning process. Your son or daughter's success in learning how to listen and talk depends on you, the parent or guardian. Following are some useful tips to help you and your child achieve his or her success with listening and talking.

When working with your child shortly after he or she receives a Nucleus® cochlear implant, it is important to keep background noise to a minimum. Sit next to your child on the side of his or her cochlear implant, speaking clearly and near the headset microphone at a normal volume. Talk in complete sentences, using speech that is repetitive. Expose your child to as many learning to listen sounds as possible. Learning to listen sounds vary in duration, intensity and pitch, making them easier to hear. They include "a(r)" for an airplane, "oo" for a train, "beep" for a car or truck, "meow" for a kitten and "bu, bu" for a bus. Continuous use of these sounds will help your son or daughter process what he or she is hearing.

To incorporate the learning to listen sounds into your daily activities, place pictures of the sounds around your house in easy-to-see places. Some ideal places include the refrigerator, placemats, mirrors, and doors. Take a walk to the park, pointing out the different sounds heard, such as birds singing or an airplane flying overhead. Or go to the zoo, listening to the different animal sounds. When drawing attention to sounds, point to your ear and say, "Listen! I hear _____."

Airplanes, cars, stuffed animals, dolls, costume jewelry, and wind-up toys are just some of the objects that can be used to help assist you in teaching your child the learning to listen sounds, while having fun at the same time! Make sure to use toys that are appropriate to the age of your child.

Singing and reading to your child are two great ways to ensure his or her success. Reading to your child at an early age will cultivate a love of books, helping to increase your child's vocabulary. Therefore, when your child is older, he or she will be a skilled reader. Singing both children's songs and what you say to your child will help your son or daughter develop natural-sounding speech.

Another great idea is to make an experience book. Include such items as pictures of the learning to listen sounds from magazines, photographs or drawings, as well as entries about your child's day, souvenirs from a trip to the park, special events, your child's drawings, stories, stickers, and photographs of family and friends. You and your child can talk about these items and experiences, plus your child can share the book with others.

An interactive, fun, and enjoyable game to play is Memory, also called Concentration. Cut note cards in half and place stickers or drawings on the cards, making pairs of key target words such as apple, hat, man, shoe, and flower. Or do themes such as holidays, cars, animals, etc. With all cards face down, select one card and try to find the match. Most likely the match won't be found on the first try, so cards are again placed down in the same spot, and the next person draws a card. The key is to remember where certain cards are in order to match the pairs. Talk about each card as it is turned up, using language appropriate for your child.

Your child will learn best through lessons that are reinforced in play and significant daily experiences. A lot of what your child sees you doing during his or her formative years, he or she will also do, so be a good role model. Above all, when teaching your child, keep things flexible and adaptable.

These are just a few tips to assist you with your child's auditory/verbal therapy at home. Speak to your child's therapist to learn more auditory/verbal therapy tips and practices that will cater specifically to your child's needs.

Resources

Estabrooks, Warren, Ed. *Auditory/Verbal Therapy for Parents and Professionals.* Washington DC: The Alexander Graham Bell Association for the Deaf, 1994.

Estabrooks, Warren, Ed. *Cochlear Implants for Kids.* Washington DC: The Alexander Graham Bell Association for the Deaf, 1998.

Source: COCHLEAR (2005).

The **Auditory/Oral** option is another approach that encourages the use of the child's residual hearing with the aid of amplification, but also stresses the use of speechreading. **Speechreading** is speech recognition using all available information, including the auditory signal, lipreading, contextual cues, facial expressions, and body language. Therefore, the Auditory/Oral option is not unisensory and encourages the use of visual cues that are available in most communication situations. Both the Auditory/Verbal and Auditory/Oral options are very appropriate for young children, particularly before the age of 2 years, receiving cochlear implants because of their emphasis on the use of residual hearing in taking full advantage of neural plasticity in the development of spoken language. **Neural plasticity** is the ability of the brain to form new connections and reorganize itself through the processing of sensory information provided by auditory experiences (Tremblay, Kraus, McGee, Ponton, & Otis, 2001). Similarly, Isabel, who developed speech and language prior to the onset of her hearing loss, would do particularly well with either approach.

Some children who receive cochlear implants may not be able to benefit from either the Auditory/Verbal or Auditory/Oral options. For example, children with prelingual hearing losses who are implanted after the age of 5 may have difficulty learning spoken language through the use of their residual hearing with or without speechreading. Other options, such as Cued Speech or Total Communication may provide the needed visual input plus access to spoken language. **Cued Speech** is a visual communication system that incorporates eight handshapes and four hand positions (cues) that represent how sounds are said while talking, providing help to the child in distinguishing sounds that look the same on the mouth. The handshapes made in various positions are not signs representing the words being said, but indicate places of articulation for sounds in the words. Children still must use their residual hearing through the use of amplification to understand spoken language. However, **Total Communication**—a philosophy supporting the use of every and all means to communicate with children who are deaf—uses simultaneous exposure of a formal sign-language system (based on English), finger spelling (manual alphabet), natural gestures, speechreading, body language, oral speech, and the use of amplification. The message can be understood on the basis of the representation of what is being said using the sign-language system. Therefore, Total Communication may be a useful option for children who need a visual representation of what the speaker is saying. **American Sign Language (ASL)**—a manual language with its own syntax, semantics, and pragmatics—is used extensively within and among the Deaf community within the United States. The use of ASL is an unlikely communication option for children with cochlear implants. Later on in the chapter, we will discuss cochlear implants and Deaf culture. The selection of a communication option should be made based on the unique needs of the child, program availability, and the amount of family commitment needed for success.

Examples of Therapy Programs/Materials

Extensive auditory rehabilitation curricula have been developed and some will be covered in the following chapters. Below, some therapy programs and materials are presented to give readers an idea of some activities to use with children and adults with cochlear implants.

For Children

Cochlear has developed some supplementary auditory habilitation materials for parents and clinicians to use with children having cochlear implants. *Listen, Learn, and Talk* is an auditory learning kit for parents of children whose hearing losses were identified prior to 1 year of age. The package consists of a book and three videotapes to be used by both parents and clinicians as a supplement to the child's auditory habilitation program. The program includes the following features:

- Auditory habilitation theory explained in everyday language
- Scales of communication development from 0 to 48 months
- Age-appropriate video demonstrations of real parents using auditory habilitation activities with their children
- Additional ideas/activities, assessment tools, and references for further explanation

Another tool for audiologists to use is *Nucleus: Here We Go*, a special software program, which permits audiologists and speech-language pathologists to make customized workbooks for teenagers with cochlear implants based on their individual interests. For example, the program contains 24 interest topics (e.g., Animals and Pets, Arts and Crafts, Ball Sports, Cars and Bikes, etc.) with three different auditory skill levels for each one. Teenagers are frequently difficult to motivate and may be more apt to get involved if *they* get to choose the topic.

Advanced Bionics also has aural habilitation therapy programs; some are free and others are available for purchase. Advanced Bionics operates The Listening Room, a free web resource providing clinicians with therapy materials and suggestions. Downloadable materials include *High Chair Theatre* by David Sindrey, a pre-meal activity for infants and toddlers seated in high chairs. Parents select and hide three toys that have associated sounds (e.g., a horse says "neigh"). The activity calls for parents to make the associated sound prior to placing the toy within the child's view. Children learn that sounds are meaningfully associated with specific objects. An activity for older children, *Pan-de-mo-nium Circle Time* by Chris Barton, provides new songs and stories each month that may be downloaded onto MP3 players. Another activity for teens and adults, *Telephone Practice Phone Sounds*, involves identifying typical sounds encountered when using the telephone such as answering-machine beeps, busy signals, dial tones, cell phone ringers, and someone saying "hello."

Med-El also provides therapy materials (e.g., *HearSay e-Newsletters*, songs, resources, clinical tools) via their BRIDGE to Better Communication Program. Some of the materials are free while others are available for purchase. *SoundScape* provides age-appropriate interactive listening activities to use with infants/toddlers, preschool/elementary school children, tweens, teenagers, and adults. Activities for infants and toddlers provide parents of children undergoing cochlear implantation information about encouraging their babies to listen, speech/language development, what to do after the first fitting, and emotional issues. An interactive activity for infants and toddlers, *Listening Fun with Music and Songs*, demonstrates via video clips how parents may engage their children in singing the "Itsy, Bitsy Spider," "The Morning Song," and "Five Little Monkeys." In addition, parents are provided with information on children's typical responses to sound and are prompted to view the video clips of the songs again to see if they can recognize specific auditory behaviors. Activities for older children increase in complexity such that the one for tweens, *Telling Tales*, requires listening to 13 different stories at three levels of difficulty and then answering questions.

For Adults

So far, we have focused on children with cochlear implants; adults who have implants also require rigorous therapy to reap the benefits of these devices. One effective technique to use is **speech tracking**, a procedure requiring a partner to read materials to the patient who is to repeat *exactly* what has been said (DeFilippo & Scott, 1978). If a passage is not repeated back verbatim, then the clinician acknowledges the error and provides clues so that the patient can figure out what the word or phrase was. The clues should not be gestural, but verbal. For example, the clinician should provide words that are opposite of the word missed or use a similar sounding word (e.g., "Sounds like _____"). The reading material may be from books, newspaper articles, and/or magazines. The activity is usually done in the following three parts (Spitzer, Leder, & Giolas, 1993):

- Without the implant (lipreading only)
- With lipreading and the implant together
- With the implant only and no other visual cues

The last part is the most difficult for adults, but develops their listening abilities the most. The main goal is to increase the number of words correctly repeated over time. At first, patients should do this activity with only one or two communication partners and should try to practice every day. A major problem with speech tracking is that it is highly individualistic due to interspeaker differences and how patients respond to these variations (Levitt, 2006). A relatively new software program, *Computer-Assisted Tracking*, has been developed that maintains the interactive nature of the technique, but reduces the sources of variation (Levitt, 2006). The program was also designed for patients to self-train at home.

Adults are busy and often do not have time off from work to go to therapy. Over the past 20 years, three computerized audiovisual speech perception training programs have been developed for both adults and children: (1) *Computer-Assisted Speech Perception Evaluation and Training* (CASPER) developed by Boothroyd and colleagues at the City University of New York (Boothroyd, 1987); (2) *Computer-Aided Speechreading Training (CAST)* by Pichora-Fuller and colleagues (Benguerel & Pichora-Fuller, 1988; Pichora-Fuller & Benguerel, 1991); and (3) a computerized videodisc system (Tye-Murray, Tyler, Bong, & Nares, 1988). More recently, Boothroyd (2006b) and his colleagues at San Diego State University have developed *Computer Assisted Speech Perception Evaluation and Training of Sentences* (CasperSent), a multimedia program with an aim to evaluate and train sentence-level speech perception.

Another program for adults developed by Cochlear is *Sound and Beyond*—an interactive, self-paced software program designed to help adults practice and develop their listening skills at home. The program has a database of over 10,000 sounds, words, and sentences that are used in listening modules to train the following skills:

- Pure tones—identifying different pitches of sound
- Environmental sounds—identifying common environmental sounds
- Male/female identification—discrimination between speakers
- Vowel recognition—vowel discrimination and identification
- Consonant recognition—consonant discrimination and identification
- Word discrimination—common word discrimination from four different topic categories
- Everyday sentences—identifying sentences with different levels of background noise
- Music appreciation—identifying musical instruments and familiar tunes as a start to music appreciation

The program has a feature in which patients can prepare and send a report to their clinician regarding their practice on *Sound and Beyond*.

Advanced Bionics also has interactive listening activities for teens and adults in their online Listening Room in a section called the Listening Gym. This area has conversation practice, discrimination activities, music appreciation, and speech tracking exercises. Most sections also offer "Thumbprints," video files of activities patients download onto their MP3 players or iPODs and "Paper Trails," printable exercises to be completed with a clinician. Discrimination interactive activities, *Clix*, provide opportunities for patients to practice listening skills at three levels of warm-up/beginner, intermediate/advanced, and expert/Olympic on their personal computers. Music appreciation has examples of musical instruments, different genres, and popular selections for listening in addition to guides for enjoying classical and popular music of the Western world.

In their BRIDGE to Better Communication Program, Med-El has an interactive activity for adults called *Sentence Matrix*. In this activity, adult cochlear implant users can specify conditions for a closed-set sentence-recognition task by selecting the type of (1) talker (male, female, or both), (2) noise (none, some, or more), (3) speed (slow, normal, or fast), and (4) number of sentences (10, 25, or 50). Adults listen to simple sentences (e.g., "John saw three books.") through computer loudspeakers and click on the words within a matrix to indicate what they heard. The program provides listeners with percent correct responses as feedback at the conclusion of training sequences. Additional downloadable materials are available for clinicians to create similar listening situations in therapy.

Assessment of Auditory Progress

Earlier in this chapter, we discussed the importance of monitoring patients' performance with cochlear implants. Communication between and among team members is essential for determining patients' use of and progress with their implants in multiple contexts. It is important to note that outcomes or **benchmarks**, or projected performance levels after cochlear implant activation, are individual to each patient, but should be comparable to others with similar histories. Benchmarks are important for parents who want to know how their child is progressing; benchmarks are important for speech pathologists and audiologists to determine whether something in the child's MAP, or intervention program, needs modification. Benchmarks are also important for adult cochlear implant recipients and their families to assist in determining if appropriate progress is being made.

The performance of patients with cochlear implants must be compared against that of their peers. The most critical factors for matching patients to appropriate peers are age at the time of implantation and the quality, type, and amount of auditory experience prior to receiving the device. Children with cochlear implants represent a very heterogeneous population, especially regarding variations in their status for the critical factors that impact prognosis. Recall that the earlier a child is implanted, the better is the prognosis for the development of age-appropriate speech and language skills and academic achievement. Further, children who have prior auditory experience, either with normal hearing or with amplification, should progress more quickly and to higher levels of performance than those without. Evidence-based practice has been a major theme of this textbook, and benchmarking of performance must be based on the results of high-quality research documenting how age of onset and amount of auditory experience influence outcomes for children with cochlear implants. **Benchmarking** is comparing a single patient's performance to evidence-based, normative outcomes.

Robbins (2005) developed her red-flag procedure for clinicians to use in benchmarking patients' progress during the first year after cochlear implant activation. **Red flags** are indications that patients are not making average progress with their implants. In other words, how does a patient's performance compare with the statistical mean of a group of his or her peers? It is important, though, to remember that in using means, half of the patients took longer to achieve a particular goal and the other half progressed more quickly. Comparing individual patients' outcomes against average performances of their peers is helpful because speech, language, and auditory development are cumulative processes; acquisition of new skills is based on mastery of earlier competencies (Robbins, 2005). Therefore, arrested development precludes timely progress, and minimal setbacks may lead to more severe delays.

Comparing individual patient outcomes to group averages is imperfect, but represents the "best guess" of appropriate postimplant performance trajectories. When groups of similar patients are assessed on benchmarks, the average or mean time required to master certain skills after implantation may be calculated and used as benchmarks. Robbins's (2005) evidence-based benchmarks arose from the results of longitudinal studies that followed patients and measured their outcomes over time (e.g., McConkey Robbins, Koch, Osberger, Zimmerman-Phillips, & Kishon Rabin, 2004; Osberger, Zimmerman-Phillips, Barker, & Geier, 1999; Waltzman & Cohen, 1999). As stated in Chapter 1, age of identification, diagnosis, and intervention of hearing loss affects speech, language, and hearing expectations and outcomes. Generally, the later the diagnosis of hearing loss, the more difficult it is for cochlear implantation coupled with auditory habilitation to exploit critical periods of auditory and linguistic development. Therefore, Robbins developed benchmarks for auditory skills for three groups of children who received an implant by (1) 4 years of age, with many prior to age 3 years; (2) 5 years of age with some development of residual hearing through hearing aid use; and (3) 5 years of age and older with little or no preimplant use of residual hearing and heavy reliance on speechreading and sign language.

Tables 8.4, 8.5, and 8.6 show the skills to be achieved as a function of months elapsed since implantation. The shaded boxes represent the average month postimplantation that skills are acquired by each group. Notice that skills are expected to be acquired earlier for the group receiving cochlear implants at younger ages. Robbins (2005) stresses that full-time use of a cochlear implant is a prerequisite for achieving expected outcomes. Therefore, all three groups are expected to have full-time cochlear implant use by one month postimplant. Recently, Archbold, Nikolopoulos, and Lloyd-Richmond (2009) investigated long-term use of cochlear implants for children who had been implanted for seven years. Although 83% were full-time implant users, nearly 20% were not. Generally, full-time users were implanted earlier, used oral rather than signed communication, and had a greater proportion in mainstreamed settings than the group who wore their devices on a part-time basis. The authors recommended monitoring children on a regular basis so that cochlear implant teams can address nonuse issues and provide support to users, families, and school personnel in a timely fashion (Archbold et al., 2009).

In tracking patients' progress, clinicians should be concerned about the number of skills and the amount of delay. Robbins (2005) provided a continuum for red flags based on the severity of the situation. She explained that a one-flag response is one skill that is delayed by three months. A two-flag response is a delay of more than six months for two or more skills. She strongly advocates addressing one-flag responses before they

table *8.4*   Tracking Auditory Progress in Children Implanted at 4 Years of Age, or Earlier With Many Prior to Age 3 Years (Shaded Boxes Indicate Time Post-Implant Child Should Demonstrate Skill)

Skill	1 Month	3 Months	6 Months	9 Months	12 Months
1. Full-time use of cochlear implant (CI)	▓				
2. Changes in spontaneous vocalizations with CI use		▓			
3. Spontaneously alerts to name 25% of the time		▓			
4. Spontaneously alerts to name 50% of time			▓		
5. Spontaneously alerts to a few environmental sounds			▓		
6. Performance in the audiometric booth consistent with what is reported at home				▓	
7. Evidence of deriving meaning from many speech and environmental sounds					▓
8. Major improvement in language					▓

Source: From "Clinical Red Flags for Slow Progress in Children with Cochlear Implants," by A. M. Robbins, 2005, *Advanced Bionics: Loud and Clear, Issue 1,* retrieved from www.advancedbionics.com/userfiles/File/Issue1-2005.pdf. Used with permission.

table 8.5 Tracking Auditory Progress in Children Implanted at Age 5 Years and Older With Some Residual Hearing, Consistent Hearing Aid Use Prior to Cochlear Implants, and Who Are Primarily Oral (Shaded Boxes Indicate Time Post-Implant Child Should Demonstrate Skill)

Skill	1 Month	3 Months	6 Months	9 Months	12 Months
1. Full-time use of cochlear implant (CI)	▓				
2. Understands some words or phrases in closed set		▓			
3. Understands many words or phrases in closed set			▓		
4. Spontaneously alerts to name 50% of time			▓		
5. Understands familiar phrases in everyday situations when listening in the auditory-only mode				▓	
6. Spontaneous recognition of own name versus other names				▓	
7. Knows meaning of some environmental or speech signals when heard in the auditory-only mode					▓
8. Major improvement in language					▓

Source: From "Clinical Red Flags for Slow Progress in Children with Cochlear Implants," by A. M. Robbins, 2005, *Advanced Bionics: Loud and Clear, Issue 1*, retrieved from www.advancedbionics.com/userfiles/File/Issue1-2005.pdf. Used with permission.

table 8.6 Tracking Auditory Progress in Children Implanted at Age 5 Years or Older With Limited or No Residual Hearing, Limited or No Hearing Aid Use, and Who Rely Heavily on Visual Cues or Signs (Shaded Boxes Indicate Time Post-Implant Child Should Demonstrate Skill)

Skill	1 Month	3 Months	6 Months	9 Months	12 Months
1. Full-time use of cochlear implant (CI)	▓				
2. Begins to discriminate patterns of speech (e.g., syllable number, stress, length, etc.)		▓			
3. Understands some words in closed set			▓		
4. Begins to spontaneously respond to name			▓		
5. Reports when device is not working (e.g., dead battery)				▓	
6. Understands many words or phrases in closed set					▓
7. Understands a few things in open set					
8. Major improvement in language					▓

Source: From "Clinical Red Flags for Slow Progress in Children with Cochlear Implants," by A. M. Robbins, 2005, *Advanced Bionics: Loud and Clear, Issue 1*, retrieved from www.advancedbionics.com/userfiles/File/Issue1-2005.pdf. Used with permission.

develop into two-flag responses. Red-flag intervention strategies should involve the parents, cochlear implant audiologist, and speech language pathologist. First, red flags should be discussed with parents and confirmation made that the child is wearing his or her cochlear implant(s) during all waking hours and if not, determine the reasons for nonuse. Adequate progress depends on consistent utilization of the cochlear implant. Parents are partners in habilitation and may provide critical information and observations regarding children's lack of progress. Consultation with the cochlear implant audiologist may be in order to determine the existence of any issues (e.g., equipment malfunction) with the device that precludes adequate progress toward these goals. Moreover, Robbins advises that a child may not have mastered a skill simply because of insufficient opportunities for mastery. Observations of a child's classroom environment may find many missed opportunities by a teacher who gains the child's attention visually, rather than by calling his or her name when the child is not looking. Therefore, intervention plans should be altered to provide specific training on certain skills. In some cases, red-flag responses may be due to developmental delays or mild cognitive impairments. Nevertheless, the red-flag procedure is a useful tool for benchmarking progress during the first year of cochlear implantation.

These benchmarks will need to be updated as outcomes from children implanted at or even before their first birthdays become available. This generation of children has two advantages over their predecessors, namely early diagnosis of hearing loss through newborn hearing screening programs and technological advancements in cochlear implants. Chapter 9 summarizes the Joint Committee on Infant Hearing Year 2007 Position Statement (JCIH, 2007) mandating that all children's hearing be screened by 1 month of age, diagnosis of loss by 3 months of age, and formal intervention initiated before 6 months of age. With recommendation for placement of hearing aids within 1 month of diagnosis, children are able to have trial periods with amplification shortly after birth. Therefore, those children who do not receive adequate benefit from hearing aids may be referred for a cochlear implant evaluation long before their first birthdays. Auditory habilitative efforts with these infants are able to harness neural plasticity during critical periods of auditory, speech, and language development. Concomitantly, improvements in implant technology have resulted in greater sophistication in processing of auditory stimuli resulting in enhanced speech recognition capabilities. In the next section, we will discuss the long-term expectations for patients after cochlear implantation.

LONG-TERM EXPECTATIONS FOR PATIENTS WITH COCHLEAR IMPLANTS

The following section describes pediatric and adults' outcomes after receiving a cochlear implant.

Pediatric Expectations

Professionals must accurately counsel parents and their children, when appropriate, regarding expected outcomes after cochlear implantation. Moreover, expectations are different for children with different patient profiles, and the parents' decision to consider cochlear implantation is most influenced by professionals' recommendations (Li, Bain, & Steinberg, 2004). Parents should be advised that children's level of achievement is inversely related to the age at implantation, namely that higher levels of performance are obtained by those children implanted early, particularly before age 2 and not after age 4 to avoid irreversible permanent performance losses (Anderson et al., 2004; Govaerts et al., 2002; O'Neill, O'Donoghue, Archbold, Nikolopoulos, & Sach, 2002). For example, growth rates in vocabulary development decline for some children when implanted after age 5 (El-Hakim et al., 2001). In addition, speech perception performance has been found to improve more for children who are implanted earlier rather than later (Zwolan, Ashbaugh, Alarfaj, Kileny, Arts, El-Kashlan, & Telian, 2004). Besides age of implantation, the appropriateness of mapping and aural habilitation services impact outcomes.

Some parents of children younger than age 2 may be concerned about the surgical risks of cochlear implantation. However, Hehar, Nikolopoulos, Gibbin, and O'Donoghue (2002) demonstrated successful surgical and functional outcomes for twelve children implanted before age 2. Six of the children acquired severe-to-profound hearing loss from meningitis and six had congenital sensorineural hearing loss. Four of the children had cochlear ossification from meningitis. Eleven children achieved complete insertion, with one child receiving partial insertion with 16 electrodes. No serious surgical complications existed and functional outcomes two years after implantation were as good or better than for children who underwent implantation between 2 and 5 years of age. More recently, Roland, Cosetti, Wang, Immerman, and Waltzman (2009) reported on the results and safety of implantation of 50 children who were implanted before the age of 1 year and followed them for 7 years. They found that the number and types of complications for these infants were similar to those for older children and adults (Roland et al., 2009). Cochlear implantation is a safe and efficacious procedure for children younger than 1 year old, yet poses unique issues (Cosetti & Roland, 2010).

Regarding language performance and literacy, much of the available data were from those who were implanted later than many of the children are today. Nevertheless, 16 children with cochlear implants in mainstreamed classes in a public school system in the Midwest were compared with 16 age-matched peers with normal hearing on measures of language and literacy (Spencer, Barker, & Tomblin, 2003). Children with cochlear implants performed within one standard deviation of their peers on language comprehension, reading, and writing accuracy, but significantly poorer on sentence formulation. Similarly, Spencer, Gantz, and Knutson (2004) retrospectively analyzed the outcomes of 27 prelingually, profoundly deaf students who received cochlear implants between 2 and 12 years of age. They found achievement scores within one standard deviation of peers with normal hearing, over 50% of college-eligible student enrollments, and a wide range of vocational outcomes. Furthermore, Waltzman, Robbins, Green, and Cohen (2003) found that children with profound congenital sensorineural hearing loss who were implanted before the age of 5 achieved some degree of fluency in learning a second oral language. In addition, Tait, Nikolopoulos, Archbold, and O'Donoghue (2001) found that prelingually deaf children with multichannel cochlear implants showed consistent improvement in their ability to use the telephone. Children with congenital hearing losses who use the latest cochlear implants have reported that they find listening to music quite enjoyable (Trehub, Vongpaisal, & Nakata, 2009). Today, it is expected that young children implanted as a result of being diagnosed with hearing loss through early hearing identification and intervention programs will be comparable to that of their peers with normal hearing.

Parents with children who have contraindicating medical conditions must carefully be counseled regarding the outcomes from cochlear implantation. Initially, it was believed that children with auditory neuropathy/dyssynchrony were not suitable candidates for cochlear implants. Recall that these children have dysfunction in that cranial nerve VIII does not transmit neural impulses generated in the periphery to the central auditory nervous system causing a neural hearing loss (Joint Committee on Infant Hearing, 2007). Some of these children have tried using hearing aids, but have found that they were of little benefit and were referred for cochlear implant evaluations. Some of these children have been found to achieve outcomes for speech production/perception and communication similar to other cochlear implant patients (Rance & Barker, 2009; Shallop et al., 2001).

Patients with cochlear malformations have also been considered poor candidates for cochlear implants. Mylanus, Rotteveel, and Leeuw (2004) advised parents of children with cochlear malformations that implantation may have uncertain results. However, others have reported successful outcomes for children with cochlear malformations (Hoffman, Downey, Waltzman, & Cohen, 1997). Similarly, parents with children that have CHARGE association (described in Chapter 9) should be counseled that variations in temporal bone anatomy found with this disorder may yield increased challenges for the surgical team and possible risk to the facial nerve (Bauer, Wippold, Goldin, & Lusk, 2002). Briefly, CHARGE association is a complex genetic disorder with major features of colomboma (type of cleft) of the eye; choanal atresia (closure) or stenosis (narrowing); cranial nerve abnormalities; and outer, middle, and inner ear malformations (CHARGE Syndrome Association, 2010). These children also have minor features manifesting in malformations in other parts of the body such as the heart. Many children with CHARGE syndrome have hearing and visual impairments. Recommendations to parents of deaf-blind children should include finding a cochlear implant clinic with low-vision rehabilitation specialists along with access to the strengths of the deaf-blind community (Saeed, Ramsden, & Axon, 1998).

Parents of children with large vestibular aqueduct syndrome should be advised that even if their hearing loss progresses to profound levels, cochlear implantation can have positive outcomes (Fahy, Carney, Nikolopoulos, Ludman, & Gibbin, 2001; Miyamoto, Bichey, Wynne, & Kirk, 2002). Greater social connectivity and environmental awareness, in addition to better speech perception and production, have been reported for children with multiple handicaps who have received cochlear implants (Hamzavi, Baumgartner, Egelierler, Franz, Schenk, & Gstoettner, 2000; Waltzman, Scalchunes, & Cohen, 2000). Similar results have been obtained for adults with other disabilities (e.g., deaf-blindness, psychopathologies, and/or mental retardation) who achieved improved listening, communication skills, and stability in familial relationships after cochlear implantation (Filipo, Bosco, Mancini, & Ballantyne, 2004). Therefore, patients with multiple disabilities need to be advised of the benefits and risks regarding cochlear implantation.

Adult Expectations

The literature contains a large number of studies documenting the outcomes for adults who have received cochlear implants during the last 30 years. Performance expectations have increased with technological advancements. For example, Kirk (2001) stated the single-channel cochlear implant systems used in the United States during the 1980s were the 3M/House device (Fretz & Fravel, 1985) and the 3M/Vienna cochlear implant

(Hochmair & Hochmair-Desoyer, 1983), which enabled patients who were completely deaf to develop some of the following auditory skills:

- Detection of speech below conversational levels (Tyler, Gantz, McCabe, Lowder, Otto, & Preece, 1985)
- Identify environmental sounds with some accuracy (Gantz, Tyler, Knutson, et al., 1988)
- Discrimination of some vowels in a closed-set format based on fundamental frequency (Gantz, Tye-Murray, & Tyler, 1989) and first formant cues (Tyler, Tye-Murray, Moore, & McCabe, 1989)
- Discrimination of some consonants in a closed-set format based on duration and voicing cues (Gantz et al., 1989)
- Better lipreading (Gantz et al., 1988; Tyler et al., 1985)

In summary, single-channel cochlear implants with only one stimulating electrode provided primarily durational and intensity cues, but limited spectral information.

Technological advancements have developed cochlear implants with multiple channels and electrodes. Kirk (2001) stated that with today's technology, the speech signal is filtered to different frequency bands to specific electrodes which, in turn, stimulate specific nerve fibers at specific frequencies. Therefore, multichannel cochlear implant systems provide users with spectral information in addition to durational and intensity cues (Kirk, 2001). In the United States, the three cochlear implant manufacturers mentioned have used multichannel cochlear implants for at least 20 years. The three manufacturers have active research and development programs for continuous quality improvement of their products and outcomes for patients.

Regardless of the cochlear implant system used, audiologists and speech-language pathologists must be able to convey what adult patients can expect after receiving a device. That question is difficult to answer because it depends on the patient. The most important determinant of adult outcomes is duration of deafness (Blamey et al., 1996). The onset of deafness may have been congenital, gradual over time, or sudden. In addition, patients with gradually progressive hearing losses may range from those who always have had amplification to some who have had no hearing aid use. Generally, the longer the adult has been deprived of sound, the poorer the prognosis. Postlingually deafened adults have better prognosis than those with prelingual hearing losses. Other factors indicative of poorer prognosis are the use of sign language for the primary mode of communication and a lack of commitment to be part of the hearing world and auditory rehabilitation. Zwolan, Kileny, and Telian (1996) found that postlingually deafened cochlear implant users outperformed those who had prelingual hearing losses, although the latter group subjectively reported regular use, satisfaction, and improved receptive and expressive communication skills with their devices. Other investigators have found similar results and stress the importance of including subjective patient-report questionnaires in reporting outcomes, particularly those pertaining to quality of life (Kaplan, Shipp, Chen, Ng, & Nedzelski, 2003). In addition, the first 12 months after implantation show the greatest improvement in performance for prelingually deafened adult patients receiving a cochlear implant (Hamzavi, Baumgartner, Pok, Franz, & Gstoettner, 2003; Teoh, Pisoni, & Miyamoto, 2004). Recently, Klop, Briaire, Stiggelbout, and Frijns (2007) found that adults with prelingual deafness have found significant improvement in speech production/perception and quality of life when implanted with state-of-the-art technology.

Why are the outcomes after cochlear implantation different for prelingually versus postlingually deafened people? Koch (1999) explained that postlingually deafened people are already "programmed" for understanding spoken language, and cochlear implants bypass the damaged peripheral auditory system, reconnecting the brain with the speech signal. On the other hand, prelingually deafened people have a limited neurological network for processing spoken language such that information provided through a cochlear implant is meaningless without extensive auditory rehabilitation (Koch, 1999).

Recall that there are no upper age limits for cochlear implantation provided that patients are in good health and satisfy candidacy criteria for implantation. The results of recent studies have shown that cochlear implantation is safe for older adults, whose results are comparable to their younger counterparts. For example, Sterkers et al. (2004) reported outcome data for 28 patients over 60 years of age with profound bilateral sensorineural hearing loss who received a cochlear implant between 1991 and 2001. Benefits in speech perception were fairly consistent across subjects; patients over 70 years old performed similarly to patients under 70 years old. Similarly, Chatelin et al. (2004) reported significant benefits in speech perception for elderly patients, but found that those over 70 years of age received slightly less benefit than individuals younger than 70. More recently, Poissant, Beaudoin, Huang, Brodsky, and Lee (2008) also found that cochlear implant users 70 years and older achieved speech recognition performance in quiet and in noise comparable to that of younger implantees. Moreover, no surgical complications were found with the elderly patients, who also reported a reduction in depression and loneliness after receiving cochlear implants. In summary, the elderly may be excellent candidates for cochlear implants, but require assessment of their physical status to determine accurate risk-to-benefit ratios (Sterkers et al., 2004).

OTHER OPTIONS FOR COCHLEAR IMPLANT WEARERS

Patients most often receive a cochlear implant on either the right or left side. However, both children and adults have other options in addition to single-sided cochlear implants. The reasons for pursuing the use of another device in the ear opposite the cochlear implant are similar to those for pursing binaural hearing aids. In Chapter 6, we discussed the benefits of hearing with two ears rather than just one. Localization and speech recognition in noise are two skills that are also important to cochlear implant users. Two options to achieve these benefits are wearing hearing aids and cochlear implants in opposite ears or having bilateral cochlear implants (i.e., cochlear implants in both ears). In addition, some patients may benefit from a new type of device, a hybrid cochlear implant.

Bimodal Stimulation

Bimodal stimulation is an arrangement of wearing a hearing aid in the ear opposite to the cochlear implant. The term *bimodal* is appropriate because the cochlear implant electrically stimulates the auditory nerve on one side and an air-conduction hearing aid provides input to the other ear. Ching, Incerti, and Hill (2004) showed that adults who wore cochlear implants and hearing aids in opposite ears demonstrated objective improvement in speech recognition and localization performance (i.e., ability to determine the direction sound is coming from), in addition to subjective patient reports of increased benefits with bimodal stimulation. The authors caution, though, that the hearing aid must be fine-tuned to suit the patient's individual needs in order to achieve maximum benefit.

What Does the Evidence Show?

Olson and Shinn (2008) conducted a systematic review to determine if there was evidence that showed that wearing hearing aids in the ears opposite to the cochlear implant improved the communication function of adults. Authors searched for evidence by submitting key words and phrases into the Cochrane Database of Systematic Reviews, PubMed, Central Index of Nursing and Allied Health Literature, and Medline. They also searched the references of textbooks and trade journals. The search yielded 187 articles, with 52 of them comprehensively reviewed, and 11 articles included in the systematic review. The authors found that adults obtained better speech recognition performance in the bimodal conditions, particularly in noise. However, they found that patients had variable performance with localization. It was found that patients had an improvement in their functional ability with bimodal stimulation. Based on the evidence, the recommendation that bimodal stimulation improves adults' communication function had a grade of B or C. The authors recommended that patients try bimodal stimulation prior to pursuing bilateral cochlear implantation.

Bilateral Cochlear Implants

Another relatively new treatment option is bilateral cochlear implants. As of 5 years ago, 4,600 individuals have received bilateral cochlear implants and that number has grown (Kirk, Firszt, Hood, & Holt, 2006). Patients pursuing bilateral cochlear implants may have one ear implanted first, and then the other, which is known as **sequential implantation**. The patient may or may not have worn a hearing aid on the previously unimplanted ear. Alternatively, some patients may elect to have both ears implanted at the same time, which is known as **simultaneous implantation**. Recall that this issue was at the center of an evidence-based problem discussed in Chapter 5.

Vermeire, Brokx, Van de Heyning, Cochet, and Carpentier (2003) presented a case study of a preschool child who received her first cochlear implant when she was 2.5 years old and then a second implant when she was 4.4 years old. The child demonstrated better thresholds and improved speech identification/recognition with two implants versus one. Similarly, Litovsky et al. (2004) demonstrated improved binaural listening skills such as localization for adults and children when using two cochlear implants rather than one. For example, localization ability has been assessed using the minimum audible angle paradigm in which the dependent variable is the smallest angular differentiation between two sounds perceived as originating from two distinct sources (Litovsky, Johnstone, & Godar, 2006; Litovsky et al., 2006). Kühn-Inacker, Shehata-Dieler, Müller, and Helms (2004) showed improved speech recognition abilities for children when using two cochlear implants rather than just one and provided important suggestions for optimizing benefit. For example, bilateral cochlear implantation must be coupled with an intensive aural habilitation program. Older children should have realistic expectations about the immediate benefits of the second implant. They may unrealistically expect that the second implant will sound just like their first implant, not realizing the amount or work and adjustment required for optimal benefit.

It is important that the second processor be fit with the first cochlear implant turned on so that patients will not be excessively discouraged about the initial sound of the second implant. Later on, auditory skill training with only the second implant turned on will assist in decreasing the difference in competence between the two implants. For example, it may be advisable for a child who has undergone a sequential implantation to work on listening activities with both implants and then with only the second implant. Some have advised removing the older implant for specified periods during the day. The most recently implanted ear and pathways should progress through the same stages of auditory development as the other with initial training sessions.

Hybrid Cochlear Implants

Another technological advancement is the **hybrid cochlear implant**, which simultaneously provides acoustic input through a hearing aid for the lower frequencies and electrical stimulation of afferent auditory nerve fibers tuned to the higher frequencies via a cochlear implant to the same ear. Typically, the device consists of an in-the-ear hearing aid and a cochlear implant. The electrode array for these devices is much shorter than typical cochlear implants and is situated at the base of the cochlea. Alternatively, the hearing-aid component amplifies the sounds that travel toward the apical region of the cochlea, preserving low-frequency hearing. The hybrid cochlear implant is particularly suited for patients with steeply sloping sensorineural hearing losses. With relatively good low-frequency hearing sensitivity, these patients may not be suitable cochlear implant candidates, but they may have difficulty getting sufficient benefit in hearing high-frequency sounds through hearing aids. Over the past 10 years, the Food and Drug Administration has conducted a clinical trial at the University of Iowa of hybrid cochlear implants manufactured by Cochlear Corporation (Dunn & Marciniak, 2009). Preliminary results have shown that these devices provide improved speech recognition in noise and greater enjoyment when listening to music (Dunn & Marciniak, 2009). Undoubtedly, hybrid cochlear implants have shown great promise as an option for some patients (Gantz, Hansen, Turner, Oleson, Reiss, & Parkinson, 2009).

AUDITORY BRAINSTEM IMPLANTS

Another type of device is the auditory brainstem implant, which is a hearing prosthesis for patients who have neurofibromatosis of which there are several types (defined previously). Neurofibromatosis Type II (NF-2), is an autosomal dominant hereditary condition with a worldwide incidence of 1 in every 30,000 to 40,000 people (Kanowitz, Shapiro, Golfinos, Cohen, & Roland, 2004). Auditory brainstem implants may also be an option for patients who have auditory nerve damage (cranial nerve VIII) from the surgery to remove bilateral tumors known as **schwannomas** (Kanowitz et al., 2004). Schwannomas are tumors arising from the nerve sheaths of cranial and spinal nerves and often invade the internal auditory canal or cerebellopontine angle in over 90% of gene carriers with NF-2 (Kanowitz et al., 2004; Wagner, 2008). Definitive diagnosis of NF-2 requires either the presence of schwannomas on cranial nerve VIII bilaterally, confirmed radiographically (e.g., magnetic resonance imaging [MRI]) *or* a first-degree relative and presence of a single schwannoma before age 30, *or* presence of two or more of the following conditions: meningioma, glioma, schwannoma, or juvenile cortical cataract (Wagner, 2008). The auditory brainstem implant may also be an option for patients who were born without auditory nerves or whose nerves have been damaged accidentally (House Ear Institute, 2006).

The auditory brainstem implant was initially developed in 1979 at the House Ear Institute and has been implanted in over 500 patients around the world (House Ear Institute, 2006). The U.S. Food and Drug Administration (FDA) approved the Nucleus 24 auditory brainstem implant system for patients 12 years and older with NF-2 (FDA, 2000). Like the cochlear implant, the auditory brainstem implant has surgically implanted, or inside, parts and externally worn parts. The outside parts include a ear-level or pocket-size speech processor worn on the body and a microphone headset in addition to an internal part implanted in the brainstem (FDA, 2000).

Patients considering an auditory brainstem implant should be counseled about its risks versus benefits. Possible risks include those normally associated with surgery and general anesthesia (e.g., infection/bleeding, numbness/stiffness around the ear, injury/stimulation of the facial nerve, taste disturbance, dizziness, increased tinnitus, neck pain, or leakage of cerebral spinal fluid, possibly causing meningitis) (FDA, 2000). Colletti (2006) found that both tumor and nontumor patients received improved communication and awareness of environmental sounds with an auditory brainstem implant. Nontumor patients achieved greater speech understanding abilities with auditory brainstem implants than those with tumors, and performed at levels similar to patients with cochlear implants (Colletti, 2006). Only a small percentage of NF-2 patients have achieved open-set speech recognition with an auditory brainstem implant (Colletti & Shannon, 2005). Open-set speech recognition is the ability to understand speech without any cues provided by multiple-choice response paradigms.

COCHLEAR IMPLANTS AND DEAF CULTURE

In Chapter 3, we discussed how audiologists and speech-language pathologists need to develop cross-cultural competence in serving patients and their family members who are members of cultural and/or ethnic minorities. Some people who are deaf or hard of hearing are members of the Deaf culture, many of whom believe that hearing loss is a biological difference, not an abnormality, and have fought for acceptance and equal rights (Tyler, 1993). **Audism** is a term that describes how the hearing establishment is perceived as imposing their values onto Deaf culture by defining its members as a group of individuals who have a common affliction needing treatment (Harlan, 1999). Some members of the Deaf culture have strong negative feelings toward cochlear implantation and view it as an attempt at ethnocide or eradication of their culture (Harlan & Bahan, 1998). In addition, some feel that subjecting a beautiful deaf child to surgery for a non–life-threatening illness is abusive (Hladek, 2002).

The National Association of the Deaf (NAD), an organization devoted to preserving the psychological integrity of children and adults who are deaf and hard of hearing, published a position statement on cochlear implants that made the following 10 recommendations (NAD, 2010a):

1. Train healthcare professionals toward a wellness model, portraying individuals who are deaf and hard of hearing as valuable and contributing members of society. Parents may be more apt to expose their children who are deaf and hard of hearing to Deaf culture if that culture were portrayed more positively by the medical establishment.
2. Adequate trial periods with the latest digital hearing aids should occur before considering cochlear implants, especially for children. How do parents and professionals determine if cochlear implants are an option without assessing outcomes with the latest technology for sufficient periods of time?
3. Cochlear implant teams should weigh the risks against the long-term benefits when reviewing the initial candidacy of patients. Moreover, other options should be provided for those patients who received limited benefits from cochlear implants.

4. Auditory habilitation should include American Sign Language (ASL) to increase the likelihood of developing age-appropriate psychological, social, cognitive, and language development in children who are deaf or hard of hearing.

5. Third-party payers should provide equal coverage for alternative treatments to cochlear implants (i.e., hearing aids) so that parents' choices are not primarily based on financial considerations.

6. The media should provide fair and unbiased coverage of all viable treatments for hearing loss when covering stories on cochlear implants.

7. Sound longitudinal research reporting outcomes for patients with *both* positive and negative outcomes from cochlear implantation are needed so that comparisons to patients receiving alternative treatments can be made.

8. Parents should carefully investigate *all* treatment options prior to making a decision concerning their children's futures, realizing that cochlear implants are not a cure for deafness.

9. Support services must be in place in the home and school environments for children and their families.

10. Educational programming should advocate for the development of auditory speech skills in a dynamic and interactive visual environment that includes sign language and English.

In summary, both hearing and Deaf worlds must work toward a resolution of their differences on issues surrounding cochlear implants. Tyler (1993) recommended three steps that audiologists and speech-language pathologists could take to try to build bridges with members of the Deaf community. First, they should try to learn about Deaf culture through reading, communicating with the Deaf, and acknowledging their feelings regarding cochlear implants. Second, fair and accurate counseling should be provided to patients and their families to include ASL and Deaf culture as a viable option for treatment. Third, members of both the hearing and Deaf communities must learn to accept diversity within and across their cultures. For example, communication sciences and disorders professionals should not prejudge those in the Deaf community who reject cochlear implants or any form of amplification. Alternatively, members of the Deaf culture should not negatively judge members of their own community who choose to try a cochlear implant. Together, audiologists, speech-language pathologists, and the Deaf community can achieve a common ground.

SUMMARY

Cochlear implant technology continues to evolve, expanding the number of those who may benefit and improving expectations for patient outcomes. This chapter reviewed how cochlear implants work, options from manufacturers, patient selection criteria for children and adults, the surgery and follow-up, therapy programs and materials, possible patient outcomes, and options of bimodal stimulation, bilateral, and hybrid cochlear implants. The chapter concluded with an introduction to auditory brainstem implants in addition to a discussion about cochlear implants and Deaf culture.

LEARNING ACTIVITIES

- Contact your nearest cochlear implant center to inquire about observing surgery for cochlear implantation.
- Go to the websites of cochlear implant manufacturers and print out all available information for parents considering a cochlear implant for their child. Obtain, organize, and develop a parent resource list using the materials you have gathered.
- Interview parents of a child or an adult who has recently received a cochlear implant. Ask about their experiences and feelings during each part of the process.

APPENDIX 8.1

Contact Information for Cochlear Implant Manufacturers

Advanced Bionics
Advanced Bionics Corporate Headquarters
28515 Westinghouse Place
Valencia, CA 91355
1 (877) 829-0026 Toll-free voice U.S. and Canada
1 (800) 678-3575 TTY
(661) 362-1503 Fax
Website: www.advancedbionics.com or www.cochlearimplant.com
Hours of operation: 5 a.m. to 5 p.m., PST

Cochlear Americas
13059 E. Peakview Avenue
Centennial, CO 80111
1 (800) 523-5798 Toll-free voice (Voice and TTY)
(303) 792-9025 Fax
Website: www.cochlearamericas.com
Hours of operation: 8 a.m. to 5 p.m., Monday through Friday, MST

Med-El Hearing Implants
MED-EL Corporation (North America)
2511 Old Cornwallis Rd., Suite 100
Durham, NC 27713
1 (888) MED-EL-CI (633-3524) Toll-free voice
(919) 572-2222 Voice
(919) 484-9229 Fax
Website: www.medel.com
e-mail: implants@medelus.com

CHAPTER nine

Auditory Habilitation for Young Children and Their Families

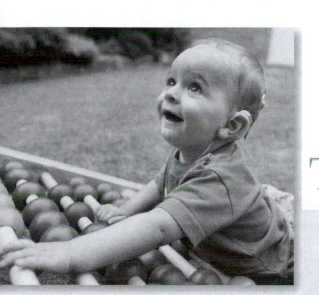

LEARNING *objectives*

After reading this chapter, you should be able to:

1. Define early hearing detection and intervention (EHDI) programs and discuss their history.

2. Describe key position statements regarding EHDI programs.

3. Compare and contrast sensorineural hearing loss and auditory neuropathy-dyssynchrony (AN/AD).

4. Describe newborn hearing screening programs (NHSPs) and their effect on parents.

5. Understand parents' informational needs and preferences when their children are diagnosed with hearing loss.

6. Compare and contrast scenarios when a deaf baby is born in a Deaf family versus a hearing family. Define and describe the importance of the medical home in EHDI programs.

7. Trace Robbins's (2002) stages from diagnosis of hearing loss to the beginning of formal communication intervention, including important steps for auditory habilitation.

8. Compare and contrast communication modes and approaches for facilitating oral language development in deaf children.

9. Describe commonly used assessment tools for infants and toddlers who are deaf and hard of hearing.

10. Discuss evidence-based practice in selection of an auditory habilitation approach.

11. Describe the basics of special education law and procurement of services for 0- to 2-year-old children who are deaf and hard of hearing and their families.

12. Recognize the importance of identification, diagnosis, and intervention of dual sensory impairment in young children.

The phrase "Congratulations, it's a boy!" signals a time for celebration and joy in any family. Parents are excited and anticipate what the future will be for their child. Will he favor his mother, will he have his father's athletic ability, or will he be the life of the party like his grandpa? These are common questions that parents may ask. However, for parents of a child diagnosed as deaf or hard of hearing, the questions they ask may break your heart. Will my child ever hear me say "I love you," will he ever talk, or learn how to read? Moreover, every year about 3 in 1,000 children are born with permanent hearing loss.

Diagnosis of hearing loss in a child is a very emotional event for the family. As communication sciences and disorders professionals, we must learn how to assist parents in their journeys through the process of identification, diagnosis, and management of their children's hearing losses. We must understand how parents feel, what information they want, and how we can help them the most at different points of time in their journeys.

EARLY HEARING DETECTION AND INTERVENTION (EHDI) PROGRAMS

Technology has enabled children to be identified with hearing loss at birth or a few days after. Communication sciences and disorders personnel must be prepared to serve these infants with hearing loss and their families. We will first discuss the history of EHDI programs; changes in recommended guidelines; and then the continuum of screening, diagnosis, and management of hearing loss in young children.

History of EHDI Programs

Newborn hearing screening is the first step in EHDI programs and has had a long history leading to the development of program standards recommended today. Table 9.1 shows a timeline of significant events, though only a few of them will be discussed here (Centers for Disease Control and Prevention, 2009).

One of the earliest events was the submission of the Babbidge Report (Babbidge, 1965) to the U.S. Secretary of Health, Education, and Welfare that recommended the development and nationwide implementation of "universally applied procedures for early identification and evaluation of hearing impairment." The Babbidge Report focused on the shortcomings of the education received by deaf and hard of hearing students mostly in residential schools (Babbidge, 1965). Two years later, on recommendation from the National Conference on Education of the Deaf, a **high-risk register** approach to hearing screening was implemented across the country, which was to assess the hearing of infants who had at least one condition (e.g., hyperbilirubinemia, birth weight less than 1,500 grams, and so on) that placed them at risk for hearing loss (U.S. Department of Health Education and Welfare, 1967). However, in 1988, the Commission on Education for the Deaf reported that the average age of identification of children with profound sensorineural hearing loss was 2½ years (Commission on Education of the Deaf, 1988). Clearly, the hearing screening programs at that time were not identifying hearing loss early enough. Screening on the basis of those identified via the high-risk registry let too many children with hearing loss "fall through the cracks."

During this time, two significant developments occurred that would change the face of hearing screening programs. First, otoacoustic emission testing was introduced as a viable means of noninvasively screening hearing loss in newborn babies. Furthermore, in 1993, the National Institutes of Health (NIH) Consensus Statement on the Early Hearing Detection of Hearing Impairment in Infants and Young Children recommended that all newborns be screened for hearing loss before leaving the hospital. These events paved the way for the current guidelines mentioned in the Joint Committee on Infant Hearing (JCIH) Year 2000 Position Statement and by the Centers for Disease Control and Prevention in Atlanta, Georgia.

The Joint Committee on Infant Hearing (JCIH) supports early detection and intervention of infants with hearing loss through integrated, interdisciplinary state and national systems of EHDI programs, evaluation, and family-centered intervention (Joint Committee on Infant Hearing [JCIH], 2000). The JCIH Year 2000 Position Statement was based on the following eight principles (JCIH, 2000):

- All infants have access to hearing screening using a physiologic measure. Newborns who receive routine care have access to hearing screening during their hospital birth admission. Newborns in alternative birthing facilities, including home births, have access to and are referred for screening before 1 month of age. All newborns or infants who require neonatal intensive care receive hearing screening before discharge from the hospital. These components constitute universal newborn hearing screening (UNHS).
- All infants who do not pass the birth admission screening and any subsequent re-screening begin appropriate audiologic and medical evaluations to confirm the presence of hearing loss before 3 months of age.
- All infants with confirmed permanent hearing loss receive services before 6 months of age in interdisciplinary intervention programs that recognize and build on strengths, informed choices, traditions, and cultural beliefs of the family.

table *9.1*   Historic Moments in Newborn Hearing Screening

1965 – Babbidge Report (Report to the Secretary of Health, Education, and Welfare)

- Recommended the development and nationwide implementation of "universally applied procedures for early identification and evaluation of hearing impairment"

1967 – Recommendations From the National Conference on Education of the Deaf

- High-risk register to facilitate identification
- Public information campaign
- Testing of infants and children 5–12 months of age should be investigated

1988 – Commission on Education of the Deaf

- Reported the average age of identification for profoundly deaf children in the United States was 2½ years

1988 – An advisory group of national experts convened by the U.S. Department of Education and Bureau of Maternal and Child Health for the purpose of advising the government about the feasibility of developing guidelines on early identification

- Recommended that the federal government fund demonstration projects to expand and document systematically the cost efficiency of proven techniques already in existence but infrequently used

1988 – Former Surgeon General C. Everett Koop issued a challenge

- That by the year 2000, 90% of children with significant hearing loss be identified by 12 months of age

1990 – Joint Committee on Infant Hearing (JCIH) Position Statement

- Recommended that high-risk infants be screened prior to their discharge from the hospital and no later than 3 months after their birth

1990 – Healthy People 2000

- Goal: To reduce the average age at which children with significant hearing impairment are identified by no more than 12 months of age by year 2000

1993 – National Institutes of Health (NIH) Consensus Development Program

- Recommended that all newborns be screened for hearing loss before leaving the hospital

1994 – The JCIH Position Statement

- Recommended that all infants with hearing loss should be identified before 3 months of age and receive intervention by 6 months of age

1999 – The American Academy of Pediatrics endorses universal newborn hearing screening

- Detection of hearing loss before 3 months of age
- Intervention services initiated by 6 months of age

2000 – The JCIH Year 2000 Position Statement: Principles and Guidelines for EHDI Programs

2007 – The JCIH Year 2007 Position Statement: Principles and Guidelines for Early Hearing Detection and Intervention Programs

2008 – The U.S. Preventive Services Task Force Recommendation on Newborn Hearing Screening

- Provided a grade of B for the recommendation of the screening for hearing loss of all newborn babies

Source: Information from *Historical Moments in Newborn Hearing Screening,* by the Centers for Disease Control and Prevention, 2009, retrieved from http://www.cdc.gov/ncbddd/hearingloss/ehdi-history.html.

- All infants who pass newborn hearing screening but who have risk indicators for other auditory disorders and/or speech and language delay receive ongoing audiologic and medical surveillance and monitoring for communication development. Infants with indicators associated with late-onset, progressive, or fluctuating hearing loss as well as auditory neural conduction disorders and/or brainstem auditory pathway dysfunction should be monitored.
- Infant and family rights are guaranteed through informed choice, decision-making, and consent.
- Infant hearing screening and evaluation results are afforded the same protection as all other healthcare and educational information. As new standards for privacy and confidentiality are proposed, they must balance the needs of society and the rights of the infant and family, without compromising the ability of health and education to provide care (American Academy of Pediatrics, 1999).
- Information systems are used to measure and report the effectiveness of EHDI services. While state registries measure and track screening, evaluation, and intervention outcomes for infants and families, efforts should be made to honor a family's privacy by removing identifying information wherever possible. Aggregate state and national data may also be used to measure and track the impact of EHDI programs on public health and education while maintaining the confidentiality of the infant and family information.
- EHDI programs provide data to monitor quality, demonstrate compliance with legislation and regulations, determine fiscal accountability and cost effectiveness, support reimbursement for services, and mobilize and maintain community support.

The JCIH Year 2000 Position Statement developed benchmarks and quality indicators for screening, evaluation, and intervention phases of EHDI programming.

Using input from the JCIH, the American Academy of Pediatrics (AAP), in conjunction with the National Center on Birth Defects and Developmental Disabilities' EHDI Program at the Centers for Disease Control and Prevention (CDCP), cooperated to develop a mission and national goals. The mission of the CDCP EHDI is for every state and territory to have a complete EHDI tracking and surveillance system that ensures that children with hearing loss achieve communication and social skills commensurate with their cognitive abilities. Their national EHDI goals are as follows:

- Goal 1: All newborns will be screened for hearing loss before 1 month of age, preferably before hospital discharge.
- Goal 2: All infants who screen positive will have a diagnostic audiologic evaluation before 3 months of age.
- Goal 3: All infants identified with hearing loss will receive appropriate early intervention services before 6 months of age (medical, audiologic, and early intervention).
- Goal 4: All infants and children with late onset, progressive, or acquired hearing loss will be identified at the earliest possible time.
- Goal 5: All infants with hearing loss will have a medical home as defined by the American Academy of Pediatrics.

- Goal 6: Every state will have a complete EHDI Tracking and Surveillance System that will minimize loss to follow-up.
- Goal 7: Every state will have a comprehensive system that monitors and evaluates the progress toward the EHDI Goals and Objectives.

The principles and goals of the AAP, JCIH, and CDCP are ideals worthy of attaining, and thus far, progress has been steady. In November 1999, the World Council on Hearing Health (WCHH) reported on data finding that only 25% of newborns were screened for hearing loss that year. In contrast, in May 2004, the Annual Hearing Healthy Kids State Report Card on Infant Hearing Screening, released by the WCHH, the AAP, and the National Center for Hearing Assessment and Management (NCHAM), reported that the percentage of babies screened for hearing loss at birth had risen to 89.8%, an increase of 64.8% increase over 1999 statistics. Furthermore, the report found a wide variation of performance among states, with unsatisfactory screening rates for California and Ohio.

The JCIH updated its recommendations with the publishing of the Joint Committee on Infant Hearing Year 2007 Position Statement (JCIH, 2007). Although the same basic principles of the earlier document are upheld, the new position statement included critical updates to improve clinical outcomes and to keep pace with technological advancements. The major changes pertained to definition of targeted hearing loss, hearing screening/rescreening protocols, diagnostic audiologic evaluations, early intervention, and surveillance/screening in the medical home, communication, and information infrastructure. Specifics of these changes are discussed later in the chapter.

Additional improvements have been reported from data aggregated and analyzed by the CDCP in 2008. They reported that although about 92% of babies born received hearing screening by 1 month of age, there are still children lost to follow-up. Nearly 65% of those babies who did not pass have no documented diagnosis. Moreover, 87% of children diagnosed with hearing loss are referred for early intervention services through Part C of the **Individuals with Disabilities Education Improvement Act** (IDEIA), but only 53% received early intervention services. The IDEA is a federal law that ensures that all children with disabilities are entitled to a free and appropriate public education in the least restricted environment. Despite a significant proportion of babies lost to follow-up, the evidence is quite good regarding the overall effectiveness of EHDI programs as summarized in the following section.

What Does the Evidence Show?

The **Agency for Healthcare Research and Quality** (AHRQ), part of the Department of Health and Human Services, is concerned with health services research and supports research to improve the quality, safety, efficiency, and effectiveness of healthcare (AHRQ, 2010). The AHRQ **United States Preventive Services Task Force** (USPSTF) analyzes scientific evidence and then grades the clinical recommendations regarding health practices. Recall that in Chapter 5 on evidence-based practice, we discussed the process of grading clinical recommendations. In 2001, the USPSTF deemed that there was insufficient evidence for either recommending or refuting universal newborn hearing screening. However, Nelson, Bougatsos, Nygren, and the USPSTF (2008), conducted a systematic review to update the latest evidence supporting newborn hearing screening. Their systematic review asked three key questions:

1. "Among infants identified by universal screening who would not be identified by targeted screening, does initiating treatment by 6 months of age improve language and communication outcomes?"
2. "Compared with targeted screening, does universal screening increase the chance that treatment will be initiated by 6 months of age for infants at average risk or those at high risk?"
3. "What are the adverse effects of screening and early treatment?"

Nelson et al. (2008) conducted a thorough literature search using the following databases: Cochrane Central Register of Controlled Clinical Trials, Cochrane Database of Systematic Reviews, Database of Abstracts of Reviews of Effects, and Ovid Medline in addition to reference lists of reviews, studies, editorials, reports, websites, and so on. Overall, two studies were included for question 1, seven studies for question 2, and 11 studies for question 3. The studies included for questions 1 and 2 were controlled trials and observational studies and those for question 3 were descriptive and comparative studies. All studies underwent quality assessment using criteria appropriate for specifics designs. Nelson et al. concluded that children with hearing loss who were initially identified through newborn hearing screening had better receptive language outcomes at 8 years of age than their peers who did not participate in these programs. However, they did not have better expressive language or speech (Kennedy et al., 2006). Moreover, these children had earlier identification, diagnoses, and referral than infants who did not participate in newborn hearing screening (Kennedy, McCann, Campbell, Kimm, & Thorton, 2005; Wessex Universal Neonatal Screening Trial Group, 1998). Furthermore, the evidence showed little or no adverse effects of screening and treatment of sensorineural hearing loss in children. After consideration of new evidence, they assigned a grade of B to the recommendation to screen for hearing loss in all newborns. Table 9.2 shows the *Clinical Summary of the U.S. Preventive Services Task Force Recommendation.*

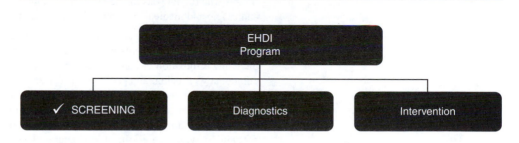

Screening for Hearing Loss

We will now discuss current recommendations for screening and parents' reactions to newborn hearing screening programs (NHSPs).

Current Recommendations for Screening

The purpose of newborn hearing screening programs (NHSPs) is to identify hearing loss at or a few days after birth so that intervention may begin (JCIH, 2000, 2007). The JCIH Year 2000 Position Statement definition of hearing loss was congenital biliateral, unilateral **sensory**

table *9.2* Clinical Summary of the U.S. Preventive Services Task Force Recommendation on Newborn Hearing Screening

Population	All Newborns
Recommendation	Screen for hearing loss in all newborn infants Grade: B
Risk Assessment	The prevalence of hearing loss in newborn infants with specific risk indicators is 10 to 20 times higher than in the general population of newborns. Risk indicators associated with permanent bilateral congenital hearing loss include: • Neonatal intensive care unit admission for two or more days • Family history of hereditary childhood sensorineural hearing loss • Craniofacial abnormalities • Certain congenital syndromes and infections Approximately 50% of newborns with permanent bilateral congenital hearing loss do not have any known risk indicators.
Screening Tests	Screening programs should be conducted using a one-step or two-step validated protocol. A frequently used two-step screening process involves otoacoustic emissions followed by auditory brainstem response in newborns who fail the first test. Infants with positive screening tests should receive appropriate audiologic evaluation and follow-up after discharge. Procedures for screening and follow-up should be in place for newborns delivered at home, birthing centers, or hospitals without hearing screening facilities.
Timing of Screening	All infants should have hearing screening before 1 month of age. Infants who do not pass the newborn screening should undergo audiologic and medical evaluation before 3 months of age.
Treatment	Early intervention services for infants with hearing impairments should meet the individualized needs of the infant and family, including acquisition of communication competence, social skills, emotional well-being, and positive self-esteem. Early intervention comprises evaluation for amplification or sensory devices, surgical and medical evaluation, and communication assessment and therapy. Cochlear implants are usually considered for children with severe-to-profound hearing loss only after inadequate response to hearing aids.

Source: From *Universal Screening for Hearing Loss in Newborns: Clinical Summary of U.S. Preventive Services Task Force Recommendation*, by the U.S. Preventive Services Task Force, AHRQ Publication No. 08-05117-EF-3, July 2008, Rockville, MD: Agency for Healthcare Research and Quality, retrieved from http://www.ahrq.gov/clinic/uspstf08/newbornhear/newbhearsum.htm. Used with permission.

table *9.3* Differences Between Children With Sensory Hearing Loss
and Auditory Neuropathy/Dyssynchrony

	Sensory Hearing Loss	Auditory Neuropathy/ Dyssynchrony
Site of Lesion	Inner and outer hair cells	Cranial nerve VIII
Pure-Tone Audiometry	Variable thresholds from slight to profound	
Otoacoustic Emissions	Absent if loss of thresholds are 30 dB HL or greater	Present
Speech Recognition Scores	Match expectations based on audiometric results	Do not match expectations based on audiometric results
Success With Hearing Aids	Consistent with degree of loss	Variable

hearing loss, or **permanent conductive hearing loss.** Recall that sensory hearing loss results from damage to the inner and outer hair cells. Permanent conductive hearing loss results from problems in the outer or middle ear that may not be completely ameliorated through medical management (e.g., congenital aural atresia). The new position statement has expanded the definition of targeted hearing loss to include **neural hearing loss**, also known as **auditory neuropathy/dyssynchrony (AN/AD)**, which is dysfunction of cranial nerve VIII that impedes the transmission of neural impulses generated in the periphery to the central auditory nervous system. In addition, there may be more than one specific site of lesion for AN/AD.

Approximately 10% of children diagnosed with hearing loss have AN/AD. Table 9.3 shows some fundamental differences between children with sensory hearing loss and AN/AD. The site of lesion for sensory hearing loss is the inner and outer hair cells; the typical site of lesion for AN/AD is cranial nerve VIII. Both sensory and neural hearing losses show air- and bone-conduction thresholds out of the range of normal with no significant air-bone gaps. However, results for **otoacoustic emissions testing** are normal for patients with neural hearing loss and absent for those with sensory hearing losses greater than about 30 dB HL. Otoacoustic emissions testing, a noninvasive assessment of outer hair cell integrity, involves presenting stimuli into the ear canal (acoustic energy) that travel through the middle ear (mechanical energy), and into the inner ear (bioelectric energy) to which the outer hair cells emit a response that travels in the reverse direction and is measured in the ear canal. There are two types of otoacoustic emission testing: (1) **distortion product otoacoustic emissions (DPOAEs)** and (2) **transient evoked otoacoustic emissions (TEOAEs)**. DPOAE testing delivers two tones (f_1 and f_2) via a probe and measures the emissions from sensory cells in the form of a distortion product ($2f_1 - f_2$). TEOAE testing delivers click stimulus via a probe and measures the emissions from sensory cells. Speech recognition scores for patients with neural hearing loss do not match the degree of hearing loss found on the

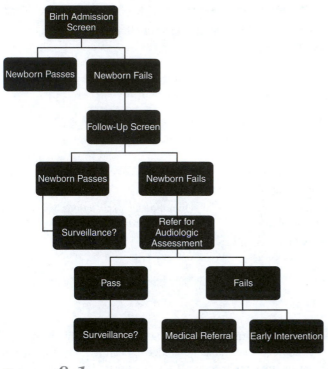

figure *9.1*

The newborn hearing screening process.

Source: Based on "The Role of the Pediatrician in Hearing Loss: From Detection to Connection," by T. Finitzo and W. Crumley, 1999, *Pediatric Clinics in North America, 46*, pp. 15–34.

audiogram. Typically, their speech recognition scores are lower than those for patients with the same degree of sensory hearing loss. Moreover, patients with neural hearing losses have variable and often poorer performance with hearing aids than their peers with the same degree of sensory hearing loss. Young children with AN/AD who do not do well with hearing aids may be suitable candidates for and may do well with cochlear implants (e.g., Shallop, Peterson, Facer, Fabry, & Driscoll, 2001). However, some may not do well with either. Teagle and colleagues (2010) are developing a stepwise management procedure using preimplant magnetic resonance imaging studies and electrophysiologic measures that are fairly accurate in determining which children with AN/AD will be successful with cochlear implants. Management of neural hearing loss is discussed more in Chapter 10.

The EHDI process is shown in Figure 9.1. The process begins before the baby is discharged from the hospital. The JCIH Year 2007 Position Statement recommended separate protocols for babies in the **neonatal intensive care unit (NICU)** versus **well-baby nurseries**. The NICU is where the most fragile and sickest babies go after birth, including but not limited to those who are premature, have multiple birth defects, or have severe medical issues (e.g., heart, lung, gastrointestinal, or other life-threatening conditions). The well-baby nursery is for babies who do not need any specialized services. The prevalence of hearing loss in the well-baby nursery is 1 per 1,000 births. However, for the NICU, the prevalence is 1 in 100 births or 10 times more common than in the well-baby nursery. It is recommended that any baby admitted to the NICU for more than five days is to receive an auditory brainstem response (ABR) test as part of the newborn hearing screening to increase the likelihood of identifying those neonates with neural hearing loss. Babies who do not pass their ABR test should be referred to an experienced pediatric audiologist for a complete diagnostic evaluation. Frequently, babies who do not pass their initial screening are tested closer to hospital discharge. Often, newborns do not pass for a variety of reasons, such as the presence of cerumen or **vernix caseosa** in one or both external auditory canals. Vernix caseosa is a fatty lipid material that is left over from the amniotic fluid on the baby's skin that can be present in the ear canal and may interfere with newborn hearing screening. Surprisingly, the chemical composition of vernix caseosa from preterm infants is different from that of full-term infants. The JCIH Year 2007 Position Statement recommended that both ears should be rescreened even if only one ear failed. Further, it is recommended that any babies with high-risk factors for hearing loss who are readmitted to the hospital within the first month of life be rescreened. For babies born in alternative facilities (e.g., at home), the initial screening should occur by 1 month of age. If the baby passes, he or she is excused from further testing. However, if the baby does not pass, then an appointment is made for an audiologic evaluation between 1 and 3 months of age. NHSPs are of little value if parents do not follow through with recommendations and follow-up appointments.

Parents' Reactions to NHSPs

Parents play a critical role in successful follow-up after screening referral. Parents' initial encounters with EHDI programs can set the tone for success or failure in auditory habilitation. Several studies have focused on the possible negative effects of NHSPs on parents. Concerns have been expressed that NHSPs may induce anxiety in and raise the stress levels of new parents, possibly affecting the bonding process with their babies. Over the past 15 years, several studies have investigated parents' reactions to NHSPs. Barringer, Mauk, Jensen, and Woods-Kershner (1997) disseminated a 10-question survey of parents' perceptions of NHSPs using evoked otoacoustic emissions (EOAE) via obstetric nurses at Logan Regional Hospital in Logan, Utah. They found that parents had essentially positive attitudes toward NHSPs. Stuart, Moretz, and Yang (2000) investigated whether there was a significant difference in the stress levels between mothers whose infants failed newborn hearing screening versus mothers whose infants passed. They found that both groups of mothers had equivalent stress levels. Similarly, Weichbold and Welzl-Mueller (2001) found no significant degree of concern between mothers whose babies did not pass the first screening and those who failed the second screening. However, Magnuson and Hergils (1999) found that parents whose infants passed either the first or second time were positive about NHSPs and not anxious. Parents whose infants failed the second screening (i.e., failed two screenings) were more ambivalent to NHSP than the other parents and had a greater degree of anxiety, suggesting that support and counseling may be beneficial at this time. However, these parents' anxiety diminished once they received the results of the audiologic evaluation, whether positive or negative. Results from a more recent study found that parental anxiety increases as the number of tests increases (Crockett, Wright, Uus, Bamford, & Marteau, 2006). Therefore, audiologists should be particularly sensitive to the needs of parents whose infants have failed two screenings and schedule the audiologic evaluation as soon as possible to reduce anxiety.

Weichbold, Welzl-Mueller, and Mussbacher (2001) in a retrospective cohort study found that mothers who were supportive of NHSPs were more likely to be well-informed about the process and know the results of the hearing assessment. Therefore, educating parents increases the likelihood that they will be advocates of NHSPs and will follow through with audiologic evaluation and recommendations for intervention. Parent education should include information about the purpose and mechanics of NHSP, but also the detrimental effects of all types of hearing loss. Parents' knowledge of and attitudes toward NHSPs may impact their adherence to recommendations provided by audiologists and other healthcare providers.

The National Institute on Deafness and other Communication Disorders of the National Institutes of Health (NIDCD) recommends five steps for improving parents' adherence to follow-up. First, audiologists need to ensure a clear presentation of information to parents. Babies are born 24 hours a day, seven days a week, and NHSPs operate on the same schedule. Therefore, NHSP managers must ensure that someone is available to explain accurate results, stress the importance of follow-up, and emphasize the deleterious effects of hearing loss using culturally sensitive materials as part of a consistent protocol. Second, audiologists should develop a "fail-safe" system for scheduling follow-up appointments, obtain families' contact information, connect with a child's primary care physician, ensure that office staff and nurse have a lead role in scheduling, and seek broad-based support from hospitals to keep all stakeholders "on-board." Third, audiologists should develop a strong alliance with nurses and adopt a commitment to training, elicit their feedback and suggestions, and retrain as often as necessary. Fourth, audiologists should minimize the number of return appointments by ensuring that a follow-up examination can be completed prior to discharge from the hospital or during the well-baby check-up. Fifth, audiologists need to empower parents in their participation in EHDI programs through their involvement in screening, provision of information for decision-making, and use of a family-centered approach. Improving follow-up rates ensures the early diagnosis for hearing loss.

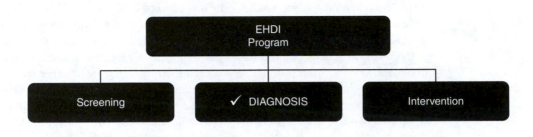

Diagnosis of Hearing Loss

We will now discuss current recommendations for and parents' reactions to diagnosis of hearing loss in young children.

Current Recommendations for Diagnosis of Hearing Loss

The JCIH Year 2007 Position Statement states that children should have hearing loss diagnosed by 3 months of age by audiologists who have experience in evaluating newborns and young children. Moreover, the JCIH Year 2007 Position Statement recommends that an ABR be conducted to confirm diagnosis of a sensory or neural hearing loss for children 3 years of age and younger. If the baby is found to have normal hearing, he or she is excused from further testing except for those who have high-risk factors who will be monitored periodically. The JCIH Year 2007 Position Statement recommends that the scheduling and frequency of hearing reevaluations be individualized and based on the likelihood of the child developing a delayed-onset hearing loss. At minimum, however, babies who have at least one high-risk factor should have a hearing reevaluation by the time they are 2 to 2½ years of age. Further, it is recommended that earlier and more aggressive evaluations should occur for babies with one or more of the following high-risk conditions:

- ECMO or chemotherapy
- Cytomegalovirus infection
- Syndromes that have progressive hearing loss
- Neurodegenerative disorders
- Trauma
- Postnatal infections associated with sensorineural hearing loss
- Caregiver concern
- Family history of hearing loss

Two terms on the previous bulleted list may be unfamiliar to readers. The first is the acronym **ECMO**, which stands for **extra corporeal membrane oxygenation**, a procedure in which a machine outside of the body delivers oxygen to a patient's blood much like the heart and lungs are supposed to do. Infants who undergo ECMO are typically those babies in NICUs who have health conditions that preclude proper functioning of the heart and/or lungs. The second term, **cytomegalovirus**, describes a member of the herpes virus family, one of the most common congenital infections and a leading cause of hearing loss present at birth. Diagnosis of hearing loss should trigger referrals to other healthcare professionals.

Babies who are found to have hearing loss are referred for medical management, and results of the screening and diagnostic evaluation are sent to the child's pediatrician or family physician. If the hearing loss is conductive, the physician may refer the child to an otolaryngologist and/or otologist for medical management. However, if the hearing loss is sensorineural, the JCIH Year 2007 Position Statement recommends that the infant be evaluated by an otolaryngologist who has an expertise in dealing with children with hearing loss. Furthermore, the JCIH Year 2007 Position Statement recommends that the infant and his or her family should be referred for a **genetics consultation** and to a pediatric ophthalmologist for a **visual acuity examination**. A genetics consultation is valuable because hearing loss may run in families who need to know the chances of having other children with the same condition. Moreover, a visual acuity examination is important because children with hearing loss may also have visual problems.

A genetic consultation is an appointment with a qualified healthcare professional (e.g., clinical geneticist, genetics counselors, or clinical molecular geneticist) that includes genetic testing and counseling. The purpose of the consultation is to provide information to the family regarding the types of hearing loss that may be hereditary by analyzing the case history information (e.g., family, pregnancy, birth, and early developmental). Laboratory testing often confirms existence of specific hereditary hearing losses, assisting in planning for appropriate treatment and estimating the chances of impairment in future offspring. Over 500 centers across the country offer these services. More than half of all cases of congenital or early-onset deafness are genetic in origin; the remaining proportion is due to nongenetic factors (Burton, Pandya, & Arnos, 2006). Approximately 25% of congenital genetic hearing losses are syndromic and 75% are nonsyndromic. **Syndromic** hearing loss occurs with other signs and sympotms; **nonsyndromic** hearing loss is that which usually occurs as the only disability. Approximately 20% of nonsyndromic hearing losses are autosomal dominant disorders, 74% are autosomal recessive disorders, 5% are **x-linked disorders**, and 1% are **mitochondrial disorders** (Kemperman, Hoefsloot, & Cremers, 2002). The discussion of x-linked and mitochondrial disorders is beyond the scope of this textbook; readers are referred to Robin (2008) for further information.

Briefly, we are born with 23 pairs of chromosomes, 22 pairs of autosomes, and 1 pair of sex chromosomes. Chromosomes are big pieces of genetic information. Chromosomal abnormalities occur when there is either too much or too little genetic information, or material that is in the wrong place. Located on the chromosomes are tinier pieces of genetic information known as genes. Burton et al. (2006) stated that each human has about 30,000 genes, of which an estimated 10% have some role in determining both the structure and function of the ear. Genetic abnormalities, also known as **mutations**, are a little more subtle than chromosomal abnormalities and may be classified based upon whether they are located on an autosome or sex chromosome. Besides location on a particular chromosome, genetic disorders may be classified by inheritance pattern. **Dominant transmission** requires only one gene for the trait to be passed on; **recessive transmission** requires that two copies of a gene are needed for a trait to be passed on. **Autosomal dominant disorders** have an inheritance pattern in which one parent has the genetic mutation, expresses the disorder, and has a 50% chance of passing it on to his or her children. When a person has a trait in his or her genes, it is called a **genotype**. However, when the person actually presents the trait, that is referred to as a **phenotype**. Autosomal dominant hearing loss often is not a mystery to families. Generally, they know that hearing loss "runs in the family." Another characteristic of autosomal dominant disorders is that they have a **variation in expressivity**, meaning that the disability may present in a mild or severe form. Therefore, the degree of autosomal dominant hearing loss may range from mild to profound. When these disorders present in their mildest forms, it is known as **decreased penetrance**. **Autosomal recessive disorders** occur when both parents are carriers of the genetic mutation, but usually do not express it and have a 25% chance of having a child with the disorder, 50% chance that their child will be a carrier, and 25% chance that their child will be normal. Because both parents are carriers of the mutation but do not express it, autosomal recessive hearing loss is more of a surprise to parents. The most common nonsyndromic cause of genetic hearing loss is a mutation on the connexin 26 gene (GJB2), which is inherited most often in the autosomal recessive mode. Mutations generally result in variable degrees of impairment and rates of progression, although most present with congenital profound sensorineural hearing loss (Burton et al., 2006). Genetic testing and counseling has an important niche in early intervention for families with young children with hearing loss.

The referral to a pediatric ophthalmologist for visual acuity screening is recommended for children diagnosed with hearing loss because of the existence of several hereditary causes of **dual sensory impairment**, which means simultaneous ocular and auditory impairment. One hereditary cause of dual sensory impairment is **Usher syndrome** (Boughman, Vernon, & Shaver, 1983). Usher syndrome is a recessively transmitted genetic condition that includes congenital hearing loss and a progressive loss of vision that become noticeable in the late teens and early 20s (Northern & Downs, 2002). There are at least three different types of Usher syndrome, and visual acuity screening of infants with hearing loss may not be adequate because of the delayed onset of ocular problems in some cases. Early identification of dual sensory impairment in infants assists in planning early intervention efforts and is discussed later in the chapter.

Parents' Reactions to Diagnosis of Hearing Loss

English, Kooper, and Bratt (2004) stated that the development of EHDI programs has moved audiology from a **parent-initiated model** to a **surprise model** of diagnosis (i.e., baby referred for a diagnostic evaluation from an NHSP). Before NHSPs, parents would often have to take the initiative of scheduling an appointment with their pediatrician if they had concerns about their child's hearing. Unfortunately, manifestations of hearing loss may not have been obvious to parents or they may have been reassured by pediatricians that any concerns regarding their child's hearing were unfounded, often delaying diagnosis until 18 months of age or later. Even today, many parents are oblivious to the fact that their child has even had a newborn hearing screening and are surprised when he or she does not pass the screening and is diagnosed with a hearing loss.

Diagnosis of Hearing Loss in a Child Born to Hearing Parents. Diagnosis of hearing loss is often a devastating and life-altering event for parents; many report that life is never the same afterward. For generations, physicians have had to give difficult diagnoses, prognoses, and have even conducted research on how best to deliver bad news to patients and their families. They have found that an insensitive approach to delivering bad news may immobilize patients and their families, affecting their ability to adapt and cope with life (Fallowfield & Jenkins, 2004). Some audiologists have wondered about the best way to deliver the news of a diagnosis of hearing loss in children to parents. Within the field of audiology, English et al. (2004) used a consensus approach and asked parents of children with hearing loss how audiologists might "break the bad news." Parents believed that the audiologist who breaks the news to the parents should either be the one who conducted the audiologic evaluation and/or will manage the auditory habilitation. Second, audiologists should plan enough time for counseling and ensure that there is privacy and no interruptions from colleagues, office staff, cell phones, or pagers. Ideally, the consultation should be conducted in a quiet room with the door closed with no physical barriers (e.g., desks, tables, other chairs, and so on) between audiologist and parents. The audiologist should begin by saying, "I'm afraid I have some difficult news," avoiding detailed explanations of test procedures.

Third, audiologists should assess parents' understanding of the situation and, after a simply stated diagnosis, should say, "I have a lot of information I will need to share with you eventually, but for now, what questions or concerns do you have?" (English et al., 2004). It was suggested that audiologists follow the parents' lead by not providing any more information than that which is specifically asked for. The rationale for this approach is that parents are in a state of shock and will not retain much of the information provided at this time (Robbins, 2002).

Fourth, audiologists should encourage parents to express their feelings (English et al., 2004). Parents react in a wide variety of ways to the news that their children have hearing losses. Some parents may cry uncontrollably; some parents may show no emotion whatsoever. Audiologists should say, "This may take a while to sink in, and when it does, it could be very upsetting. I hope you will keep talking to me about it" (English et al., 2004). Above all, parents should get their feelings out in the open to reduce the likelihood of the development of maladaptive behaviors, such as nonadherence to hearing healthcare professionals' recommendations and denial. Nonadherent behaviors may include failing to keep follow-up appointments; denial of children's hearing losses may manifest in parents' discounting the validity of audiologic test results. **Maladaptive behaviors** are those actions that interfere or sabotage the auditory (re)habilitation process.

Fifth, audiologists should respond with warmth and empathy, accepting parents' reactions with **unconditional positive regard**, and believing that they can manage their own lives (Clark & English, 2003; English et al., 2004). Recall from Chapter 2 that unconditional positive regard is accepting patients and their reactions to diagnosis of hearing loss, "warts and all." Audiologists may be uncomfortable with parents who show deep sadness, but should resist the temptation to trivialize the situation by saying something like, "Well at least it isn't cancer," in an attempt to rescue families from their feelings (English et al., 2004). However, parents may use this strategy as a defense mechanism against facing the reality of the situation, possibly impeding taking the necessary steps toward habilitation of their child's hearing loss (English et al.).

Sixth, audiologists should provide a reasonable time frame for parents to make important decisions, being careful not to push, though, until they are ready (English et al., 2004). Instead, audiologists may gently suggest that parents *start* thinking about when they would like to begin fitting amplification on their child (English et al., 2004). Parents differ in their readiness to begin the process. For example, some parents may want to begin immediately by having the audiologist make earmold impressions. Alternatively, some parents may desire to wait a few days before scheduling a follow-up appointment. Moreover, audiologists may provide contact information of other parents of children with hearing loss at this time. Some parents may prefer to talk to peers who have gone through diagnosis of hearing loss in their children. Parent-to-parent support is powerful and may instill confidence in those just beginning their journeys, knowing that others have gone through this process, survived, and have positive outcomes for their children. Audiologists may also ask if parents would like their pediatrician or family physician notified of the results of the hearing evaluation. Parents gain confidence when allowed to make some decisions early on in the process.

Seventh, audiologists should provide parents with specific objectives to accomplish while waiting for follow-up appointments (English et al., 2004). Some parents may want direction from audiologists in getting started even before the follow-up appointment. Some of the activities may include providing parents with written materials to read and appropriate videotapes to view on hearing loss, explaining their child's hearing loss in relation to the **Familiar Sounds on the Audiogram Chart** (Northern & Downs, 2002; see Chapter 1), or asking them to pick three sounds in their home environment that they want their child to hear (English et al., 2004). English et al. (2004) suggested providing parents with a notebook to record their child's behavior in answering the following questions: What soothes or delights your baby? How does your child tell you that he or she is sleepy? What is your child's body language while he or she watches your face? Parents should also write down any questions they have, which may reduce their anxiety while waiting for follow-up appointments.

Eighth, audiologists should schedule a follow-up appointment and provide contact information if the parents should have questions before that time (English et al., 2004). It is not unusual for audiologists to give parents their cell phone numbers should they have additional questions or just want to talk (English et al., 2004).

Ninth, at the follow-up appointment, audiologists should begin auditory habilitation by reviewing and expanding on information during the initial counseling session. Parents are now more able to be presented with details about the audiologic evaluation and in-depth explanations of the auditory habilitation process. Audiologists may want to use some of Margolis's (2004) informational counseling tips discussed in Chapter 2.

Tenth, audiologists should document the information provided to parents at specific points in time in addition to any counseling. Audiologists may start off on the right foot with parents by following suggestions for "breaking the news" to parents based on a consensus of those parents who have been there.

OK now, let's see if you can find things that may be improved in the following scenario. As you recall from Chapter 2, Leon and Debbie Washington felt a little uneasy about Joshua failing his birth admission hearing screening. The Washingtons made a follow-up appointment in the audiology department of the hospital for a rescreen and auditory brainstem response. Debbie arrived at a busy waiting room with Joshua in his car seat while Leon went to park the car. They were called back for the rescreen, which Joshua did not pass. Debbie watched Dr. Trenoth's face during the test that she did over and over again with the same results. She then said that she would perform an auditory brainstem response test that would be helpful in diagnosing a hearing loss. Joshua was fast asleep and the test was completed without incident. Debbie could tell that the results of the ABR were not good.

Let's look at several different ways the audiologist might have proceeded with the news she had to deliver to the Washingtons.

Casebook Reflection

What's Wrong With This Picture?

Dr. Trenoth had a concerned look on her face while she removed the electrodes from Joshua's head. She looked at her watch and was running behind schedule. She had two more patients scheduled before lunch. Dr. Green had just had a cancellation and was available to counsel the Washingtons on the results of the ABR.

"Mrs. Washington, I'm going to ask the receptionist to call your husband back into Dr. Green's office so that he can explain the results of the test," said Dr. Trenoth in a hurried voice. "Please, Mrs. Washington, have a seat, and it was a pleasure to meet you. Dr. Green will be with you shortly."

Leon was escorted to Dr. Green's office and sat next to his wife. He could tell that his wife was very upset because she had tears in her eyes. Before they could speak, Dr. Green entered the office and took a seat behind his enormous desk.

"Hello, I am Dr. Green and have reviewed the results of your son's ABR," he said, reaching across the desk to shake hands with Leon. All of a sudden, a loud beeping sound could be heard from Dr. Green's pager. Instinctively, he looked at it and then shut it off. "Oh, excuse me. . . ."

"Let me first explain what has been done thus far. As you recall, Joshua did not pass his in-patient hearing screening using transient otoacoustic emissions in which a probe is placed into his ear canal that presented a click sound that went through the middle ear into the inner ear, and. . . . What's the matter, Mrs. Washington?" asked Dr. Green, noticing tears in Debbie's eyes.

Can you understand why Mrs. Washington was so upset? Yes, that's right! First, Mrs. Washington puts her trust into Dr. Trenoth, who completed the ABR test, but then Debbie was passed along to Dr. Green because of scheduling difficulties. It must have been especially torturous to see the concerned look on Dr. Trenoth's face during the ABR and have no explanation of what was going on. Second, the Washingtons felt insignificant and powerless when seated on the other side of the doctor's desk. Third, the Washingtons were offended when Dr. Green looked at his pager during a very difficult moment for them. Fourth, Dr. Green's detailed explanation of transient-evoked otoacoustic emissions was the last thing Mrs. Washington wanted to hear. Let's go back in time and do this the right way!

Casebook Reflection

What's Right With This Picture?

At the end of the ABR, Dr. Trenoth seated Mrs. Washington and her sleeping son in the counseling room, which was comfortable and looked like a typical living room.

"Mrs. Washington, I'll go into the waiting room to get your husband," Dr. Trenoth said. On the way to the waiting room she told the receptionist, "I'll be in the counseling room with the Washingtons. Please, no interruptions. . . . Please ask Dr. Green to see my 10:00 appointment for me. I'll explain later."

"Mr. Washington, hello, my name is Dr. Trenoth," she said, shaking Leon's hand. "Please come this way and I'll explain the results of this morning's test. Have a seat next to your wife."

"I'm afraid I have some difficult news," said Dr. Trenoth, sitting down next to the Washingtons. "I'm afraid that Joshua has a severe to profound sensorineural hearing loss, bilaterally. I have a lot of information I will eventually need to share with you, but what questions or concerns do you have at this time?"

Debbie couldn't believe what she had just heard. She felt numb, in a state of shock. All she could do was look down at the floor. She wanted to say something, but the words weren't coming out.

Leon, on the other hand, was quick to ask a question. "Is there some type of treatment that can correct the problem?"

"No, Mr. Washington, there is not," explained Dr. Trenoth. "The hearing loss is permanent, affecting the inner ear."

"Do you mean my son is deaf and will have to use sign language?" asked Leon.

"No, not necessarily. Through the use of hearing aids and early intervention, Joshua can most likely use the hearing he has left to learn speech and language, but he most likely will need special services in the schools. I'd like to say that diagnosing Joshua's hearing loss at such an early age puts us at an advantage. It wasn't long ago that children were most often diagnosed with hearing loss at 2 to 3 years of age or even older."

Leon just rubbed his chin and Debbie was still looking down; both were emotionless. Dr. Trenoth knew that parents vary in their response to news that their child has a hearing loss. She was careful not to judge parents on the basis of their initial reactions. She gently placed a box of tissues on the table.

"Thank you," said Debbie, looking at Dr. Trenoth and wiping the tears from her eyes.

"When you're ready, I'd like for you to talk with me about how you feel," requested Dr. Trenoth. "If you don't want to talk to me, talk to each other. It is important to express your feelings. The most important thing is that I don't want to rush you into making any decisions, but I do want you to think about when you'd like to start the hearing aid selection, evaluation, and fitting process. We can start today by making ear impressions for the earmold, or the part that will connect Joshua's ears to his hearing aids."

"Dr. Trenoth, I think we need to wait a week or so. We're very tired and overwhelmed right now," admitted Debbie.

"I can understand that," said Dr. Trenoth. "Would you like to talk to some other parents who have children with hearing loss?"

"I think in time. Right now, I think that we will make an appointment next week," Leon said. "Thank you, Dr. Trenoth."

"Thank you," said Dr. Trenoth, shaking Leon's hand.

"Dr. Trenoth, is there anything that we might do before we see you again?" asked Debbie, surprising her husband.

"Yes, there is. I have a videotape that you can watch about hearing loss and hearing aids. I also would like for you to write down three sounds in your home that you would like Joshua to hear. I would also like you to keep a diary of Joshua's behavior. What soothes or makes Joshua happy? How does he tell you he's hungry or tired?" suggested Dr. Trenoth. "These worksheets tell you exactly what to do. Also, write down questions as you think of them to bring with you next time. Let's go to the receptionist and make a follow-up appointment. Also, here is a card with my home phone number in case you have any questions *before* then."

"Thanks again, Dr. Trenoth," Debbie said as she went out the door.

Outcomes for parents may seem more attainable to them when audiologists thoughtfully approach the diagnosis of hearing loss in their children. Breaking the news to parents in a sensitive manner may minimize the trauma they may experience, paving the way for timely intervention. As stated earlier, audiologists should not expect any particularly stereotypical responses from parents resulting from a diagnosis of hearing loss in their children. In fact, parents who are Deaf are happy when they find out that their children have a hearing loss.

Diagnosis of Hearing Loss in a Child of Deaf Parents. Communication sciences and disorders professionals need to consider cultural differences in families' responses to a diagnosis of hearing loss. The most obvious difference is the reaction to diagnosis of hearing loss in a child of deaf parents. The following Casebook Reflection describes how the birth of a deaf child is viewed by Deaf parents.

Casebook Reflection

The Birth of a Deaf Baby to Deaf Parents

The reactions of Deaf parents on learning that their child is Deaf are as diverse as the parents themselves. In general, however, many members of the DEAF-WORLD would prefer having a Deaf child to having a hearing child, and those whose happiness at the advent of a Deaf child is tinged with sadness (after all, that child will face many extra challenges) commonly overcome their reservations quickly. If you belong to a hearing culture, you may find such Deaf preferences hard to understand; yet all cultures have preferences about children: some prefer male babies, others fair-skinned or dark-skinned babies. Of course, Deaf parents' preference for Deaf children does not mean that they love their hearing children less, only that the birth of a Deaf baby in a Deaf household signifies that the Deaf heritage of the family will be secure. Deaf families with many Deaf members are commonly proud of their genealogy.

In other words, when a Deaf infant of Deaf parents is diagnosed as Deaf, the joy of the parents reflects the fact that most Deaf parents, like parents generally, look forward to having children who are a reflection of themselves. . . . Deaf parents bring their Deaf baby home to a nurturing environment in which communication is naturally dependent on visual, not auditory, cues. Almost all use the signed language of the DEAF-WORLD (American Sign Language in the U.S. and most of Canada) to interact with their child. Their home is already functioning as an environment conducive to using vision as the main means of learning and development. The house is wired to respond to environmental signals with visual ones. For example, doorbells and telephones don't ring. Instead, they flash lights, each with its own pattern. Deaf parents usually have a TTY so they can communicate over the telephone.

Like the hearing child born to a well-functioning hearing family, the Deaf infant in a Deaf family . . . is immediately exposed to a world suited to maximizing his or her social, emotional, psychological, cognitive, and linguistic development. Social development is assured through exposure to adults who function normally as models for the child. Emotional development is encouraged by the positive responses of the family to its new member. Psychologically, Deaf parents treat their Deaf child as an extension of themselves. Cognitively, parental expectations are high: with proper nurturing, there are no Deaf-dependent limits on intellectual development. Finally, and most importantly . . . the child will enjoy a full command of language through exposure to ASL, allowing him or her to grasp the idea of communication, its purpose, and its form.

Source: Reprinted with permission from Lane, H., Hoffmeister, R., & Bahan, B. (1996) *A Journey Into the Deaf-World,* San Diego, CA; DawnSignPress.

Lane et al. (1996) stated that being deaf is viewed negatively in the hearing society resulting in complicated interactions between hearing healthcare professionals and deaf parents of a deaf newborn. Lane et al. (1996) advised that deaf parents do not respond well to two common recommendations provided by audiologists. First, audiologists sometimes recommend that deaf parents not use sign language with their hearing children because it may delay auditory speech and language development. Such recommendations may make deaf parents feel guilty, angry, and mistrustful. Second, audiologists recommend that deaf parents have hearing aids fit on their deaf babies with the rationale that some auditory experience and exposure to spoken language is better than nothing (Lane et al., 1996). Because sound has little meaning to deaf parents, they often ignore audiologists' recommendations and raise their deaf children in the Deaf world.

Communication sciences and disorders professionals should respect the views and beliefs of other cultures, including the Deaf culture. Audiologists' efforts may be viewed negatively by the Deaf culture. In fact, some believe that hearing parents of deaf children are made to feel that they have produced genetically inferior offspring resulting in feelings of inadequacy (Lane et al., 1996). Some members of the Deaf culture believe that early auditory habilitation is viewed as a professionally driven process in the "creation of a hearing-impaired person" (Lane et al., 1996). The process sets up a "deficit model" of deafness and the "deaf-child as patient" who needs the assistance of a team of professionals to mitigate the disability (Lane et al., 1996). In an era of empowerment through information, parents are rarely exposed to avenues explored by the Deaf culture, which include the early use of American Sign Language (ASL), hiring of deaf babysitters, and day caretakers (Lane et al., 1996).

Lane et al. (1996) stated that the lack of exposure of hearing parents of deaf children to the Deaf culture is due, in part, to two reasons. First, most hearing parents are completely unaware of options for exposure to Deaf culture. Second, hearing healthcare professionals seek to establish a partnership with the parents of a deaf child, possibly viewing Deaf culture as a threat to that relationship. Development of cross-cultural competence, discussed in Chapter 3, increases the likelihood of expanded options for parents of deaf children. An awareness of how our professions are viewed by members of the Deaf culture is the first step in correcting injustices of the past. In addition to respecting the Deaf culture, communication sciences and disorders professionals must be sensitive to how families of different cultural and ethnic minorities may react to the diagnosis of hearing loss in the family. Different ethnic and cultural groups may view disabilities differently than does the clinician. Therefore, clinicians must be open to a wide variety of responses and accept families with unconditional positive regard.

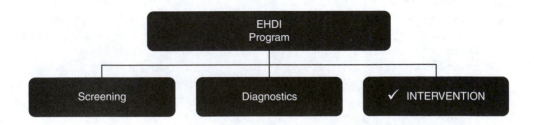

Early Intervention

According to the JCIH Year 2007 Position Statement, the fitting of amplification should occur within 1 month of diagnosis of hearing loss, with early intervention services to be in place by 6 months of age. The primary role of the family of a child with hearing loss is to

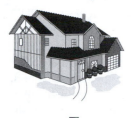

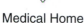

Medical Home

- Accessible
- Compassionate
- Comprehensive
- Coordinated
- Culturally sensitive
- Family-centered
- Individualized care

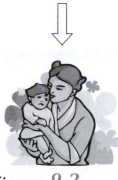

figure *9.2*

The concept of a medical home.

love, nurture, and communicate with the infant (JCIH, 2007). Early intervention can begin as soon as the audiologist has told parents that their child has a hearing loss. In addition to their roles in screening and audiologic evaluation, audiologists can supply parents with critical information facilitating the initiation of early intervention and serve as a conduit for families' communication with other service providers. Parents should be asked if they want test results to be sent to their children's pediatrician or family physician who serves as the medical home provider. The American Academy of Pediatrics (1997) established the concept of a **medical home**, shown in Figure 9.2, which is a high-quality and cost-effective approach to providing accessible, family-centered, ongoing, comprehensive, coordinated, and compassionate care to children through assignment of a primary healthcare provider who knows the child on an individual basis, and acknowledges any special needs and cultural background for achievement of maximum potential (JCIH, 2007). Usually, the pediatrician or family's general practitioner serving as the child's medical home provider coordinates the early intervention process. The JCIH Year 2007 Position Statement recommends that the birth hospital along with the state EHDI coordinator ensure that the parents and medical home provider receive the newborn hearing screening results. Moreover, the medical home provider should communicate with the audiologist about the results of diagnostic evaluations and any auditory habilitative efforts.

It is important that the medical home provider be prepared to meet the needs of children with hearing loss and their families. In general, some parents do not feel that they receive enough guidance from pediatricians, the recognized authorities on child care (Young, Davis, Schoen, & Parker, 1998). Parents of children with hearing loss are no different and will expect medical home providers to answer questions about the impact of and treatments for hearing loss. However, medical home providers, usually pediatricians or family physicians, must keep current on a plethora of topics. Hearing loss is but one of many health issues that these physicians have to deal with. Audiologists and speech-language pathologists may need to provide physicians with current information on auditory habilitation.

Several investigations have administered surveys and assembled focus groups of physicians at local, state, and national levels to assess their preparedness to participate in EHDI programs and serve as medical home providers for children with hearing loss and their families. The results of these studies found that although most physicians knew what EHDI programs were, they needed information about benchmarks for screening, diagnosis, and intervention; specifics about diagnostic protocols; and up-to-date information about treatment options (Brown, James, Liu, Hatcher, & Li, 2006; Carron, Moore, & Dhaliwal, 2006; Danhauer, Johnson, Finnegan, Hansen, et al., 2006; Danhauer, Johnson, Finnegan, Lamb, et al., 2006; Dorros, Kurtzer-White, Ahlgren, Simon, & Vohr, 2007; Moeller, White, & Shisler, 2006; Wall et al., 2001; Wall, Senicz, Evans, Woolley, & Hardin, 2006). In particular, physicians were deficient regarding their knowledge about technological advancements in diagnostic audiology and realistic benefits to be derived from the use of amplification (Dorros et al., 2007). Similarly, they were unsure of patient selection criteria for pediatric cochlear implantation (Mathews, Johnson, & Danhauer, 2009; Moeller et al., 2006). Parents may become distressed if they receive conflicting information from their child's audiologist and medical home provider. Therefore, audiologists need to form a partnership with children's medical home providers and anticipate their informational needs so that they may provide consistent and coordinated care, particularly in light of the relatively new recommendations in the JCIH Year 2007 Position Statement.

In Chapter 4, we discussed **cross-professional competence** in which audiologists and speech-language pathologists provide services within their scopes of practice in collaboration with other healthcare professionals toward achieving positive patient outcomes. Moreover, in EHDI programs, services are provided by a team of professionals who often must establish lines of communication to ensure that babies and their families are not lost to follow-up. Teamwork involves members helping each other, sometimes requiring not only anticipating, but meeting each other's needs. Audiologists and speech-language pathologists need to realize that medical home providers may not know what they need to know to serve children with hearing loss and their families. Munoz, Shisler, Moeller, and White (2009) found that physicians need informational outreach in five areas: overview of the EHDI process; newborn screening and referral for audiologic assessment and medical evaluation; amplification; referrals for early intervention; and family support and ongoing surveillance. Appendices 9.1 and 9.2 contain some resources for physicians and a checklist for audiologists in meeting the informational needs of medical home providers of their patients (adapted from Munoz et al., 2009).

Informational outreach to parents is also an important part of EHDI programs. Parents have many needs after diagnosis of hearing loss in their child. Clinicians are very valuable in guiding parents through the process. Moreover, parents not only need information, but to have opportunities to *discuss* issues with clinicians. Parents need to be frequently asked the following questions (English et al., 2004; Robbins, 2002):

- What are the goals for your child?
- What do you need to know now?
- What would you like me to discuss now?
- What do you need to know next week?
- What would you like me to discuss with you next week?

In other words, parents should be provided with information and then be allowed to discuss any questions or concerns about it.

Parents' informational needs change over time, meaning that what is of interest at the time of diagnosis may not be a priority during early intervention. For example, Roush and Harrison (2002) mailed 600 questionnaires to parents of children with hearing loss who received an introductory subscription of *Volta Voices* from the Alexander Graham Bell Association. The questionnaire was designed to elicit parents' informational needs at the time of diagnosis of hearing loss and during the first months of the auditory habilitation process. Specifically, the questionnaire had two lists of topics that parents were to rate as low, medium, and high priority in addition to rank ordering the most popular topics. The rank order of topics from most important to least important by parents at the time of diagnosis was (Rousch & Harrison, 2002): (1) causes of hearing loss, (2) coping with the emotional aspects of hearing loss, (3) understanding the audiogram, (4) learning to listen and speak, and finally, (5) understanding the ear and hearing. At the time of diagnosis of hearing loss, parents focus on causes of and coping with their emotional reactions to hearing loss. They also want to understand their child's audiogram. Parents of children with AN/AD may have a particularly difficult time understanding their child's hearing disorder. They need to be provided with accurate information and told of the variable prognoses for their child. Parents may grow anxious when talking with parents of children with sensorineural hearing losses that may have more definitive plans for habilitation. The parents were requested to do the same thing a few months after diagnosis of their child's hearing loss. The rank order of topics from most important to least important was (1) learning to listen and speak, (2) realistic timelines for learning to listen and speak, (3) cochlear implants, (4) communication systems, (5) responsibilities of early intervention agencies, followed by (6) legal rights of children with hearing loss. Later on, parents shift their attention to intervention and want information about timelines for speech and language development and treatment options such as cochlear implants.

Timeline for Intervention

Robbins (2002) stated that audiologists and speech-language pathologists serve an advisory role for parents during the six months following the diagnosis of the child's hearing loss. The first six months are tough for parents who are both trying to adjust to and accomplish initial tasks toward habilitation of their child's hearing loss. Robbins has divided up this period of time into three phases as shown in Figure 9.3.

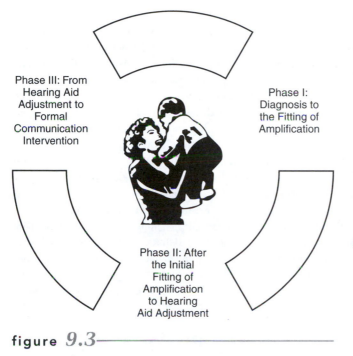

figure *9.3*

Robbins's (2002) phases of early intervention.

Source: Based on "Empowering Parents to Help Their Newly Diagnosed Child Gain Communication Skills," by A. M. Robbins, 2002, *The Hearing Journal, 55 (11),* pp. 55–56, 59.

Phase I: Diagnosis to the Fitting of Amplification.
Period Immediately After Diagnosis. The first phase encompasses the period from diagnosis to the fitting of amplification. During the first few weeks, some parents, immobilized by the diagnosis of hearing loss in their child, may feel a sense of empowerment by taking steps toward helping their child, no matter how small. Parents may begin to feel some sense of control over the situation through participation; they need to realize that they are their child's most important teacher. Robbins (2002) suggested giving parents some activities to do before the beginning of intervention that may be helpful in developing their child's communication skills. First, parents should be advised to continue to talk to their child (regardless of the degree of hearing loss) and ensure that they speak close to the face, use animated facial expressions and gestures, sing songs, and recite nursery rhymes. Second, Robbins suggested that parents keep a journal regarding experiences they are having, focusing on feelings, emotions, as well as observations about their child's hearing and responses to environmental sounds. The journal serves two purposes: (1) an outlet for parents, and (2) documentation of children's development (Robbins, 2002). Third, Robbins (2002) suggested that parents contact the John Tracy Clinic (www .johntracy-clinic.com) to enroll in a home correspondence course that includes videotapes, written information, and lessons to work on with their children. Parents send their completed lessons back to the John Tracy Clinic for feedback and receive encouragement throughout the auditory rehabilitation process.

Issues with Hearing Aid Selection, Evaluation, and Fitting on Infants. The Pediatric Amplification Protocol (American Academy of Audiology [AAA], 2003) states that hearing aids should be considered for any child who presents with a significant hearing loss whether it is conductive, sensorineural, or mixed of any degree. The AAA protocol recommends that the age of onset and configuration contribute to audiologists' strategy in fitting children with hearing aids. In addition, audiologists must also consider other factors such as a child's health status, cognitive functioning, and functional needs when developing an amplification plan. Aural habilitation plans for parents should be individualized based on the unique needs of the child and family.

Issues for prescribing and verifying the electroacoustic characteristics of hearing aids for newborn babies, infants, and toddlers are critical and are discussed in Chapter 6 on amplification. Briefly, electroacoustic characteristics include how much gain at each frequency hearing aids provide and determine the sound pressure levels going into children's ears. Prescribing the appropriate amount of gain and need for compression at each frequency is based on data from audiologic evaluations. Unfortunately, newborns and infants under the developmental age of 6 months cannot provide reliable hearing threshold levels. Therefore, estimates of hearing sensitivity must be obtained from electrophysiological measures such as the auditory brainstem response (ABR) test that was defined in Chapter 1. The ABR is a nonbehavioral assessment of how the auditory nerve conducts impulses from the periphery to the auditory brainstem pathway in response to an acoustic stimulus. Prescribing the appropriate gain and output of a hearing aid requires frequency-specific information about the child's hearing sensitivity. For example, in order to determine how much gain is needed at 1000 Hz in the right ear requires knowledge of the child's air-conduction threshold at 1000 Hz in the right ear. If at all possible, frequency-specific air- and bone-conduction thresholds should be obtained bilaterally for each child. However, for children under the developmental age of 6 months, physiologic testing using frequency-specific ABRs may aid in estimating the degree and configuration of hearing loss. The AAA protocol also advised audiologists to use other physiologic measures including immittance testing and otoacoustic emissions (OAEs) to aid in determining type and degree of hearing loss.

New electrophysiological procedures such as the auditory steady-state response technique (ASSR) shows promise in providing reasonable estimates of air- and bone-conduction thresholds (Herdman & Stapells, 2001; Roberson, O'Rourke, & Stidham, 2003; Stueve & O'Rourke, 2003; Vander Werff, Brown, Gienapp, & Schmidt Clay, 2002) and even estimation of air-bone gaps (Jeng, Brownt, Johnson, & Vander Werff, 2004) in young children under 6 months of age. Currently, the minimal amount of information required to prescribe hearing aid parameters on infants under 6 months of age is low- and high-frequency estimation of hearing loss in each ear (AAA, 2003).

The AAA protocol suggests that behavioral thresholds should be obtained for children using a method that is appropriate for the child's developmental levels. For example, visual reinforcement audiometry (VRA) and/or conditioned oriented response audiometry (COR) can be used for infants older than 6 months, or conditioned play audiometry (CPA) can be used with children 2 years and older (Northern & Downs, 2002). Audiologists should seek to use procedures that result in frequency-specific air- and bone-conduction thresholds required for valid hearing aid fittings (Pediatric Working Group, 1996).

Prescriptive methods for determining gain and output for hearing were described in Chapter 6. One approach is the National Acoustics Laboratory NL1 (NAL-NL1: Byrne, Dillon, Ching, Katsch, & Keidser, 2001), which aims to make the output comfortable; gain is based on patients' audiometric thresholds. NAL-NL1 is most frequently used with adults, but is also used for children (Ching, Scollie, Dillon, & Seewald, 2010; Scollie, Ching, Seewald, Dillon, Britton et al., 2010). Another method, the Desired Sensation Level (DSL) (Scollie, Seewald, Cornelisse, Moodie, & Bagatto, 2005), is used most often with children and ensures that conversational speech is audible while avoiding loudness discomfort. The DSL method uses the **real-ear-to-coupler difference** (RECD) to predict how much gain and output a hearing aid is providing inside a baby's ear canal from measurements made in a 2-cc coupler. The RECD is the measurement that compares what the hearing aid does in the child's ear and what it does in a 2-cc coupler. Growth of and other changes in infants' ears require monitoring of hearing aid function by audiologists so that appropriate adjustments can be made.

The AAA protocol advises that additional factors should be considered when determining candidacy for amplification. Specifically, middle ear pathology should be a consideration when fitting children with amplification. Chronic or recurrent otitis media can affect hearing sensitivity and may interfere with a child's ability to wear an earmold and a hearing aid. In addition, the presence of other disabilities besides hearing loss should be a factor in considering children's candidacy for amplification. For example, Pappas, Flexer, and Shackelford (1994) found that amplification was a major factor in an aggressive multidisciplinary habilitative program for children with Down syndrome that also included reconstruction of the external auditory canal and speech-language intervention that emphasized Auditory-Verbal therapy (A/V).

The style of choice for infants and toddlers is the behind-the-ear hearing aid because it is durable and can accommodate rough-and-tumble play of young children. Second, the behind-the-ear hearing aid is suitable for different styles of earmolds that may provide additional opportunities to shape the frequency response. For example, use of a special tubing called a **libby horn** (see Chapter 6) may provide additional high-frequency spectral energy that may enhance children's speech and language development (Stelmachowicz, Pittman, Hoover, & Lewis, 2001; Stelmachowicz, Pittman, Hoover, Lewis, & Moeller, 2004). Third, the ability to remake earmolds can accommodate the rapid growth of children's ears during infancy and early childhood alleviating the need to re-case the hearing aid (Kalcioglu, Miman, Toplu, Yakinci, & Ozturan, 2003). Fourth, behind-the-ear hearing aids are easier for parents to clean, care for, handle, and adjust than other styles of hearing aids. Fifth, behind-the-ear hearing aids can accommodate extra circuitry such as telecoils, direct-audio input (DAI), or snap-on FM receivers. Hearing aid manufacturers do make small BTE cases to accommodate infants' tiny little ears! Parents may use **Huggies**, a plastic loop that is attached to the hearing aid case, surrounds the ear, and snugly holds the BTE in place.

Parents and hearing healthcare professionals must also decide if hearing aids are to be worn on one ear (i.e., monaural amplification), or both ears (i.e., binaural amplification) for young children with bilateral sensorineural hearing loss. Although difficult to believe, binaural fitting of hearing aids was considered to be a misuse of amplification by some audiologists during the 1970s (Peck, 1980). Binaural amplification of children was hypothesized to result by some in overamplification, placing the child at risk for additional hearing loss (Madell, 1978). One solution was to switch the hearing aid alternatively from one ear to the other to allow each ear a rest period from amplification. However, even the majority of studies at that time showed that the thresholds of unaided ears actually deteriorated when compared with ears that received amplification (Markides & Aryee, 1978, 1980). Today, hearing healthcare professionals recognize the need for binaural amplification in order to avoid the effect of auditory deprivation including a loss of hearing sensitivity and a decrease in speech recognition ability (Gelfand, Silman, & Ross, 1987; Gelfand & Silman, 1993). The advantages of binaural amplification are reviewed in the chapter on amplification. However, for some situations, such as a chronically draining middle ear, some periods of monaural amplification may be recommended for some children.

Parents should be advised that not all children benefit from amplification, but may receive better outcomes from **cochlear implants**, surgically implanted cochlear prostheses that bypass the damaged peripheral auditory system to directly stimulate nerve VIII for hearing (see Chapter 8 for a detailed explanation). Most children undergo a three- to six-month trial period with hearing aids prior to considering cochlear implants. Later in the chapter, a separate section discusses assessment tools that may be used for determining infants' and toddlers' initial progress with hearing aids and candidacy for cochlear implantation. Usually, a **cochlear implant team**, composed of a group of healthcare professionals, is involved in the cochlear implantation of patients, from candidacy to rehabilitation. Parents should talk to as many professionals as possible who are experienced with cochlear implants in order to make informed decisions for their children. Informed decision-making requires input from a variety of sources, including parents of children with cochlear implants (Boys Town National Research Hospital, 2010). Parents should also talk with members of the Deaf community regarding their view of cochlear implantation (National Association of the Deaf, 2010a). Additional considerations include which ear to implant, whether to wear a hearing aid on the other ear (Ching, Psarros, Hill, Dillon, & Incerti, 2001; Litovsky, Johnstone, & Godar, 2006), or whether to implant both ears (Litovsky et al., 2006; Litovsky, Johnstone, Godar, Agrawal, et al., 2006).

Phase II: After the Initial Fitting of Amplification to Hearing Aid Adjustment. It is important for parents to receive a thorough hearing aid orientation and delivery of their children's hearing instruments. Due to the hustled and harried lifestyle of today's families, the hearing aid orientation and training may include multiple family members and caregivers outside the home. For example, Grandma and daycare workers may need to know how to change a battery on a child's hearing aids.

Parents should be taught how to care for the hearing aid, be advised of the importance of keeping the earmold bores free of cerumen, and of minimizing moisture in the hearing aid. Parents may be advised to purchase a dehumidifier that draws the moisture out of the hearing aid. Several dehumidifiers are available on the market and were discussed and shown in Chapter 6. For example, recall the super Dri-Aid Kit that consisted of a jar of blue and white pellets made of silicagel, a desiccant. At the end of the day, parents should open the battery compartments, place the hearing aids on top of the sponge, and then replace the lid on top of the jar. The pellets absorb the moisture out of the hearing aids during the night. When the blue pellets turn white, the directions for reactivating the desiccant should be implemented such that some of them turn back to blue. Similarly, the more expensive dehumidifier, the Dry 'N Store, also discussed and shown in Chapter 6, has to be plugged in to work. The Dry 'N Store requires a power source to dehumidify and clean hearing aids.

Young children should wear their hearing aids during all waking hours. Audiologists should require that parents demonstrate mastery in the insertion and removal of their child's hearing aids. Furthermore, parents should be instructed on battery insertion/removal, life, storage, and disposal, and their toxicity. Parents should know that all batteries have a positive and negative side and that the side with the plus sign always faces up. In general, hearing aid batteries last from a week to 10 days; their useable life varies, based on the power of the hearing aid the number of hours per day the device is worn. Hearing aid batteries should be stored in a safe place because they may cause damage if swallowed. Parents should always be given the Battery Ingestion Hotline: (202) 625-3333.

Parents should purchase a hearing aid check kit and be taught to perform a visual and listening check, and basic troubleshooting of the hearing aid. Figure 9.4 shows a basic hearing aid check kit consisting of a battery tester, two listening stethoscopes, forced-air bulb, wax pick, and soft brush. Ideally, parents should perform the check once a day and document its results on a checksheet provided in Appendix 9.3. The visual check consists of inspecting the case for cleanliness and ensuring that it is not cracked. Dirty hearing aid cases can be cleaned with a soft, dry towel. Cracked cases may expose the electrical components of the hearing aid to moisture, dust, and debris. Furthermore, a crack in the hearing aid may cause

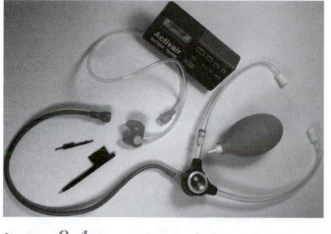

figure *9.4*

A hearing aid visual and listening check kit.

sound to escape and to be re-amplified, resulting in feedback. Cracked hearing aid cases must be sent back to the manufacturer for repair. The battery must be checked for adequate charge and the battery compartment for corrosion. Batteries having a charge of less than 1.2 volts should be changed and any corrosion should be cleaned by the audiologist with battery contact spray. The earmold, or the part that couples the hearing aid to the child's ear, should have a sound bore that is free of cerumen and moisture, and the tubing should be undamaged. Cerumen can be removed using a wax loop, and moisture can be dried using a forced-air bulb. Earmold tubing that has discolored and become brittle must be replaced by an audiologist.

The listening check of the hearing aid should be completed with the suction tip of the stethoscope over the sound bore of the earmold. If problems are noted, the parent can check to see if the problem is isolated to the earmold or hearing aid. For example, parents may find that the hearing aid is distorted only when connected to an earmold with moisture in the tubing. In addition, the volume control wheel should move smoothly and no unusual sounds should be audible. The Hearing Aid Checksheet (Appendix 9.3) has spaces and boxes for parents to record the date and check off items, respectively. In addition, a comments section allows parents to record unusual findings or questions that they have for the audiologist. Daily visual and listening checks of hearing aids ensure children's hearing aids are working.

Some infants and toddlers may use hearing assistive technology (HAT) defined and discussed in Chapter 7. Even though young children may not be in preschool, they may benefit from the use of remote microphone HAT (RMHAT) (AAA, 2009d). Young children with hearing loss deserve access to as many opportunities for learning speech and language as their peers with normal hearing. Young children learn language through listening in a variety of situations. Older children and adults may not think that a young child sitting in the backseat of a car listens to their conversations (Moeller, 2010). However, young children learn a lot from eavesdropping on others' conversations as part of **incidental learning**, which is unplanned learning or natural acquisition of information (Moeller). However, young children with hearing loss may not be able to do this even when wearing hearing aids. Therefore, use of an FM system may increase opportunities for learning speech and language.

Dispensing of HAT requires adequate orientation to parents regarding the care and use of devices. As discussed in Chapter 7, at minimum HAT delivery should consist of ensuring that the parent can install the device, turn it on or off, change batteries, if applicable, and clean and care for the device. Parents should also know how to couple their child's hearing aid to the HAT device and be aware that those using it must be close to the microphone for improvement in signal-to-noise ratio. Furthermore, parents must be able to explain to others (e.g., the speech-language pathologist, Grandma, and the daycare worker) what the HAT device is, what it does, and what the speaker needs to do to be able to use it. Parents should also be able to recognize appropriate situations in which to use the HAT device and be able to troubleshoot the device regarding its installation, coupling to hearing aids, and operation.

As mentioned in Chapter 7, documentation of the HAT device selection, evaluation, and fitting protocol should include its make, model, and serial numbers; the rationale for the device; counseling provided; procedures used for assessment; parent and child's response to the device; prognosis for benefit; and plans for orientation, monitoring, reassessment, and final disposition (ASHA, 2006b). For information about current clinical practice guidelines, see *Remote Microphone Hearing Assistance Technology for Children and Youth from Birth to 21 Years* (AAA, 2009d).

Earlier in the chapter, we discussed what parents want to know at diagnosis and during the first year. Hearing instrument and training coincides with Robbins' (2002) Phase II in auditory habilitation just after the initial fitting of amplification. Robbins suggested that parents must make the connection between full-time use of hearing aids and the development of spoken language. It has been suggested that children who inconsistently use amplification have limited opportunities for incidental learning (Moeller, 2010). Parents have found that it is more difficult to achieve amplification compliance in those situations that are hard to monitor (e.g., going to the zoo, school) (Moeller, Hoover, Peterson, & Stelmachowicz, 2009). Additionally, it has been found that some families are better at ensuring that their children wear hearing aids than others (Moeller et al., 2009). It is important for audiologists and parents to realize that the reasons why children do not wear hearing aids change over time (Moeller, 2010). For example, 12-month-olds simply do not like wearing hearing aids and may pull them out. Other reasons for noncompliance include that they are teething and do not feel good. Alternatively, Moeller (2010) stated that 15-month-olds have learned that taking out their hearing aids results in attention from Mom and Dad. Therefore, children's consistent use of amplification must be monitored over time (Moeller, 2010). Audiologists should ask parents about consistency of amplification during routine hearing aid checks. Moreover, speech-language pathologists should note whether children consistently wear their hearing aids to therapy. Parents should keep a dedicated weekly hearing calendar recording such things as the number of hours the hearing aid is worn each day, equipment problems, children's resistance to hearing aid use and attempts at removal, and children's responses to sound and nature of response (e.g., startle, cessation of activity, or eye widening). It is suggested that in some cases, the calendars should be faxed to the audiologist to hold parents accountable for tracking aspects of their children's use of amplification (Robbins, 2002). The calendars should be reviewed by audiologists during follow-up appointments. See Appendix 9.4 for an example of such a calendar.

During this stage, audiologists may introduce other goals to parents to promote communication (Robbins, 2002). For example, parents may teach children to recognize their own name in as many contexts as possible (e.g., when face-to-face say, "Hi Bobby . . . There's Bobby . . . I love you, Bobby"), but only calling the child's name for clear purposes. Parents can teach their children to attend to auditory stimuli by using a hands-to-ears response to sound by pointing to ears with an animated expression saying, "I hear that!" (Robbins, 2002). Parents should be encouraged to carefully listen to variations in their child's vocalizations (Robbins, 2002). For example, is their child's fussy cry different from his or her cry of pain? Does their child make mostly consonant or vowel sounds during vocal play? Does their child squeal or scream? Does their child imitate others' speech? Does their child sing along to music? Are there sounds that will calm or soothe their baby? Parents need to know that their journal entries may provide important information to audiologists and speech-language pathologists about the child's benefit derived from the use of amplification.

Phase III: From Hearing Aid Adjustment to Formal Communication Intervention.
Robbins's (2002) Phase III involves the period of time from completion of the hearing aid adjustment to formal communication intervention. By this time, parents and children have adjusted to amplification and no longer struggle with mechanical issues. The hallmark of this stage is a focus on communication development. The audiologist and speech-language pathologist should encourage parents to stimulate communication in their young child by (Robbins, 2002):

- imitating their vocalizations, including intonation patterns and sounds
- teaching turn taking (e.g., encouraging the child to wait for his turn to talk by waiting for your turn, and so on)
- pretending that vocalizations have meaning (e.g., if the child says, "Ere idy idy," respond with "Yes, here kitty, kitty!")
- encouraging an anticipatory response to sound by:
  - maximizing opportunities for events based on hearing alone (e.g., speak from behind the child and say, "Where's Mr. Bear?" and then showing the bear)
  - selecting three sounds in the home (e.g., the doorbell/telephone ringing and dog barking), and then drawing a child's attention to it (e.g., "I hear the doggy barking" when the dog barks)

It is not unusual for speech-language pathologists to go into the home to observe and provide coaching to parents on **facilitative language techniques**, or things that caregivers can do to enhance children's communication. In the following Casebook Reflection, Stacy Metcalf, Joshua Washington's speech-language pathologist, is making a home visit to provide coaching to Debbie and Leon about how they can enhance their son's language learning. Stacy had videotaped Leon and Debbie's interactions with their son and had prepared a series of clips to illustrate how they might use facilitative language techniques.

Casebook Reflection

Coaching the Washingtons on Facilitative Language Techniques

Debbie: "Leon, hurry downstairs, Stacy is here. Hi, Stacy, how are you?"

Stacy: "I'm fine. Thanks for your directions. I had no problem finding your house."

Leon: "Hi Stacy. How are you?"

Stacy: "I'm fine. Have you had the opportunity to read the handout I provided based on the works of Tye-Murray and DesJardin and Eisenberg?"

Debbie: "Yes, we did. . . ."

Stacy: "Great! I've brought my computer to show you some clips of both of you playing with Joshua to show where facilitative language techniques could have been used. Let's sit around the table so that we all can see the screen on my laptop."

Debbie: "OK, sounds good."

Stacy: "OK, first let me show you a situation in which you could've used the **comment technique**. Looking at your handout, what is the comment technique?"

Leon: It is saying something that keeps the conversation going or encourages a child."

Stacy: "Right. Let's watch the clip. . . ."

Debbie: "Oh, Joshua looks so cute. . . ."

Stacy: "Yes, you see, Leon, when Joshua put the block in the bucket and looked at you, you could have said, 'Good job, Joshua!' What else could you have done to keep the sequence going?"

Leon: (Looks over at Debbie. . . .)

Debbie: "He could've asked, 'Do you want another block?'"

Stacy: "Yes, very good! . . . OK, here is another clip with the block falling on the ground and Joshua saying 'Uh-oh . . . bahhhh.' How could you have used **expansion and modeling** here? Remember, expansion and modeling is repeating what the child says and adding more to it."

Leon: "Debbie could've said, 'Uh-oh, the block fell on the floor.'"

Stacy: "Very good!" OK, here is another clip in which you might have used **linguistic mapping**, which is saying what you think the child is trying to say using what is around you or the context to convey meaning. See how Joshua has eaten his last Goldfish cracker and reaches for more and says, 'Uh . . . uh. . . .'"

Debbie: "I could've said, 'Joshua, wants another Goldfish' when giving him another one to eat."

Stacy: "Yes, very good! OK, let's go discuss **parallel talking**, which is simply using words to describe what the child is attending to or doing. Let's look at this clip where Leon is sitting on the floor stacking the blocks. . . . How could you have used parallel talking?"

Leon: "I could've said, 'Joshua is stacking the blocks. . . . One, two, and three blocks.'"

Stacy: "Excellent!"

Leon: "Well, sometimes I feel silly saying those things. Does it really help him learn?"

Stacy: "Yes, it does. I know it is hard not to feel self-conscious talking like that when you're not at home or when other adults are around."

Debbie: "C'mon Leon, it's for Joshua!"

Leon: "I know, I know."

Stacy: "OK, you're doing great. And Leon, I appreciate you discussing your feelings about using these techniques. It is important to say what you feel and get issues out in the open. OK, **recasting** is simply restating a child's statement as a question. Alternatively, it can be the restating of a question into a statement. OK, let's look at a clip of the block falling on the ground and Joshua saying, 'Uh-oh. . . . bahhhh.' How could you have recast what Joshua said?"

Debbie: "'Did the block fall on the floor?'"

Stacy: "Very good! Please note though, that several language facilitation techniques may be appropriate for the same situation."

Debbie: "Stacy, how do we know which technique is the best?"

Stacy: "Debbie, your question brings up an important point and that is that parents shouldn't think too much about this. Parents should practice a little, and then try to be as spontaneous and natural as possible. It is like riding a bike. Before you know it, you're off and rolling with it. . . . OK, two more techniques, one is **self-talk** and the other is **signaling expectation** or **time delay**. Self-talk is simply talking about what you're doing like, 'Mommy is dusting the furniture' . . . or 'Daddy is washing the car'. . . ."

Leon: "Debbie ought to be good at this. . . ."

Debbie: "Stop. . . ."

Stacy: "OK, you two. Signal expectation and time delay is showing the child that you are waiting for their response. Let's look at this clip. . . . Tell me how Leon could have used the technique with Joshua who is holding the ball."

Leon: "I could've said, 'You have the ball. . . . It's my turn' and hold up my arms anticipating that he will throw it to me."

Stacy: "Yes, very good! Do you have any questions?"

Debbie: "I don't."

Leon: "I don't either."

Stacy: "What I'd like you to do is practice these at home."

Debbie: "Should I share these with his grandma and grandpa? They stay with Joshua during the day while we work. . . ."

Stacy: "Absolutely. . . ."

Debbie: "Thank you, Stacy, for coming to our home."

Leon: "Yes, thank you!"

Stacy: "You are welcome. Please write down any questions you may have. And practice these techniques. Next time you come to therapy, I will watch you two play with Joshua and provide some more coaching on the use of these techniques."

Parents should engage their children in **preliteracy activities** to prepare them for reading and writing. Parents should develop rituals around joint book-reading with their children at specified times during the day, such as at bedtime. Sitting in parents' laps provides children with a special sense of belonging and security. Having Mom or Dad point to words while orally reading helps children to associate orthographic symbols with meaningful words. Many of the same language facilitation techniques presented in the previous Casebook Reflection can be used in joint book-reading activities between parent and child. Children tend to mimic their parents by retelling their own versions of stories, developing narrative abilities and auditory memory span. Moreover, having children copy letters with a pencil and paper are precursors for learning how to write. Some experts have felt that so much emphasis has been placed on facilitating spoken oral language in children with hearing loss that the development of preliteracy skills has been neglected.

ASSESSMENT FOR TREATMENT PLANNING AND PROGRESS

After initial fitting with hearing aids, infants' progress must be assessed to provide an indication of whether adjustments need to be made on the hearing aid or whether a cochlear implant should be considered by the family. Because 40% of children with hearing loss have other disabilities, assessment often is multidisciplinary, involving professionals from a variety of disciplines. Audiologists and speech-language pathologists are responsible for assessing communicative function of children with hearing loss. In a multidisciplinary team assessment, it is important to determine how hearing loss impacts other areas of development. Assessment is particularly important to determine initial level of functioning and then to gauge progress with amplification.

In other chapters of this book, we defined **outcome measures** as data collected to determine the benefit of treatment and frequently involve the use of self-assessment scales. Audiologists can easily use self-assessment scales with older children and adults. Similarly, speech-language pathologists can administer standardized tests of speech and language development with these same populations. However, with infants, clinicians often must rely on interviewing parents or other caregivers to complete the assessment of children's speech, language, and auditory behaviors. Typically, these measures are made before and after the fitting of hearing aids to determine the amount of benefit and estimate the child's prognosis with amplification. Lack of progress with hearing aids may indicate that a family may consider cochlear implantation for their child. Clinicians must ensure that children have worn their hearing aids during all waking hours for the adjustment period for a valid assessment of outcomes. Table 9.4 lists assessment tools that can be used for infants and toddlers with hearing loss.

Speech-language pathologists may employ either informal or formal assessments. Informal assessment includes obtaining and analyzing speech and language samples. A **language sample** is an exact transcription of a patient's use of language including what is communicated by all participants along with notation of relevant context. Speech-language pathologists perform specific analyses of the sample to obtain important indices of language competence. One measure is the **mean length of utterance** (MLU), which is the average number of morphemes used per utterance. Children's performances may be compared against normative data of peers of the same chronological age with normal hearing. Speech-language pathologists may also find using standardized tests such as the *Reynell Developmental Language Scales* (Reynell & Gruber, 1990) useful in assessing children's verbal

table *9.4*   Examples of Assessment Tools to Use With Infants and Toddlers With Hearing loss

Informal Assessment

Language sample

Formal Assessment

Receptive and expressive language

- *Reynell Developmental Language Scales* (Reynell & Gruber, 1990)
- *Receptive-Expressive Language Test, Third Edition* (REEL-3) (Bzoch, League, & Brown, 2003)
- *Preschool Language Scale, Fourth Edition* (PLS-4) (Zimmerman, Steiner, & Pond, 2002)

Auditory skills

- *Functional Auditory Performance Indicator: An Integrated Approach to Auditory Skill Development.* (FAPI) (Stredler-Brown & Johnson, 2004)
- *Infant-Toddler Meaningful Auditory Integration Scale* (IT-MAIS) (Zimmerman-Phillips, Robbins, & Osberger, 2000)
- *Client Oriented Scale of Improvement for Children* (COSI-C) (National Acoustics Laboratories, 2009)
- *Early Listening Functiont Test* (ELF) (Anderson, 2007)

comprehension and expressive language. The *Receptive-Expressive Language Test, Third Edition* (REEL-3) (Bzoch, League, & Brown, 2003) is for infants and toddlers with developmental delays or other disabilities, such as hearing loss, that may impact language development. The test is normed allowing for comparisons of children's performances based on age, gender, race, ethnic group, and geographic location. Another instrument, the *Preschool Language Scale, Fourth Edition* (PLS-4) (Zimmerman, Steiner, & Pond, 2002), is also appropriate for young children providing specific items for infants and toddlers that target interaction, attention, and vocal/gestural behaviors. In addition, the test has a caregiver questionnaire that asks about children's communicative behavior displayed in the home.

Audiologists and speech-language pathologists may find the following four tools useful in the evaluation of infant and toddlers' auditory development:

1. ***Functional Auditory Performance Indicator: An Integrated Approach to Auditory Skill Development* (FAPI) (Stredler-Brown & Johnson, 2004).** *Functional Auditory Performance Indicator* (FAPI) tracks auditory skills that are interdependent and hierarchical, from simple to complex. The seven auditory skill levels are:
   - Awareness and Meaning of Sound: Child knows the sound is present and has meaning (e.g., loud environmental sounds, noisemakers, music, vocalizations, and speech).
   - Auditory Feedback and Integration: Child is aware of and modifies his or her vocalizations according to changes in auditory input (e.g., modifications when hearing instrument is turned on, using voice to monitor amplification, or noticing his or her own vocalizations).
   - Localizing Sound Source: Child seeks and succeeds in finding auditory stimuli in the environment.

- Auditory Discrimination: Child can determine if two sounds are the same or different (e.g., environmental sounds, suprasegmentals [pitch, loudness, and duration], and words).
- Auditory Comprehension: Child knows the meaning of linguistic stimuli (e.g., identifying auditory stimuli or following directions).
- Short-Term Auditory Memory: Child is able to remember, repeat, and/or recall a sequence of items (e.g., objects, colors, or numbers).
- Linguistic Auditory Processing: Child uses auditory information for language processing (e.g., understands a story or participates in a conversation).

The FAPI is used to profile children's functional auditory skills by administering all items on the test. The results of the test show what the child can do and are useful for planning therapy. Some clinicians mistakenly believe that each level of the FAPI must be completed in succession and must be mastered before moving on to the next. However, working on 4 to 8 levels at the same time for the integration of auditory skill development is both appropriate and helpful to the child.

The FAPI is to be administered over time because it is doubtful that clinicians could observe all of the skills in a single session. Each level has specific skills to be evaluated in a variety of situations. For example, Awareness and Meaning of Sound is evaluated in the following modes: auditory-only, with visual cues, close (3 feet), far, in quiet, in noise, prompted, or spontaneous. The clinician creates opportunities to observe and score children's auditory behaviors. Items are scored according to their frequency of occurrence out of the total number of opportunities for: (a) "not present" (NP) having 0–10% occurrence and 0 points, (b) "emerging" (E) having 11–35% occurrence and 1 point, (c) "in process" (P) with 36–79% occurrence and 2 points, and (d) "acquired" (A) with 80–100% occurrence and 3 points. Scores for each indicator in all situations are tallied, weighted, and added together for an overall skill score. Skills scores are added together and then divided by a perfect score to yield a percent of mastery for an overall category. For example, an overall category score of 81% achieved in the Awareness and Meaning of Sound level indicates that the skills have been acquired. Overall scores for each of the seven auditory skill areas are shaded to create an individual performance profile for each child.

As alluded to earlier, the FAPI is not just an assessment tool, but is excellent for developing a specific auditory rehabilitation curriculum for children. Not only are the levels hierarchically arranged, but the skills within each are assessed in situations that range from easy to more difficult. For example, if the skill "Responds to loud environmental noisemakers" from the Awareness and Meaning of Sound level is "IP" or "in process" at a distance of 3 feet, then clinicians know to not only work toward a child's acquisition of this behavior at 3 feet but then at far distances (e.g., 10 feet). By determining children's performance profiles, clinicians can determine both long- and short-term goals.

2. *Infant-Toddler Meaningful Auditory Integration Scale* (IT-MAIS) (**Zimmerman-Phillips, Robbins, & Osberger, 2000**). The *Infant-Toddler Meaningful Auditory Integration Scale* (IT-MAIS) is a parent-report scale consisting of 10 items that assess children's (1) vocalization behavior, (2) alerting to sounds, and (3) deriving meaning from sound. Clinicians are to administer the IT-MAIS in an interview format so parents are not led into responding in any particular way. For example, item 1 says "Is the child's vocal behavior affected while wearing his/her sensory aid (hearing aid or cochlear implant)?" However, instead of asking this question directly, clinicians are instructed to interview parents by asking them to "describe_____'s vocalizations when you first put his/her device on each day. . . .," which elicits a more valid description of behavior. Each

item comes with several questions increasing in depth of probing so that if parents do not provide enough information from one question, another one may be used to obtain an adequate description for scoring. Each of the 10 items are scored on a 0 to 4 scale indicating the frequency of occurrence for behaviors with a score of 0 for "Never" (approximately 0%), 1 for "Rarely" (approximately 25%), 2 for "Occasionally" (approximately 50%), 3 for "Frequently" (approximately 75%), or 4 for "Always" (approximately 100%). In addition, each item contains specific scoring criteria. For example, for item 1 a score of 0 is warranted when there is no difference between the child's vocalizations with the device turned on or off. Similarly, a score of 4 means that the child's vocalizations increase 100% with the device turned on. Credit is to be given only if parents respond to the questions in a spontaneous fashion without direct prompting from the audiologist or speech-language pathologist. Furthermore, children's auditory responses elicited in a structured listening task (e.g., within a therapy session) do not receive credit. Because there are 10 items, scores on the IT-MAIS range from 0 to 40. Obviously, the higher the overall score, the better are children's auditory skills. In addition to scoring, parents' verbal responses should also be recorded on the test booklet. Clinicians are reminded that the IT-MAIS is *not* to be given to parents to fill out, but must be administered in an interview format.

3. ***Client Oriented Scale of Improvement for Children* (COSI-C) (National Acoustics Laboratories, 2009).** Another outcome measure is the COSI-C, which is an adaptation of the *Client Oriented Scale of Improvement* (COSI) (Dillon, James, & Ginis, 1997). The COSI-C is similar to measures used with the 0- to 2-year-old population in that it is completed by parents with assistance from clinicians. The main goal of the COSI-C is to document parents' goals/needs for their children and measure the amount of benefit from hearing aids. On the COSI-C score sheet, parents, with assistance from audiologists, list and prioritize from one to five goals/needs to target and then possible strategies for their achievement. On the National Acoustics (the test's publisher) website are two handouts, "Goals for Promoting Hearing in Infants: A Guide for Audiologists," and "Goals for Promoting Hearing in Toddlers: A Guide for Audiologists" with suggested goals and strategies for infants and toddlers. For example, one goal suggested for infants is consistent hearing aid use with numerous strategies, such as discussing the relationship between full-time amplification use and speech-language development with parents and providing the contact information for families that have achieved this goal. Similarly, a goal for toddlers may be to indicate feedback and a possible strategy to reinforce this behavior. COSI-C goals/needs may also be classified into one of the 16 general categories from the regular COSI. In addition, the date for review of progress on the goals/needs should be planned after children's initial adjustment to amplification. Assessment of postamplification progress is indicated through responses of "no change," "small change," "significant change," or "goal achieved." It is suggested that parents and audiologists dialogue regarding changes in strategies or expectations for goals/needs labeled either "no change" or "small change." The COSI-C is more than an outcome measure; it is a habilitative tool, assisting in the setting of and methods for attaining appropriate goals.

4. ***Early Listening Function* test (ELF) (Anderson, 2007).** Not all outcome measures are completed through interview formats nor require the audiologist or speech-language pathologist to complete the questionnaire. For example, caregivers may complete the *Early Listening Function* (ELF) test on their own. One fundamental goal of the ELF is to determine children's **listening bubbles**, or proximities for communication, indicated by the distances at which they consistently respond to quiet, typical, and loud sounds. This idea is based on the premise that the farther away the sound source, the lower is the sound

pressure level of the signal. The **inverse square law** describes how the sound pressure level of a signal changes as a function of distance from the source. For every doubling of distance from the sound source, the sound pressure level drops 6 dB. It follows then that children with hearing impairment do not respond to sounds at distances as do children with normal hearing. However, placement of a hearing aid or cochlear implant may increase distances from which children with hearing loss can consistently respond to sounds.

The ELF has explicit instructions for parents who will be watching how their children respond to 12 different listening activities in the home environment and will write results on the ELF Listening Activities Sheet. Four listening activities are found in each of the three categories of quiet, typical, and loud. For example, two of the activities in the quiet category are, "Mommy saying 'sh, sh' quietly," and "Hands together, palms rubbing together briskly." Similarly, two of the activities in the loud category are, "Loud door knock with knuckles," and "Hitting a frying pan or pot with a metal or wooden spoon." Across the top of the ELF Listening Activities Sheet are listening distances of 6 inches, 3 feet, 6 feet, 10 feet, and the next room (15 feet). A final column on the sheet asks for the farthest distances at which children respond to listening activities in noise. Parents are instructed to indicate at what distances they have observed their children responding in each of the listening activities. A "Y" is put in the box for "yes" to indicate consistent responding (e.g., 4 out of 5 times), an "M" for "maybe" (e.g., 2 or 3 out of 5 times), and "N" for "no" (e.g., no certain responses). Parents are advised that they need not assess all listening activities at all distances. For example, if a child responds consistently to quiet activities at 10 feet, it can be assumed that he or she will respond to the typical and loud ones at that distance as well.

Another component of the ELF is the Infant and Young Child Amplification Use Checklist that parents should complete each time children are provided with new hearing aids, settings, cochlear implants, or assistive listening devices. The checklist asks parents to describe children's current amplification situation and indicate the number of times a visual/listening check is performed each day, the number of hours devices are worn during waking hours, and their comfort level with the system and its maintenance. In addition, parents mark the degree of agreement regarding the improvement in their child's auditory skills (e.g., awareness of parent's voice/environmental sounds, localization of parent's voice), increases in babbling/talking, greater interest in communicating, and increases in the listening bubble for a variety of stimuli in ELF listening activities (e.g., quiet, typical, and loud sounds/voices), and improvement for listening in background noise. Parents also are to describe specific situations where they have noticed improvements in their children's listening abilities.

The ELF also comes with a detailed Early Listening Function Score Sheet for clinicians who want to quantify children's performances. The scoresheet concludes with a section called Hearing Loss Management Considerations Discussed by Audiologists/ Interventionists in making recommendations based on performance on the ELF. Audiologists/interventionists simply mark appropriate recommendations and fill in needed information such as the size of the listening bubble (e.g., distance) in quiet, with and without amplification. In addition, audiologists/interventionists may indicate the need to control background noise when communicating with the baby at certain distances and beyond. If a child had particular difficulty listening in noise and to speech at a distance, audiologists/interventionists may consider that a child may be a potential FM system user. Based on ELF performance, audiologists/interventionists may consider that a child may be a potential cochlear prosthesis user and suggest parents contact an implant team for more information. In summary, the ELF is a useful outcome measure that can measure the benefit of amplification and other sensory devices, but provides avenues for planning aural habilitation with parents.

EARLY SPEECH AND LANGUAGE DEVELOPMENT OF CHILDREN WITH HEARING IMPAIRMENT

Babies make a lot of different vocalizations that develop in an orderly fashion, from vegetative sounds to the use of words (Stoel-Gammon & Otomo, 1986). Vocalizations of babies with hearing loss and their hearing peers do not differ much during prelinguistic development. From birth to 2 months, all babies' vocalizations include fussing, burping, sneezing, and crying (Stoel-Gammon, 1998). From 2 to 3 months of age, babies do a lot of cooing that consists of vowels, velars (e.g., /k/ and /g/), and nasals (e.g., /n/). Later, from 4 to 6 months of age, babies expand their vocalizations to include playful productions of sounds including vowels, raspberries, squeals, and yells (Stoel-Gammon, 1998). However, at about 6 to 8 months of age, babies start listening to the speech of others around them and begin to self-monitor. Up until this point, the early vocalizations of babies with normal hearing and hearing loss are similar and do not resemble any particular language. However, soon linguistic environment becomes important, and infants' vocalizations have language-specific characteristics. DeBoysson-Bardies, Halle, Sagart, and Durand (1989) found that 10-month-olds' vowel productions showed first- and second-formant language-specific characteristics. Children with hearing impairment display both quantitative and qualitative differences from their peers with normal hearing in speech and language development. It was found that even temporary conductive hearing losses in children with otitis media resulted in qualitative restrictions in front-to-back tongue movement in vowel production compared with their peers without middle-ear disease (Rvachew, Slawinski, Williams, & Green, 1997, 1999).

The results of a case study show the effects of profound sensorineural hearing loss on early speech and language development. Kent, Osberger, Netsell, and Godschmidt-Hustedde (1987) compared and contrasted the phonetic development of twin boys at 8, 12, and 15 months of age. One twin had normal hearing and the other had a profound sensorineural hearing loss. They found that the difference in the speech between the two boys increased with age. The twin with hearing loss demonstrated restricted formant space and variations in vowel production in comparison with the boy with normal hearing. He also produced less fricatives, affricates, trills, and used fewer types of syllables than the twin with normal hearing. Similarly, in comparing prelinguistic consonant inventories, researchers found that infants with hearing loss produced more labials, but fewer alveolar sounds and nonsyllabic affricates than babies with normal hearing (Stoel-Gammon & Otomo, 1986). The results of this case study concur with Stoel-Gammon and Otomo (1986), who found less syllabic variation in infants with hearing loss than those with normal hearing. The results of these studies show qualitative and quantitative differences in the prelinguistic vocalizations of infants with hearing loss compared with their peers. However, these studies and others like them were conducted before the development of EHDI programs.

More recent research has suggested that if hearing loss is identified and amplification is provided early on, the difference in speech and language development of children with hearing loss will not differ greatly from and may even parallel their peers with normal hearing. Mary Pat Moeller and colleagues at the Boys Town National Research Hospital are currently investigating the speech and language outcomes of children with early identified hearing losses. They conducted a longitudinal investigation of prelinguistic vocalizations and the early use of words in children whose hearing losses were identified, diagnosed, and managed via hearing aids or cochlear implants through EHDI programs. They followed 21 infants with normal hearing and 12 with hearing loss from ages 10 to 24 months, videotaping their mother-child interactions in a laboratory setting. One consistent finding was that there was no difference in the amount of vocalizations between the two groups from 8.5 to 12 months. However, some of the infants with hearing loss were delayed in the development of **canonical babbling**. Briefly, early babbling consists of children's experimentation with vocalizations made up of mostly vowels or even noises like raspberries. Canonical babbling is an advanced form, consisting of consonant-vowel (e.g., CV like /ba/) or consonant-vowel-consonant-vowel (e.g., CVCV like /baba/) syllables. It was found that those infants with moderately severe hearing losses were not delayed in their babbling, but that those with more severe degrees of hearing loss were. However, these children started babbling between two and six months after receiving their cochlear implants. Similar to previous findings, the children with hearing loss did not have as many consonants in their inventories, particularly in the use of fricative and affricates. Moeller et al. (2007) hypothesized that the children's delay in fricative acquisition may be due to several factors: (1) their hearing losses; (2) limitations in high-frequency spectral energy accessed via their hearing aids and/or cochlear implants; and/or (3) masking of cues by noise and reverberation.

Babbling behaviors set the foundation for the use of single words in meaningful speech at about 1 year of age. Early syllabic productions pave the way for a baby's first words (McCure & Vihman, 2001). Their vocalizations transition from jargon, to babble, to attempts at words, and then to intelligible speech at about 12 months of age. Children's **lexicons**, or sets of words, expand from just a few at 12 months of age to more than 50 items at 18 months (Moeller, 2010). Between 18 and 22 months of age, children have a "growth spurt" in their vocabularies, doubling to 100 words by 21 to 23 months (Moeller, 2010). Nott, Cowan, Brown, and Wigglesworth (2009) found that children with profound hearing losses who were identified early and fit with cochlear implants were delayed in vocabulary development. These results are consistent with earlier studies that found that children with varying degrees of hearing loss were about 6 months delayed in their vocabulary "growth spurts" (Mayne, Yoshinaga-Itano, Sedey, & Carey, 2000).

At around 2 years of age, only about 50% of children's speech is actually intelligible because of immature phonological systems and language abilities (Stoel-Gammon, 1998). Slowly the data regarding the changes in developmental trajectories for graduates of NHSPs are becoming available. In a companion study to the one discussed in the previous paragraph, Moeller and colleagues (2007) expanded their longitudinal study and analyzed children's vocalizations on communicative intent and intelligibility. Both groups of children increased their use of purposeful speech, but those with hearing impairment used fewer intelligible words than their peers with normal hearing who were already using two-word phrases by 2 years of age. Moreover, the words of the children with normal hearing were judged to be more complex on several measures than those uttered by toddlers with hearing loss. Overall, these children were more delayed in their transition from babbling to word use, but demonstrated parallel trajectories of development to their peers with normal hearing. Ultimately, however, these delays in development impacted their spoken language development. Nevertheless, these later studies of children who have gone through EHDI programs are showing better speech and language outcomes than their predecessors.

The results of other studies, however, have shown that early diagnosis of hearing loss is not enough and that careful selection of the type of early intervention can impact outcomes.

For example, McGowan, Nittrouer, and Chenausky (2008) compared the vocalizations of 12-month-olds with and without hearing loss for syllable shape, consonant type, and formant frequencies of vowels. The infants with hearing loss had participated in EHDI programs with diagnosis of hearing loss by 3 months and intervention started by 6 months of age. Surprisingly, they found similar results to studies conducted before NHSPs, with the infants with hearing loss producing fewer fricatives, alveolar/velar stops, and multisyllabic utterances. Although both groups had similar use of tongue height, infants with hearing loss had a more restricted lingual movement in the front-to-back dimension during vowel production. McGowan et al. (2008) stated that appropriate amplification, selection of communication mode, and method of facilitating development of oral language with exposure to an abundance of linguistic experiences are paramount in closing the gaps in speech and language development between children with hearing loss and their peers with normal hearing. The next two sections discuss selection of communication mode and approaches to oral language development in children with hearing impairment.

SELECTION OF COMMUNICATION MODE

One of the most important decisions for parents is selection of a communication mode for their children. All too often, parents are rushed into making a decision before they are emotionally ready and fully knowledgeable about the strengths and weaknesses of various options (Gravel & O'Gara, 2003). Audiologists and speech-language pathologists may be biased in their presentation of various communication modes to parents. However, the JCIH Year 2007 Position Statement recommends that families should be aware of all options and that the information they receive should be presented in an unbiased manner. It is important to realize that no one approach works for everyone and that the decision is a highly personal one. There are three major communication modes for parents to consider: Auditory-Oral approach, Total Communication, and American Sign Language.

The **Auditory-Oral** or **Aural-Oral** communication mode stresses the development of spoken English (oral) through the use of amplification (aural), the learning of speechreading, and the discouragement of signing (English, 2002). The oral-aural approach was supported by Alexander Graham Bell. Pure oralism, or the auditory stimulation approach, developed at the Clarke School for the Deaf in Northampton, Massachusetts, strongly discourages the use of sign language and advocates that children have abundant auditory stimulation and exposure to spoken language progressing from individual speech sounds to syllables, words, and sentences (Northern & Downs, 2002). The goals for the preschool program are for children to develop sensory awareness, age-appropriate gross/fine motor, cognitive, and social skills with an emphasis on educating family members (Clarke Schools for Hearing and Speech [CSHS], 2010a). Today, the Clarke Schools for Hearing and Speech are leaders in auditory-oral deaf education, providing both campus-based and outreach services. Early intervention, kindergarten, and preschool programs exist on the Northampton Campus in addition to satellite programs at the Clarke School East in Boston, Clarke Jacksonville in Florida, Clarke New York City, and Clarke Pennsylvania in Philadelphia. For example, the Clarke Pennsylvania Auditory/Oral Center's staff of audiologists, certified deaf educators, early childhood educators, and speech-language pathologists have developed early intervention programs to demonstrate to families from the time of their children's diagnosis of hearing loss, how they may enrich their children's lives with meaningful sounds, language, and play (Clarke School for Hearing and Speech [CSHS], 2010b). Staff work with families in home environments; conduct biweekly meetings for families to provide information on topics such as hearing loss, child development, and ways to stimulate emerging spoken language skills; and create opportunities for toddlers to interact with each other to develop preschool readiness skills (CSHS, 2010b). Children attend the preschool and kindergarten classes five days a week that offer typical curricula developing pre-academic skills with an emphasis on the development of sensory awareness, age-appropriate fine and gross motor skills, cognition, and social skills (CSHS, 2010b). The mission of these auditory/oral programs is to provide children who are deaf and hard of hearing the self-confidence and skills to participate as independent, contributing members of society.

The Auditory-Oral method has been criticized for its emphasis on lipreading because many sounds of the English language look the same on the mouth (e.g., *b*an, *m*an, and *p*an), many sounds cannot be seen, and most talkers do not speak clearly (Northern & Downs, 2002). To improve on traditional oral methods, Doreen Pollack developed the Acoupedic Approach, which is today known as the Auditory-Verbal approach (Pollack, 1983). The Auditory-Verbal approach is a **unisensory approach** emphasizing the use of audition for the development of spoken language while discouraging the reliance on speechreading. The Auditory-Verbal approach is based upon a logical and critical set of guiding principles that enable children who are deaf and hard of hearing to use even minimal amounts of residual hearing provided by hearing aids or hearing through cochlear implants to listen, to process verbal language, and to speak (AG Bell Academy for Listening and Spoken Language [AGBALSL], 2010). The guiding principles of the Auditory-Verbal approach are as follows (AGBALSL, 2010):

- To detect hearing impairment as early as possible through screening programs, ideally in the newborn nursery and throughout childhood.
- To pursue prompt and vigorous medical and audiologic management, including selection, modification, and maintenance of appropriate hearing aids, cochlear implants, or other sensory aids.
- To guide, counsel, and support parents and caregivers as the primary models for spoken language through listening and to help them understand the impact of deafness and impaired hearing on the entire family.
- To help children integrate listening into their development of communication and social skills.
- To support children's Auditory-Verbal development through one-to-one teaching.
- To help children monitor their own voices and the voices of others in order to enhance the intelligibility of their spoken language.
- To use developmental patterns of listening, language, speech, and cognition to stimulate natural communication.
- To continually assess and evaluate children's development in the preceding areas and, through diagnostic intervention, modify the program when needed.
- To provide support services to facilitate children's educational and social inclusion in regular education classes.

Auditory-Verbal is a family-centered program; parents are taught how to integrate the principles of the approach into their everyday lives (Estabrooks, 1994). Mealtime, bath time, and getting dressed are transformed into contexts for auditory learning. Children are constantly stimulated with sounds, with a focus on the development of their auditory abilities. A **"hand cue"** in which clinicians and parents cover their mouths while speaking is frequently used, eliminating visual cues and encouraging children to rely on and develop their auditory skills (Pollack, 1993).

The main goal of Auditory-Verbal is to integrate hearing into the identities of children who are hard of hearing or deaf so that they may be fully functioning and contributing members of society (Goldberg, 1996). Auditory-Verbal is discussed in greater detail in Chapter 10.

Parents who select the Auditory-Oral mode of communication must commit to ensuring that their children consistently wear amplification, attend auditory habilitation therapy, and create a home environment for the maximization of auditory skill and spoken language development. Parents should be open to other modes of communication such as Total Communication or the use of American Sign Language when the Auditory-Oral mode does not meet their children's communication needs.

Total Communication (TC) is the use of any form of communication to teach English to children who are deaf, including sign language, voice, fingerspelling, lipreading, amplification, vibrotactile stimulation, gestures, or even pictures. The type of signing that accompanies spoken messages varies with the speaker who may use American Sign Language or a signed system such as Signing Exact English (SEE), or a combination of ASL and SEE called **Pidgin Sign** (English, 2002). **Signing Exact English** is a manual communication system that aims to represent spoken English on the hands as accurately as possible. One advantage of TC is that it provides the child with both an auditory and visual message; the meaning is understood regardless of individual preferences in communication modality. Alternatively, there are several criticisms of TC. First, providing a child with both auditory and visual representations of a message may result in "sensory overload." Second, advocates of American Sign Language (ASL) advise that when SEE is used, children are exposed to neither English nor ASL, but to something that only partially resembles English (Bowe, 2004). Third, TC may place children at a disadvantage because the vast majority of society does not use TC as a communication mode. Moreover, families must make a strong commitment to learn and use the type of signing. Learning a sign system is not easy, and may require taking classes and extensive practice to accommodate and facilitate their children's rate of acquisition. Fourth, the effectiveness of TC in the classroom depends on the skills of the teacher, the number of students in the class, their learning styles, hearing levels, and age of onset of deafness (Ogden, 1996). For example, teachers must struggle to meet the linguistic needs of each student while involving the entire class in a single activity. Let's look in on Jessie Baxter, teacher of the hearing-impaired class at Brice Elementary during her meeting with her principal, Dolores Vasquez.

Casebook Reflection

Difficulty in the Classroom

Ms. Vasquez: "Hi Jessie, how has it been going?"

Ms. Baxter: "Pretty well, but I'm having difficulty in my classroom with the addition of Bobby Owen. He is the boy from Baldwin County with the profound sensorineural hearing loss. His parents are deaf and he is fluent in ASL, but his English skills are far behind those of the other children in the class. He is very frustrated and seems like he is giving up. When I simplify the material for Bobby, the others get bored, act out, or tune out."

Ms. Vasquez: "Jessie, what do you think may help?"

Ms. Baxter: "I think that a paraprofessional skilled in TC could assist in the adaptation of the material to his level so that I could continue with the others."

Ms. Vasquez: "I'll come in and observe your class. We will be having Bobby's initial IEP meeting in a few weeks."

Ms. Baxter: "Thanks, Ms. Vasquez."

Ms. Vasquez: "Thanks for keeping me informed, Jessie."

After Ms. Vasquez observed Jessie's classroom, she saw how a paraprofessional was needed to support Bobby in the classroom, which was written into his individualized education program. The addition of the paraprofessional immediately resulted in Bobby's engagement in classroom activities without impeding the others' progress.

American Sign Language (ASL) is the language of the Deaf community with an estimated user population of 500,000 to 2,000,000. In fact, ASL is the fifth leading minority language in the United States after Spanish, Italian, French, and German. The population of ASL users has transmitted their language from generation to generation by various means, assuring a rich culture for the Deaf (Lane, Hoeffmeister, & Bahan, 1996). As any language, ASL has its own grammar. Bilingual-biculturalism is an approach that advocates teaching deaf children American Sign Language as a primary language and English as a second language. Advocates of the bilingual-bicultural education believe that American Sign Language can serve as a basis for building knowledge about both conversation and school language (Lane et al., 1996). However, ASL has been criticized because it has no written form, delaying the learning of reading and writing until children have mastered their native language to serve as a basis for literacy (Bowe, 2004). Families considering ASL as an option must develop a bilingual-bicultural environment by becoming fluent in another language and assimilating into the Deaf community. A bilingual-bicultural approach mandates that children have access to the Deaf community and its members who may serve as role models. Parents may experience some skepticism from some members of the Deaf community and should be counseled on the origins of their mistrust of the hearing establishment.

Some programs have been developed to implement a bilingual-bicultural home environment. For example, the Deaf-Mentor Outreach Project of the SKI-HI Institute (i.e., Sensory Kids Impaired Home Intervention) assists families with deaf children in implementing a bilingual-bicultural, home-based program (Deaf Mentor, 2006). The program provides the family opportunities for scheduling regular visits by a deaf adult or mentor who interacts with the child using ASL, shows how to implement the language within the home, and fosters an appreciation for Deaf culture (Deaf Mentor, 2006). The program has a strong commitment to the training of Deaf mentors and parent advisors. A *Deaf Mentor Curriculum Manual* has been published and is available from HOPE, Inc. Contact information for this program and HOPE, Inc. is provided in Appendix 9.1. Other types of manual communication invented for educational purposes are covered in Chapter 10.

METHODS OF FACILITATING ORAL LANGUAGE DEVELOPMENT IN CHILDREN WHO ARE DEAF AND HARD OF HEARING

Selection of a communication mode is different than selection of an auditory habilitative approach that facilitates oral language development of children who are deaf and hard of hearing. In most cases, parents select the communication philosophy first, and if they select an aural/oral philosophy, they then select an auditory habilitative approach. An **auditory habilitative approach** is a particular methodology used to develop the auditory, speech, and language skills through a child's use of his or her residual hearing. Auditory habilitationists may use **specific** or **eclectic approaches** to auditory habilitation. Several specific auditory habilitative approaches have been developed over the years such as the Auditory-Verbal Approach, the Ling Method, and Verbotonal Method. Auditory habilitationists may use a specific approach reflecting their clinical training or place of employment. For example, the Dade County Public School System in Miami, Florida, uses the Verbotonal Method in its program for students who are deaf and hard of hearing. However, the majority of communication and sciences and disorders professionals providing auditory habilitation use an eclectic or a combination of techniques that are common to several of these approaches.

Another excellent program is the previously mentioned SKI-HI Program, which was the first program of the SKI-HI Institute located within the Department of Communication Disorders and Deaf Education at Utah State University (SKI-HI Institute, 2010). The Institute provides outreach to families with children who have hearing, visual, and/or other disabilities within the United States and Canada. The SKI-HI Institute is based on the premise that the family is the most important factor in a child's development and that the home is the most natural learning environment, with intervention implemented in other important settings such as preschool and daycare centers. The SKI-HI Institute provides a plethora of resource materials for each of its projects. For example, the SKI-HI resource manual provides details on individualizing home-based programs to meet the needs of each child and family and provides information and activities on early communication, audition, hearing aids, ASL, aural-oral languages, total communication, and psycho-educational support (SKI-HI). In addition, the manual assists in the implementation of information gathering, assessment, and planning needed for the development of the Individual Family Services Plan (IFSP) (SKI-HI).

Readers might be wondering, which approach is the best? The same question is asked by parents of deaf and hard-of-hearing children. As with any health problem, parents want to know the best treatment that is available for their child. Communication sciences and disorders professionals should encourage parents to use an evidence-based approach when considering auditory habilitative approaches for their children.

What Does the Evidence Show?

Parents of children with hearing loss have several auditory habilitation approaches to choose from. Which one is best? Which one has the best outcomes? Unfortunately, no double-blinded, randomized controlled clinical trials have been conducted to establish the efficacy of one approach over another. Nevertheless, although parents can't wait for research to be done, they can be taught to be critical consumers of information that they may read in the newspaper and see on television by recognizing characteristics of treatments for hearing loss that have yet to be substantiated by research.

Tharpe (1998) warned that fad or alternative treatments have four recognizable characteristics. First, fad treatments are often based on *concepts outside the mainstream*. Frequently, parents do not have the sophistication of recognizing concepts out of the mainstream, but they can be told that if a treatment sounds too good to be true, then it probably is. Second, a fad treatment usually has an *initial burst of popularity prior to demonstrated effectiveness*. Parents should be wary in accepting enthusiastic clinician recommendations and parental reports as a substitute for empirical evidence. Third, most of the articles on fad treatments are published in *nonrefereed publications.* Nonrefereed publications are those that do not require a review by an author's professional peers prior to publication. For example, every article published in the *Journal of Speech-Language-Hearing Research* has undergone a critical scientific review process by three reviewers, an associate editor, and the editor of the journal. Examples of nonrefereed publications in the field include *The Hearing Journal, The Hearing Review, Hearing Loss,* and so on. Parents should seek out articles that have been published in peer-reviewed journals when evaluating various approaches for their children.

Tharpe (1998) demonstrated how ineffective treatments can demonstrate improvement in patients due to several possible phenomena. First, she explains that the severity of symptoms for patients with chronic healthcare conditions fluctuates, and when left untreated, tends to return to some average level or state. For example, patients may seek medical treatment for their health conditions when symptoms are at their greatest severity. The physician may prescribe some treatment that may or may not be effective, but the condition may get better with or without the treatment due to the natural course of the disease process. Similarly, even though sensorineural hearing loss is not a "disease" that benefits from medical intervention per se, intervention approaches can be used to improve a child's communication skills, but advancement in speech and language development may be due to the child's maturation and not necessarily to the specific treatment approach.

The other three phenomena resulting in patient improvement with ineffective treatments are inherent to interventional research that are not double-blinded, randomized controlled clinical trials (DBRCT). Recall that DBRCT requires that subjects are randomly assigned to treatment or control groups reducing selection bias. In addition, in these studies, both experimenters and the participants are unaware of the assignment to treatment or control groups, reducing the experimenter and subject bias on the results. Unfortunately, few if any DBRCTs have been done assessing the efficacy of auditory habilitation methods. Therefore, ineffective treatments may show improvement in results due to experimenter and subject and/or expectation bias. **Experimenter bias** is anything that investigators do, either consciously or subconsciously, that may affect the results of a study. For example, all researchers have some bias or hypothesis that they want to test in an experiment. A researcher investigating the efficiency of Auditory-Verbal Therapy over Total Communication may provide more praise and support to children and their families receiving their favorite approach versus the other. Similarly, **subject bias** is anything that participants do consciously or subconsciously to affect the results of a study. For example, parents may work harder with their children if they are enrolled in a study to assess the effectiveness of an intervention in which they have made considerable investment. **Expectation bias** is anything that may be done by researchers or participants who expect certain results in an experiment that actually influences the outcomes of a study. Even without any bias toward a particular intervention, the **Hawthorne effect**, or the tendency for participants to act differently when they know they are part of a research experiment, is a common occurrence in studies. In summary, parents need to be careful consumers of auditory habilitation methods by keeping watch for characteristics of fad treatments and realizing that even ineffective treatments can show positive outcomes under certain conditions.

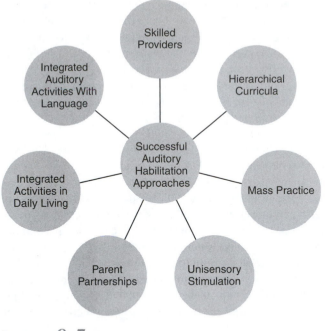

As in many areas of auditory rehabilitation, no double-blinded, randomized controlled clinical trials have been done to suggest the efficacy of one approach over another. However, as mentioned previously, parents can be advised to be wary of fad treatments and realize that even ineffective treatments can and do show promising results. Parents should also be skeptical of programs that strongly encourage a "one-size-fits-all" approach to auditory habilitation. Children who are deaf and hard of hearing and their family members are unique individuals with regard to their strengths and weaknesses. Auditory habilitation approaches should be flexible enough to accommodate individual needs of children and their families.

Yoshinaga-Itano (2000) stated that successful auditory habilitation approaches share seven common characteristics as shown in Figure 9.5. The first characteristic is that clinicians are *skilled providers* of auditory habilitation services. Direct service providers should have the necessary training, certification, and/or licensure in providing auditory habilitation to young children. Preferably, parents should ask how much experience practitioners have in providing services to infants and toddlers

figure *9.5*—

Characteristics of effective aural habilitation approaches.

Source: Based on "Preschool Children Who Are Deaf and Hard of Hearing," by C. Yoshinaga-Itano, 2000, in J. G. Alpiner and P. A. McCarthy (Eds.), *Rehabilitative Audiology: Children and Adults,* (pp. 140–177), Philadelphia: Lippincott Williams & Wilkins.

who are deaf and hard of hearing. For example, Auditory-Verbal International has specific requirements for practitioners to become certified therapists that involve attending workshops, mentoring, and clinical clock hours. Moreover, the JCIH Year 2007 Position Statement recommended that early intervention services should be provided by professionals who have knowledge, skills, and experiences in working with children with hearing loss and their families. Second, auditory habilitation approaches should have *hierarchical curricula* based on sound scientific evidence. Parents should be able to understand how their children will progress in therapy and what outcomes may be expected. Third, auditory habilitation approaches must incorporate *mass practice* of auditory, speech, and language skills. Children who are deaf and hard of hearing require conscious practice of skills that children with normal hearing develop naturally. Fourth, auditory habilitation approaches that promote *unisensory stimulation* requiring children to develop their residual hearing seem to have better outcomes than those programs that do not. Fifth, successful auditory habilitation approaches work closely not only with children but their *parents as partners* in the process. Sixth, auditory habilitation approaches should *integrate auditory training into activities of daily living* and seventh, *integrate auditory activities with language training*. For example, auditory training should be incorporated into common activities (e.g., getting dressed, mealtime, going to the store, and so on) such that each and every opportunity for receptive and expressive language development is exploited to the greatest possible extent.

Some recent studies have shown that auditory habilitation approaches with these principles have positive outcomes. For example, Nittrouer and Burton (2001) found that children who were provided with intensive preschool oral education performed similarly to their peers with normal hearing on a variety of speech perception and linguistic processing tasks. Alternatively, children who had been placed in general special education preschools performed much more poorly, even though their degree of hearing loss and other characteristics were comparable to the group receiving an oral education. Similarly, Tobey, Rekart, Buckley, and Geers (2004) found that after cochlear implantation, higher achievement in speech intelligibility scores was associated with placement in educational settings focusing on oral education. Furthermore, the earlier children who are deaf and hard of hearing are fit with either hearing aids or receive a cochlear implant, the better chance they have of acquiring communication skills commensurate with their peers with normal hearing (McConkey Robbins, Koch, Zimmerman-Phillips, & Kishon-Rabin, 2004).

Brackett (2002) states that audiologists and speech-language pathologists should form a collaborative partnership with parents in selecting an auditory habilitation program for their children. She believes that these practitioners can serve as "independent" listeners and reactors that can discuss, guide, lead, inform, and review information with the parents. She listed the following possible multifaceted roles of audiologists and speech-language pathologists:

- Serve as information sources
- Facilitate the parental network
- Collaborate with professionals
- Help with parental review of information and options
- Review family communication assets
- Review child's skills/assets
- Discuss future desires/outcomes
- Help parents ask questions

In summary, audiologists and speech-language pathologists should build partnerships with parents through all phases of EHDI programming: screening, diagnosis, and intervention. Advocating for parents requires knowledge of special education and the process to initiate services under the Individuals with Disabilities Education Improvement Act (2004).

SPECIAL EDUCATION SERVICES FOR CHILDREN WITH HEARING LOSS

Early intervention services for children between 0 and 2 years of age and who are deaf and hard of hearing are mandated by special education law. We will begin with a brief review of special education law and then discuss receiving services.

Special Education Law

Special education for children with hearing loss is governed by the Individuals with Disabilities Education Act, the IDEA. On November 19, 1975, Congress passed the Education for All

Handicapped Children's Act, or Public Law 94-142, in order to accomplish specific goals that are cited in the current Implementing Regulations, at 34 CFR 34 CFR 300.1:

> The purposes of this part of IDEA are:
>
> (a) to ensure that all children with disabilities have available to them a free appropriate public education that emphasizes special education, designed to meet their unique needs and prepare them for employment and independent living,
> (b) to ensure that the rights of children with disabilities and their parents are protected,
> (c) to assist States, localities, educational service agencies, and Federal agencies in providing for the education of all children with disabilities, and
> (d) to assess and ensure the effectiveness of efforts to educate children with disabilities.
>
> (Authority: 20 U. S. C. 1400 note)

Prior to 1975, many students with disabilities were provided with inadequate education or no education at all. Johnson (2000) stated that numerous states permitted schools to exclude students with disabilities from their mandatory attendance laws; the only options for deaf and hard of hearing was a state school for the deaf. Three important Supreme Court decisions helped pave the way for PL-94-142. First, in 1954, the Supreme Court stated in its decision in *Brown v. the Board of Education of Topeka, Kansas* (1954) that a separate education is unequal. Johnson stated that although *Brown vs. the Board of Education* was based on racial segregation, parents of children with disabilities began filing suit against their school systems for their children to receive equal educational opportunity. In 1972, the Supreme Court stated that public education must include children with disabilities in its decisions on the following two landmark cases:

* *Pennsylvania Association for Retarded Citizens (PARC) v. Pennsylvania,*334 F. Supp. 1257 (Pa. 1972)
* *Mills v. Washington D.C. Board of Education,* 348 F. Supp. 866 (D.C. 1972)

Public Law 94-142 was a funding statute stipulating that in order to receive federal funding, each state must develop a plan to ensure requirements of the law. PL-94-142 has been amended at least seven times, most recently on December 3, 2004, when President George W. Bush signed the legislation that is now Public Law 108-446.

The IDEA has some important underpinnings that serve as fundamental principles regarding the education of children with disabilities. Two fundamental principles are *Zero Reject* and *Free and Appropriate Public Education.* The principle of **zero reject** is that schools cannot refuse to provide a program for a child, regardless of the disability (Johnson, 2000). The explanation of **free and appropriate public education** requires analyzing the phrase part by part. "Free" means educational programs and services (e.g., evaluations, transportation, and related services) must be provided at no cost to parents (Johnson, 2000). For children with hearing loss, the public agency should pay for audiologic evaluations in addition to FM systems and other assistive listening devices, if it is "appropriate" for the child. Other accommodations that are covered include the use of interpreters for extracurricular activities. "Public education" means that IDEA applies to all public educational agencies and charter schools.

Another fundamental principle of the IDEA is the concept of the **least restrictive environment** (LRE), which means that to the greatest extent possible, children with hearing loss should be educated with their peers who are nondisabled. The LRE concept has been associated with **mainstreaming**, which is educating children with disabilities with their nondisabled peers. Mainstreaming is not an all-or-nothing situation, but consists of a series of options along a continuum from the least (i.e., integrated) to most (i.e., segregated) restrictive.

Another fundamental principle of the IDEA is **procedural safeguards**, which help ensure protections of the rights of children with disabilities and their families. Parents have rights such as (Johnson, 2000; Wrightslaw.com, 2010):

- to give informed consent
- to examine any records pertaining to their child
- to expect confidentiality of personally identifiable information
- to disagree with a proposed individualized education plan (IEP) or its implementation

Parents also have the right to be involved in all meetings, to prior written notice concerning matters related to their child, to obtain an independent evaluation, and to file a complaint (Johnson, 2000; Wrightslaw.com, 2010). The foundational principles of the IDEA are covered in more detail in Chapter 10.

Receiving Special Education Services Through the IDEIA (2004)

Children with hearing loss may begin to receive special education services via a special education referral. According to the IDEA, state educational agencies have a responsibility to identify children with disabilities. In all 50 states, referral for an evaluation must be made to a public agency (e.g., Health Department) within two working days of identification (Roush, 2000). For hearing loss, over 45 states have mandated NHSPs that can identify children at birth for hearing loss with diagnosis by 3 months of age, hearing aid fitting within 1 month of diagnosis, and intervention by 6 months of age (JCIH, 2007). The initial evaluation determines whether a child's disability would qualify the child for special education services. The law defines deafness as "a hearing impairment that is so severe that the child is impaired in processing linguistic information through hearing with or without amplification, [and] that adversely affects a child's educational performance." Moreover, the law defines hearing impairment as "an impairment in hearing, whether permanent or fluctuating, that adversely affects a child's educational performance, but that is not included under the definition of deafness in this section." Each state defines a minimum decibel loss for a classification of hearing impairment.

For children 0 to 2 years of age who qualify for special education services, the public agency will assign families a service coordinator, preferably in the area pertaining to the child's disability, who assists the family through the screening, diagnosis, and intervention of the child's hearing loss (JCIH, 2007). Parents should have access to the state's central directory, which contains information on available early intervention, service providers, and resources. Early intervention programs may provide services from both the public agencies and service providers in the private sector. The role of service coordinator is to schedule testing of the child and to organize the development, review, and implementation of the **individual family service plans** (IFSPs) reflecting the family preferences for communication options (JCIH, 2007). Infants and toddlers and their families must have an IFSP developed by an interdisciplinary team within 45 days of receiving a referral (Roush, 2000). An IFSP is a written document developed by a team of professionals that states the programs, services, and equipment that the public agency must provide to the child and his or her family. The IFSP team frequently includes the parent; other family members; the service coordinator; the evaluation team; professionals providing services, including audiologists; and any others that the family may request. The goal of the IFSP is to create a way for professionals and families to meet intended goals. An important part of the IFSP is to discuss transition planning for children and their families from IDEA Part C, infant/toddler early intervention, to Part B services involving preschool and public school programs. Each child and his or her family should have a plan with activities designed to ease the transition to a new school and to ensure that appropriate accommodations are planned for and services are in place. Activities may include, but are not limited to talking with parents about the transition, a visit by the child and family to the new school, practice of skills needed for success in the next placement, and so on. Transition planning is critical for the success of young children who are deaf and hard of hearing in preschool settings; this concept will be discussed in the next chapter.

DUAL SENSORY IMPAIRMENT IN YOUNG CHILDREN

Dual sensory impairment is present when a person has concurrent visual and hearing impairment, which may be the result of any or a combination of over 70 known causes such as prematurity, viral infections, brain diseases, Usher, and CHARGE syndromes. For example, **Usher syndrome** is the most common condition that causes concurrent hearing and vision (e.g., retinitis pigmentosa) problems that get worse over time (National Institute on Deafness and other Communication Disorders [NIDCD], 2009). It is estimated that 3% to 6% of children who are deaf and hard of hearing have Usher syndrome (NIDCD, 2009). Similarly, **CHARGE syndrome**, a recognizable and often life-threatening birth defect, occurs in approximately 1 in every 9,000 to 10,000 births and may cause craniofacial anomalies, complex heart and breathing problems, as well as vision, hearing, and balance impairments (CHARGE Syndrome Association, 2010).

All children under 3 years of age should have their vision screened, but particularly children with hearing loss. As discussed earlier in the chapter, the JCIH Year 2007 Position Statement recommends that all children diagnosed with hearing loss be referred for a visual acuity screening performed by a pediatric ophthalmologist. It is estimated that 1 in 10 to 1 in 20, or between 5% and 10%, of all preschool children have undetected visual impairment. Three common types of visual impairment in young children include amblyopia, strabismus, and abnormal refractive errors. **Amblyopia** is also known as "lazy eye" and is the result of one eye failing to develop normally, but can be corrected during infancy or early childhood (University of Michigan Kellogg Eye Center [UMKEC], 2006a). **Strabismus** is known as "cross eye" or wall eye, meaning that patients cannot align their eyes at the same time under normal conditions, with one of the eyes turning in, up, or out (UMKEC, 2006b). **Abnormal refractive errors** include astigmatisms, hyperopia, and myopia. **Astigmatism** is a condition in which there is an irregular curvature of the cornea causing problems in how light is focused within the eye and occurs frequently with hyperopia or myopia (UMKEC, 2006c). **Hyperopia** is known as farsightedness, is usually inherited, and may result in blurred vision, difficulty seeing objects close up, and/or crossing of the eyes in children (UMKEC, 2006d). Alternatively, **myopia** is known as nearsightedness, is usually inherited, and is frequently diagnosed in childhood, causing blurred vision and difficulty seeing distant objects (UMKEC, 2006e).

The American Academy of Pediatrics Eye Evaluation Guidelines (2003) suggest obtaining children's ocular history, vision assessment, external inspection of the eyes and lids, ocular motility assessment, pupil examination, and red reflex examination. The American Academy of Ophthalmology supports screening of young children because impairments may interfere with developing normal vision, good health, and academic skills. In fact, untreated visual disorders can lead to permanent impairment (Giangiacomo & Morey, 2005; Jakobsson, Kvarnström, Abrahamsson, Bjernbrink-Hörnblad, & Sunnqvist, 2002; Simon & Kaw, 2001). For example, untreated amblyopia presents a risk for visual impairment if vision is lost in the better eye (Good-Lite, 2006). Healthcare professionals, including audiologists and speech-language pathologists, should ask parents about any vision screenings or presence of any visual disorders in their young children or their families. Furthermore, it is important to know the visual developmental milestones for children birth to 5 years of age that are shown in Table 9.5.

Early identification of dual sensory impairment is necessary for referring these children and their families with critical early intervention services. Some early intervention programs are available for these families. For example, the SPARKLE (**S**upporting **P**arent **A**ccess to **R**esources, **K**nowledge, **L**inkages, and **E**ducation) program is offered through the SKI-HI Institute discussed earlier and is for families with young children who are deaf and blind. SPARKLE is a training program provided to parents via DVD technology, a parent guidebook, and website (SPARKLE, 2010). The website has a Family Room where parents can receive important information and inspirational stories about other families in addition to an Internet listserv for discussion on deaf-blind topics (SPARKLE). We will discuss the impact of dual sensory impairment across the lifespan in subsequent chapters.

table *9.5*   Vision Developmental Milestones for Children

0 to 3 Months
- Turns eyes and head to look at light sources
- Briefly holds gaze on bright lights or objects
- Stares at surroundings
- Blinks at camera flash
- Moves eyes and head together
- Tracks vertically and horizontally
- Begins eye contact at 6 to 8 weeks

3 to 6 Months
- Follows moving objects with eyes across midline
- Begins moving eyes with less head movement
- Watches own hands before face
- Looks at hands, food, or bottle when sitting
- Watches face when spoken to
- Briefly fixates on still objects
- Reaches for small objects

7 to 12 Months
- Orients to objects in home
- May turn eyes inward when looking at hands or toys
- Notices small objects, like cereal
- Interested in pictures
- Enjoys hide-and-seek (recognizes partially hidden objects)
- Inspects toys held in hands
- Responds to smiles and voices
- Sweeps eyes across room

1 to 2 Years
- Uses "pincer grasp" to hold objects between forefinger and thumb
- Looks for toys that fall out of sight
- Builds tower with 3 blocks
- Enjoys pictures books and points to pictures
- Uses both hands
- Holds objects close to eyes to inspect

(*Continued*)

table *9.5*   *(Continued)*

2 to 3 Years

- Builds towers with 6 blocks
- Imitates vertical line
- Recognizes people in photographs
- Begins to inspect objects without touching objects
- Smiles and brightens face when looking at favorite people or objects
- Likes to watch movement of object, such as wheels on a toy vehicle
- Watches and imitates other children
- "Reads" pictures in books
- Begins to control hand movement while coloring or drawing

4 to 5 Years

- Copies a cross, square, and triangle
- Draws a person with head, trunk, and limbs
- Draws recognizable person and house and names pictures
- Uses eyes and hands together with increasing skill
- Moves and rolls eyes expressively
- Can place small objects into small openings
- Demonstrates visual interest in new "stuff"
- Cuts and pastes simple projects

3 to 4 Years

- Copies a circle
- Begins to know colors
- Cuts with scissors
- Brings head and eyes close to page of a book
- Can close eyes on request and may be able to wink

Source: Pediatric Vision Screening from Good-Lite, by Good-Lite, 2006, Author: Elgin, IL.

SUMMARY

This chapter addressed the continuum of hearing healthcare through EHDI programs consisting of screening, diagnosis, and intervention with particular emphasis on parental preferences and experiences. Early intervention with young children who are deaf and hard of hearing begins after the initial diagnosis of hearing loss. Audiologists and speech-language pathologists serve an important role in the transition from initial diagnosis of hearing loss to early intervention. One important task for parents is to select a communication mode. This chapter also reviewed reasons why parents should partner with audiologists for evidence-based decision-making in selecting an auditory habilitation approach by focusing on characteristics of fad treatments and ways that even ineffective interventions can show promising results. The characteristics of successful auditory habilitative approaches were reviewed along with some basics on special education law and early intervention services. The chapter concluded with a discussion of dual sensory impairment in young children.

LEARNING ACTIVITIES

- Investigate whether your state has mandated universal newborn hearing screening. What types of early intervention services are available for infants and toddlers who are deaf and hard of hearing in your community?
- Interview a parent of a child who was diagnosed with a hearing loss. Ask him or her what was particularly difficult in receiving the diagnosis. Ask him or her, "If you could change anything about the way you were told, what would it be?"
- Develop two skits with your classmates illustrating the right way and the wrong way of breaking the news of a child's diagnosis of sensorineural hearing loss to parents. Video-tape the two skits and see if others in the class can pick out what's right and wrong in each scenario.
- Assemble a Parent Resource Notebook by visiting the websites of organizations listed in Appendix 9.1 and printing out free materials available to the public. Use dividers and organize the material so that it will be helpful to you or a professional in working with parents.

APPENDIX 9.1
Parent Resources

Alexander Graham Bell Association for the Deaf and Hard of Hearing
3417 Volta Place, N.W.
Washington, DC 20007-2778
(202) 337-5220 Voice
(202) 337-5221 TTY
(202) 337-8314 FAX
www.agbell.org/

American Academy of Audiology
11730 Plaza America Drive, Suite 300
Reston, VA 20190
1 (800) AAA-2336 Voice
(703) 790-8631 FAX
www.audiology.org/

American Society for Deaf Children
800 Florida Ave NE, #2047
Washington, DC 20002-3695
1 (800) 942-2732 Voice and TTY
1 (866) 895-4206
(410) 795-0965 FAX
www.deafchildren.org/

American Speech-Language-Hearing Association
2200 Research Boulevard
Rockville, MD 20850-3289
1 (800) 638-8255
(301) 296-5650 TTY
(301) 296-8580 FAX
www.asha.org/

American Tinnitus Association
P.O. Box 5
Portland, OR 97207-0005
(503) 248-9985 Voice
1 (800) 634-8978 Toll Free
(503) 248-0024 Fax
www.ata.org/

Beginnings for Parents of Hearing-Impaired Children
302 Jefferson Street, Suite 110
Raleigh, NC 27605
1 (800) 541-4327 Voice and TTY (NC only)
(919) 715-4092 Voice/TTY (Outside NC)
(919) 715-4093 FAX
www.ncbegin.org/

Better Hearing Institute (BHI)
1444 I Street NW
Suite 700
Washington, DC, 20005
(202) 449-1000
www.betterhearing.org/

Canadian Hard of Hearing Association/ L'Association des malentendants canadiens
2415 Holly Lane, Suite 205
Ottawa, Ontario, Canada, K1V 7P2
1 (800) 263-8068 Toll Free/sans frais (Canada only)
(613) 526-1584 Voice/voix
(613) 526-2692 TTY/ATS
(613) 526-4718 Fax/télécopieur
http://chha.ca/chha/

DEAFPRIDE, INC
1350 Potomac Avenue SE
Washington, DC 20003-4426
(202) 675-6700 Voice and TTY

Hearing Loss Association of America (HLAA)
7910 Woodmont Avenue, Suite 1200
Bethesda, MD 20814
(301) 657-2248
www.hearingloss.org/

HEAR NOW-PART OF STARKEY HEARING FOUNDATION
6700 Washington Avenue, South
Eden Prairie, MN 55344
1 (800) 328-8602 Voice
(952) 828-6900 FAX
www.starkeyhearingfoundation.org/hear-now.php

HOPE, Inc
1856 North 1200 East
North Logan, UT 34341
(435) 245-2888
www.hopepubl.com

John Tracy Clinic
806 West Adams Blvd.
Los Angeles, CA 90007–2505
1 (800) 522-4582 (Toll Free)
(213) 748-5481 Voice
(213) 747-2924 TTY
(213) 749-1651 Fax
www.jtc.org

Marion Downs National Center for Innovation in Hearing
1793 Quentin Street, Unit 2
Aurora, CO 80045
(720) 848-3042 Voice
(720) 848-2979 TTY
(720) 848-2976 FAX
www.uch.edu/conditions/ear-nose-throat/hearing-loss/marion-downs-hearing-center.aspx

National Association for the Deaf (NAD)
8630 Fenton, Suite 820
Silver Spring, MD 20910
(301) 587-1788 Voice
(301) 587-1789 TTY
www.nad.org/

National Cued Speech Association
5619 McLean Drive
Bethesda, MD 20814-1021
1 (800) 459-3529 Toll Free
(301) 915-2009
www.cuedspeech.org/

National Deaf Education Center-Laurent Clerc
Gallaudet University
800 Florida Avenue N.E.
Washington, DC 20002-3695
(202) 651-5206 Voice
(202) 250-2761 Video phone
(202) 651-5646 FAX
www.clerccenter.gallaudet.edu

Signing Exact English Center for the Advancement of Deaf Children
P.O. Box 1181
Los Alamitos, CA 90720
(562) 430-1467 Voice and TTY
(562) 795-6614 FAX
www.seecenter.org

Starkey Foundation
6700 Washington Avenue South
Eden Prairie, MN 55346
1 (800) 328-8602 Voice
www.starkeyhearingfoundation.org/

APPENDIX 9.2

Checklist for Audiologists to Support Medical Home Providers' Informational Needs

---

Overview of EHDI Process

_____ Distill and disseminate relevant guidance from Joint Committee on Infant Hearing Year 2007 Position Statement

---

Newborn Screening and Referral for Audiological Assessment

Encourage Physicians to:

_____ Obtain hearing screening results by contacting birth hospitals or their state EHDI program

_____ Modify standard history forms to ask parents the results of newborn hearing screening and follow-up testing

_____ Use evidence-based diagnostic protocols

_____ Consult local pediatric audiologists who have the equipment, expertise, and experience to conduct a comprehensive diagnostic evaluation

---

Referral for Medical Evaluation

_____ Provide list of local otolaryngologists who have expertise with infants

_____ Supply information about need for, and importance of, referral to medical specialists

_____ Provide list of local medical specialists, including geneticists and ophthalmologists who have expertise with infants

---

Amplification

_____ Provide list of local pediatric audiologists who can fit hearing aids

_____ Provide list of pediatric cochlear implant teams in the area

_____ Reference evidence-based amplification protocols

Referral for Early Intervention and Family Support

_____ Provide list of local early interventionists and speech-language pathologists skilled in working with infants with hearing loss

_____ Disseminate parent-friendly materials for physicians to use in counseling and supporting families

---

Ongoing Surveillance

_____ Provide list of local resources where infants/toddlers can receive hearing screening

_____ Provide training materials and support to physicians who want to do early childhood screening as a part of well child visits

---

Source: Based on "Improving the Quality of Early Hearing Detection and Intervention Programs through Physician Outreach," by K. Munoz, L. Shisler, M. P. Moeller, and K. R. White, 2009, *Seminars in Hearing, 30(3),* pp. 184–192.

Hearing Aid Checksheet

Child: _____

Make/Model of Aid: _____

Serial Number: _____ **Right or Left**

INSTRUCTIONS: *Please complete the visual and listening check by recording the date of the check and circling "yes" or "no" for each test. Write down any pertinent comments or questions for the audiologist.*

Visual Check							
Date							
Case clean	Yes No	Yes No	Yes No	Yes No	Yes No	Yes No	Yes No
Case uncracked	Yes No	Yes No	Yes No	Yes No	Yes No	Yes No	Yes No
Undamaged tubing	Yes No	Yes No	Yes No	Yes No	Yes No	Yes No	Yes No
Uncorroded battery contacts	Yes No	Yes No	Yes No	Yes No	Yes No	Yes No	Yes No
Battery charged	Yes No	Yes No	Yes No	Yes No	Yes No	Yes No	Yes No
No sign of moisture	Yes No	Yes No	Yes No	Yes No	Yes No	Yes No	Yes No

Comments or Questions:

Listening Check							
Date							
Adequate volume	Yes No	Yes No	Yes No	Yes No	Yes No	Yes No	Yes No
Good sound quality	Yes No	Yes No	Yes No	Yes No	Yes No	Yes No	Yes No
No unusual sounds	Yes No	Yes No	Yes No	Yes No	Yes No	Yes No	Yes No

Comments or Questions:

APPENDIX 9.4

Calendar for Recording Infant's Reaction to Amplification

INSTRUCTIONS: *Please fill in the month and days on the calendar. Each day, record the time hearing aids are put on and taken off the child. Circle "Yes" or "No" as to whether resistance to hearing aids was encountered and write down notes for the audiologist.*

Month _____

Sunday	Monday	Tuesday	Wednesday	Thursday	Friday	Saturday
_____ On_____ Off_____ Resistance Yes No Notes?	_____ On_____ Off_____ Resistance Yes No Notes?	_____ On_____ Off_____ Resistance Yes No Notes?	_____ On_____ Off_____ Resistance Yes No Notes?	_____ On_____ Off_____ Resistance Yes No Notes?	_____ On_____ Off_____ Resistance Yes No Notes?	_____ On_____ Off_____ Resistance Yes No Notes?
_____ On_____ Off_____ Resistance Yes No Notes?	_____ On_____ Off_____ Resistance Yes No Notes?	_____ On_____ Off_____ Resistance Yes No Notes?	_____ On_____ Off_____ Resistance Yes No Notes?	_____ On_____ Off_____ Resistance Yes No Notes?	_____ On_____ Off_____ Resistance Yes No Notes?	_____ On_____ Off_____ Resistance Yes No Notes?
_____ On_____ Off_____ Resistance Yes No Notes?	_____ On_____ Off_____ Resistance Yes No Notes?	_____ On_____ Off_____ Resistance Yes No Notes?	_____ On_____ Off_____ Resistance Yes No Notes?	_____ On_____ Off_____ Resistance Yes No Notes?	_____ On_____ Off_____ Resistance Yes No Notes?	_____ On_____ Off_____ Resistance Yes No Notes?
_____ On_____ Off_____ Resistance Yes No Notes?	_____ On_____ Off_____ Resistance Yes No Notes?	_____ On_____ Off_____ Resistance Yes No Notes?	_____ On_____ Off_____ Resistance Yes No Notes?	_____ On_____ Off_____ Resistance Yes No Notes?	_____ On_____ Off_____ Resistance Yes No Notes?	_____ On_____ Off_____ Resistance Yes No Notes?
_____ On_____ Off_____ Resistance Yes No Notes?	_____ On_____ Off_____ Resistance Yes No Notes?	_____ On_____ Off_____ Resistance Yes No Notes?	_____ On_____ Off_____ Resistance Yes No Notes?	_____ On_____ Off_____ Resistance Yes No Notes?	_____ On_____ Off_____ Resistance Yes No Notes?	_____ On_____ Off_____ Resistance Yes No Notes?

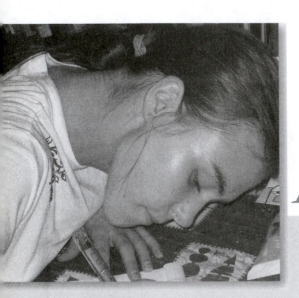

CHAPTER ten

Auditory Habilitation for School-Aged Children

LEARNING *objectives*

After reading this chapter, you should be able to:

1. Describe the effects of hearing loss on the speech, language, and psychosocial development of school-age children.

2. List the four main principles of the Individuals with Disabilities Education Improvement Act (2004) and discuss them in relation to children with hearing impairment.

3. List two other federal laws used in securing children with disabilities access to an education.

4. Define the roles of audiologists and speech-language pathologists in serving children with hearing impairment in the school setting.

5. List and describe possible areas of accommodation for children with hearing impairment.

6. Sequence the steps and use techniques for personal adjustment counseling of children with hearing impairment.

7. Discuss direct service delivery and compare and contrast the following approaches facilitating the oral spoken language use of children with hearing impairment: Auditory-Verbal, the Verbotonal method, and the Erber method.

8. List and describe assessment tools for children with hearing impairment.

9. Define, list characteristics, and describe management of children with (central) auditory processing disorders ([C]APD).

10. Explain the auditory disorders of auditory neuropathy/dyssynchrony (AN/AD) and tinnitus in school-age children.

11. Discuss dual sensory impairment in school-age children.

12. Define child abuse and neglect and describe how it may apply to children with hearing impairment.

13. Describe transition services for children with hearing impairment.

From ages 3 to 18, children undergo a tremendous amount of growth and development on their way to adulthood. In the last chapter, we discussed the importance of early identification, diagnosis, and management of hearing loss through early hearing detection and intervention programs. The sense of urgency must continue through the school-age years for these children to reach their full potential. Hearing impairment afflicts more children than what statistics may show. It is estimated that 14.9% of children 6 to 19 years of age have hearing threshold levels of at least 16 dB HL in one or both ears (Niskar et al., 1998). More recently, it has been estimated that one in five U.S. teenagers have some degree of hearing loss (Shargorodsky, Curhan, Curhan, & Favey, 2010). Even children with minimal amounts of hearing loss experience more educational and psychosocial difficulties than their peers with normal hearing (Bess, Dodd-Murphy, & Parker, 1998).

The preceding chapter ended by discussing the basic principles of the Individuals With Disabilities Education Improvement Act (IDEA, 2004). Federal law defines *hearing impairment* and *deafness* as follows:

> **Hearing impairment** is "an impairment in hearing, whether permanent or fluctuating, that adversely affects a child's educational performance but that is not included under the definition of deafness in this section" (300.7[c][5]).

> **Deafness** is "a hearing impairment that is so severe that the child is impaired in processing linguistic information through hearing, with or without amplification, [and] that adversely affects a child's educational performance" (300.7[c][3]).

Friend (2005) stated that the definitions created by the National Center for Education Statistics (2002), which follow, improved on the federal law definitions by further clarifying hearing impairment and adding the term hard of hearing, although most educators still do not agree on their appropriateness:

> **Hearing impairment**—An impairment in hearing, whether permanent or fluctuating, that adversely affects a child's educational performance, in the most severe case because the child is impaired in processing linguistic information through hearing. (p. 546)

> **Deafness**—Having a hearing impairment which is so severe that the student is impaired in processing linguistic information through hearing (with or without amplification) and which adversely affects educational performance. (p. 546)

Hard of hearing—Having a hearing impairment, whether permanent or fluctuating, which adversely affects the student's educational performance, but which is not included under the definition of "deaf." (p. 546)

It is important to note that these definitions do not include specific audiometric criteria to be met or specific types of auditory disorders. Moreover, the IDEA is a federal law, and individual states determine specific criteria for qualifications for special education services. Therefore, the quality of services and accessibility for children with hearing impairment vary widely from state to state and from school district to district. Therefore, audiologists and speech-language pathologists must be prepared to see that the public agency (school) meets the needs of these children. It is important that teachers understand the educational needs of children with hearing loss and realize that some students with similar audiograms may have very different needs, particularly when comparing those with sensory versus neural hearing varieties. Recall that children with sensory hearing losses are those with damage primarily in the cochlea, and more specifically, to the inner and outer hair cells. Children with neural hearing losses, or auditory neuropathy/auditory dyssynchrony (AN/AD), have problems with the auditory nerve (cranial nerve VIII) in its transmission of electrical signals generated in the periphery to the central auditory nervous system, although there may be multiple sites of lesions. Children with sensory hearing losses typically do well with hearing aids and accommodations that schools and teachers provide to facilitate their learning. Alternatively, children with neural hearing losses have rather unpredictable benefit from hearing aids and accommodations in the classroom. **Accommodations** are adjustments in procedures or rules that permit students' with disabilities access to an education. Teachers may be confused when students with AN/AD do not benefit from typical accommodations provided to others with similar degrees of sensory hearing loss. Audiologists and speech-language pathologists can assist teachers to understand the unique needs of these children. Similarly, school personnel may be baffled by children with **(central) auditory processing disorders ([C]APD)**, who have who have normal audiograms yet poor performance in certain auditory skills (American Speech-Language-Hearing Association, 2005a, 2005b). In this chapter, we will discuss the effects of hearing impairment on speech, language, and psychosocial development; the IDEA, aspects of educational audiology; roles of audiologists and speech-language pathologists; classroom accommodations; personal adjustment counseling; direct service provision; assessment tools; management of (C)APD, AN/AD, and tinnitus; dual sensory impairment in school-aged children; child abuse; and transition planning.

EFFECTS OF HEARING IMPAIRMENT ON SPEECH, LANGUAGE, AND PSYCHOSOCIAL DEVELOPMENT

Prior to discussing auditory habilitation of school-age children, readers must review the effects of hearing loss on speech, language, and psychosocial development.

Effects of Hearing Loss on Speech Production

Hearing loss impacts not only articulation, but manifests itself in every aspect of speech production including respiration, phonation, and resonance. Because the anatomical and physiological function of speaking is a process, it is necessary to discuss the impact of hearing loss from its beginning, highlighting how problems early in the chain of events impact those at the end.

Speech scientists have studied the speech of individuals who are deaf and hard of hearing both acoustically and perceptually. Acoustic assessments have involved using **spectrographic analyses**, or the use of computers, in digitizing and analyzing the duration, frequency, and intensity characteristics of speech. Perceptual analyses have involved naïve and expert listeners in either identifying abnormalities or making judgments about the speech of the hearing impaired. The expert listeners most often include speech-language pathologists who judge aspects of **voice quality**, which includes the degree of breathiness, roughness, strain, and overall noise during speech production (Monsen, 1979). Another avenue for investigation has been assessing the relationship between speakers' degree of hearing loss and deviancy of their speech. Generally, it has been found that the speech of children with mild-to-moderate hearing losses is both quantitatively and qualitatively different than those with severe-to-profound impairment.

Speech begins with respiration, or the act of inhaling and exhaling, for the purpose of exchanging carbon dioxide for oxygen involving the lungs, trachea, and bronchial tubes (MedicineNet.com, 2010). During this process, enough air must be brought into the lungs for breathing and speaking. When we breathe, a large muscle in our chest, the **diaphragm**, contracts and moves downward to create negative air pressure in the lungs relative to the outside of the body, causing air to rush in. Speakers with profound hearing loss were found to have some abnormalities in respiration affecting speech production. For example, Forner and Hixon (1977) measured how the rib cage and abdomen moved for respiration and speaking tasks in a group of adults with profound sensorineural hearing loss. The investigators found that although their rib cage and abdominal movement were within normal limits for breathing, significant differences from speakers with normal hearing were found in their respiration for speech. Specifically, they found that deaf speakers had a more restricted range of rib cage and abdominal movement and, therefore, brought in an insufficient volume of air into their lungs for speech. In addition, these speakers tended to misuse the limited air that they did have in that they controlled it poorly, uttering fewer syllables for each breath. The deaf speakers also used approximately three times the amount of air (e.g., 100 cubic centimeters [cc]) for each syllable compared with normal speakers (e.g., 20 to 40 cc). Forner and Hixon (1977) surmised that these differences resulted in lack of normal auditory sensations and inadequate speech, language, and hearing therapy. Children with mild-to-moderate hearing losses have been found not to have these abnormalities.

Phonation is the second process involved in speaking, and it involves the larynx, glottis, and vocal folds. The wastage of air during speech has a great deal to do with the inability of deaf speakers to control the laryngeal musculature for appropriate valving of air through the glottis. Deaf speakers have been found to have either hyper- (i.e., too much) or hypo- (i.e., too little) valving, resulting in abnormalities in **phonation**, or the vibration of the vocal folds. One important term to know is **fundamental frequency (Fo)**, which is the number of times that the vocal folds open and close per second. A speaker's Fo is the pitch of his or her voice that varies according to sex and age. For example, the average Fo for an adult male is about 125 Hz, and for an adult female about 250 Hz, or about one octave higher. The Fo for a young child is about 350 Hz, with sex not being much of a factor until puberty. **Intonation** is the use of fundamental frequency over time. Intonation, along with rhythm, are part of **suprasegmentals**, or the prosodic aspects of language that convey meaning in speech. For example, sentences that have a rising intonation signify that a question has been asked. Alternatively, intonation may also indicate **sarcasm**, such as when someone's words have one meaning, but convey the opposite when said with a particular intonation.

Monsen (1979) had a panel of expert listeners judge the voice quality of children with normal hearing and those who were deaf when producing consonant-vowel syllables. He found that children with the most deviant intonation patterns were judged to have the worst voice quality, displaying breathiness and diplophonia. **Breathiness** is the perception that too much air is being expended during speech; **diplophonia** is the perception of two fundamental frequencies occurring simultaneously during phonation. Similarly, Monsen, Engebretson, and Vemula (1979) found that adolescents with hearing impairment also displayed diplophonia and "creaky-voice" episodes during the onset or middle of phonation. It has also been found that the more harshness or tension in a speaker's voice, the more noise there is in the speech spectrum (Whitehead & Whitehead, 1985). However, the voice quality of children with mild-to-moderate sensorineural hearing losses is closer to that of their peers with normal hearing.

Regarding the suprasegmentals, deaf speech is not only slower, but is lacking in rhythm when compared with that of speakers with normal hearing (John & Howarth, 1965). The slow rate of speech has been attributed to excessive pausing and the insertion of adventitious, or extra, sounds that have nothing to do with the message (Osberger & Levitt, 1979). Adventitious sounds have been found to affect intelligibility the most, followed by excessive phoneme duration and inappropriate pitch breaks (Parkhurst & Levitt, 1978). Their intonation has been described as monotone and lacking in variation, although the opposite, excessive variability, has also been found (Angelocci, Kopp, & Holbrook, 1964). In one study, Hood and Dixon (1969) found that although the intonation patterns were similar to their peers with normal hearing, deaf speakers' range of Fo was much more restricted. In addition, the intensity level of speech has been found to be inappropriate, either too soft (Calvert & Silverman, 1975), too loud (Penn, 1955), or inappropriate for certain social situations. The use of suprasegmentals by children who have mild-to-moderate sensorineural hearing losses is closer to that of their peers with normal hearing.

When describing the intelligibility of speech of the hearing impaired, it is important to remember to separate performances of children who are deaf and those who are hard of hearing in addition to considering school placement (Levitt, Stromberg, Smith, & Gold, 1980). The intelligibility of deaf speech has been found to be 20% or less, and in general, the poorer the child's voice quality, the poorer is the intelligibility of his or her speech (Smith, 1975). Children with severe to profound hearing loss have been found to have omissions, distortions, and substitution of both vowels and consonants resulting in errors in voicing, manner, and place. Class error patterns include *vowel substitution* and *neutralization, diphthongalization,* and *diphthong distortions* (Seyfried, Hutchinson, & Smith, 1989). **Vowel substitution** is using one vowel in place of another, and in the case of **neutralization**, most vowels are substituted for the neutral vowel *schwa*. Other substitutions are using a lax vowel in place of a tense one (e.g., /I/ for /i/), or vice-versa (e.g., /i/ for /I/). Another error pattern occurs with the use of **diphthongs**—a vowel that is a combination of two vowels, resulting in movement of the second formant (e.g., /a/ + /I/ = /aI/). **Diphthongalization** is changing a regular, single vowel, or monothong, into a diphthong (e.g., /e/ into /eI/). An example of **diphthong distortion** is doing the reverse, changing a diphthong into a monothong (e.g., /e/ into /eI/). Difficulty in correctly positioning the tongue in the oral cavity is a major factor in the vowel errors of children who are deaf. Nasalization of vowels results from inappropriately opening the **velopharyngeal port** (opening between the oral and nasal cavities) resulting in a **cul-de-sac resonance**—the nasalization of speech sounds—during vowel production. Children with mild-to-moderate hearing loss rarely make these errors in vowel production.

The voicing errors of children who are deaf include voice and voiceless confusion, frequently resulting in devoicing of voiced consonants (e.g., /t/ for /d/), particularly in the final positions of words (Smith, 1975). Regarding place of articulation, errors on phonemes that are more visible (e.g., bilabials) are less common than those that are not (e.g., fricatives) (Tye-Murray, Spencer, & Woodworth, 1995). Consonants are more likely to be omitted if they appear in the middle or at the ends of words than those in the initial position. Phonemes occurring at the ends of words include suffixes that convey meaning (e.g., -s for plurality). Some of these errors may be perceptual in that the sound pressure level of speech decreases toward the end of utterances. Sounds that are not heard are not produced. However, some believe that some of these errors may be due, in part, to lack of linguistic knowledge. Trends in manner of production include more accurate production of plosives than nasals, affricates, fricative, glides, or laterals (Osberger et al., 1986). Speakers who are deaf tend to have difficulty in producing **blends** (e.g., /br/) and **clusters** (e.g., /skr/), often omitting consonants. Moreover, as with vowels, these speakers tend to nasalize consonants, although the opposite has also been found. Alternatively, children with mild-to-moderate sensorineural hearing losses do not display the severe articulation errors of their peers who are deaf, but have patterns similar to younger children with normal hearing (Seyfried et al., 1989).

Effects of Hearing Loss on Language Development

Children who acquire hearing loss before the development of spoken language, generally before the age of 3, are at a severe disadvantage and are continually trying to "catch up." These children struggle to learn what just comes naturally to their normal hearing peers. The more severe the hearing loss, the greater is the impact on language development. For the most part, children with pre- or even peri lingual hearing losses lag behind their peers in the development of oral language, both spoken and written (Svirsky, Robbins, Kirk, Pisoni, & Miyamoto, 2000). These lags in development can be seen in the following four components of language:

- **Phonology:** how sounds come together to form words
- **Syntax:** how words come together to form sentences
- **Semantics:** the meaning of words
- **Pragmatics:** the use of language in context

Hearing loss impacts each area of language development in unique ways. Regarding phonology, it is obvious that if words cannot be adequately perceived, then children with hearing loss cannot adequately learn phonological processes, a prerequisite for reading and writing. They cannot rely on their auditory memory as do children with normal hearing who sound out words when reading or spelling. Children with hearing loss frequently must rely on remembering what a word looks like rather than what it sounds like.

Children with normal hearing enter school with an internal set of rules for how words come together to form sentences, and they can produce an infinite number of word combinations for communication. Deaf and hard of hearing children have difficulty with English syntax, and degree of hearing loss influences the amount of trouble they experience. Bishop (1983) found that 8- to 12-year-old children with profound hearing loss comprehended English syntax at a level below that has 4-year-old hearing children. Additionally, the syntax of children trained in aural-oral has been assessed via their spontaneous language samples and in structured tasks (Friedmann & Szertman, 2006). It has been found that children with hearing impairment lag in their learning of syntactic structures and rules (Pressnell, 1973). Essentially, these studies found that these children produced more ungrammatical sentences than their peers with normal hearing in addition to using more simple structures; they also had more difficulty comprehending complex syntax (Pressnell, 1973; Geers & Moog, 1978). Friedman and Szertman (2006) stated that the three structures providing the most difficulty for these children were:

1. the passive voice (e.g., active: The car hit the curb; passive: The curb was hit by the car) (e.g., Power & Quigley, 1973).
2. *Wh* questions (i.e., questions that start with who, what, where, when, and why) (e.g., de Villiers, de Villiers, & Hoban, 1994).
3. object-relative clauses (e.g., This is the boy that the girl kissed) (e.g., de Villiers, 1988).

Children with hearing loss tend to overuse the subject + verb + object syntactic structure, and frequently omit smaller function words (e.g., adjectives, adverbs, auxiliaries, and so on) (Seyfried et al., 1989). Children with severe-to-profound sensorineural hearing losses show not only delay in these skills, but a plateau and deviation in their syntactic development, whereas those with mild-to-moderate losses are simply delayed.

Children who are hearing impaired also have semantic and vocabulary delays, most likely as a direct result of restricted use of word classes. Curtiss, Prutting, and Lowell (1979) found that young children who were deaf had restricted knowledge and use of semantic functions compared with preschoolers with normal hearing. Children with severe-to-profound hearing loss identified between 10- to 12-months of age demonstrated a reduced use of vocabulary compared with peers with normal hearing (Nicholas, Geers, & Sedey, 2003). Standardized tests such as the *Peabody Picture Vocabulary Test* (PPVT) (Dunn, Dunn, Robertson, & Eisenberg, 1979) and the *Boehm Test of Basic Concepts* (Boehm, 1971) have been used to compare deaf children's performance with peers having normal hearing. Brenza, Kricos, and Lasky (1981) found that 80% of 13- and 14-year-old deaf children scored below the 10th percentile and 66% below the 1st percentile for normal-hearing second graders on the *Boehm Test of Basic Concepts.* Davis, Elfenbein, Schum, and Belter (1986) found not only severe delays, but a plateauing of vocabulary development. Delay and plateauing of vocabulary development impacts the ability to read, placing these children at a severe academic disadvantage when compared with their peers with normal hearing (Paul, 1996). In addition, Ross, Brackett, and Maxon (1991) stated that it is not just these quantitative differences that pose problems, but these children's difficulty in understanding idioms, casual expressions, and slang are important in communicating with their peer group.

Children who are deaf and hard of hearing also have difficulties with pragmatics, or the use of language in context, which includes a variety of behaviors: use of speech functions, turn taking, eye gaze, conversational fluency, and so on. Previous research with mother-child dyads has shown that preschoolers with hearing loss were less spontaneous in their use of speech, were less able to comply with commands, and could not stay on topic when compared with peers with normal hearing (e.g., Cross, Nienhuys, & Kirkman, 1985). Similarly, Nicholas et al., (2003) analyzed language samples from similar dyads of caregivers and their 1- to 4-year-old children who had severe-to-profound hearing loss.

They found that these children used a reduced range of pragmatic functions (e.g., requesting, calling attention, directing, and so on). Furthermore, young children with hearing loss do not take into consideration what their communicative partner knows or does not know, a situation frequently providing insufficient information as well as a restricted range of topics (e.g., Day, 1986). Pragmatic deficiencies become more pronounced the older the child gets. Children with hearing loss do not know how to enter conversations, and if they do, they have a difficult time with fluency partly due to not being able to hear subtle acoustic cues. As a result, some children with hearing loss stay to themselves, rather than risking communication breakdowns, thus avoiding embarrassment (English, 2002).

Effects of Hearing Loss on Psychosocial Development

In the previous chapter, the importance of parents' acceptance of their children's hearing losses was discussed. If parents are not accepting, their child may absorb some of their negativity about having offspring with hearing impairment, precluding development of a positive self-concept. Therefore, early intervention should assist parents in coming to terms with hearing loss, setting the stage for positive coping strategies for disability. Moreover, parents who fail to come to terms with their child's hearing loss may develop **maladaptive behaviors** that may actually sabotage aural habilitative efforts. Parents do not have to tell their young children about their unresolved feelings about hearing loss; children can feel it in their caregivers' actions. Parents may be overwhelmed with feelings of anger, doubt, guilt, fear, and resentment in addition to not being able to communicate with their preschooler. Young children do not have the ability to understand parents' feelings and are frustrated in not being able to communicate their needs. Parents may overreact and become too restrictive or overprotective, discouraging children's attempts at trying new activities or exerting independence, resulting in learned helplessness (Rall, 2007). Children's helplessness may change into passivity, a tendency to withdraw, an unwillingness to try new things, or to reach out to others. As a result, young children with hearing loss may be difficult to place in preschool or daycare settings.

These characteristics continue into formal school settings in that children with hearing loss demonstrate less independence in the classroom (Johnson, Benson, & Seaton, 1997). Some children with normal hearing feel that students with hearing loss do not work as hard as they do and may be better off placed in special schools (Cambra, 2002). However, some studies have shown that Swedish children with hearing loss who are mainstreamed in regular schools have better self-images and social access than their peers at schools for the deaf (Mejstad, Heiling, & Svedin, 2009). Moreover, if children with normal hearing are exposed to others with hearing loss in educational settings, they tend to be more understanding and accepting of the disability (Bowen, 2008). Parent involvement in their children's educations has been found to enhance their children's academic performance (Calderon, 2000). Alternatively, it is important to remember that children who are deaf in deaf families and are part of the Deaf community have stronger self-concepts and have been known to thrive in schools for the deaf (Lane, Hoffmeister, & Bahan, 1996). In addition, future research should focus on the psychosocial development of children whose hearing losses were identified in newborn hearing screening programs (Moeller, 2007). It is predicted that this generation of children who have benefited from early detection and intervention of hearing loss may have fewer psychosocial adjustment issues than their predecessors.

What Does the Evidence Show?

The previous section presented what were typical benchmarks of these patients prior to the development of early hearing detection and intervention programs and the advancement in technology of hearing aids and cochlear implants. Indeed, the graduates of early intervention programs represent a new generation of students who are expected to shatter past trends in performance. This issue was discussed a bit in Chapter 9 along with a presentation of the results of the systematic review supporting the United States Preventive Services Task Force (USPSTF) recent grading of the efficacy of newborn hearing screening programs in advancing the speech and language development for children having hearing loss. Recall that the USPSTF provided a grade of B for the evidence supporting early hearing detection and intervention programs. When reviewing the literature in this area, it is exciting to see active investigators such as Mary Pat Moeller, Mary Jo Osberger, Nancy Tye-Murray, and Christine Yoshinaga-Itano, who during the course of their careers have witnessed the beginning of the closing of the developmental gaps between children with hearing impairment and their peers with normal hearing. Indeed, the futures of the graduates of early hearing detection and intervention programs look bright!

FEDERAL LAWS

Individuals With Disabilities Education Improvement Act

The Individuals With Disabilities Education Improvement Act (IDEA, 2004) was introduced in the preceding chapter, particularly those components pertaining to Part C of the law for children 0 to 2 years of age and their families. Part B has to do with children 3 to 21 years of age. Recall that the IDEA has several fundamental principles that were introduced in the last chapter, as follows:

- Zero reject
- Free and appropriate public education
- Least restrictive environment
- Procedural safeguards

The first principle is *zero reject*, which states that the public agency must provide an educational program for all children, regardless of the type or severity of a child's disability.

The second principle is that the public agency must provide the child a *free and appropriate public education* (FAPE), meaning that the program should be provided at no cost to the family. However, the terms *free* and *appropriate* require qualification. According to the law, "free" means that special education and related services should be provided at the public's expense without charge. A child's family should not have to pay for an audiologic evaluation or for the use of hearing assistive technology (HAT) (e.g., FM systems) during school hours or sponsored events. However, the IDEA stipulates that the school does not have to pay for cochlear implant mapping. "Appropriate" means that the educational program must conform to requirements set forth in the IDEA and its Implementing Regulations, the specific state's special education rules, and must meet the individual needs of the child (Johnson, 2000).

The third principle is that the educational program should be carried out in the *least restrictive environment* (LRE) or to the extent possible with the child's nondisabled peers.

The concept of LRE goes along with the concept of *mainstreaming*, or the placement of children with disabilities into the regular education stream with nondisabled peers. As discussed in the previous chapter, mainstreaming is not an all-or-nothing concept, but rather consists of a continuum of options for placement of children who are deaf and hard of hearing. The placement options for preschool are different than for older children.

Children 3 to 5 years of age who have one of the following disabling conditions may qualify for preschool special education: speech-language impaired, other health impaired, hearing impaired, visually impaired, orthopedically impaired, cognitively delayed, multiply disabled, deaf/blind, seriously emotionally disturbed, learning disabled, autistic, or traumatic brain injured. Many children will transition from Part C to Part B of the IDEA; some may acquire hearing losses after passing their newborn hearing screening. Qualification requires the determination of the existence and extent of a child's disability. Children with suspected hearing loss typically undergo a complete audiologic evaluation to determine the type, degree, and configuration of hearing loss so that appropriate referrals (e.g., physician) can be made. Assessment also includes areas impacted by hearing loss such as speech, language, and academic achievement. Once qualified, an individualized education plan is established as discussed in Chapter 9. Preschool special education is highly variable from district to district because many schools do not have classes for 3- to 5-year-olds with normal hearing. Therefore, educating children with disabilities in the LRE may not always be possible.

Some possibilities include serving a child in a special education program for children with a variety of disabilities in an elementary school, or in another setting operated by private or public agencies (e.g., Head Start), or even in a preschool program for hearing impaired children. Ideally, the placement should meet the unique needs of the child, but frequently students and their families must make the best use of resources available to them. Some educators may feel that mainstreaming children with hearing loss into regular preschool classes provides the best preparation for the school years to come. However, some believe that placing young children into preschool programs for the hearing impaired provides the opportunity for intensive aural habilitation, ensuring a greater likelihood of successful mainstreaming into regular kindergarten classrooms. A relatively new concept called **reverse mainstreaming**, or including children from regular education in special education programs, may provide intensive aural habilitation and exposure to peers with normal hearing. Indeed, preschool children should have a selection of alternative placements, particularly those that expose them to peers with normal hearing that can serve as good speech and language models (Ross, Brackett, and Maxon, 1991). Heavner (2007) advised that children with hearing loss need to be able to maintain their attention, follow directions, initiate/respond to greetings, and ask for assistance in order to be mainstreamed into a regular preschool classroom. Young children need to have adequate language skills to understand typical routines, correctly answer questions (e.g., How are you?), and benefit from **incidental learning**, or that which occurs naturally within the classroom (Heavner). Once children reach school age, more options for mainstreaming are available and become more consistent across schools and districts. Figure 10.1 shows one continuum of possible placements, which may vary from district to district.

Possible placements involve different schools and classrooms. At one end of the continuum is complete segregation at a residential school for the deaf. States often have residential schools for the deaf where children live in dormitories with house parents, attend classes on campus, and go home for weekends and holidays. Let's look in on Brooke, a student at a residential school for the deaf.

COMPLETE SEGREGATION

- Residential school for the deaf
- Centralized school with a program for the hearing impaired
  - Self-contained classroom
  - Self-contained classroom with social mainstreaming
  - Self-contained classroom with mainstreaming for some academic subjects
- Neighborhood school
  - Special educational categorical classroom
  - Special educational categorical classroom with social mainstreaming
  - Regular classroom and special education categorical classroom
  - Regular classroom with related services
  - Regular classroom

COMPLETE INTEGRATION

figure *10.1*

Continuum of mainstreaming.

Source: Based on *How the Individuals with Disabilities Education Act (IDEA) Applies to Deaf and Hard of Hearing Students,* by C. Johnson, 2000, Washington, DC: Laurent LeClerc National Deaf Education Center, Gallaudet University.

Casebook Reflection

Brooke

Brooke, a ninth grader, has a severe-to-profound sensorineural hearing loss and two hearing parents. Her hearing loss was identified at age 2; she has worn bilateral hearing aids ever since and has lived in a dormitory at the state school for the deaf for as long as she can remember. The school has both day and residential school programs. Children who live within commuting distance attend the day school. Because Brooke's family lives more than 50 miles away, she lives in the dormitory as part of the residential program. She goes home on the weekends and holidays. Brooke gets homesick from time to time, but she loves her school. She has had the same roommate for two years. Everyone on campus uses American Sign Language and most of her teachers are deaf. Brooke enjoys being in class and being part of a community in which everyone is just like her. Her school follows the same curriculum as other public schools in the state, and she must pass the state high school graduation examination to receive her academic diploma. Her school is accredited by the state department of education, the Southern Association of Colleges and Schools, and the Conference of Educational Administrators Serving the Deaf. Her mentor is Ms. Crawford, her English teacher, who is also deaf. Brooke aspires to be a teacher just like her mentor and plans to attend Gallaudet University in Washington, DC Brooke has speech-language therapy two times a week from Ms. Bishop, the speech-language pathologist. Brooke enjoys her classes and all of the other activities available to her like hiking, boating, skating, and arts and crafts. Some weekends, the school takes trips to Six Flags over Georgia and in the summer, they will go to Disney World in Orlando. Brooke is also going to try out for cheerleading.

Larger school districts frequently have centralized programs for children with hearing impairment that are contained within regular schools, providing an opportunity for various degrees of mainstreaming. Let's look in on Javier, a 10th grader.

Casebook Reflection

Javier

Javier, a 10th grader, attends a high school that has a centralized program for students with hearing impairment. He has a severe bilateral sensorineural hearing loss and wears bilateral behind-the-ear hearing aids. It isn't the same high school that his friends in his neighborhood attend, but it isn't that far and his mother drops him off on her way to work each morning. Javier likes the school, and it has the necessary programming for Javier to succeed. Each morning, he goes to his homeroom and puts on his FM receiver provided by the school so that he can hear his teachers better. While Javier relies on his FM system, some of his peers in the centralized program don't like the device; they associate with the Deaf community, mostly sign to their peers, and do not interact much with hearing students. Javier has friends who are normal hearing and hearing impaired. The program for hearing impaired students has self-contained classes, but many of the students are mainstreamed into regular education classes. Javier is mainstreamed into math, science, shop, and gym classes. However, for language arts and history, he remains in the self-contained classroom where the teachers use total communication. Javier receives speech-language therapy two times a week for 30 minutes. Javier expects to graduate with an academic diploma with a goal of attending a vocational-technical school to study drafting.

In smaller school systems, children with hearing impairment may attend their neighborhood schools that may not have centralized programs for the hearing impaired, but have categorical special education classrooms in which many children with various disabilities are placed for all or part of the day. Class sizes may be small with sufficient opportunities for small-group or one-on-one teaching with teachers and/or **paraprofessionals** with opportunities for mainstreaming into regular classes. Paraprofessionals are teachers' aides who provide valuable support, but frequently need special instruction on how to use FM systems and other tips on interacting with children having hearing loss. **Co-teaching** frequently involves regular and special education teachers teaming up to teach specific subjects to children with and without disabilities. Some children with hearing loss, like Jade, are mainstreamed for all academic subjects, but rely on related-services support.

Casebook Reflection

Jade

Jade is an 11th grader, has a bilateral moderate-to-severe sensorineural hearing loss, and is in the college preparatory program at her neighborhood high school. She was just fitted with bilateral open-ear digital hearing aids and was pleased to transition from wearing in-the-ear hearing aids. Jade is an A-student and plans to go to college as a premed student majoring in biology. Jade uses an FM system in the classroom and has speech-language therapy twice a week.

Although her speech is very intelligible, most people can tell she has a hearing loss. Jade is on the swim team, very active in extracurricular activities such as yearbook, and was elected student body president. She is very popular and credits her parents and speech-language pathologist, with whom she has worked since preschool. Her parents have always encouraged her and been very involved with her schooling and in designing her individualized education plan with school personnel. Early on, Jade required special education services in elementary school, but through hard work and with the aid of extensive tutoring and involved teachers, she was able to perform at grade level and is now excelling and achieving her dreams.

Mainstreaming does not always occur, nor is it always successful. Ross et al. (1991) have listed successful characteristics of the educational setting and the child that facilitate mainstreaming, which are shown in Figures 10.2 and 10.3, respectively. Optimal mainstreaming depends on a supportive educational setting in which the teacher, the class, the environment, and the administration meet certain criteria. Mainstreaming is always easier with receptive teachers who have an understanding of children with hearing loss and a willingness to use technologies and teaching strategies conducive for learning. Children with hearing impairment benefit from classrooms that are adequately staffed with teachers and paraprofessionals, resulting in a manageable number of children. Moreover, mainstreaming is facilitated if other children in the classroom have an understanding of their peers with hearing loss. In addition, the environment should have optimal acoustics, adequate lighting, and HAT to maximize children's speech recognition. School administrators should understand how deficiencies impact students' learning and be willing to provide resources for improvements.

Teacher
- Receptive to having children with hearing impairment in his or her classroom
- Willingness to use an FM system
- Willingness to adapt teaching style
- Recipient of adequate inservice training

Class
- Relatively small class size
- Adequate staffing with teachers and paraprofessionals
- Adequate instruction of peers regarding hearing loss

Environment
- Favorable acoustic conditions with minimal noise and reverberation
- Adequate lighting
- Availability of adequate technology (e.g., FM systems [individual or group], closed-captioning, and so on)

Administration
- Willingness to fund necessary services and technology
- Role of case manager legitimized
- Availability of speech-language pathologist for intensive therapy and assistance with educational programming

figure *10.2*

Classroom characteristics that facilitate mainstreaming.

Source: Based on *Assessment and Management of Mainstreamed Hearing-Impaired Children,* by M. Ross, D. Brackett, and A. Maxon, 1991, Austin, TX: Pro-Ed.

Social
- Age-appropriate behaviors
- Fits into peer group

Auditory
- Coordinates auditory input via personal hearing aids and FM systems with visual cues

Behavioral
- Comparable academic and language performance to children in the class
- Uses intelligible speech with teachers, paraprofessionals, and peers
- Has receptive language skills to keep up in the classroom
- Has expressive language skills to competently communicate with teachers, paraprofessionals, and peers
- Can self-advocate on educational matters
- Is adaptable and flexible to changing classroom contexts

Attitudinal
- Wants to fit into a mainstream classroom
- Has parents who want their child to be in a mainstream classroom

figure *10.3* ———————————————————————

Child characteristics that facilitate mainstreaming.

Source: Based on *Assessment and Management of Mainstreamed Hearing-Impaired Children,* by M. Ross, D. Brackett, and A. Maxon, 1991, Austin, TX: Pro-Ed.

Mainstreaming is easier for children if they possess the social, auditory, behavioral, and attitudinal characteristics listed in Figure 10.3. Ideally, children should display age-appropriate behaviors and fit socially into their peer groups. Similarly, they need intelligible speech and adequate receptive and expressive language to keep up with classroom discourse involving teachers, peers, and paraprofessionals. Dialogue is frequently fast-paced among participants located at various locations throughout the classroom, and participation requires the coordination of auditory and visual input through the use of hearing aids and HAT. Mainstreaming requires the individual's flexibility to adapt to ever-changing educational contexts and the confidence to self-advocate. Students need to feel comfortable enough to request clarification to repair conversational breakdowns. Additionally, children and parents with positive attitudes have an easier time adapting to mainstreaming.

The demands placed on children with hearing loss are considerable; they have to adapt to an ever-increasing complexity of information during the course of a school year. At times, they may feel like they are walking a tightrope—one false move and they'll fall to the ground (English, 2002). English (2002) uses the **safety-net metaphor** in describing all of the services (protections, professionals, and accommodations) provided that decrease the degree of risk a child must take in attempting to succeed in the class room.

A fourth fundamental principle of the IDEA (2004) introduced in the last chapter is that of *procedural safeguards*, which has the intent of ensuring that the rights of children with disabilities and their families are protected; each state must develop a system guaranteeing those rights (IDEA, 2004; Johnson, 2000). Parents must be provided with written notification in their native language of their procedural safeguards, at least at the occurrence of the following events (IDEA, 2004; Johnson, 2000):

- When their child is referred for an evaluation to determine eligibility for special education services
- When they are notified that their child's Individualized Education Plan Team (IEPT) is going to meet
- When their child is going to be reevaluated
- When the parents file a complaint or requests a hearing about their child's evaluation, identification, aspects of the FAPE, or placement

The first procedural safeguard is the right of informed consent regarding aspects of their child's education. The public agency must clearly explain exactly what they need the parents' consent for in writing and that legal guardians understand the matter for their consideration. Another safeguard is that parents have the right to examine any records pertaining to their child and that any personally identifiable information must remain confidential. Parents also have the right to disagree with any aspect of their child's individualized education plan (IEP) (discussed in the next section) or implementation of that program. If disagreement cannot be settled between parents and the public agency, parents have the right to mediation or due process. Both parents and the public agency have the following rights (IDEA, 2004; Johnson, 2000):

- To be represented by legal counsel and to be accompanied by experts with special knowledge about disabilities or special education
- To present evidence
- To confront, examine, cross-examine, and request the presence of witnesses
- To present arguments verbally or in writing
- To obtain a free transcript of the hearing
- To receive the findings of the decision
- To prohibit the presentation of evidence that was not provided at least five days before the hearing
- To appeal any decisions

The **stay-put principle** mandates that children remain in their current educational placement during mediation processes. Furthermore, parents have the right to be involved in the development of their child's IEP and to be involved in all meetings. Parents also have the right of prior written notice before any change in plans of the public agency is implemented in any aspect of the child's educational programming. Finally, procedural safeguards afford the parents the right of filing a complaint.

Individualized Education Plans

The IDEA (2004) requires that each child over the age of 3 years with a qualified disability is to have an **individualized education plan** (IEP), which is a written document that stipulates the special education programs and services, long-term goals, short-term objectives, and any accommodations and related services provided by the public agency. The IEP is developed after a meeting is held involving the parents; the child (if appropriate); the child's regular education teacher, if the child participates in the general education curriculum; the child's special education teacher; a representative of the public agency; evaluation personnel, such as the school psychologist or any professional who can interpret how the evaluation results impact the educational program; translators or interpreters; transition personnel; or other individuals who have an expertise in the area of the child's disability. For example, ideally an audiologist, speech-language pathologist, or teacher of the deaf should attend IEP meetings of children who are deaf or hard of hearing.

By law, the IEP meeting should be convened within 30 days after the child has established eligibility for special education services. Parents must be given written notice of the date, time, and place of the meeting so that they may make appropriate arrangements to attend and not have to forfeit wages from their jobs to do so. The school must notify parents why the meeting is taking place and those attending. Parents have the right to invite people who have special areas of expertise or who may offer support. Parents may be intimidated by the process, but they should know that they are a very important part of the IEP team, and should not be afraid to ask questions or share their concerns. Parents know their children better than anyone else and their input is critical to the success of an IEP meeting. They may provide the results of any private evaluations in addition to information about their child's strengths, weaknesses, needs, goals, effective rewards, and work habits. Parents can also provide examples of behaviors that confirm results of formal diagnostic evaluations. For example, parents' observation of auditory behaviors at home may confirm results of audiologic testing. The IEP should contain the child's strengths; current educational status; present level of functioning; participation in general education curriculum; long-term goals and short-term objectives; evaluation tools, activities, procedures, and criteria; how parents will be regularly notified; explanation of why a child will not participate with nondisabled students; explanation of participation in assessments; statement of frequency and duration of services; explanation of program options; placement considerations; transition plans; and description of related services, supplementary aids and services (IDEA, 2004).

Related Services and Supplementary Aids and Services

Audiology and speech-language pathology are **related services**, which means they are in a category that includes anything from transportation to developmental, corrective, or other supportive services that are needed for the child to benefit from special education. Related services are provided by audiologists, educational interpreters, school counselors, school nurses, school psychologists, school social workers, and speech-language pathologists (IDEA, 2004).

Supplementary aids and services are those things that support a child with disabilities in general education such as interpreters and assistive technology that are discussed in Chapter 7. Specifically, the IDEA (2004) defines these as follows:

> PART B INTERPRETING SERVICES 34CFR300.34(c)(4)
> *Interpreting services* includes
>
> (i) The following when used with respect to children who are deaf or hard of hearing: oral transliteration services, cued language transliteration services, and sign language transliteration and interpreting services, and transcription services, such as communication access real-time translation (CART), C-Print, and TypeWell; and
> (ii) Special interpreting services for children who are deaf-blind.   (Authority: 20 U.S.C. 1401(26))
>
> PART B ASSISTIVE TECHNOLOGY 300.105(a)(2)
> On a case-by-case basis, the use of school-purchased assistive technology devices in a child's home or in other settings is required if the child's IEP Team determines that the child needs access to those devices in order to receive FAPE. Authority: 20 U.S.C. 1412(a)(1), 1412(a)(12)(b)(i)

Classroom teachers need to understand how to meet the needs of students who are deaf and hard of hearing. Teachers need to know what assistive technology is, the types that are available, and how to integrate them into the classroom. Educational audiologists and speech-language pathologists help teachers accomplish these goals; their roles are discussed after this brief explanation of two additional federal laws.

Other Laws

Two other federal laws, Section 504 of the Rehabilitation Act of 1973 and the Americans with Disabilities Act (1990), may also be used to secure accommodations for children with hearing impairment.

Section 504 of the Rehabilitation Act of 1973 is a federal law that protects otherwise qualified individuals from discrimination based on their disabilities. The law defines those with disabilities as individuals with physical or mental impairments that substantially limit one or more major life activities (e.g., walking, sitting, breathing, learning, working, sleeping, speaking, hearing, eating, reading, concentrating, etc.). Section 504 is often used in schools to ensure that children with disabilities have equal access to an education. Children who have disabilities, but not the type or to the degree necessary to meet state guidelines for special education under the IDEA, may seek accommodations through a Section 504 Plan. For example, a child with a minimal hearing loss who does not qualify as having a hearing impairment according to state guidelines may receive equal access to an education through use of a personal FM system.

The Americans with Disabilities Act (1990) is a far-reaching piece of legislation that prohibits private employers, state, and local governments and others from discriminating against otherwise qualified individuals with a disability. A person with a disability is defined as follows (ADA, 1990):

- Has a physical or mental impairment that substantially limits one or more major life activities;
- Has a record of such an impairment; or
- Is regarded as having such an impairment.

The ADA (1990) can be used to gain access to an education for students with disabilities who may not qualify for services under the IDEA (2004).

ROLE OF AUDIOLOGISTS

The IDEA (2004) defined audiology in this manner:

PART B - DEFINITION OF AUDIOLOGY 34CFR300.34(c)(1)
Audiology includes

(i) Identification of children with hearing loss;
(ii) Determination of the range, nature, and degree of hearing loss, including referral for medical or other professional attention for the habilitation of hearing;
(iii) Provision of habilitation activities, such as language habilitation, auditory training, speech reading (lipreading), hearing evaluation, and speech conservation;
(iv) Creation and administration of programs for prevention of hearing loss;
(v) Counseling and guidance of children, parents, and teachers regarding hearing loss; and
(vi) Determination of children's needs for group and individual amplification, selecting and fitting an appropriate aid, and evaluating the effectiveness of amplification.

Educational audiologists are hearing healthcare professionals who provide services to children in schools. Johnson et al. (1997) stated that there were two service delivery

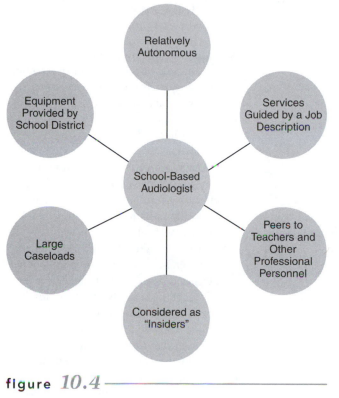

figure *10.4*

Characteristics of a school-based audiologist.

Source: Based on *Educational Audiology Handbook, by* C. D. Johnson, P. V. Benson, and J. B. Seaton, 1997, San Diego, CA: Singular.

models for educational audiologists. The first, the **school-based model**, occurs when audiologists are full-time employees of the school district or educational agency. Figure 10.4 displays the characteristics of audiologists in school-based service delivery models.

School-based audiologists are relatively autonomous employees who are often "on-the-go," traveling from school to school, providing comprehensive services stipulated by their job description. School-based audiologists are considered peers of and "insiders" by other professional personnel. School-based audiologists use equipment provided by the public agency and are more common in large school systems with many children on their caseloads.

The second, the **contract-for-service model**, occurs when audiologists are hired by school systems to perform duties as specified in a contract. Figure 10.5 illustrates the characteristics of audiologists in contract-for-service delivery models.

Contract-for-service audiologists are autonomous employees who are also "on the go," traveling from school to school; however, the services they provide are limited and specified by a contract. Contract-for-service audiologists are viewed as part-time employees and even as "outsiders" by school personnel. Contract-for-service audiologists must supply equipment and materials and are more common in smaller, rural school systems with limited caseloads.

Regardless of service delivery model, there is a severe shortage of educational audiologists. Although Johnson et al. (1997) recommended an audiologist-to-student ratio of 1:12,000, recent estimates have stated that there are approximately five times fewer educational audiologists than are needed to adequately serve the needs of school-aged population. More recently, the Educational Audiology Association recommended a target ratio of one full-time audiologist for every 10,000 students in a local school agency (Educational Audiology Association, 2009). For school-based audiologists, only one or two audiologists may be employed per school district, resulting in huge caseloads. Contract-for-service audiologists frequently are hired to cover only the most necessary audiologic services involving screening, diagnosis, and determining the needs for group and individual amplification. Shortages of hearing healthcare professionals require that speech-language pathologists fill in the gaps in meeting the needs of children with hearing loss. We will now discuss various service delivery functions performed by educational audiologists.

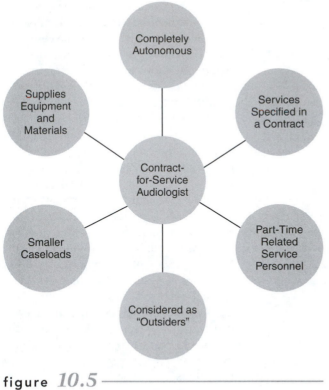

figure *10.5*

Characteristics of a contract-for-service audiologist.

Source: Based on *Educational Audiology Handbook*, by C. D. Johnson, P. V. Benson, and J. B. Seaton, 1997, San Diego, CA: Singular.

Identification of Children With Hearing Loss

According to the IDEA (2004), audiology services include identification of or screening of children for hearing loss. **Screening** is a short process that serves to identify persons who may have a condition (e.g., hearing loss) needing further evaluation from those who do not. In the last chapter, we discussed the developments in universal newborn hearing screening programs. Educational audiologists direct hearing screening programs in the public schools in order to identify those children who may have been missed or who have developed a hearing loss during early childhood. These programs often include pure-tone audiometry and assessment of middle ear function. Screening should be done in preschool and periodically throughout the school-age years. The *Guidelines for Audiology Service Provision in and for Schools* (ASHA, 2002) suggests that screening should be done liberally, "needed, referred, requested, and/or required by federal, state, and local mandates as well as for all children on initial entry into school and annually in kindergarten through 3rd grade, and in the 7th and 11th grades." Children who fail the hearing screenings should be scheduled for a complete audiologic evaluation. Moreover, educational audiologists should ensure that the screening tools used are appropriate for children both developmentally and culturally (Educational Audiology Association, 2009). In addition, educational audiologists should participate in the assessment and documentation of the effectiveness of screening programs. Periodically, *sensitivity* and *specificity* measures should be obtained to determine the validity of screening programs. **Sensitivity** is the accuracy with which screening protocols identify those who actually have a disorder. **Specificity** is the accuracy with which screening protocols accurately dismiss those individuals who, in fact, do not have a certain disorder. Both measures are scored in percent; the higher the percent, the more accurate the screening protocol. Screening programs that have marginal sensitivity and/or specificity require assessment to determine what areas need improvement. One area that may affect the validity of protocols is the use of inappropriate screening techniques. Educational audiologists do not have time to conduct each and every screening and must rely on others, such as school nurses and speech-language pathologists. Therefore, audiologists should provide training and support for educational personnel performing hearing screenings (Educational Audiology Association, 2009).

Some children are referred for hearing screening by teachers who observe inconsistent auditory behaviors or problems with comprehension in the classroom. In Chapter 1 and earlier in this chapter, we defined an auditory condition called **(central) auditory processing disorders ([C]APD).** Children with these disorders have normal hearing sensitivity, but have problems with the central nervous system that are exemplified by poor performance in one or more auditory behaviors or skills, such as the ability to locate the origin of a sound in the environment or difficulty understanding speech in noise. Children with (C)APD appear to teachers as having a hearing loss, so naturally they are referred for hearing screenings. However, for children who display behaviors common to children with hearing loss and pass the hearing screening, further evaluations are warranted. Bellis (2003) recommended that school systems develop a program specifically for screening (C)APD, discussed later in the chapter.

Diagnosis of Hearing Loss

The IDEA states that audiology services include audiologic evaluations to determine the type, degree, and configuration of hearing loss in addition to appropriate referrals for medical or other appropriate professional services. However, it is recommended that the evaluation be multidisciplinary and measure the impact of hearing loss on communication function, academic performance, and psychosocial development (ASHA, 2002). Moreover, audiologic testing should include a variety of procedures appropriate for the child's developmental level and be conducted with calibrated equipment in appropriate acoustic environments (Educational Audiology Association, 2009). In Chapter 9, we discussed the role of the *medical home* in the auditory habilitation of young children. Recall that the medical home is a high-quality and cost-effective approach to providing accessible, family-centered, ongoing, comprehensive, coordinated, and compassionate care to children through assignment of a primary healthcare provider who knows the child on an individual basis, acknowledging any special needs, and cultural background for achievement of maximum potential (American Academy of Pediatrics, 1997). The educational audiologist must refer children with hearing loss to their medical home providers for treatment. Children with conductive hearing losses can be treated and reevaluated. Those with sensorineural hearing losses or AN/AD are referred for habilitative services to include the selection, evaluation, and fitting of appropriate amplification. Many families may not be able to afford hearing aids for their children, and social workers may need to be involved to assist parents in applying for public healthcare assistance for obtaining hearing aids.

Selecting, Fitting, and Managing Amplification

Another major area of audiologists' work is the determination of children's need for group and individual amplification, selecting and fitting appropriate hearing aid or HAT (Defined as hearing assistive technology in chapter 7), and evaluating the effectiveness of these devices. Educational audiologists should have the equipment and testing environment appropriate for conducting hearing instrument selection, verification, and fitting procedures. Essential equipment includes hearing aid analyzers, real-ear probe-tube microphone measurement capabilities, and methods for testing speech recognition performance in quiet and noise. Most public agencies do not directly supply personal hearing aids to children, although it could be argued that they are needed for access to a FAPE in the LRE. However, the public agency is not obligated to provide personal hearing aids.

The agency should provide amplification to be worn during the school day, usually in the form of personal and group FM amplification systems. These systems are important for overcoming *noise* and *reverberation* that are common in most classrooms (Knecht, Nelson,

Whitelaw, & Feth, 2002). **Noise** is any unwanted sound; **reverberation** is the continuation of acoustic energy due to the reflections of that energy off room surfaces after the source has been terminated. Classroom acoustics will be discussed in more detail later in this chapter.

Educational audiologists also take the lead in managing **hearing assistive technology (HAT)** or **assistive listening devices (ALDs)**, which are defined in Chapter 7 as a range of devices, services, strategies, and practices that are conceived and applied to ameliorate the hearing problems faced by individuals who have hearing loss. Hearing assistive technology in schools includes **remote microphone hearing assistive technology** (RMHAT) that includes personal FM systems, group/individual sound-field systems, and induction loop systems, also discussed in Chapter 7. Determination of children's need for group and individual amplification involves candidacy for RMHAT, which not only includes children with hearing loss, but students with (C)APD, learning disabilities, AN/AD, language deficits, attention deficit disorders, and non-native speakers of English (AAA, 2009d). The FM-receivers can be tiny and connect directly to hearing aids or they can be larger body-worn devices. These devices also help to overcome the deleterious effects of reverberation and noise. Audiologists should advocate for children with hearing loss for getting access to these devices (AAA, 2009d).

Chapter 8 discussed important school follow-up for children with cochlear implants. School personnel, particularly the educational audiologist, must communicate with professionals at the cochlear implant center regarding children's school performance and need for HAT (Educational Audiology Association, 2009). In particular, audiologists and speech language pathologists consult with the hearing healthcare professional who maps students' cochlear implants. Performance in speech-language therapy and in the classroom helps determine the need for checking and/or adjustment of cochlear implants used with HAT devices.

A specific part of the IDEA (2004) that pertains to amplification systems including surgically implanted medical devices such as cochlear implants states as follows:

PART B ROUTINE CHECKING OF HEARING AIDS AND EXTERNAL COMPONENTS OF SURGICALLY IMPLANTED MEDICAL DEVICES 34CFR300.113

(a) *Hearing aids.* Each public agency must ensure that hearing aids worn in school by children with hearing impairments, including deafness, are functioning properly.
(b) *External components of surgically implanted medical devices.*
    (1) Subject to paragraph (b)(2) of this section, each public agency must ensure that the external components of surgically implanted medical devices are functioning properly.
    (2) For a child with a surgically implanted medical device who is receiving special education and related services under this part, a public agency is not responsible for the post-surgical maintenance, programming, or replacement of the medical device that has been surgically implanted (or of an external component of the surgically implanted medical device). (Authority: 20 U.S.C. 1401(1), 1401 (26) (B))

This part of the law states that school systems must make sure that the hearing aids, FM systems, and cochlear implants are functioning properly. Audiologists who manage the amplification device maintenance programs need to ensure their effectiveness in meeting student's needs. Reichman and Healey (1989; p. 43) stated that adequate programs follow these five preferred practices:

- Daily visual and listening inspections of hearing aids and FM systems
- Periodic electroacoustic analysis of hearing aids and FM systems (two times per year)

- Availability of hearing aids and FM systems as loaners on the day a malfunction is detected
- Procedures for replacing earmolds and other accessories, including equipment provisions and fiscal responsibility
- Teacher, parent, and student instruction in amplification device monitoring and maintenance

Chapter 9, Appendix 9.3 contains a checklist for a daily visual and listening check of hearing aids that could be used for this purpose. Documentation of these checks is critical and becomes part of children's permanent records. Educational audiologists frequently require assistance in hearing aid monitoring and must train others on how to participate in these programs (Johnson, 1999). Educational audiologists must also be trained specifically in RMHAT, including how to perform visual and listening checks. Kooper (2009) advised that a person must be designated to take responsibility for RMHAT, who will learn how to check, troubleshoot, send for repair, order extended warranties, and send in for routine maintenance. Just as with hearing aids, educational audiologists should delegate some of the responsibilities for visual and listening checks to those having the most contact with students who can fix minor problems and know when to refer a unit for repair.

According to the law, the external parts of children's cochlear implants must also be checked and maintained. However, the law is clear in stating that the public agency is not responsible for the postsurgical maintenance, programming, or replacement of the medical device that has been surgically implanted or its external parts. In Chapter 8, it was stressed that school personnel should have a good working relationship with cochlear implant centers in the event that problems arise for children with these devices. In particular, audiologists should closely communicate with teachers and speech-language pathologists, advising them to report equipment problems and to monitor children's sound awareness, classroom behaviors, and speech production and recognition (Advanced Bionics, 2009). Problems in any one of these areas may signal that adjustments of the cochlear implant are needed.

In addition to checking the functioning of hearing aids, RMHAT, and cochlear implants, audiologists should measure the effectiveness of amplification. Assessment of amplification devices includes performances with individual technologies in addition to their use in combination. For example, assessment of children's performance with their hearing aids and when coupled to RMHAT is required according to recommended guidelines. Measures of effectiveness should include objective clinical measures, input from stakeholders, and use of paper-and-pencil outcome measures. Assessment tools for this purpose are discussed later in the chapter.

Prevention of Hearing Loss

Audiologists also develop and maintain programs for the prevention of hearing loss. Hearing loss is something that most people associate with aging. However, hearing loss from overexposure to noise is insidious, and damage frequently begins in childhood. Teachers and children may be exposed to potentially hazardous sound levels in certain classes at school (e.g., shop) or when involved in certain activities (e.g., band) (Behar MacDonald Lee, Cui, Kunov, & Wong, 2004). Therefore, audiologists should conduct **sound surveys** or sound measurements in noisy areas to determine the amount of risk for developing noise-induced hearing loss. If so, baseline audiograms should be obtained for those at risk, with audiologic reevaluations each year, and education provided on preventing noise-induced hearing loss as part of a hearing conservation program. (Chapter 11 has additional information regarding these programs.)

A national prevalence study found that approximately 12.5% of children aged 6 to 19 years in the United States have signs of a noise-induced hearing loss in one or both ears (Niskar et al., 2001). Namely, they had noise-induced threshold shifts at 4000 Hz, demonstrating that school-age children are vulnerable to excessive exposure to loud sound levels. More recently, the prevalence of hearing loss has been estimated to be one in five (Shargorodsky, Curhan, Curhan, & Eavey, 2010). Niskar et al. (2001) recommended that programs for preventing noise-induced hearing loss be administered to school-age children. Ideally, these programs may be implemented and directed by educational audiologists who partner with health educators to teach school-age children about the dangers of noise on hearing health. Successful hearing loss prevention programs not only educate school-age children, but convince them to change their behaviors. However, encouraging children to change their present behavior is extremely difficult because it is hard for youngsters to imagine how hearing loss may negatively affect their quality of life in the future. Daniel (2007) advised that audiologists and health educators must identify and address ways to encourage children to wear devices to protect their hearing and to avoid listening to excessively loud music.

One recent source of concern has been the possibility of noise-induced hearing loss from listening to **personal listening devices** (PLDs) in the form of MP3 players and iPods. As of 2010, Apple, Inc. has sold in excess of 280 million iPods around the world. iPods are especially popular with high school and college students, although a growing number of younger students also own iPods (Danhauer, Johnson, Byrd, DeGood, Meuel, Pecile, & Koch, 2009; Torre, 2008; Zogby International, 2006). Fligor and Cox (2004) found that PLDs can produce sound pressure levels in excess of 130 dB, which can damage hearing even for short listening periods. These authors suggested a **60/60 rule**, which is that people should limit their listening to compact disc players for no more than 60% of full volume for 60 minutes per day. Later, however, Fligor and Ives (2006) modified those recommendations to listening to iPods with stock earphones for no more than 70% of full volume for 4.6 hours per day. It has been estimated that less than 10% of young people seem to have iPod listening behaviors that put them at risk for hearing loss (e.g., Danhauer et al., 2009). Nevertheless, children and young adults are exposed to other sources of potentially hazardous sound levels. Hearing loss prevention programs are useful in teaching that the effects of noise are cumulative, symptoms of overexposure, and ways to protect hearing. For example, if students experience ringing in their ears during noisy activities, it is a clear sign that they are overdoing it (Johnson, Stein, Gorman, & Tracy, 1997).

The Educational Audiology Association (2009) listed the roles of audiologists in developing hearing loss prevention programs:

1. Determining the content and making the curriculum relevant for the various age groups
2. Identifying existing courses where noise education may be infused
3. Identifying who will teach the various modules and the role of the audiologist in the management and delivery of the program.

The audiologist is best suited to assist general education teachers in integrating the critical information into their own health, science, or vocational education courses.

Counseling and Guidance

Another area of educational audiology is counseling and guidance of children, parents, and teachers regarding hearing loss. Guidance and counseling are important because children with hearing loss need an adult who understands what they are going through and can foster opportunities for development of self-awareness and self-efficacy. Growing up to be responsible and well-adjusted adults is a challenging task for all children, but especially for those with hearing loss. These children have difficulty in academic performance and often feel socially isolated from their peers.

Audiologists and speech-language pathologists frequently provide counseling to these children, either in the form of informational counseling and/or personal adjustment counseling, which were discussed in Chapter 2. **Informational counseling** for children consists of providing factual information to a child. Types of information may include how to take care of hearing aids, personal FM systems, or other HAT, as well as how to use compensatory strategies in the classroom. **Personal adjustment counseling** consists of assisting children to cope with and solve problems caused by the secondary emotional and social effects of hearing loss. Specific techniques for counseling will be discussed later in this chapter.

Educational audiologists should partner with parents and teachers in order to best meet the needs of children with hearing impairment. Parents and teachers may not fully understand the impact of hearing loss on children's ability to learn or on their self-esteem. Audiologists and speech-language pathologists must partner in providing *inservices* to teachers and other school personnel to raise awareness levels about educational consequences of hearing loss and what must be done to best accommodate students' needs. **Inservices** are continuing education opportunities to teach knowledge and skills on selected topics. Figure 10.6 shows typical topics of inservices provided to teachers and other educational personnel.

In the public school setting, because staff time and resources are scarce, inservices must be well-planned. Figure 10.7 shows characteristics of effective learning opportunities.

- Accommodations for children who are deaf and hard of hearing
- Auditory neuropathy/dyssynchrony
- Auditory processing disorders
- Care and maintenance of hearing aids and sound-field amplification
- Classroom acoustics
- Cochlear implants
- Communication tips
- Screening for hearing loss
- Transition planning

figure *10.6*

Typical topics for inservices to school personnel.

Source: Based on *Guidebook for Support Programs in Aural Rehabilitation, by* C. E. Johnson and J. L. Danhauer, 1999, San Diego, CA: Singular.

Educational audiologists, speech-language pathologists, and teachers of the deaf are the experts best qualified to provide inservices about the educational needs of children who are deaf and hard of hearing. School personnel time is valuable, and inservices should have well-defined behavioral objectives with specific knowledge and skills for outcomes. Inservice providers should be respectful of others' time and provide participants with instruction on what they need to know and do. For example, an inservice on how to perform visual and listening checks on hearing aids should specifically cover the types of hearing aids most often encountered in the school setting. Adequate planning is necessary to ensure that the inservice is well-equipped for the number of participants involved. In using our example, there should be

- Directed by licensed and certified audiologists and speech-language pathologists
- Well-defined and specific to limited tasks
- Appropriate to the scope and intensity of training
- Competency based
- Well equipped
- Both informal and formal in format
- Ongoing and current
- Rigorous in evaluating participants' skills

figure *10.7* —————————————————

Characteristics of successful inservices.

Source: Based on *Guidebook for Support Programs in Aural Rehabilitation, by* C. E. Johnson and J. L. Danhauer, 1999, San Diego, CA: Singular.

enough listening stethoscopes, batteries, and hearings aids for all participants to practice visual and listening checks. Inservices should have formal or group instruction, in addition to informal, one-on-one practicum instruction with participants. Inservices should be ongoing and planned in such a way that they are not vulnerable to turnover in staff. The topics of inservices should be current, such as about the latest developments in new, open-ear hearing aids. Lastly, inservices should keep careful track of who has had training, in addition to assessing what attendees have learned and their impressions of the experience. Inservices that directly relate to the quality of education for children with hearing impairment should be a top priority.

ROLE OF SPEECH-LANGUAGE PATHOLOGISTS

As previously stated in this book, the roles of audiologists and speech-language pathologists are complementary and overlapping in providing auditory rehabilitation. The same holds true for serving children who are deaf and hard of hearing in the public schools. In Chapter 4, the knowledge and skills required for speech-language pathologists providing auditory rehabilitation services were listed, and many of them apply to the school setting. Unlike audiologists, speech-language pathologists are usually employees of the school system. Speech-language pathologists may be placed at a particular school or may be **itinerant**, traveling from school to school to provide services to children. Speech-language pathologists may also supervise **speech-language pathology assistants** in the provision of services to children with hearing loss (ASHA, 2007). As suggested by the Joint Committee on Infant Hearing Year 2007 Position Statement (JCIH, 2007), professionals serving children who are deaf and hard of hearing should have expertise on the effects of and interventions for hearing loss, particularly in the educational milieu. Speech-language pathologists providing direct services to these children should have training and received certification, if applicable, in aural habilitative approaches such as Auditory-Verbal therapy.

Speech-language pathologists work closely with audiologists and teachers of the deaf to ensure that the goals and objectives of children's IEPs are met. Speech-language pathologists provide feedback to educational audiologists regarding the child's use of individual/group amplification and progress in therapy. Speech-language pathologists and audiologists may collaborate in providing inservices to school personnel. The speech-language pathologist is a conduit for communication with children's classroom teachers, including those in regular and special education. Speech-language pathologists consult with regular education teachers regarding specific areas of children's needs and facilitate learning by preteaching concepts that have yet to be introduced in the classroom. Like audiologists, speech-language pathologists may suggest possible strategies for teachers to use in the classroom to facilitate children's learning. They may also collaborate about service delivery with teachers of the deaf and hard of hearing who are at schools containing specialized training to deliver children's educational programs. These programs include developing communicative competence in a variety of social, linguistic, and cognitive/academic contexts in the following settings (ASHA, 2004d):

- Schools for the deaf
- Other schools that serve hearing, deaf, and hard-of-hearing children to include:
  - Self-contained classrooms
  - Resource rooms
  - Regular education classrooms
- Itinerant-, home-, or community-based programs

As discussed in Chapter 1, some teachers of the deaf and hard of hearing have specialized training to provide aural habilitative therapy.

Figure 10.8 lists collaborative responsibilities between speech-language pathologists and teachers of the deaf and hard of hearing. Together, when planning programs for children, they should consider students' background information, including family history, medical profile, any prior assessments, previous reports, and any direct observations of the child. Chapter 3 stressed that the child's cultural background should be considered in educational programming. Of particular importance is the communication and linguistic history of the child and family, including modalities and languages. Assessment should include a variety of measures to determine communicative strengths and weaknesses for the establishment of appropriate long-term goals and short-term educational objectives for the IEP. Speech-language pathologists must monitor how children's language abilities impact academic performance in the classroom. It is also important that communicative goals and objectives reflect educational goals that have been established from input of multiple stakeholders such as the family and members of the IEP team. The child, related services, and the educational programs should be monitored for continuous quality improvement.

Collaborative efforts should also include the generation of regular progress reports to relevant professionals in accordance with Part B of the IDEA (2004). Speech-language pathologists and teachers may be the only personnel who may directly observe the child and have regular contact with the family to determine success with HAT. In addition to audiologists, these professionals should provide consultation, guidance, and education to children with hearing loss and their families. For example, some parents may want additional information regarding possible referral sources for pursuing cochlear implants for their children. In addition, these professionals may serve a supportive role for other school personnel involved in the auditory habilitation of students. For example, they may need to take the time to show how to change a battery on a child's hearing aid.

Speech-language pathologists and teachers of the deaf and hard of hearing are critical in reviewing children's overall strengths and weaknesses and determining what problems, if any, are related to issues other than hearing loss. For example, children with hearing loss, like their peers with normal hearing, may have issues that require referral to another professional (e.g., psychologist). Moreover, the collaboration of these two professionals is critical for transition planning to postsecondary educational training or career planning in addition to developing self-advocacy skills for the future.

- Consider relevant background information (family history, medical information, previous assessments, reports, and observations) for the purposes of program planning.
- Obtain a comprehensive description of communicative and linguistic abilities and needs of the child, history of communication modalities and languages (signed and/or spoken) used and/or tried, family preferences, and concerns related to communication.
- Administer and interpret appropriate formal and informal standardized and nonstandardized assessments of all areas of communicative competence.
- Develop communicative competence goals and objectives that address the general curriculum for the child; incorporate recommendations and findings of the family and interdisciplinary team.
- Identify individuals responsible for the design and implementation of an instructional program and related services to assist the child in achieving the identified goals and objectives.
- Evaluate the child's progress as related to the goals.
- Evaluate the program or related services provided.
- Provide progress reports to families on a regular basis and other professionals as consistent with IDEA Parts B and C.
- Determine the effectiveness of assistive technologies for the child in collaboration with the family and interdisciplinary team.
- Facilitate the development of social aspects of communication.
- Provide consultation, guidance, and education to children and young adults who are deaf or hard of hearing and to their families.
- Provide consultation and support to and/or collaborate with professionals and paraprofessionals involved in the habilitation/educational program of the child.
- Consider overall learning strengths, weaknesses, differences, and/or delays that may be unrelated to hearing status for appropriate referral and/or educational planning.
- Collaborate with families and children regarding communicative and linguistic strengths and needs in planning appropriate educational, vocational, and/or career transitions.
- Assist families in receiving appropriate access to communicative and linguistic services for the child.
- Assist students in developing the skills and knowledge necessary for self-advocacy.

figure *10.8*

Collaborative responsibilities of speech-language pathologists in working with teachers of the deaf in the public schools.

Source: From *Roles of Speech-Language Pathologists and Teachers of Children Who Are Deaf and Hard of Hearing in the Development of Communicative and Linguistic Competence* [Guidelines], 2004, by the American Speech-Language-Hearing Association, retrieved from www.asha.org/policy. All rights reserved. Reprinted with permission.

ACCOMMODATIONS FOR CHILDREN WHO ARE DEAF AND HARD OF HEARING

The academic success of children with hearing impairment depends on the availability of accommodations in the classroom. English (2002) used a safety net metaphor to describe accommodations needed by these children who find themselves in precarious learning classroom environments. Friend (2005) identified the following seven areas requiring accommodations for students who are deaf and hard of hearing: (1) environmental, (2) input, (3) output, (4) evaluation, (5) grading, (6) behavioral, and (7) social.

Environmental Modifications

Environmental modifications involve changing aspects of the learning environment to maximize the reception of auditory and visual information, including the acoustic environment and classroom set-up.

Acoustic Environment

The American Speech-Language-Hearing Association wrote a position statement in 2005 recommending an appropriate acoustical environment for all students in educational settings and endorses *ANSI S12.60-2002 Acoustical Performance Criteria, Design Requirements and Guidelines for Schools* (ANSI S12.60-2002), a national standard for classroom acoustics. The *Acoustics in Educational Settings: Position Statement* cites three acoustical factors in classrooms: (1) the level of the ambient noise, (2) the relative intensity of the teacher's voice to that of the background noise or signal-to-noise ratio (SNR), and (3) the reverberant characteristics of the room. ASHA's position statement recommends tolerances for each of these factors (ASHA, 2005d).

First, they recommended that the level of ambient noise should not exceed 35 dB A. These measurements should not be done when the classroom is empty, but during the regular school day. The measurements are made with a **sound level meter**, which is an instrument that measures the levels of various sounds. The sound level meter has different weighting scales to measure decibel values. Note that the abbreviation "dB" is followed by an "A," meaning that these measurements are made on the A-weighting scale. The A-weighting scale represents how well humans hear across the frequency range for sounds of moderate levels. Sound level meters range in price, varying from less than $100 to tens of thousands of dollars. These measures can be made with a sound level meter that can be purchased from Radio Shack for around $100. Sound level meters are discussed more in Chapter 11.

Second, ASHA's position statement recommended that the SNR be at least +15 dB at the child's ears. Note that no letter appears after "dB" in this example because we are talking about relative values. In other words, the level of the teacher's voice must be 15 dB greater than the noise level in the classroom. For example, if the level of the background noise is 50 dB A, the level of the teacher's voice must be 65 dB A or greater. Determining the SNR requires at least three steps and must be completed during a normal school day during regular classroom activities. The first step is to measure the teacher's voice at the child's ear. Next, the noise in the classroom should be measured at the same location and compared with that of the background noise. If the S/N is not +15 dB or greater at the child's ear, then acoustic modification or use of RMHAT is warranted.

Third, ASHA (2005d) recommends that the reverberation time of unoccupied classrooms should not exceed 0.6 seconds in small classrooms (i.e., smaller than 10,000 ft^3) or 0.7 seconds in larger classrooms (i.e., 10,000 ft^3 or larger, but less than 20,000 ft^3). Recall that reverberation is the continuation of acoustic energy due to the reflections of that energy off the room surfaces after the source of the sound has been terminated (Crandall & Smaldino, 2005). The extent of reverberation is signified by the **reverberation time**, which is the time it takes for the root mean square sound pressure level of the sound to decrease 60 dB after the source has been terminated. The longer the reverberation time, the greater are the effects of smearing and other distortions to the speech signal. Larger rooms with hard surfaces have longer reverberation times than smaller rooms with more absorptive surfaces. Reverberation time is somewhat more difficult to obtain than SNR, requiring special equipment.

Scientifically, reverberation time is the time it takes for the root mean square of the sound to decrease 60 dB after termination of the stimulus. However, due to relatively high ambient noise levels in a room, usually it is not possible to measure the 60 dB of decay, so estimates are made based on measureable values, like 20 dB. Reverberation times exceeding recommended values warrant the acoustical treatment of classrooms. Classroom acoustics provide an excellent example of how school personnel, audiologists, and other professionals can collaborate toward enhancing the educational experiences of individuals who are deaf and hard of hearing.

Acoustical Treatment

Acoustical treatment of classrooms includes minimizing three potential sources of noise. **External noise** is that which comes from outside of the school (e.g., playground noise and traffic noise). Crandell and Smaldino (2005) provided several suggestions for reducing external noise. First, it can be reduced by locating classrooms away from high-noise sources such as air-conditioning units. They also suggested using building materials with a *sound transmission loss* (STL) of at least 45 to 50 dB. **Sound transmission loss** is the number of decibels that are attenuated from one side of a partition to another. In addition, they suggested ensuring that exterior walls and windows are free from cracks and openings and are properly limiting possible pathways for noise. In addition, they suggested using either natural landscaping (e.g., shrubbery) or concrete walls to serve as barriers between a school and noise sources such as a nearby highway.

Internal noise is that which comes from inside the school, but outside the classroom (e.g., hallway noise and noise from the cafeteria). Crandell and Smaldino (2005) also provided suggestions for reducing internal noise, beginning with placement of classrooms in quiet areas of the school away from gymnasiums. Second, they suggested placing lead sheets or fiberglass installations in the plenum between classrooms with drop ceilings and using double or thick wall constructions for interior walls of a classroom. Moreover, high-mass-per-unit doors that are acoustically treated can attenuate and prevent sound in the hallway from entering the classroom. In addition, the hallways outside of the classroom should be carpeted and/or have acoustic ceiling tile. Finally, they suggested the acoustical treatment of heating/cooling ducts and permanently mounted blackboards to reduce sound transmission from adjacent rooms.

Classroom noise comes from inside the classroom (e.g., children talking and computer noise). Crandell and Smaldino (2005) also provided suggestions for reducing classroom noise, such as moving children away from high-noise sources (e.g., fans, air conditioners, and heating ducts). Much of the noise from these sources can be minimized through adequate maintenance of fluorescent lights, educational equipment (e.g., fans on overhead projectors), and heating and air-conditioning units. Like the hallways, classrooms should have thick, wall-to-wall carpet installed and acoustic paneling placed on the walls, curtains covering windows, and rubber tips on the legs of desks and chairs. They also suggested lowering noise from computer stations by placing rubber pads under keyboards.

Crandell and Smaldino's (2005) suggestions for reducing reverberation are similar to those for classroom noise: hard surfaces should be covered with sound-absorptive materials, floors should be covered with thick carpeting, windows and unused blackboards should be covered with curtains, and artwork should be placed on the walls. They also suggested that blackboards should be placed at angles rather than parallel to each other to reduce the chance of "**flutter echo**," or the ricocheting of reflected sound bouncing between two parallel structures.

Classroom Type and Teaching Style

An important part of environmental modifications includes classroom type and teaching style and their impact on the educational experiences of children who are deaf and hard of hearing. **Classroom types** involve the formats for teaching and include (1) closed classrooms, (2) open area concepts, (3) split grades, and (4) portable classrooms (Edwards, 2005). **Closed classrooms** are traditional classrooms in which teachers and students are in a completely enclosed space. Edwards (2005) describes **open area concepts** that allow for up to eight classes to be located in the same space, permitting team teaching and cross-grouping of children who can move easily from class to class (Edwards, 2005). She defines **split-grade classrooms** as the combination of children from two or more grade levels into a single classroom resulting in two or more activities occurring within the same enclosure. **Portable classrooms** are moveable educational enclosures that are typically used when the number of children exceeds the capacity of the school (Edwards, 2005).

Edwards (2005) also discussed five different teaching styles: (1) didactic, (2) interactive, (3) small group, (4) team teaching, and (5) independent work periods. **Didactic teaching**, the most traditional method, usually involves a teacher standing and talking to students seated at their desks. **Interactive teaching** styles involve teacher-to-student and student-to-student dialogue and may be appropriate for small or large groups. **Small-group instruction** is one teacher instructing 10 students or fewer. **Team teaching** is two or more teachers combining their classes together in one classroom. Edwards (2005) says that teachers may have older students concentrate on assignments during **independent work periods**.

In today's economy, many schools have to get by with the facilities that they have. The type of classroom may not always be the best for children who are deaf and hard of hearing. Obviously, closed classrooms seem like the best option for them because noise and other distractions are minimized. Open area concept, split-grade, and team teaching classrooms frequently have more than one learning activity going on at the same time. Multiple group activities can cause classroom noise levels to spiral out of control, resulting in a negative SNR.

Classroom type is not completely independent of teaching style. The type of classroom, its size, seating arrangement, and the number of children influence teaching style. The greater the number of teachers, grade-levels, and children that utilize a single space, the larger the classroom has to be. Larger classrooms allow for greater **square-foot-to-student ratios**, or the number of square feet per child. Larger classrooms with appropriate numbers of students afford teachers and paraprofessionals the opportunity of isolating small groups of children for small-group work, when needed. Teachers often have to adapt and do more things with less space and higher teacher-to-student ratios. However, the situation becomes more complicated when children who have special needs, particularly those who are deaf and hard of hearing, are added to the class rosters.

School administrators and IEP teams need to consider classroom type and teaching style when determining the placement for children with hearing impairment. Audiologists and speech-language pathologists are invaluable for making recommendations regarding optimal learning environments for these children. They frequently teach groups of educators via inservices or consult directly with teachers about the needs of students with hearing loss. Edwards (2005) believes that inservices should not only tell, but provide simulations of hearing loss to educators so that they may *experience* obstacles to listening encountered by these children in the classroom. Individual consultation with teachers may involve explaining why interactive activities may be difficult for particular students, especially when class discussions are often fast-paced and involve several speakers at different locations within the classroom. It is also important for teachers to realize that students can be easily distracted by background noise when trying to complete individual work at their seats such as in *e-learning*, in which student(s) interact with multimedia computers in learning new material.

Other environmental changes include seating the student in the best position for attending to instruction and class participation, and using semicircular arrangements for group work (Friend, 2005). For example, optimal seating for a child who is deaf or hard of hearing should minimize any visual distractions, limit glare, and enable the visibility of the teacher to all children in the group. The student should be able to clearly see and hear all children in the group. Friend suggested giving the student a swivel chair with coasters, thus enabling proper positioning to see any student in the class. Finally, any auditory signals alerting students to class schedules or potential hazards (e.g., fire alarms) should have visual warnings (e.g., blinking lights) (Friend, 2005).

Accommodations for Input of Information

Input is how information gets into the child's brain. Accommodations for input of information begin with considering the use of hearing assistive technology (HAT) to overcome any remaining acoustic barriers. For example, the use of sound-field amplification or personal FM systems can help. A sound-field amplification system consists of a wireless microphone worn by the teacher that transmits his or her voice to a main unit that sends the information to strategically-placed loudspeakers within the classroom. At most, these units improve the SNR about 10 to 15 dB. For example, if the SNR at a child's desk was +5 dB, use of a sound-field amplification system could improve it to +15 to +20 dB. Figure 10.9 shows a young teacher using a portable sound-field amplication system.

Selection and implementation of appropriate sound-field amplification systems in classrooms require close collaboration between audiologists knowledgeable in this area and teachers. First, the classroom style needs to be considered in the process and may be simpler for one type of classroom than another. For example, closed classrooms under the control of one teacher and a single group of students may be served with the use of only one wireless microphone and a single loudspeaker mounted on the ceiling. However, classrooms utilizing team teaching may require the use of two wireless

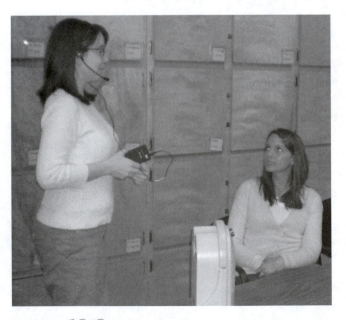

figure *10.9* ——————————————

A young teacher using a sound-field amplification system.

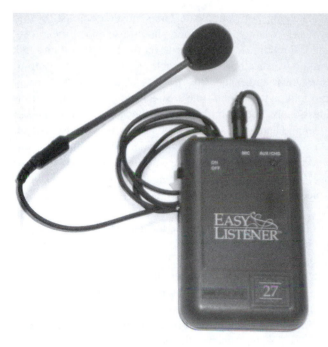

figure *10.10* —————————————————

Phonic Ear Easy Listener Transmitter.

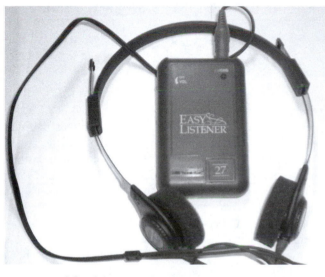

figure *10.11* —————————————————

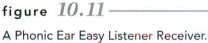

A Phonic Ear Easy Listener Receiver.

microphones simultaneously. Second, the classroom design (e.g., space utilization and classroom seating) may determine the type of sound-field systems used and loudspeaker placement. For example, teachers who may frequently rearrange their classrooms throughout the school year may need portable systems to use in different areas for different activities. Moreover, teaching style (e.g., didactic approaches, interactive activities, small-group activities) may influence the type of microphones and accessories used by teachers. For example, children can participate in group interactions by speaking into pass-around microphones that are patched into the teacher's transmitter (Edwards, 2005).

Personal FM amplification systems can improve SNR by 20 to 30 dB. The system consists of a wireless microphone worn by the teacher that transmits his or her voice to students' FM receivers. Personal FM amplification systems are used by children with significant hearing loss in addition to children with normal hearing sensitivity having auditory processing difficulties. Figures 10.10 and 10.11 show the transmitter and receiver of the Phonic Ear Easy Listener, respectively, for children with minimal hearing loss or auditory processing difficulties.

In this scenario, teachers wear the FM transmitter (upper left) that broadcasts to the FM receiver worn by students. The FM receiver can be coupled to children's ear via headsets or ear buds. Similarly, the Phonic Ear Solaris, a personal FM system for children with significant hearing loss, was shown in Chapter 7 on HAT. Similarly to the Easy Listener, teachers wear the transmitter, which sends their voices to students' FM receivers. Technology has enabled the miniaturization of FM receivers to behind-the-ear models, or even to FM receivers that plug directly into the direct-audio-input (DAI) jack of children's hearing aids. In fact, an entirely new generation of FM systems have been developed.

Communication tips for teachers and children can also improve input of information for children who are deaf and hard of hearing. For example, teachers must consciously ensure that students can see their faces clearly when speaking, and should use an overhead projector (Friend, 2005). For example, sometimes teachers write on the blackboard and talk with their back to students. Use of an overhead projector enables teachers to write important information visible to the entire class and ensure the visibility of articulatory cues.

Ensuring optimal input of information to students who are deaf and hard of hearing may require the services of other professionals. For example, regular educators should consider team teaching with a teacher of deaf and hard of hearing students who has expertise in techniques and adaptation of curricula. Similarly, teachers might consider the use of interpreters in the classroom for students who are deaf. **Interpreters** are professionals who translate what is said into another language, such as American Sign Language. In addition, teachers should consider asking another student in the class to provide notes to students who are deaf and hard of hearing.

Maximizing the child's input may involve changing the manner and form of the presentation of the information. Teachers should be creative in adapting their lessons to provide information through other sensory modalities such as vision and tactile senses. For example, elementary school teachers could supplement lessons about the weather with frozen snowballs, captioned videos showing lightning and tornadoes, and charts showing different types of clouds. Similarly, teachers could use cotton balls to show students the softness of clouds. Teachers can change their manner of presentation to include cueing to indicate when someone is talking, repeat statements by other students, and demonstrate directions showing what needs to be done.

Finally, teachers can exploit input of information by directly checking and teaching skills to students. For example, periodically checking comprehension of information keeps students who are deaf and hard of hearing current with the rest of the class. Similarly, teachers and students working together can develop simple strategies that increase the likelihood of achievement. For example, writing down due dates for assignments, along with with frequent reminders, assists students in timely completion of work. In addition, teaching students organizational skills and providing opportunities for practice develops personal mastery of the academic milieu.

Accommodations for Output of Information, Evaluation, and Grading

Output of information is how the child expresses what he or she has learned in the classroom in the form of performance on tests, class assignments, and contributions to group discussions. Friend (2005) suggested that students who are deaf and hard of hearing should be allowed such accommodations as additional time to complete assignments to demonstrate what they know, and the opportunity to use computers/word processors. For example, some students who are deaf and hard of hearing may feel self-conscious about speaking in class or may be difficult for others to understand.

Students who are deaf and hard of hearing benefit from multiple ways of modifying examinations and grading. For example, examinations can be allowed to be given by teachers or paraprofessionals who can sign test items to students who are deaf. Other tests adaptations may include the following (Friend, 2005):

- Modified vocabulary
- Graphic cues (e.g., stop signs or arrows)

- Alternative forms (e.g., matching, multiple choice, fill-in-the-blank)
- Reduced length

Teachers can also work with students who are deaf and hard of hearing to develop their test-taking skills. Moreover, projects or portfolios should be considered in lieu of tests. Alternative grading may include any one or a combination of the following approaches (Stewart & Kluwin, 2001):

- **IEP grading** involves using IEP long-term goals and short-term objectives for criteria for grading, complete with descriptive narratives about students' performance and a checklist of competencies mastered for each course (Friend, 2005).
- **Contract grading** is based on a signed agreement between the teacher and the student on the criteria for which work is to be evaluated.
- **Multiple grading** involves dividing a unit into parts for specific evaluation (e.g., participation, achievement, progress).
- **Level grading** breaks assessment into two parts—letter grades (e.g., A, B, C, and so on) and degree of difficulty (e.g., 1, 2, and 3).
- **Narrative grading** is writing a descriptive evaluation of the student's work, along with strengths and weaknesses.

Behavioral and Social Accommodations

Students who are deaf and hard of hearing, particularly young children, may have behavioral problems in the classroom. Classroom teachers should establish a code of respect between and among students. For example, Friend (2005) suggested that teachers place general rules and behavioral expectations on charts for all students to see. Strong collaboration between the children's teachers and parents is particularly powerful in establishing consistent ground rules of behavior at school and at home. Teachers can establish a rewards program (e.g., extra time playing video games) or a home-school contract with a child's parents that can reinforce appropriate behaviors. Consistent, descriptive, and constructive feedback is the key to success. For example, every time a child displays inappropriate behavior, teachers should consistently provide descriptive and corrective feedback (e.g., "I would have preferred that you waited for your turn to look at the pictures rather than taking them from Charles before he was finished").

Teaching about hearing loss and the Deaf community can assist students who are deaf and hard of hearing to socially integrate with their peers. Understanding what hearing loss is and its impact may reduce animosity between students. Students are often afraid of or may react negatively to things that they do not understand. Special lessons on sign language, books about hearing loss, and guest speakers from the Deaf community for an assembly are a few examples of opportunities to inform students about the topic (Friend, 2005). In addition, students who are deaf and hard of hearing can be selectively paired with hearing students for class assignments to facilitate social interactions. Teachers and other school personnel must be vigilant regarding any bullying of children with hearing loss. **Bullying** is demeaning, threatening, intimidating, physically harming, or abusing someone in any way (Smith & Monks, 2008). Little research is known about the prevalence or long-term effects of bullying children with hearing loss by their peers (Weiner & Miller, 2006). However, any suspicion of it should be reported and handled immediately. Teachers, audiologists, and speech-language pathologists can assist children who are deaf and hard of hearing to develop social skills through direct instruction and personal adjustment counseling.

PERSONAL ADJUSTMENT COUNSELING FOR SCHOOL-AGED CHILDREN

Part of audiologists' and speech-language pathologists' duties may include providing guidance on personal matters to children with hearing loss. Earlier in this chapter, personal adjustment counseling was redefined and placed within a context of the types of services provided by audiologists and speech-language pathologists. Related services personnel that have ongoing professional relationships with students may be sought out for help in handling challenging situations in school. Students may need help with approaching a teacher about changes in accommodations or with interactions with peers. Often, specific situations can be addressed using the following process (Egan, 1998; English, 2002, pp. 8–9):

- Help students tell their stories
- Help students clarify their problems
- Help students to challenge themselves in solving their problems
- Help students set goals
- Help students develop action plans
- Observe the students as they implement their plans
- Help students evaluate their plans
  - Did it accomplish their goal?
  - Is more consideration needed?
  - Did a new goal emerge?

Helping Children Tell Their Stories

Children who are deaf and hard of hearing may be too shy to openly ask for help from adults, particularly about personal topics involving fitting in and making friends. English (2002) uses a door metaphor for describing a communication barrier that may exist between the communication sciences and disorders professionals and students and their families. English (2002) believes that audiologists and speech-language pathologists must *listen* carefully for "knocks at the door" that invite adults into a child's world. Listening must be done with the brain *and* the heart. Knocks on the door often come in the form of **affective statements** that express a child's social and emotional concerns regarding hearing loss. Careful listeners catch these statements during the course of a conversation and use them as opportunities for children to tell their stories.

Let's look in on Dr. Kenneth Bright, an educational audiologist in the Tempe, Arizona, school district, on a consult with Bobby Blackhorse, a seventh grader with a moderately severe sensorineural hearing loss. Bobby had some difficulty in his world history class with Mr. Jackson's style of presentation and keeping up with the class notes. Dr. Bright and Bobby spoke with Mr. Jackson, who was eager to do anything he could to help. Mr. Jackson selected Crystal Matthews as a buddy to assist Bobby with class notes and assignments. Mr. Jackson and Dr. Bright had no idea that Crystal was the most popular girl in the seventh grade!

Casebook Reflection

Bobby and the School Dance

Telling the Story – Take 1

1. **Dr. Bright:** "Hi, Bobby, how are you doing in your history class? Has Mr. Jackson been ensuring that you see him when he lectures?"
2. **Bobby:** "Yes."
3. **Dr. Bright:** "Has working with a buddy helped, too, with taking notes?"
4. **Bobby:** "Yes. Crystal helps me a lot. I get nervous talking to her, especially because of my hearing loss."
5. **Dr. Bright:** "Well, remember what I told you about being an assertive communicator, and tell her when you don't understand something."
6. **Bobby:** "Sometimes, I feel so dumb asking her a question. I freeze up."
7. **Dr. Bright:** "If you're not sure what she said to you, ask her to repeat. Remember how important it is to be able to detect and repair communication breakdowns?"
8. **Bobby:** "Yeah, right . . . Thanks, Dr. Bright. I need to get to my math class."

Can you see the breakdown in communication? Dr. Bright doesn't know it, but he missed Bobby's knock at the door. Can you find which of Bobby's statements were affective or knocks at the door? Yes, statements 4 and 6, respectively, expressing nervousness and feeling dumb when talking to Crystal, contained the affective statements. What did Dr. Bright do in response to Bobby's affective statements? He made statements that were informational in nature, reminding Bobby to be an assertive communicator and about the importance of detecting and repairing conversation breakdowns, resulting in a communication mismatch. A **communication mismatch** is responding to patients' affective statements with informational statements. Communication mismatches create barriers to understanding and signals to patients that professionals are not really listening to their concerns. Dr. Bright had two communication mismatches in the conversation in statements 5 and 7. The last thing that Bobby wanted to hear was that he should be an assertive communicator and that conversational repair is important. Let's try this again and see what happens when Dr. Bright listens with his brain and his heart.

Casebook Reflection

Bobby and the School Dance

Telling the Story – Take 2

1. **Dr. Bright:** "Hi, Bobby, how are you doing in your history class? Has Mr. Jackson been ensuring that you see him when he lectures?"
2. **Bobby:** "Yes."
3. **Dr. Bright:** "Has working with a buddy helped, too, with taking notes?"
4. **Bobby:** "Yes. Crystal helps me a lot. I get nervous talking to her, especially because of my hearing loss."
5. **Dr. Bright:** "Mr. Jackson and I didn't know that. Tell me about that. What makes you feel nervous?"
6. **Bobby:** "Sometimes, I feel so dumb asking her a question when I've missed something. Getting a copy of her notes really helps me with getting what I need for homework. Crystal even writes down exactly what the assignment is, but I can't get the words out to ask her about something I don't understand. I freeze up. Crystal is the most popular girl in the seventh grade. . . ."

How different was the conversation when Dr. Bright was listening with both his brain *and* his heart? Dr. Bright was able to hear the knock at the door, using heart-to-heart communication, and encouraging Bobby to share his feelings. Dr. Bright accomplished the first step in personal adjustment counseling, helping Bobby to tell his story. However, Dr. Bright is not clear on exactly what the problem is. In fact, Bobby may need help in clarifying exactly what the problem is.

Helping Children Clarify Their Problems

After communication sciences and disorders professionals help children tell their stories, they now must assist them in clarifying their problem(s) (Egan, 1998; English, 2002, pp. 8–9).

Helping children clarify the situation is the initial step in developing self-mastery in problem solving. Dr. Bright is not really sure if the problem has to do with Crystal or if the problem is with Bobby's perception of the situation. Let's see how Dr. Bright can assist Bobby clarify the problem.

Casebook Reflection

Bobby and the School Dance

Clarifying the Problem

1. **Dr. Bright:** "Does Crystal get impatient when you ask her a question? If so, we can get another buddy for you."

2. **Bobby:** "Oh no, Crystal is so nice to me. She always asks me if I have any questions. I just can't get the words out."

3. **Dr. Bright:** "So, you've never asked Crystal any questions that you had about class work."

4. **Bobby:** "No, I haven't. I get so nervous. . . ."

5. **Dr. Bright:** "What do you think might happen if you did ask her a question?"

6. **Bobby:** "I'm afraid she might laugh at me or think I'm dumb."

7. **Dr. Bright:** "You said that Crystal has been so nice to you. Do you really think that would happen?"

8. **Bobby:** "Well, I guess not. . . ."

9. **Dr. Bright:** "Do you think maybe you're not being entirely fair to Crystal in not giving her a chance? What makes you think she might laugh at you?"

10. **Bobby:** "Well, sometimes kids in my classes have laughed at my questions."

11. **Dr. Bright:** "Wow, I understand why you feel the way you do. So, it is your fear of being laughed at that prevents you from asking Crystal any questions."

12. **Bobby:** "Exactly."

Dr. Bright has assisted Bobby in clarifying what the problem is; particularly in statements 1, 3, 5, 7, and 9. Both realized that the current problem is not with Crystal, but in Bobby's fear of being laughed at. The next step in the process includes challenging Bobby to solve his problems, set some goals, and develop an action plan.

Helping Children Problem Solve, Set Goals, and Develop Action Plans

Once a child's problem has been clarified, the next steps in the process include assisting the child to look within for possible solutions and having them set goals and develop action plans (Egan, 1998; English, 2002, pp. 8–9).

Casebook Reflection

Bobby and the School Dance

Solving Problems, Setting Goals, Developing Action Plans

1. **Dr. Bright:** "Can you describe for me how your fear is interfering with the success of the buddy system?"
2. **Bobby:** "Well, I'd sure like to have some of my questions about Crystal's notes answered."
3. **Dr. Bright:** "Uh-huh, go on. . . ."
4. **Bobby:** "Also, I'm not being fair to Crystal by assuming that she will be mean to me and laugh."
5. **Dr. Bright:** "So, what I hear you saying is that you'd really like to be able to ask Crystal questions and that maybe you're not giving Crystal enough credit."
6. **Bobby:** "Yes, that's right."
7. **Dr. Bright:** "What can YOU do to change the situation?"
8. **Bobby:** "Well, I can get up the courage to ask Crystal a question."
9. **Dr. Bright:** "How does that make you feel?"
10. **Bobby:** "Nervous!"
11. **Dr. Bright:** "You say that you feel nervous about talking to Crystal?"
12. **Bobby:** "Yes, so nervous I can't find my words."
13. **Dr. Bright:** "Do you see any other solutions to change the situation other than giving it a try?"
14. **Bobby:** "Not really."
15. **Dr. Bright:** "OK, what can you specifically do to get past your nervousness?"
16. **Bobby:** "Maybe I can get comfortable in just talking to Crystal. Maybe, if I feel comfortable talking to her, asking questions can be easier."
17. **Dr. Bright:** "So, you feel if you could successfully 'break the ice' with Crystal, you could overcome your uneasiness. Is there any opportunity for you to talk to Crystal about other stuff than class work?"
18. **Bobby:** "She sits next to me in class. We both usually get to class early. Maybe, I could try talking to her then. I just don't know how to start a conversation!"
19. **Dr. Bright:** "Why don't you ask her about any movies she's seen?"
20. **Bobby:** "OK, that sounds good. I'll try that."
21. **Dr. Bright:** "When? Let's set a goal. Can you try this soon?"
22. **Bobby:** "I think so."
23. **Dr. Bright:** "This week?"
24. **Bobby:** "Yeah, I guess so."
25. **Dr. Bright:** "OK, can you tell me your goal?"
26. **Bobby:** "By the end of the week, I will start a conversation with Crystal before history class starts."
27. **Dr. Bright:** "That sounds great. Come see me a week from today and let me know how it goes."
28. **Bobby:** "OK, see ya next week!"

Let's look in on Dr. Bright and see how he accomplishes the next steps of the process.

Dr. Bright was very effective in challenging Bobby to find a solution to his problem. He accomplished this with a technique called **surrendering the role of expert**, which is allowing children to find their own answers instead of telling them what to do (English, 2002). For example, note how Dr. Bright directly asks Bobby what he can do to solve his problem. Surrendering the role of expert empowers children to develop self-mastery over their own problems and keeps the door of communication open.

Communication sciences and disorders professionals need to not only hear knocks at the door, but be diligent in keeping that door open. English (2002) illustrated how the use of six basic listening skills can keep the door of communication open. One skill is the **use**

of minimal encouragers and verbal followings, which means simply saying short phrases (e.g., "Uh-huh," "Go on," and so on) to show the speaker that his or her communication partner is listening and that the speaker should continue talking. For example, in statement 3, Dr. Bright uses this skill quite effectively. Another skill is **paraphrasing**, or restating what the speaker has just said, which accomplishes two goals. First, it shows that the listener is involved, and second, it shows that what has been said has been understood. For example, Dr. Bright uses this skill quite effectively in statement 5 by restating what Bobby had said. A third skill is **acknowledging and reflecting feelings** in which the audiologist reflects on what the patient may be feeling about a particular issue. For example, in statement 11, Dr. Bright hears how Bobby feels about an issue and asks for verification of his perceptions. A fourth listening skill is **providing feedback**, which consists of making descriptive and specific statements to the patient to ensure accurate communication. For example, Dr. Bright effectively provides feedback to Bobby about a possible solution to his problem in statement 17. A fifth listening skill is to be comfortable with silence through the realization that periods of quiet assist conversational partners to reflect on what has been said.

Adults can innocently make mistakes that can sabotage the counseling process. For example, if Dr. Bright failed to relinquish the role of expert by declaring what specifically should be done to solve the problem, Bobby may have resented being told what to do and would not have an opportunity to gain confidence in his own problem-solving skills. In addition, English (2002) says that two common pitfalls in counseling are **reassurance** and **persuasion**. Reassurance is telling the child that he or she should not feel a certain way and that the situation is not as bad as it seems. For example, if Dr. Bright told Bobby that he was a capable young man who should not feel nervous about asking questions, the door of communication would close. Another error is persuasion, when adults to try and persuade children to see things their way. For example, Dr. Bright might have tried to persuade Bobby what a cool guy he was (e.g., "You're funny, good at sports, have lots of friends," and so on) to reduce his nervousness and fear.

Another behavior that slams the door of communication is competing with the child for "talk time." Frequently, adults who identify with a child's problem will tell the child about similar experiences they had when they were their age. Adults may so identify with the situation that they may go into great detail about their experiences to the point of dominating the conversation and pushing the child out of the spotlight (English, 2002). Identifying too closely with a child's issue may result in the adult **listening through filters** and interpreting the situation through his or her own life experiences rather than remaining objective. These behaviors may result in daydreaming such that although the adult may be in the same room with the child, his or her mind is somewhere else. Children can tell when adults are not "plugged in," closing down the lines of communication.

Observing the Implementation of the Plan

Once an action plan has been developed, the next step in the process is to observe the child implement the plan (Egan, 1998; English, 2002, pp. 8–9). In our scenario, Bobby had developed an action plan with the assistance of Dr. Bright. Without violating Bobby's confidentiality, Dr. Bright had asked Mr. Jackson to observe Bobby and Crystal's classroom interactions. The next day, right before class was about to begin, Mr. Jackson observed the following interaction.

Casebook Reflection

Bobby and the School Dance

Observing Implementation of Plans

1. **Bobby:** "Crystal, have you heard anything about any new movies this week showing at the mall theatre?"
2. **Crystal:** "Yes, the new Harry Potter movie is out and I heard it was awesome!"
3. **Bobby:** "I've read the entire Harry Potter series!"
4. **Crystal:** "Me too, and the movie is supposed to follow the book pretty well."
5. **Bobby:** "I'm going to check it out on Saturday."
6. **Crystal:** "Tell me Monday if you liked it. . . . Have you started your class project yet?"
7. **Bobby:** "Not yet, but I'm going to. . . ." [Bell rings.]
8. **Mr. Jackson:** "OK, class, settle down. . . ."

Later in the Teacher's Lounge

9. **Mr. Jackson:** "Glad I caught up with you. . . . What were your concerns about Bobby and Crystal? They seem to get along well. Before class, they were talking about the latest Harry Potter movie. Is there a problem?"
10. **Dr. Bright:** "Oh no, not at all. I was just wondering how they were doing after setting Bobby up with Crystal as study buddies. Thanks for the information! See you next week!"

Dr. Bright was proud of Bobby for successfully implementing his plan.

Helping Children Evaluate Their Plans

After observing children implementing their plan, communication sciences and disorders professionals should help them evaluate how it went (Egan, 1998; English, 2002, pp. 8–9). Dr. Bright looked forward to his meeting with Bobby, who came to his appointment with a big smile on his face.

Casebook Reflection

Bobby and the School Dance

Evaluating Plans

1. **Bobby:** "Hi, Dr. Bright!"
2. **Dr. Bright:** "Hi, Bobby, how are you?"
3. **Bobby:** "Great!"
4. **Dr. Bright:** "How did your plan go?"
5. **Bobby:** "Awesome! I was afraid at first, but then I just went ahead and asked Crystal if she knew anything about the new movies playing. We talked about the new Harry Potter movie! Ya'know what else?"
6. **Dr. Bright:** "What?"
7. **Bobby:** "Crystal texted me later that day and said she thought I didn't like her because I never really talked to her! We now instant message back and forth at night when we do our homework!"
8. **Dr. Bright:** "So, your plan worked?"
9. **Bobby:** "Definitely!"
10. **Dr. Bright:** "So, you feel comfortable asking her questions about Mr. Jackson's class? Are you having any other issues?"
11. **Bobby:** "Yes, I feel nervous asking Crystal to the homecoming dance. . . ."

Dr. Bright assisted Bobby in evaluating his plan, which turned out to be successful. Furthermore, evaluating one goal provides opportunities to focus on other issues that are of concern to the child. For example, Bobby did not have any concerns about the study-buddy arrangements for Mr. Jackson's class. However, he was uneasy about asking Crystal to the dance. Bobby and Dr. Bright can use the same process in tackling this new problem.

English's (2002) approach in personal adjustment counseling children who are deaf and hard of hearing and their families can be used with many different issues ranging from acceptance of amplification to making friends. Occasionally, communication sciences and disorders professionals may face issues that are beyond their scopes of practice requiring referral to mental health professionals, child protective services, or law enforcement officials. These situations may include chronic depression in children, the impact of parents' marital problems, and child abuse. Child abuse is discussed later in this chapter.

DIRECT SERVICE DELIVERY

Direct service delivery is therapy provided by related-services personnel. Audiologists and speech-language pathologists provide direct service delivery for children who are deaf and hard of hearing. Under Part C of the IDEA, therapy is provided to students from ages 3 to 21 years. The settings for direct service provision are primarily school-based. At the age of 3, children with disabilities transition from Part C of the IDEA to Part B. Children with hearing loss transition from early intervention services stipulated by their individual family services plan to preschool placement, stated in their individualized education plan. As stated earlier, there is considerable variation in the types of preschool placements available to young children with hearing impairment. Some children are fortunate to be able to attend a preschool program for children with hearing impairment. Some of these programs are based on a particular approach for facilitating spoken language in group and individual therapy. Alternatively, some programs may have professionals using an **eclectic approach**, consisting of a conglomeration of techniques based on the needs of the child. Audiologists, speech-language pathologists, and teachers of the deaf can be found teaching in these programs.

By age 3 years, children should be wearing their hearing aids full time and be stimulable for aural habilitative therapy. **Stimulable** means the child is primed to respond when presented with a particular stimulus (e.g., imitating a clinician's model, pointing to a particular picture when hearing the name of an object, and so on). The **stimulus-response paradigm** (S-R paradigm) is the basic unit of auditory habilitative therapy in which the clinican provides a stimulus for a child to respond to, which is subsequently reinforced. It is based on the premise that a child's response directly represents his or her auditory perception of the clinician's stimulus. The clinician must have a trained ear to judge the appropriateness of the response. If the response is a close match to the stimulus, the child is positively reinforced and the clinician may decide to move on to more difficult tasks. However, if the response is incorrect, then the clinician must present the next stimulus in such a way as to shape the child's perception toward a more appropriate response. Clinicians must quickly decide what should be done to assist the child in his or her perception. Should the stimulus be presented in a louder voice? If initially presented without visual cues, should cues now be provided? If a child's error persists, perhaps adjustments must be made with the child's hearing aids or cochlear implant(s)? As discussed in Chapter 9, the approaches for facilitating spoken language differ in the types of techniques to be used in shaping children's perception.

Some clinicians strictly adhere to specific approaches; other clinicians who use more eclectic approaches may base their use of techniques on the needs of the child.

McConkey-Robbins (1998) advised that young children with hearing impairment need to be taught via didactic and incidental learning methods. As described earlier in this chapter, *didactic* approaches are highly structured in that children are directly taught to master specific skills in sequence according to a hierarchy of auditory development. Alternatively, **incidental learning** occurs when skills are learned naturally as they occur in the environment. It is important that the preschool programs offer opportunities for both didactic and incidental learning. As stated earlier, children with hearing impairment miss out on early learning experiences and require didactic learning of tasks to make up for lost opportunities. However, direct training of skills in highly structured situations does not represent the real world. Therefore, preschool environments should also use incidental learning to promote generalization of skills by teachers who are trained in using these techniques. It has been hypothesized that children whose hearing losses are identified early through newborn hearing screening programs will need less didactic training than their predecessors.

In Chapter 9, we introduced a few approaches for facilitating spoken language in children who are deaf and hard of hearing. Although the approaches have some fundamental differences, they all use the S-R paradigm as the basic unit for auditory training in teaching the perception and production of oral speech and language. Yoshinaga-Itano (2000) stated that effective approaches for facilitating the use of spoken language for children with hearing impairment have the following characteristics: (1) skilled providers, (2) unisensory stimulation, (3) mass practice, (4) parent partnerships, (5) hierarchical curricula, (6) integration of auditory training into daily living, and (7) language training. We will now compare and contrast how three approaches fulfill each of these criteria.

Auditory-Verbal

The Auditory-Verbal approach was based on the work of Helen Beebe and Doreen Pollack in the United States and Daniel Ling in Canada (Beebe, 1953; Pollack, 1993). In 1969, Doreen Pollack started using the Acoupedic approach in Denver, Colorado. Later, the name was changed to the Auditory-Verbal approach, which is used in the United States and throughout the world. An organization called Auditory-Verbal International developed certification standards for professionals and later interfaced with the Alexander Graham Bell Association in 2005 to form the independently governed subsidiary entitled the Alexander Graham Bell Academy of Listening and Spoken Language. The academy established standards of excellence through the certification of clinicians as Listening and Spoken Language Auditory-Verbal Therapists or Listening and Spoken Language Auditory-Verbal Educators. Professionals earning these certifications have met numerous eligibility requirements (i.e., academic, credential/licensure, postgraduate study, written description of auditory-verbal practice, supervision of practicum, additional monitored activities, supervisory evaluations, and parents' letters of recommendation) and passed a written examination. In Chapter 9, you learned that the main goal of the Auditory-Verbal approach was to have children with hearing impairment participate in the hearing world, particularly in school learning environments, and to develop into an independent, contributing member of society.

Auditory-Verbal is truly a **unisensory approach**, emphasizing the use of audition for the development of spoken language while discouraging the reliance on speechreading. Auditory–Verbal accomplishes its goals through five basic practices of maximizing parental participation, audition, spoken language, communication as a social act, and ongoing diagnostic teaching (Perigoe, 2009). A major component of Auditory-Verbal therapy is the guiding and coaching of parents, their children's first teachers. Parents directly participate in therapy sessions, both learning from clinicians and assisting in adapting play situations to maintain their children's interests, interpret meanings of vocalizations, model appropriate communication behaviors, and so on. Clinicians first model therapeutic techniques and then have parents try it with their own children, providing feedback and encouragement.

Much of the instruction focuses on maximizing audition in a variety of ways beginning with the acoustic environment. Noise and reverberation should be minimized and children's audibility maximized through the appropriate fitting of hearing aids, cochlear implants, and/or RMHAT systems. Clinicians ensure that amplification is functioning properly through visual and listening checks. In addition, clinicians ensure that children have sufficient audibility with amplification devices by conducting the LingSix SoundTest. Briefly, the test involves determining whether a child can detect the phonemes /u/, /a/, /i/, /sh/, /s/, and /m/, which span the speech spectrum. If the sounds cannot be detected, then the child does not have adequate audibility for therapy, and adjustments in amplification are suggested.

Once therapy begins, some clinicians prefer to sit side-by-side with children, omitting direct visual cues and requiring reliance on the auditory sense to understand what is being said. This strategy is complemented by other techniques such as cueing. For younger children, clinicians frequently use the hands-to-ears cue similar to the one mentioned in the previous chapter involving signaling the child to "listen!," presenting a stimulus, and then reacting with an "I heard that!" Moreover, some clinicians use a hand or a screen in front of their mouths to eliminate visual aspects of the message and to signal to children that they are to listen. Clinicians must be careful, however, not to distort the acoustic aspects of utterances with their hands or other barriers. The so-called "**hand cue**" has a secondary function when placed near children's mouths indicating that it is their turn to speak. The hand cue can be used to develop the stimulus-response paradigm, the basis for auditory training. Using the stimulus-response paradigm enables children to receive lots of practice in the perception and production of spoken language, a necessity for reaching therapeutic outcomes.

From the beginning, audition is emphasized and integrated into the child's personality, priming the future for integration into the hearing world through the use of spoken language. Maximizing the use of spoken language is based on normal developmental models and hierarchies of skill acquisition. Auditory-verbal therapists remind parents to always speak in full sentences, rich with suprasegmentals, and to be careful not to use telegraphic speech, thinking that it may be easier for children to understand. Moreover, although therapy occurs in natural play situations, reinforcement is carefully tied to children's responses. For example, activities frequently involve waiting until a child vocalizes prior to giving them a desired object or turn in a game. Stimuli are always presented auditorally first and if the child is not successful, other strategies are used such as **acoustic highlighting** or emphasizing certain words through the use of suprasegmentals. For example, words that are "helping words" such as adjectives, adverbs, and articles are often of lower sound pressure level than nouns and verbs. Emphasizing these words may help children with hearing loss hear them more readily. Once the child is successful, then stimuli are presented through audition once again, without additional cues. In addition to basing outcomes on normal child language development, Auditory-Verbal teaches auditory skills according to the following hierarchy shown below, along with examples of training activities (Caleffe-Schenck, 2005):

Skill	Description	Activity
Auditory Awareness and Perception	Child indicates the presence or absence of sound	Child raises hand when he or she hears a noisemaker
Auditory Attention and Inhibition	Child pays attention to auditory information, for an extended period of time	Child listens to story or music for a specified duration
Distance Hearing	Child can hear sound from a distance	Child indicates hearing a noise-maker at increasing distances
Localization	Child finds the location of a sound source	Child is blindfolded and points to the location of the sound source
Discrimination	Child differentiates and identifies sounds and words that are acoustically similar or different	Child points to cards that say "same" or "different" when presented with pairs of auditory stimuli
Auditory Feedback and Monitoring	Child listens to auditory information, repeats it, and modifies his or her production, if necessary, to match the auditory model	Child imitates the clinician with the goal of trying to closely mimic everything that is said
Auditory Memory	Child stores and recalls auditory stimuli	Child attempts to retell a story that has just been told by the clinician
Auditory Memory Span and Sequencing	Child remembers varying lengths of auditory information in exact order	Child correctly recalls a recipe of 10 steps in the correct order
Auditory Processing	Child makes cognitive judgments about auditory information	Child is able to determine if statements made about a story are correct
Auditory Understanding	Child comprehends auditory information in any situation	Child is able to have a conversation with almost anyone on age-appropriate topics

Moreover, auditory training objectives are integrated with age-appropriate speech and language goals that occur both in therapy and during children's activities of daily living and social interaction. Activities often involve the clinician, parent, and child jointly focusing on a task or situation. Frequently, clinicians and parents follow the child's lead to maintain his or her interest. Turn-taking is emphasized, laying the foundation for the development of pragmatic skills and conversational competence. The goal of therapy is for the child with hearing impairment to be fully integrated into the hearing world and mainstreamed into regular education with his or her peers.

The Verbotonal Method

The **Verbotonal Method** (VM) was developed by Professor Petar Guberina first as a method of teaching foreign language that was adapted for use for children with hearing loss. Dr. Guberina came to the United States with some of his clinicians to the Ohio State University at the invitation of his friend and colleague, Dr. John Black. A study group was formed that took faculty and students from Ohio State to Yugoslavia, now Croatia, to learn about this approach. A member of the group, Dr. Carl W. Asp, accepted a position at the University of Tennessee at Knoxville and introduced VM to that region of the country in the 1970s. Currently, VM is used at the Hearing and Speech Foundation/Blount Hearing and Speech Center in Maryville, Tennessee; in Knox County Schools in Knoxville, Tennessee; and in Dade County Schools in Miami, Florida. The American Verbotonal Society developed a rubric for certification of clinicians; however, the society is not active anymore. Clinicians may still seek training from the Hearing and Speech Foundation in Maryville, Tennessee, from John Berry.

The Verbotonal method has mistakenly been labeled a **multisensory approach** in that vibrotactile stimulation has been used as a stepping stone for further development of residual hearing (Pratt & Tye-Murray, 2009). Quite the contrary, VM is a strongly auditory approach, but it does not advocate unisensory perception as strongly as the Auditory-Verbal approach does. The Verbotonal method does not eliminate all visual cues, although clinicians have been known to limit them during auditory training. Clinicians who practice VM do not teach speechreading, but neither do they routinely discourage the use of visual cues in auditory training. Moreover, VM advocates the mass practice of speech, language, and auditory skills, because it has been estimated that preschoolers require about 3,000 hours of group and/or individual therapy for successful mainstreaming into kindergarten. Parents are key players in the overall aural habilitation of their children, but they do not routinely participate in therapy.

VM has a hierarchical curriculum that increases in difficulty in several domains: body movements, amplification, targeted phonemes, distance perception, and auditory memory span. Clinicians use dramatic movements with very young children with the aim that the qualities of whole-body movements (**macromovements**) will generalize to speech musculature (**micromovements**). As the child matures, the body movements become less dramatic, mostly involving arm and hand movements. These movements are not signs or symbols, but are simply intended to emphasize and provide children with kinesthetic information about appropriate respiration, phonation, and articulation. Although VM is not a multisensorial approach, one of its amplification sensing tools used with young children is that they are placed on vibratory floor panels for the development of appropriate rhythm and intonation of speech (Pratt & Tye-Murray, 2009). The vibratory floor panels are connected to special desktop auditory trainers, Systems Universal Verbotonal Audiometry Guberina (SUVAG I or II) that provide extended low-frequency amplification. As the child progresses, the child wears circumaural headsets and wrist vibrators, advancing to headsets, and then finally to wearable hearing aids. The frequencies that are amplified change, beginning with extended low-frequency wideband amplification with very young children, culminating in the use of frequency responses of conventional hearing aids for older children. The low frequencies convey the suprasegmentals, which are taught first, followed by the **segmentals** of speech. Recall that the suprasegmentals are the prosodic aspects of speech (e.g., rhythm and intonation) that often extend across words and sentences. For example, **intonation**, or the variation of fundamental frequency over time, is very powerful in conveying whether an utterance is a statement or a question. Intonation can also convey speakers' emotions. The segmental aspects of speech, or phonemes, are based on **tonality**, or the spectral pitch of sounds. Young children first learn low-tonality phonemes (e.g., /p/, /b/, and /m/), then progress to middle (e.g., /t/ and /d/), and then to high (e.g., /s/, /ch/, and /sh/) tonality sounds. The development of appropriate suprasegmentals serves as a foundation for appropriate temporal aspects of speech. Auditory training increases in clinician-to-child distances from speaking directly into the ear progressing to presenting sentences from across the room. Finally, the children's auditory memory span is first developed using stimuli consisting of a few elements (e.g., boo, boo, ba, boo) to elaborate nursery rhythms (e.g., "Apples, bananas, peaches, and plums; Momma is at the food store; Oh what fun! Put it in the basket. Push it all around. Take out your money and put it down!" etc.). VM integrates auditory training into everyday activities and language training through the use of **situational teaching**, or relating therapy to meaningful contexts. The goal of VM is to prepare children with hearing impairment to be mainstreamed into regular education classrooms with minimal support.

The Erber Approach

The Erber approach was developed by Norman Erber and is an auditory method. As with VM, there is no certification program for this approach. The program is based on mass practice using stimulus-response paradigms to shape children's auditory perception and comprehension. As with VM, parents are key players in the overall auditory habilitation of their children, but they do not routinely participate in therapy.

The Erber auditory training method has a simple rubric based on a hierarchy of the response task and speech element shown in Figure 10.12. The vertical dimension is based on a response task beginning with **detection** (i.e., being able to tell the presence or absence

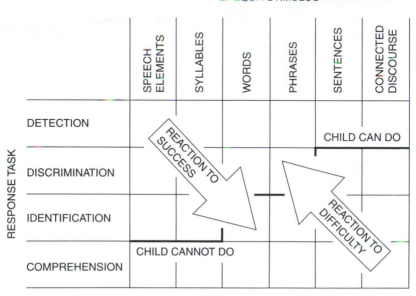

figure *10.12*

Stimulus response matrix.

Source: Based on *Auditory Training*, by N. P. Erber, 1982, Washington, DC: A.G. Bell Association.

of an auditory stimulus), and progressing to **discrimination** (i.e., being able to tell whether two auditory stimuli are the same or different), to **identification** (i.e., being able to label an auditory stimulus) and then to **comprehension** (i.e., being able to make meaning of an auditory stimulus). The horizontal dimension is for the type of speech stimulus, beginning with speech elements or phonemes, progressing to syllables, words, phrases, sentences, and ending with connected discourse. The upper right-hand square of the matrix represents the easiest auditory skill, the detection of phonemes. Alternatively, the lower right-hand square represents the most sophisticated level of the comprehension of connected discourse. In other words, the ability of comprehending connected discourse is predicated on the success at previous levels. Furthermore, Erber suggests using an index card to cover the clinician's mouth, eliminating visual cues and forcing children to develop their auditory skills. Auditory training is dynamic, with the clinician being sensitive to what the child can and cannot do, progressing onward with optimal performance and adapting the situation to increase the likelihood of a child's successful response. For example, the clinician may use an adaptive strategy by focusing on a phrase within a sentence that the child is having trouble with and then, once successful, presenting the entire sentence again.

The Erber approach easily incorporates language training into everyday activities. Erber has three general auditory training methods: (1) the natural conversational approach, (2) the moderately structured approach, and (3) practice on specific tasks. The natural conversational approach is the most flexible and may be incorporated into academic lessons or language therapy sessions. Movement about the matrix may involve any cell. The teacher or clinician uses an index card to eliminate visual cues, requiring the child to use his or her residual hearing. If the child makes an error in perception, the teacher or clinician simply modifies his or her presentation to increase the likelihood of a correct response. The clinician may work on a specific task with a child until successful and then go back to the lesson. The moderately structured approach employs the use of a closed-response task (e.g., pictures of farm animals) that is associated with a speech production and language comprehension goal (e.g., say and correctly point to pictures of animals from teacher's verbal descriptions). The clinician uses an index card to eliminate visual cues and typically works with just a few cells within the matrix (e.g., identification of words and sentences). Practice on specific tasks is the most rigid type of perceptual training in which clinicians work on tasks from one or two cells within the matrix. Practice with specific goals is limited to particular listening skills typically not involving language goals.

ASSESSMENT TOOLS

The IDEA (2004) requires that children are evaluated to determine presence of a disability, develop an IEP, and assess progress on short- and long-term goals. Assessments are multidisciplinary and may involve a variety of methods, tests, and materials. Audiologists and speech-language pathologists provide some of the most important diagnostic information for children who are deaf and hard of hearing. As discussed earlier in the chapter, the former conduct audiologic evaluations and assess children's performance with individual and group amplification. The latter conduct speech and language evaluations. Together they provide insight to others on IEP teams on how hearing loss impacts performances in other areas of evaluation (e.g., reading). The following table shows some examples of assessment tools for speech, language, auditory skills, and classroom behaviors to be used with school-age children who are deaf and hard of hearing.

Assessment Tools

Informal

Language Sample: *Systematic Analysis of Language Transcripts* (SALT) (Miller, 2010)

Formal

Articulation

Arizona Articulation Proficiency Scales, Third Revision (Arizona-3) (Fudala, 2000)
Goldman-Fristoe Test of Articulation Competence, Second Edition (G-FTA-2) (Goldman & Fristoe, 2000)
Identifying Early Phonological Needs in Children With Hearing Impairment (Paden & Brown, 1992)

Language
Vocabulary
Carolina Picture Vocabulary Test (Layton & Holmes, 1985)
Peabody Picture Vocabulary Test, Fourth Edition (PPVT-4) (Dunn & Dunn, 2007)

Syntax
Grammatical Analysis of Elicited Language- Pre-Sentence Level (GAEL-P) (Moog, Kozak, & Geers, 1983)
SKI-HI Language Development Scale (Watkins, 2004)
Teacher Assessment of Grammatical Structures (TAGS) (Moog & Kozak, 1983)
Test of Syntactic Abilities (TSA) (Quigley, Steinkamp, Power, & Jones, 1978)

Global Measures
Clinical Evaluation of Language Fundamentals, Second Edition (CELF-2) (Semel, Wiig, & Secord, 2003)
The Oral and Written Language Scales (OWLS) (Carrow-Woolfolk, 1995)

Auditory Skills

Auditory Behavior in Everyday Life (ABEL) (Purdy, Farrington, Moran, Chard, & Hodgson, 2002)
Children's Abbreviated Profile of Hearing Aid Performance (CA-PHAP) (Kopun & Stelmachowicz, 1998)
Child's Home Inventory of Listening Difficulties (CHILD) (Anderson & Smaldino, 2000)
Client Oriented Scale of Improvement for Children (COSI-C) (National Acoustics Laboratories, 2009)
Parents' Evaluation of Aural/Oral Performance of Children (PEACH) (Ching & Hill, 2007)
Teachers' Evaluation of Aural/Oral Performance of Children (TEACH) (Ching & Hill, 2005)

Educational Tools

Screening Instrument for Targeting Educational Risk (SIFTER) (Anderson, 1989)
Screening Instrument for Targeting Educational Risk in Preschool Children (Preschool SIFTER) (Anderson & Matkin, 1996)

Tools for Speech-Language Pathologists

Speech-language pathologists can use informal or formal assessment tools. Moreover, measures obtained may be be *norm-* or *criterion-referenced*. **Norm-referenced measures** compare children's performances against those of a group of peers such that students may be ranked. **Criterion-referenced measures** compare a student's performance against themselves, which is useful to determine if they are meeting their IEP goals. Both types of measures are important in the evaluation of children who are deaf and hard of hearing. For norm-referenced measures, it is helpful to compare performances of children with hearing loss to their peers and to children with normal hearing. Unfortunately, the majority of speech-language assessment tools have norms for hearing children only. As stated in Chapter 9, language samples are a type of informal assessment requiring an exact transcription of a child's use of language, including what is said by all participants along with relevant context. It is important to obtain a digital audiovisual recording of a session structured to elicit adequate representation of the child's communicative competence. One useful software program, the *Systematic Analysis of Language Transcripts* (SALT) (Miller, 2010), provides resources on the elicitation, transcription, and analysis of language samples. Measures are made on children's syntactic, morphologic, and lexical aspects of language that can be compared against norms of age-matched peers. SALT also provides assessment of speakers' fluency/rate (use of fillers, repetitions, and reformulations: words per minute) and discourse (speakers' turns) (Miller, 2010).

Assessment of articulation may be done with tests normed on children with normal hearing and hearing impairment. The *Arizona Articulation Proficiency Scales, Third Revision* (Arizona-3) (Fudala, 2000) is normed on children with normal hearing and assesses all speech sounds, including initial and final consonants, blends, vowels, and diphthongs. The value of using tests for children who are deaf and hard of hearing is that they can focus on problems inherent to this population. For example, the *Identifying Early Phonological Needs in Children With Hearing Impairment* (Paden & Brown, 1992) assesses phonological processes used by these children. The test uses 25 line drawings to elicit children's spontaneous productions of single words. Clinicians phonetically transcribe children's utterances and score them for word patterning (accuracy in syllable number and stress), vowels (tongue height and place accuracy), and consonants (manner, place, and voicing).

Assessment of language also involves tests normed on normal hearing children and those with hearing impairment. Two tests for vocabulary include the *Peabody Picture Vocabulary Test, Fourth Edition* (PPVT-4) (Dunn & Dunn, 2007) and the *Carolina Picture Vocabulary Test* (CPVT) (Layton & Holmes, 1985). The PPVT-4 assesses patients' vocabulary and was normed on those with normal hearing. Alternatively, the CPVT was normed on patients who were deaf and hard of hearing.

Many language tests target more than one area. The *Clinical Evaluation of Language Fundamentals, Second Edition* (CELF-2) (Semel, Wiig, & Secord, 2003) assesses 3- to 6-year-old children's competencies on 9 different subtests of sentence structure, word structure, expressive vocabulary, concepts, following directions, sentence recall, basic concepts, word classes, and phonological awareness. Two examples of language assessment tools normed on children with hearing loss are the *Grammatical Analysis of Elicited Language-Pre-sentence Level* (GAEL-P) (Moog, Kozak, & Geers, 1983) and the *SKI-HI Language Development Scale* (Watkins, 2004).

Tools for Audiologists

Audiologists' assessment tools focus on evaluating the effectiveness with amplification and the need for accommodations in the classroom setting. The examples include those for assessing auditory skills and classroom behaviors. Frequently, audiologists need to document pre- and postfitting measures to assess the effectiveness of group and individual amplification. These assessment tools identify strengths, weaknesses, and needs of children with hearing impairment. Some of the tools are for parents to complete, some for educators, and some for children. Some deal specifically with auditory behaviors, while others probe behaviors in the classroom.

Auditory Skills

One tool is the *Child's Home Inventory of Listening Difficulties* (CHILD) (Anderson & Smaldino, 2000), which is one of the only family-centered instruments that assesses auditory behavior in the home environment for children 3 to 12 years of age. The CHILD consists of

15 different assessments for a parent to complete. For example, item 7 requires that parents call their child's name from another room when the child cannot see the parent and then rate how difficult it seems for the child to hear and realize that he or she is being summoned. Parents use an 8-point rating scale on the Understand-O-Meter: (1) "Huh?" (2) "Tough Going," (3) "Sometimes Get It, Sometimes Don't," (4) "It Takes Work But Usually Can Get It," (5) "Okay but Not Easy," (6) "Pretty Good," (7) "Good," and (8) "Great." Older children who are at least 7 to 8 years old can complete the CHILD and can compare their ratings to those of their parents. Both total (i.e., sum of ratings for 15 items) and average (i.e., sum of the ratings divided by the number of items completed) scores are computed and recorded for the child and parent. The total score may range from 15 to 120, with average scores ranging from 1 to 8. Possible applications of the CHILD include the following (Anderson & Smaldino, 2000):

- Helping concerned parent and audiologist identify problems
- Serving as a pretest measure in a hearing aid evaluation
- Counseling parents using the results of the assessment
- Addressing HAT needs
- Measuring if improvements have been made in communicative behavior

As with many of Karen Anderson's tools, there is a section that educates parents and children about the importance of critical factors for listening such as distance, noise, visual cues, strategies for alerting listeners, and available assistive technology.

Other tools include the *Parents' Evaluation of Aural/Oral Performance of Children* (PEACH) (Ching & Hill, 2007) and the *Teachers' Evaluation of Aural/Oral Performance of Children* (TEACH) (Ching & Hill, 2005). Both tools are for evaluating the efficacy of amplification using questionnaires that elicit parents' and teachers' observations of children's functional performance with hearing aids or cochlear implants. These evaluation tools are different from other questionnaires because in addition to scoring items, evaluators are to write down their observations. Parents are supposed to observe their children for at least one week. The PEACH has 13 questions that query the following topics:

- Use of amplification and loudness discomfort
- Listening and communicating in quiet
- Listening and communicating in noise
- Telephone usage
- Responsiveness to sounds in the environment

For example, question 1 on the use of amplification and loudness discomfort section, the interviewer states to the parent, "I would like to know how often the child is wearing his/her hearing aids/cochlear implant. Can you tell me about the child's routine for wearing his/her hearing aids/cochlear implant during the past week?" The score sheet is actually a booklet that is called a "diary" that parents can complete on their own. A nice feature of the PEACH is that it provides suggestions, alternatives, and examples for parents. The TEACH is very similar to the PEACH, except that the TEACH has 11 questions in the same topic areas listed above. After completion of the diaries, audiologists work closely with parents and teachers in scoring the PEACH and TEACH, respectively. By reviewing evaluators' qualitative responses, items are scored for frequency of reported behavior assigning points as follows: (1) "Never" for 0 points (i.e., no examples are given); (2) "Seldom" for 1 point (i.e., one or two examples are given and the behavior occurs 1% to 25% of the time); (3) "Sometimes" for 3 points (i.e., three or four examples are given and the behavior occurs 26% to 50% of the time); (4) "often" for 3 points (i.e., five or six examples are given and the behavior occurs 51% to 75% of the time); and (5) "Always" for 4 points (i.e., more than six examples are given and the behavior consistently occurs greater than 75% of the time). Raw scores are summed, and the percent of consistency is calculated for listening in quiet, noise, and overall. Another scoring rubric is used to compare the current amplification situation to previous ones and rate the performance of each item as: (1) "Much worse" for –2 points; (2) "Worse" for –1 point; (3) "Same" for 0 points; (4) "Better" for 1 point; and (5) "Much better" for 2 points. The raw scores for the items and average comparison score are obtained. Applications of the PEACH and TEACH are to evaluate the effectiveness of amplification (e.g., unaided to aided conditions) or changes within devices (e.g., old to new settings). These tools may also be used in counseling parents and teachers about how hearing loss creates problems for children at home and at school.

In Chapter 9, *Client Oriented Scale of Improvement for Children* (COSI-C) (National Acoustics Laboratories, 2009), an adaptation of the *Client Oriented Scale of Improvement* (COSI) (Dillon, James, & Ginis, 1997) was discussed for use with infants and toddlers. The COSI-C for preschool, primary, and secondary students is similar to the versions used with the 0- to 2-year-old population in that it is completed by parents with assistance from clinicians. The main goal of the COSI-C is to document goals/needs for their children and measure the amount of benefit from hearing aids. On the COSI-C score sheet, parents, teachers, and, when appropriate, children with assistance from audiologists list and prioritize from one to five goals/needs to target and then possible strategies for their achievement. On the National Acoustics Laboratories website (www.nal.gov.au/), a hand-out entitled "Goals for Promoting Hearing in Preschool, Primary, and Secondary School Children" lists suggested goals for each group of children that may be appropriate for targeting on children's IEPs. For example, one goal for a primary-school child is to be aware of environmental factors that impair the child's ability to hear and how to manage these situations. Similarly, a goal for secondary-school children and their parents is to be aware of options available to assist with entering the workforce or tertiary education to indicate feedback, and a possible strategy is to reinforce this behavior. COSI-C goals/needs may also be classified into one of the 16 general categories from the regular COSI. In addition, the date for review of progress on the goals/needs should be planned after children's initial adjustment to amplification. Assessment of post-amplification progress is indicated through responses of "No change," "Small change," "Significant change," or "Goal achieved." It is suggested that parents and audiologists discuss any changes in strategies or expectations for goals/needs labeled either "No change" or "Small change." The COSI-C is more than an outcome measure; it is a habilitative tool, assisting in the setting of and methods for attaining appropriate goals.

The COSI-C is not the only tool that is appropriate for children and adolescents from 0 to 22 years of age. The *Developmental Index of Auditory and Listening* (DIAL) (Mormer & Palmer, 1997) provides functional auditory milestones for infants, toddlers, preschoolers, elementary–middle schoolers, and older adolescents. Audiologists and parents can use this tool to see if children are reaching appropriate milestones. For example, middle-school students, ages 10 to 14 years, should be using the telephone for communication with peers, attending movies/plays, and watching television with family and friends. The milestones may be targeted for goals in auditory habilitation and be used for consideration in the procurement of HAT. A middle-school child may need a cell phone that is compatible with his hearing aids, or may need an infrared TV listening system.

Two other tools are the *Auditory Behavior in Everyday Life* (ABEL) (Purdy, Farrington, Moran, Chard, & Hodgson, 2002) questionnaire and the *Children's Abbreviated Profile of Hearing Aid Performance* (CA-PHAP) (Kopun & Stelmachowicz, 1998). The ABEL is a 24-item questionnaire for parents regarding the consistency of their children's auditory behaviors. For example, for item 1, "Initiates spoken conversations with familiar people" parents rate as occurring "Never" for 0 points; "Hardly ever" for 1 point; "Occasionally" for 2 points; "About half the time" for 3 points; "Frequently" for 4 points; "Almost always" for 5 points; or "Always" for 6 points. Each of the 24 items is assigned to one of three factors: "Aural-Oral," "Auditory Awareness," or "Social/Conversational Skills." Scores for items for each factor and overall are added together, and then a mean score is obtained for each.

The CA-PHAP (Kopun & Stelmachowicz, 1998) consists of 24 items probing difficult listening situations that parents or children rate with and without their hearing aids. For example, on item 1 on the parents' version, "When we are in a crowded store talking with the cashier, my child can follow the conversation," parents rate the situations as either "Always" (99% of the time); "Almost always" (87% of the time); "Most of the time" (75% of the time); "Half of the time" (50% of the time); "Once in a while" (25% of the time); "Hardly ever" (12% of the time); or "Never" (1% of the time). The situations and scoring on the child's versions are the same, but the wording of the items is directed to the student. The tool can be used to determine the degree of difficulty children are having in listening situations and to measure improvement derived from the use of amplification.

Classroom Behavior

For children 3 to 5 years of age, Anderson and Matkin (1996) developed the *Screening Instrument for Targeting Educational Risk in Preschool Children* (Preschool SIFTER) to identify children who were at risk for developmental or educational problems due to hearing problems. The Preschool SIFTER has 15 items with three items in each of five areas: preacademics, attention, communication, class participation, and school behavior. Using a 5-point scale, teachers answer three questions in each of the five areas. An example of an item from the preacademics area asks teachers, "How well does the child understand basic concepts when compared with classmates (e.g., colors, shapes, etc.)?" to which they must respond on a scale of 1 to 5 (e.g., 1 = Below, 3 = Average, and 5 = Above). In addition, the score sheet has a space for teachers to write down pertinent comments concerning whether students have had frequent absences, health problems, or other problems or handicaps in addition to hearing. The Preschool SIFTER has a two-step scoring process. The first step involves summing responses for the six questions (i.e., items 7, 8, 9, 10, 11, and 14) for the expressive communication factor and the same for the four questions (i.e., items 4, 5, 6, and 13) for the socially appropriate behavior factor; recording the results; and classifying performance in these areas as either passing or at risk. The second step involves summing the scores for each of the three items in the five areas (i.e., preacademics, attention, communication, and so on), recording the results, and classifying performance in those areas as either passing or at risk. Anderson and Matkin stated that the area scores might assist teachers in developing a profile of the preschooler's strengths, weaknesses, and particular needs.

Similar to the Preschool SIFTER, but for children 6 years and older, the *Screening Instrument for Targeting Educational Risk* (SIFTER) (Anderson, 1989) is a screening instrument consisting of 15 items in which teachers rate students' behavior by responding to three questions in areas concerned with academics, attention, communication, class participation, and school behavior. An example of an item from the academics area asks teachers,

"What is your estimate of the student's class standing in comparison to that of his/her peers?" The teacher answers the question by selecting a number on a scale of 1 to 5 (e.g., 1 = Lower, 2 = Middle, and 5 = Upper). In addition, the score sheet has a space for teachers to write down pertinent comments concerning such issues as whether a student has repeated a grade, was frequently absent, or ill, or had special support services within the classroom. Teachers' ratings on the three items for each area are summed resulting in a score that can be recorded on a grid. The sums for each of the five areas are plotted on the grid forming a profile for each student. The sums for each area can fall into three ranges on the grid of pass, marginal, and fail. The SIFTER is meant to be a screening tool only, and students who fail a particular area should be further evaluated. For example, failure in the academic area suggests educational assessment, failure in the communication area recommends that the child receive audiologic and speech-language evaluations, and failure in the area of school behavior suggests a referral for appraisal by a psychologist or social worker (Anderson, 1989). Although the purpose of both versions of the SIFTER is to identify children at educational risk, both tools can be used to assess the effectiveness of intervention efforts, such as the use of hearing aids, preferential seating, sound-field amplification systems, and so on (Stelmachowicz, 1998).

Another pre- and post-intervention listening questionnaire that can document the effectiveness of intervention efforts is the *Listening Inventory for Education: An Efficacy Tool* (LIFE) (Anderson & Smaldino, 1998). The LIFE has two inventories: (1) the Student Appraisal of Listening Difficulty, and (2) Teacher Appraisal of Listening Difficulty. The Student Appraisal of Listening Difficulty consists of 15 situations described by pictures; items 1 through 10 are Classroom Listening Situations and 11 through 15 are Additional Listening Situations. For example, one for classroom situation is a picture of a teacher talking in front of the room. Students rate their degree of difficulty by selecting one of the following descriptors for classroom listening situations 1 through 10: "Always easy" for 10 points; (2) "Mostly easy" for 7 points; (3) "Sometimes difficult" for 5 points; (4) "Mostly difficult" for 2 points; and (5) "Always difficult" for 0 points. The scales for the additional listening situations 11 through 15 are the same, except their point values are doubled. The total number of points possible for classroom and additional listening situations is 100 for a total score of 200 points. The Student Appraisal of Listening Difficulty may be used as a pre- versus post-intervention measure to determine efficacy of hearing aids, FM systems, or use of assistive listening technology. The inventory also comes with suggestions for the student to improve classroom listening.

The Teacher Appraisal of Listening Difficulty, a post-intervention measure, consists of 16 statements for which instructors rate their degree of agreement: "Agree" for 2 points, "No change" for 0 points, and "Disagree" for –2 points. Item 16 has a different rating scale in which "Agree" receives 5 points, "No change" receives 0 points, and "Disagree" receives –5 points. An example of a statement is item 1, which states, "The student's focus on instruction has improved (more tuned in to instruction)." All of the statements are positive and the best outcome is if teachers' observations are in agreement. Therefore, the higher the score, the better is the overall outcome for the student. The scores for all 16 statements are summed and highly successful outcomes have scores ranging from 26 to 35, successful outcomes have scores from 16 to 25, and minimally successful outcomes have scores from 5 to 15 points. Similar to the student's inventory, the teacher's version has suggestions for accommodating students with hearing impairment. The Teacher Appraisal of Listening Difficulty is ideal as a post-intervention measure of the efficacy.

CHILDREN WITH (CENTRAL) AUDITORY PROCESSING DISORDERS

Earlier in the chapter, we stated that children with *(central) auditory processing disorders* ([C]APD) who have normal hearing sensitivity but have problems with the central auditory nervous system are exemplified by poor performance in one or more auditory behaviors or skills, such as the following:

- **Sound localization** is locating the origin of a sound source (e.g., "Can you point to where the sound is coming from?") and **sound lateralization** is placing of sound perception in the head (e.g., "Where does the sound seem to be coming from inside of your head? Do you hear it in the left ear, right ear, or the center of your head?").
- **Auditory discrimination** is the ability to differentiate between types of auditory stimuli (e.g., "Are /pa/ and /ba/ the same or different?").
- **Auditory pattern recognition** is the ability to recognize patterns in acoustic stimuli (e.g., "Can you recognize patterns in sequences of low- and high-pitched tones?").
- Temporal aspects of hearing include the following:
  - **Temporal resolution** is the ability to detect very fine temporal aspects of an auditory signal (e.g., "Can you detect the tiny gaps in the burst of noise you are about to hear?").
  - **Temporal masking** is the ability to detect or recognize acoustic signals that have been masked by sounds that either come before or after them in time (e.g., "Can you still identify the consonant that is being masked by a noise that comes before it?").
  - **Temporal integration** is the ability of the auditory system to integrate acoustic energy over time (e.g., "Can you still detect the tone at the same sound pressure level even though it is only half of its previous duration?").
  - **Temporal ordering** is the ability to sequence the order of items presented auditorily (e.g., "Can you repeat the numbers in the order you just heard them?").
- **Auditory performance decrements with competing acoustic signals** is the tendency for the ability to understand speech to decrease with increasing distortion (e.g., "Can speech continue to be understood even though the signal-to-noise ratio decreases and reverberation time increases?").
- **Auditory performance decrements with degraded acoustic signals** is the tendency for the ability to understand speech to decrease when some of its **redundancy** is reduced, such as speech that has had some of its acoustic energy removed through filtering (e.g., "Can you understand these words that have most of their spectral energy above 600 Hz filtered out?"). Redundancy is the multiple ways that meaning is coded in the speech signal.

An auditory processing disorder is difficulty in making complete sense out of what is heard, particularly when the message is distorted. We discussed earlier that noise and reverberation can add distortion to speech. Definitive diagnosis of (C)APD requires confirmation of a deficit in neural processing of auditory stimuli that is not due to higher order, language, cognitive or other factors, but co-occurs with deficits in other modalities leading to difficulties in learning (e.g., spelling and reading), speech, language, attention, social, and related functions, and understanding speech in noise (ASHA, 2005a, 2005b). Audiologists are uniquely qualified to diagnose (C)APD because it is primarily an auditory disorder (ASHA, 2005a, 2005b; Bellis, 2003). Audiologists use a test-battery approach involving behavioral nonbehavioral tests, and checklists. Most (C)APD behavioral tests consist of audio-cassette tape or compact disk recordings of tests that are designed to assess various auditory processing skills. Test stimuli are delivered to patients' earphones via an audiometer. Children's performances are compared against their peers of similar ages. Nonbehavioral assessment includes electrophysiological testing of the *neuromaturation* and *neural plasticity* of the central auditory pathways. **Neuromaturation** is the development of the nervous system; **neural plasticity** is the ability of the brain to form new connections and reorganize itself through the processing of sensory information (Tremblay & Kraus, 2002). Checklists completed by parents and teachers provide additional information about children's auditory processing skills. Speech-language pathologists are uniquely qualified to determine the cognitive-communicative and/or language factors that may be related to (C)APD (ASHA, 2005a, 2005b). The details of testing for (C)APD are beyond the scope of this textbook; see Bellis (2003), Musiek and Chermak (2007), and Chermak and Musiek (2007).

The following characteristics are typical of children with auditory processing disorders (National Institutes of Deafness and other Communication Disorders, 2004):

- Have trouble paying attention to and remembering information presented orally
- Have problems carrying out multistep directions
- Have poor listening skills
- Need more time to process information
- Have low academic performance
- Have behavior problems
- Have language difficulty (e.g., they confuse syllable sequences and have problems developing vocabulary and understanding language)
- Have difficulty with reading, comprehension, spelling, and vocabulary

Sometimes it is difficult for teachers and other school personnel to understand this disorder because the child seems to hear just fine, but has difficulty understanding speech in noisy classrooms, or remembering what the teacher said, or following directions. Teachers are the first to notice these behaviors, triggering notes home to parents and referrals to educational audiologists for hearing screening, audiologic evaluation, and (C)APD evaluation. Let's look in on concerns that Jimmy Jones's mother has about her son.

Casebook Reflection

Jimmy Jones

Ms. Jones was concerned about her son, Jimmy, who was in the second grade. Jimmy is a popular and cooperative child, but his teacher had sent several notes home during the grading period stating that he seems to be daydreaming, acting out in class, and not following directions. His spelling grades have deteriorated and his reading comprehension has started to lag behind his peers. Ms. Scort, Jimmy's teacher, has recommended that Jimmy have his hearing tested to determine if he has a hearing loss. Dr. O'Neill, the educational audiologist, found that Jimmy's hearing was within normal limits and explained to Ms. Scort and Jimmy's mother that his behaviors suggest that he might have an auditory processing disorder. He explained that during the audiologic evaluation, he administered the *SCAN-C: Test for Auditory Processing Disorders in Children, Revised* (Keith, 1999), which identifies children who may be at risk for auditory processing disorders and may benefit from additional evaluation. Jimmy was referred for a complete auditory processing evaluation that confirmed (C)APD. Dr. O'Neill worked with Jimmy's mother, teacher, and speech-language pathologist in developing an intervention plan involving classroom modification, amplification, direct treatment, and compensatory strategies. Within six months, Jimmy was performing satisfactorily in his academic subjects and was no longer disruptive in the classroom.

There are four areas for educational management of (C)APD, including classroom modification, amplification, compensatory strategies, and direct service treatment. Classroom modifications and use of personal and sound field amplification systems were described earlier in the chapter. **Compensatory strategies** are efforts made to overcome processing disorders and obtain information when the comprehension of auditory signals are compromised due to factors external or internal to the child. Compensatory strategies may involve tape recording lectures; having a study buddy; writing down main points rather than copying down everything the teacher says; chunking of information for memorization, and so on. Moreover, some things the teacher can do to facilitate learning include reducing distractions, minimizing multiple commands, cueing instructional transitions, using visual aids, checking for comprehension, and avoiding auditory exhaustion by providing short breaks (Bellis, 2003).

Direct service involves therapy provided by an audiologist or speech-language pathologist. A few computer programs have been developed for children with (C)APD. One program is **Fast ForWord** by Scientific Learning that develops and strengthens memory, attention, processing rate, and sequencing, all of the cognitive skills essential for learning and reading success (Scientific Learning, 2010). The program uses adaptive strategies in that the difficulty of each lesson is based on the child's current performance. **Fast ForWord** has a variety of activities in which children listen to auditory stimuli, make judgments, and then respond using the computer mouse within the context of a game. Active learning makes auditory training fun. Another program, **Earobics,** is a multisensory reading intervention for students from kindergarten through third grade (Earobics, 2010). **Earobics** intervention has four major areas: (1) implementation training for teachers, (2) interactive software for individualized instruction on reading skills, (3) resources to enrich and engage students, and (4) teachers' guides for seamlessly integrating the program into classroom curricula (Earobics, 2010). Direct therapy with a clinician involves working on skills using different activities such as auditory closure (e.g., filling in the blank with appropriate vocabulary words: "Mr. Smith drives a _____"), auditory figure ground (e.g., understanding speech in noise, such as reading a story in background noise and then asking students questions), noise desensitization (e.g., increasing tolerance of background noise, such as progressively increasing levels of background noise during listening activities), discrimination (e.g., identifying sounds as same or different, such as labeling "same" or "different" to pairs of words that differ by one phoneme), auditory memory (e.g., recalling sequence of items, such as playing Simon Says with multipart instructions), and temporal processing (e.g., recognizing temporal aspects of speech, such as imitating intonation patterns).

Designing specific intervention plans for students diagnosed with (C)APD is difficult due to the heterogeneity of the population. Several experts have tried to come up with categories based on diagnostic profiles and behavioral manifestations of (C)APD (e.g., Bellis, 2003; Bellis & Ferre, 1999; Medwetsky, 2002). The Colorado Department of Education's guide on screening, diagnosis, and intervention of (C)APD provides a summary of behavioral manifestations, typical test results, and possible interventions for different types of the disorder. Table 10.1 shows classic categories of (C)APD, their behavioral

table *10.1* (C)APD Behavioral Manifestations, Classroom Modifications, Amplification, Compensatory Strategies, and Direct Service Treatement.

Profile	Behavioral Manifestation	Classroom Modification	Amplification	Compensatory Strategies	Direct Service Treatment
Auditory Decoding	Unable to discriminate the fine acoustic details of speech, manifesting as problems in language, spelling, and listening fatigue	Reduce background noise and provide preferential seating	Remote microphone hearing assistive technology (RMHAT)	Using visual cues to augment auditory, providing lectures in written form	• Multisensory approach working on discrimination, vocabulary building, auditory closure, noise tolerance, speechreading, and critical listening skills • Use of computer programs (Earobics, FastForward, LIPS, etc.)
Auditory Integration	Difficulty with tasks involving multi-modality information input and output, manifesting as problems with reading, writing, spelling, understanding speech in noise or interactions with multiple speakers, and poor music skills	• Classroom with an animated teacher who over-exaggerates in rhythm and intonation • Use of demonstration, experiential, and "hands-on" learning	RMHAT	Providing ample repeated practice and concentrating on information presented in only one modality at a time	• Practice in extracting key words from complex passages • Practice in listening, and labeling of tactile stimuli
Auditory Temporal Processing	Difficulty managing the stream of speech, manifesting as problems in attaching meaning to timing cues (e.g., segmentation) resulting in problems in reading, spelling, speech recognition in noise, following directions, and understanding sarcasm and nonverbal cues	• Classroom with an animated teacher who over-exaggerates in rhythm and intonation • Use of demonstration, experiential, and "hands-on" learning	RMHAT	Using: • Spell checkers • Tape recorders • Study and communication buddies	• Practice in extracting key words from complex passages; prosody training; and frequently reading aloud with emphasis on intonation, stress, and rhythm

Profile	Behavioral Manifestation	Classroom Modification	Amplification	Compensatory Strategies	Direct Service Treatment
Organization	Difficulty with organization, manifesting as problems in poor note-taking, completion of assignments, planning, following directions, spelling/writing, listening, and deficits in motor planning	• Highly structured, rule-based environment	RMHAT	• Using external devices to aid in planning (e.g., lists, planners, iPhones, etc.) • Avoiding strategies involving self-monitoring of learning behaviors • Break information into smaller units • Relying on written and spoken information	Training and practice in: • Organization skills • Note-taking • Study skills • Test taking Speech and language therapy working on receptive and expressive language
Auditory Memory	Difficulty in remembering auditory messages, manifesting as problems in following directions, reading comprehension, spelling, receptive language, and has a tendency to be over stimulated and sensitive to loud sounds	• Improve signal-to-noise ratio • Preferential seating • Note-taker availability	RMHAT	Using strategies to improve memory such as: • Chunking • Verbal chaining • Mnemonics • Rehearsing • Reauditorizating • Paraphrasing • Summarizing Using tape recorder, note-taking, or asking for teacher's notes	• Work on developing auditory memory and sequencing • Preteach concepts prior to introduction into the classroom
Auditory Attention	Difficulty choosing what to attend to, manifesting as problems in attention, listening, understanding speech in background noise, taking notes, following directions, and so on	Preferential seating	RMHAT	• Maintaining eye contact • Eliminating distractions • Clarifying directions and checking comprehension • Requesting for clarification	Work on: • Metacognitive strategies or attending skills • Identifying internal and external distracters • Following directions

Source: Information from *Central Auditory Processing Deficits: A Team Approach to Screening, Assessment, and Intervention Process*, by the Colorado Department of Education, 2008, retrieved from http://www.cde.state.co.us/cdesped/download/pdf/APDGuidelines2008.pdf.

manifestations, and possible interventions including classroom modifications, compensatory strategies, use of amplification, and direct service therapeutic techniques (based on Colorado Department of Education, 2008).

Bellis (2003) believes that management of (C)APD requires a multidisciplinary team approach to include audiologists, speech-language pathologists, teachers, administrators, other professionals, parents, and the child, if appropriate. Auditory processing disorders can affect children's speech-language development, academic achievement, psychosocial well-being, and overall quality of life. With multidisciplinary teaming, each professional provides his or her expertise in identifying, diagnosing, and remediating this disorder and minimizing its impact on children's lives.

CHILDREN WITH OTHER AUDITORY DISORDERS

In Chapter 1, we stated that auditory rehabilitation includes serving children who have other auditory disorders. Two prevalent auditory disorders that may affect school-age children are auditory neuropathy/dyssynchrony (AN/AD) and tinnitus.

Auditory Neuropathy and Auditory Dyssynchrony (AN/AD)

AN/AD was defined in Chapter 9. Briefly, it is dysfunction of cranial nerve VIII that impedes the transmission of neural impulses generated in the periphery to the central auditory nervous system, resulting in a neural hearing loss. Management of children with AN/AD can be challenging because of the unique behavioral manifestations within and across patients (Berlin, Hood, Morlet, Rose, & Brashears, 2003). Moreover, some patients get better over time, some get worse, and others may stay the same (Berlin et al., 2003). Fortunately, the Joint Committee on Infant Hearing Year 2007 Position Statement (JCIH, 2007) focuses on identifying children with AN/AD through early hearing detection and intervention programs. Many children with AN/AD entering school have had IFSPs documenting what has worked and what has not, guiding professionals in transition planning from Part C to Part B of the IDEA. Therefore, at least for these children, IEPs will not have to be written "from scratch."

Nevertheless, developing an IEP is challenging because AN/AD is a relatively new disorder for many healthcare professionals and school personnel (Stredler-Brown, 2004). Assessment should focus on obtaining a comprehensive developmental profile for children with AN/AD to include communication, language, auditory skills, speech, and cognition (Stredler-Brown, 2004). It is important for IEP teams to know that it is difficult to predict which treatment options, educational placements, and accommodations work best for children with AN/AD. Hearing aids and cochlear implants have been found to be effective for many children with AN/AD (Cone-Wesson, Rance, & Sininger, 2001; Shallop, Peterson, Facer, Fabry, & Driscoll, 2001). It is important that children with AN/AD are fitted with hearing aids that have the latest digital noise reduction algorithms by audiologists experienced with this pediatric population (Zeng & Liu, 2006). Moreover, children's progress with amplification should be monitored closely so that referrals for cochlear implant centers may be provided, if necessary.

Other effective treatment options have included the use of visual communication in the form of American Sign Language, Cued Speech, and speechreading. Recall that ASL is a manual language with its own syntax, semantics, and pragmatics; it is used extensively within and among the Deaf community within the United States. Use of ASL in regular schools would require the use of an interpreter. Cued Speech is a visual communication system that incorporates eight handshapes and four hand positions (cues) that represent how sounds are said while talking, providing help to the child in distinguishing sounds that look the same on the mouth. Similarly, use of this technique would require the use of a **Cued Speech transliterater**—a professional who cues what is said in a classroom, for example. Use of either an ASL interpreter or Cued Speech transliterator in the classroom must be specified in a child's IEP. Use of these professionals can be costly, but necessary, if they are appropriate for a child to receive a FAPE in an LRE.

Speechreading, a skill introduced in Chapter 6 and covered in more detail in Chapters 11 and 12, may be developed in direct service provision by audiologists or speech-language pathologists. It is defined as a process by which listeners put together information from a variety of sources (e.g., lipreading; facial expressions; gesture, posture, and movement; situational cues; the topic of conversation; rules of the language; news of the day; motivation to understand; and residual hearing) to derive meaning (Cherry & Rubenstein, 1988). Speechreading includes **lipreading**, which is watching the speaker and deriving meaning from recognition of the visible aspects of articulation. Speechreading has been an effective strategy for adults with acquired hearing losses who have prior knowledge of language, enabling them to fill in inaudible parts of the acoustic message.

Clinicians who use the Auditory-Verbal approach may discourage the use of speechreading, but some children with AN/AD may benefit from it, particularly when the unisensory approaches have been found to be ineffective. Incorporation of speechreading into auditory habilitation should begin with referring children for visual acuity screenings. Children may benefit from an explanation of how some sounds look similar on the mouth. Moreover, coaching on self-advocacy skills to request optimal distances (e.g., 3 to 5 feet), adequate lighting, and avoidance of glare will enhance visual communication. Generally, the light source should shine on the speaker's face, not come from behind, casting a shadow. Preteaching concepts prior to their presentation in the classroom provides students with prior knowledge of the topic to aid in speechreading. Another beneficial accommodation includes preferential seating to optimize visibility of the teacher and minimize distraction.

Tinnitus

In Chapter 1, tinnitus was defined as sounds or noises in the head. Tinnitus is caused by a variety of things, from excessive cerumen in the external auditory canal to a tumor on cranial nerve VIII. Although the condition is more prevalent in adults, it has been estimated that 12% to 36% of children with normal hearing and about 66% of youngsters with hearing loss experience tinnitus (Sheyte & Kennedy, 2010). The prevalence of tinnitus has been found to be high in children with cochlear implants who experienced it most often when their implants were removed at bedtime, although most were not bothered by it (Chadha, Gordon, James, & Papsin, 2009). Despite relatively high prevalence rates, only 3% to 10% of children actually complain about their tinnitus (Sheyte & Kennedy, 2010). It has been hypothesized that many children do not complain because they consider it normal, particularly if it has been present since birth. A survey of children with normal hearing and hearing impairment who presented to a psychology clinic for tinnitus found that the problems caused were similar to those reported by adults and included insomnia, emotional distress, and listening and attention difficulties (Kentish, Crocker, & McKenna, 2000).

Children's complaints of tinnitus should be taken seriously, triggering a referral to a physician. In many cases, no reason can be found for the tinnitus, precluding amelioration through medical interventions (Academy of Otolaryngology, Head, and Neck Surgery [AAO-HNS], 2010). Fortunately, children do not have many psychological issues associated with their tinnitus (Shayte & Kennedy, 2010). As with adults, treatment begins with a demystification of tinnitus and a reassurance to the child that they are not alone (AAO-HNS, 2010). Children with hearing loss may find that their tinnitus is not as noticeable when they wear hearing aids and/or if they have cochlear implants (AAO-HNS, 2010; Chadha et al., 2010). Use of noise generators as described in Chapter 11 may assist children in their habituation of their tinnitus (AAO-HNS, 2010). School personnel should be told about children with severe cases of tinnitus so that accommodations may be provided, if needed. Teachers unknowingly may doubt children who complain of tinnitus interfering with their concentration at school.

CHILDREN WITH DUAL SENSORY IMPAIRMENT

In Chapter 9, dual sensory impairment in the 0- to 2-year-old population was discussed in reference to early identification, diagnosis, and management. Recall that *dual sensory impairment* is present when a person has concurrent visual and hearing impairment. It includes four heterogeneous categories of disability: (1) **deaf-blind**, (2) **deaf and visually impaired**, (3) **hard of hearing and blind**, and (4) **hard of hearing and visually impaired**. In addition, very few children are completely deaf and blind, that is, essentially not functioning in hearing and vision. *Hard of hearing* has been defined in earlier chapters as loss of hearing sensitivity that is still functional for the purposes of communication with amplification without visual cues. **Visually impaired** means having visual acuity less than 20/70 that cannot be corrected by conventional eyeglasses (University of Michigan Kellogg Eye Center, 2007). Most children fall into the hard of hearing and visually impaired group.

Preschool- and school-age children with dual sensory impairment may have had little opportunity to explore their environments and try new things. Dual sensory impairment may impact a child's psychosocial development more so than the effect of either impairment when considered separately. How parents of children with hearing impairment may be overprotective to the point of instilling a learned helplessness in their offspring was discussed earlier in the chapter. Parents may have similar reactions to dual sensory impairment by severely restricting their child's attempts at independence, resulting in a lack of self-confidence. Regardless of the availability of early intervention services for these children, many parents do not have the resources to manage young children who are deaf-blind. These parents need support and ways of communicating with their child.

Providing a child with dual sensory impairment with a FAPE in the LRE may be difficult because many schools may lack the resources and trained professionals for adequately serving this population. Children with dual sensory impairment are considered to have **multiple disabilities**. One option is state residential schools for the deaf and blind. Let's look in on the Helen Keller School for the Deaf and Blind in Talladega, Alabama.

Casebook Reflection

The Helen Keller School for the Deaf and Blind

The Helen Keller School for the Deaf and Blind opened in 1955. It is a residential school where children 3 to 21 years of age with dual sensory impairment from Alabama can attend at no cost to their families. The school, a part of the Southern Association of Colleges and Schools (SACS), also serves as a training center for teachers of children with multiple disabilities. The Helen Keller School focuses on providing an individualized education plan for each child, based on his or her individual needs using a multidisciplinary approach involving audiologists, occupational therapists, physical therapists, physicians, psychologists, social workers, speech-language pathologists, and so on. Parents' expectations for their children are critical for the development of an appropriate program. Because children live in dormitories, educational programming occurs 24 hours a day with development of self-care skills and enrichment opportunities in residence hall programming, including outings. Educational programming includes Braille, language, math, art, and other academic subjects.

Children must first learn how to express themselves to communicate with others, which may involve American Sign Language to communicate with sighted peers or through use of the **Tadoma method.** This method involves the person who is deaf-blind placing his or her thumb on the speaker's lip and their other three fingers along the jaw line to understand what someone is saying through the tactile sense. Reading may involve use of large-print texts or Braille. Math focuses on computational skills as in balancing a checkbook or determining a monthly budget. Students who are deaf-blind children may need to work with mobility environment. Physical therapy is provided in a variety of settings both on and off campus. The Hackney Play Therapy Center is a special facility that provides deaf-blind children with exercises that develop their coordination. Assistive technology specialists work with students in using support equipment for further academic work or employment. Graduates of the Helen Keller School may go on to the Alabama School for the Deaf or Blind or may go home to live with family to attend regular school providing special education services. Some may go on to live in group homes and attend vocational or technical training.

Most children with dual sensory impairment live with their families and receive special education services in the public schools. Individualized education plans are developed to meet their unique needs with the aim of developing their full potential. Audiologists may have to adapt service delivery by using special techniques in audiometric testing, hearing aid/FM system evaluations, and deliveries. It may be necessary to have the teachers and parents come to the evaluation because they are the most knowledgeable about how to communicate with the child. It is important to assist the children with dual sensory impairment into the test booth and explain its purpose, and let them know that they will be heard at all times in case they have questions or want a break. It is important that children know exactly what is expected of them. They may not understand what "raise your hand when you hear a tone" means. Physically raising the child's hand, showing the desired response, increases the likelihood of obtaining valid thresholds. It is also important to tell children what is going to happen prior to abruptly placing insert earphones into their ears. Hearing aid deliveries may require the use of large-print instructional materials and using the sense of touch in teaching children how to manage their hearing instruments. Children with dual sensory impairment may need extensive instruction on how to manipulate these devices. These skills may need to be targeted in their individualized education programs.

Children with dual sensory impairment will have delay in speech and language skills resulting from their hearing loss. Their concomitant visual impairment may preclude the use of speechreading. Speech-language pathologists may need to work a little more on the pragmatic aspects of communication with these children. Most of us know that when someone comes toward us and makes eye contact, he or she wants to initiate a conversation with us. Children with dual sensory impairment may not receive the visual cues that people who are sighted receive. Speech-language pathologists may need to work with students in developing ways for their peers and teachers to initiate communication. Once engaged in conversation, children with dual sensory impairment may need instruction on looking at their communicative partners even though they may not be able to make eye contact or obtain any cues from speechreading. Furthermore, they may need instruction on the use of appropriate posture to use with their communicative partners. The management of dual sensory impairment is discussed in greater detail in the next two chapters.

ABUSE AND NEGLECT IN SCHOOL-AGED CHILDREN WHO ARE DEAF AND HARD OF HEARING

Child abuse and neglect are, unfortunately, very common in today's society. Nightly news reports often contain horrific stories of the maltreatment of children. A few examples of abuse and neglect include children who have visible bruises, or are left unsupervised for days, or come to school without shoes or coats in winter. Children who are deaf and hard of hearing may be more prone to abuse than their peers simply because frustrated caretakers may be unable to communicate with them. For example, parents who are struggling to survive may not have the patience or the skills to discipline their children who are deaf or hard of hearing other than with physical violence. Similarly, deaf children in institutional settings are at risk for abuse by their caretakers who are foster parents or institutional care workers (Brookhouser, 1987). In today's world, communication sciences and disorders professionals should know the definitions of child abuse (e.g., sexual, physical, substance, and emotional), abandonment, and neglect. Moreover, healthcare workers must take an active role in identifying signs and symptoms of abuse (Brookhouser, 1986).

Defining Abuse, Abandonment, and Neglect

Official definitions of abuse and neglect appear in federal and state laws. For example, the Child Abuse Prevention and Treatment Act (CAPTA) is federal legislation that provides standards for states in how they define child abuse and neglect. The definitions are important because they determine grounds for intervention by the state in protecting children. Under this legislation, states should, at a minimum, define abuse as "any recent act or failure to act on the part of a parent or caretaker, which results in death, serious physical or emotional harm, sexual abuse, or exploitation, or an act or failure to act which presents an imminent risk of serious harm." Many states have definitions for sexual, physical, substance, and emotional abuse. Similarly, many states define neglect as "deprivation of adequate food, clothing, shelter, or medical care." Some states stipulate that the failure to provide these necessities due to financial inability is not neglect. Many states have included abandonment in their definition of neglect and consider that it is "when the parent's identity or whereabouts are unknown, the child has been left by the parent in circumstances where the child suffers serious harm, or the parent has failed to maintain contact with the child or to provide reasonable support for a specified period of time."

Recognizing Abuse, Abandonment, and Neglect

Public school personnel frequently have inservices about how to recognize and what to do in cases of suspected abuse, neglect, and/or abandonment. However, related services personnel, such as audiologists and speech-language pathologists, may not receive this training. It is important that these professionals recognize the different types of abuse, neglect, and abandonment, especially because they work closely with children who are deaf and hard of hearing.

What are the signs of child abuse or neglect? The signs may be exhibited by a child, parent, or by both. Figure 10.13 lists common signs of abuse and neglect shown by the child, parents, or by the parent and the child (NAIC, 2005). Concern should be noted if a child has sudden changes in behavior or school performance. School personnel should be concerned if children lack supervision or adult response to issues brought to the parents' attention regarding help needed for physical or medical needs. Similarly, if children have learning problems, difficulty concentrating, or are overly watchful, compliant, passive, or withdrawn, concern should also be noted. However, communication sciences and disorders professionals may be invaluable in differentiating typical behavior from signs of abuse in children who are deaf and hard of hearing. For example, sometimes children who are deaf and hard of hearing are overly watchful because they cannot hear what is going on around them. Moreover, children who are deaf and hard of hearing are often compliant, passive, and/or withdrawn. The important thing to remember is to look for changes in behavior in each child.

Parents can also display signs of possible child abuse or neglect. For example, some signs include those parents who are overly critical of or show little concern for their child, or blame him or her for problems at home or in the school. These parents may be harsh disciplinarians and expect other adults (e.g., teachers or coaches) to physically discipline

---

The Child
- Shows sudden changes in behavior or school performance
- Has not received help for physical or medical problems brought to parents' attention
- Has learning problems (or difficulty concentrating) that cannot be attributed to specific physical or psychological causes
- Is always watchful, as though preparing for something bad to happen
- Lacks adult supervision
- Is overly compliant, passive, or withdrawn
- Comes to school or other activities early, stays late, and does not want to go home

The Parent
- Shows little concern for the child
- Denies the existence of—or blames the child for—the child's problems in school or at home
- Asks teachers or other caretakers to use harsh physical discipline if the child misbehaves
- Sees the child as entirely bad, worthless, or burdensome
- Demands a level of physical or academic performance the child cannot achieve
- Looks primarily to the child for care, attention, and satisfaction of emotional needs

The Parent and Child
- Rarely touch or look at each other
- Consider their relationship entirely negative
- State that they do not like each other

---

figure *10.13*

Common signs of child abuse and neglect.

Source: Based on *Child Welfare Information Gateway*, 2008, retrieved from www.childwelfare.gov/pubs/factsheets/signs.cfm.

their child. Furthermore, these parents often view their child as bad, worthless, or as a burden, as well as having unrealistic expectations regarding his or her performance. When observing the parent and child together, they seem disconnected and may openly admit disdain for each other. However, it is important to realize that presence of a single sign of abuse or neglect does not prove that something is happening to the child. However, experts say when a sign appears over and over or in combination with other manifestations of abuse, a report should be made through the proper channels.

TRANSITION PLANNING

All children go through changes during the school-age years. Change is hard for everyone, but it may be particularly difficult for children with disabilities. **Transition services** consist of the efforts made to assist children with disabilities and their families with changes in educational programming. Changes may be from coverage under one part of the IDEA to another (e.g., changing from Part C to Part B), or progressing from junior high to high school. One of the most important transitions for children with disabilities is planning for what follows after high school.

An IEP should contain information about transition service needs for children with disabilities beginning at 14 years or younger (if deemed appropriate) and planning should begin no later than age 16 (IDEA, 2004; Johnson, 2000). Usually, the IEP team meets to develop a transition plan, notifying and inviting children and their parents to attend. One of the important realizations is that the legislation protecting access to an education changes when the child turns 21 years old. From birth to age 21 years, the IDEA (2004) ensures that each child with a disability receives a FAPE in the LRE. However, when a young person graduates from high school or turns 21, he or she is no longer protected by the IDEA, and should become familiar with the Americans with Disabilities Act (ADA) (1990) and Section 504 of the Rehabilitation Act of 1973. Students entering college, vocational/technical schools, or the world of work must qualify and document their disabilities to receive accommodations through these laws.

Let's look in on Bruce Chow, an educational audiologist, talking with Stacy Sinclair, a talented high school student with a moderate to-severe bilateral sensorineural hearing loss, and her mother regarding transition plans for college. Dr. Chow has worked with Stacy, her family, and teachers since she was in kindergarten. Stacy has done exceptionally well in high school and has aspirations of becoming a nurse. Dr. Chow, Mr. Anderson, her guidance counselor, and Stacy identified local universities with strong programs in both nursing and for students with disabilities. Dr. Chow was very proud of Stacy and wanted her to continue to succeed. Unfortunately, many students who are deaf and hard of hearing do not utilize accommodations in college, and in many cases they fail to perform up to their potential. Some students may have grown weary of being "the kid with the hearing loss," do not want to register with programs for students with disabilities, and yearn to be just a face in the crowd. However, they need to realize that actions needed for assistance are prospective, not retrospective, meaning that disabilities must be documented prior to the initiation of accommodations. Students need to know that if they do poorly all semester long, they cannot present documentation of a disability to bail them out. More detail regarding the timing and procedures for requesting accommodations is presented in Chapter 11. Let's look in on Dr. Chow and his meeting with Stacy and her mother.

Casebook Reflection

Stacy Sinclair: Soon-to-Be College Student

"Stacy and Mrs. Sinclair, please come in and have a seat. So nice to see you!" said Dr. Chow, the educational audiologist from the local school district. "I bet you're busy with your senior year, preparing for graduation in a few months."

"Yes, Dr. Chow," offered Mrs. Sinclair. "We are very proud of Stacy. She's been accepted at several universities that you and Mr. Anderson have suggested. She's trying to decide on which one to go to."

"It has been a pleasure working with Stacy over the past 12 years," remarked Dr. Chow.

"Thank you, Dr. Chow, for all that you have done for us. You've played a major role in Stacy's academic success," said Mrs. Sinclair.

"Yes, Dr. Chow, I really appreciate all of your help! You've really helped me a lot!" agreed Stacy.

"Thanks! It's really been a pleasure and I'm very proud of you," said Dr. Chow. "The reason I wanted you to come in today is to talk about some things to consider in your transition to college. I want to make sure that you receive all of the accommodations needed for you to do your best. I wanted to explain to you the changes in service provision from high school to college."

"Thank you, Dr. Chow," said Mrs. Sinclair, sitting intently and glancing over to Stacy, who nodded in agreement.

"One important change is that in public school, the Individuals With Disabilities Education Act protected your right to a free and appropriate public education in the least restrictive environment. Remember all of those annual meetings to plan Stacy's IEP?"

"Yes, I was so relieved to know that the school made sure that Stacy had everything she needed in the classroom, including speech-language therapy," added Mrs. Sinclair.

"Well, in college, everything changes, including the applicable laws. Instead of the IDEA, Section 504 of the Rehabilitation Act of 1973 and also the Americans With Disabilities Act are the laws that provide your rights to an education regardless of having a hearing loss," explained Dr. Chow. "In addition, Stacy, you have to be proactive documenting your disability and insisting that you are provided with the necessary accommodations."

"Won't Stacy automatically receive accommodations in college because she received them in high school?" asked Mrs. Sinclair.

"No, I'm afraid not, but necessary accommodations can be obtained once documentation of Stacy's hearing loss has been provided to a university's program for students with disabilities," explained Dr. Chow. "Are you going to visit all of the universities that accepted you before making a decision? Most colleges and universities appreciate at least one semester notice of an enrollment of a student with a disability in order to make adequate preparations."

"Yes, in fact, we are going to State University next week," Stacy said with excitement.

"You should make an appointment with the director of the program for students with disabilities to inquire about how many students with hearing loss are currently enrolled, what types of accommodations are provided, and assess their apparent willingness to serve students with disabilities," advised Dr. Chow, noticing a look of disappointment on Stacy's face.

"Dr. Chow, I've worked very hard to get accepted into college. I just want to be like everyone else for a change. Do I have to make a big deal about my hearing loss? I'm tired of feeling different . . . ," explained Stacy. "Can't I just see how it goes and then get accommodations if I need them?"

"Well, not exactly. Why not register with the university's program for students with disabilities and then see how it goes?" asked Dr. Chow. "If you don't document your disability up front, it is no one else's fault but yours if you don't succeed."

"We really appreciate your advice, Dr. Chow. Stacy will register with the program for students with disabilities," said Mrs. Sinclair in a stern voice to her daughter, who looked out the window and felt very much like a little girl.

Dr. Chow could tell that Stacy felt embarrassed. He got up from behind his desk, walked over to where Stacy was sitting, and sat on the edge of his desk. "Stacy, you're an adult now. No one can make you do anything you don't want to do. Your mother and I won't be there looking over your shoulder. We won't be scheming for ways to make you wear your hearing aids. Do you remember the contract you made with your parents that if you wore your hearing aids every day from the time you got up until you went to sleep that you'd get that brand new bicycle for Christmas?"

"Oh, Dr. Chow, did you have to bring that up?" asked Stacy with a big grin, looking at Dr. Chow and then at her mother who had tears in her eyes with her realization that her daughter was all grown up.

"OK, I promise we'll visit the programs for students with disabilities at each university," Stacy said reassuring her mother.

"Great! Which schools that we talked about are you favoring?" Dr. Chow asked.

"I've been accepted at the University of Tennessee, the University of Georgia, and State University," said Stacy proudly. "However, State so far is my first choice. Granddad went there, I love the atmosphere, and they have a great nursing school. We're visiting State first."

"She favors State because Pete Johnson, her boyfriend, is going to State," added Mrs. Sinclair.

"Oh, Mother," remarked Stacy, rolling her eyes and blushing.

"Well, I'd like you to visit me after your visit to State," requested Dr. Chow, getting up from the side of his desk.

"I will, Dr. Chow," promised Stacy as she stood up and gave Dr. Chow a great big hug.

"Thank you, Dr. Chow, for all you have done for us," said Mrs. Sinclair, embracing Dr. Chow.

"Yes, Dr. Chow, you're awesome!" remarked Stacy, going out the door with her mother.

Dr. Chow walked over to his window that overlooked the parking lot and watched the Sinclairs walk to their car.

We will follow Stacy and how she meets the challenges of going to college in the next chapter, which focuses on the auditory rehabilitation of young to middle-aged adults.

SUMMARY

This chapter summarized the auditory habilitation of preschool and school-aged children who are deaf and hard of hearing. The basic principles of the Individuals With Disabilities Education Act were discussed, particularly how it relates to ensuring that these children receive a free and appropriate public education (FAPE) in the least restrictive environment (LRE). The complementary roles of audiologists and speech-language pathologists were discussed within the context of contemporary service delivery models. In particular, the chapter featured accommodations for children with hearing impairment, personal adjustment counseling, direct service delivery, assessment tools, auditory processing disorders, auditory neuropathy/auditory dyssynchrony (AN/AD), tinnitus, dual sensory impairment, and child abuse.

LEARNING ACTIVITIES

- Interview and then shadow an audiologist and a speech-language pathologist who work in the school setting. What do they enjoy most and what are their greatest challenges?
- Observe a self-contained classroom for children with hearing impairment. Interview the teacher about his or her interactions with the educational audiologist and speech-language pathologist. In what ways do communication sciences and disorders professionals support the teacher in the classroom?
- Plan to tour a residential school for the deaf, and interview the teachers and students.
- Talk to regular education teachers about their thoughts and feelings about children with hearing loss in their classes. How prepared do they feel in teaching the child? What questions do they have?

CHAPTER eleven

Auditory Rehabilitation for Young to Middle-Aged Adults

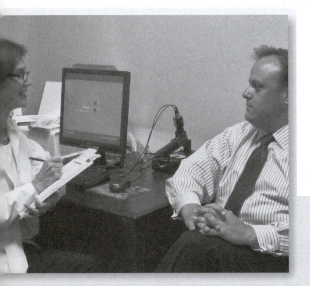

LEARNING *objectives*

After reading this chapter, you should be able to:

1. Define health-related quality of life (HRQoL) and how it is affected by hearing impairment in adults in the areas of personal achievement, physical/material well-being, and adult role fulfillment.

2. Describe federal mandates for young adults' transition to the world of work or enrollment in postsecondary educational institutions.

3. Explain the role of vocational rehabilitation (VR) in assisting adults who are deaf and hard of hearing in securing and maintaining gainful employment.

4. Explain how programs for students with disabilities, various accommodations, and sources of support assist college students with hearing impairment to achieve access to an education.

5. Define tinnitus, list causes, and explain various treatments, including tinnitus retraining therapy.

6. Compare and contrast various types of dual sensory impairment and their effects on adults.

7. Discuss various types of and treatments for vestibular disorders (e.g., benign paroxysmal positional vertigo, vestibular neuritis, and labyrinthitis).

8. Define and describe traumatic brain injury and related auditory disorders.

9. Explain commonalities and differences in the causes and preventions of noise-induced hearing loss.

Young adulthood is a challenging time of life. Teenagers are finding out who they are; they try out different roles. They move in and out of different social groups. They date. They are in a state of transition from the carefree world of childhood to the adult world of responsibility. This period of life can be uncertain at times, but exciting. Young adults who are deaf or hard of hearing experience the same challenges as their peers with normal hearing. They want to know where they belong. They wonder what the future holds. High school students must make important decisions that can affect the course of their lives: What do I want to do when I graduate? Should I further my education? What college do I want to attend? Unfortunately, studies of students with disabilities have found that they have greater difficulty transitioning from adolescence to adulthood and from school to work than do their non-disabled contemporaries (Hallahan & Kauffman, 2006). Communication sciences and disorders professionals can play a significant role in these students' transition from high school to work and/or postsecondary educational institutions. Transition planning should begin long before the senior year of high school and should involve the student, parents, and school officials.

Young adulthood sets the stage for middle-aged pursuits such as raising a family, developing a career, and preparing for retirement. Middle-aged adults can develop acquired sensorineural hearing loss in addition to other auditory disorders such as tinnitus, balance disorders, and vestibular dysfunction that can affect their health-related quality of life (HRQoL). Audiologists and speech-language pathologists are involved in the rehabilitation of adults with hearing loss and the prevention of hearing loss in adults during the most productive years of their lives. The purpose of this chapter is to discuss auditory rehabilitation in relation to critical life transitions of young and middle-aged adults who are deaf and hard of hearing.

EFFECTS OF HEARING IMPAIRMENT ON THE HEALTH-RELATED QUALITY OF LIFE OF YOUNG TO MIDDLE-AGED ADULTS

It has been estimated that 3.8 million adults between 18 and 64 years of age are hard of hearing while about 440,000 are functionally deaf (Mitchell, 2006). Most all of these adults experience some reduction of HRQoL resulting from their hearing losses, which is defined in different ways and encompasses a variety of domains (see Table 11.1).

A simple definition of HRQoL includes the following domains: (1) personal fulfillment (e.g., psychosocial well-being), (2) physical and material well-being (e.g., health and

table *11.1*   Definitions and Domains of Health-Related Quality of Life

Croog (1993)	National Institutes of Health (1993)	Revicki (1989)	Spilker (1996)
Totality of an individual's way of life: • Cognitive function • Emotional health • Life satisfaction • Social role performance • Well-being Objective conditions • Environmental stressors • Existence • Living conditions	• Cultural • Financial • Interpersonal • Philosophical • Political • Psychological • Spiritual • Temporal	• Emotional • Physical • Social	• Physical status and functional abilities • Psychological status and well-being • Social interaction • Economic and vocational status • Religious and spiritual

Source: Information from *Audiology and Quality of Life: Is There a Connection?*, by H. B. Abrams and T. H. Chisolm, 2007, retrieved from www.audiologyonline.com/articles/pf_article_detail.asp?article_id=1816.

living arrangements), and (3) adult role fulfillment (e.g., education and employment) (Halpern, 1993).

Personal Fulfillment (Psychosocial Well-Being)

In Chapter 2 on the psychosocial impact of hearing loss, Erikson's (1968) stages of development were reviewed. From ages 18 to 35, young adults face the challenge of intimacy versus isolation in which the major life tasks are to bond with peers, find a mate, and start a family. Young adults who are deaf and belong to the Deaf community may have higher senses of self-esteem than their peers who are hard of hearing. These young adults may feel that they are part of neither the hearing world nor the Deaf community. In fact, 95% of adults who are deaf select deaf spouses (Buchino, 1993). In particular, young adults who are deaf and have attended residential schools have had extensive exposure to peers and adult role models who are deaf (Scheetz, 2004). However, two drawbacks of residential school placements are the removal of children from their home environments and limited academic offerings. Alternatively, although mainstreamed settings offer better academic programs, many students who are deaf and hard of hearing are socially isolated and their relationships with hearing peers are often considered "acquaintances" rather than true friendships (Foster & Brown, 1989). Mainstreaming does not seem to promote the identification of children who are deaf and hard of hearing with their hearing peers (Stinson, Chase, & Kluwin, 1990). In fact, many college students with hearing impairment are lonely when mainstreamed at postsecondary institutions with peers who have normal hearing (Murphy & Newlon, 1987). Similarly, academic integration does not guarantee social interaction with hearing students at postsecondary institutions. For example, Brown and Foster (1991) found at the Rochester Institute of Technology that academically integrating a group of students who were deaf with their hearing peers did not result in social integration.

Erikson's (1968) stage of psychosocial development for middle-aged adults, 35 to 60 years of age, is called Generativity versus Stagnation (Erikson, 1968). The period is exemplified by peak performance levels in the workplace. The development of a hearing loss represents a psychological trauma for the middle-aged individual because it represents a loss of self. It is not uncommon for these patients to go through a grieving process for the way they used to be (Van Hecke, 1993). Middle-aged patients who acquire a hearing loss have an incongruence between their old reality and current status with hearing loss.

A recent study found that some adults with sudden severe-to-profound loss were so distressed that they needed support services (Hallam, Ashton, Sherbourne, & Gailey, 2006). We will discuss differences between these two types of hearing losses later in the chapter. Moreover, those with severe-to-profound acquired sensorineural hearing losses who have full-time employment had a higher HRQoL than peers who had part-time employment or were on disability (Ringdahl & Grimby, 2000). Although these patients appreciated audiologic and medical treatment, they felt that counseling and support services were lacking (Hallam et al., 2006).

Adults with hearing loss may find that the best support comes from groups started by their peers. Some groups for the hearing impaired include the Association of Late-Deafened Adults (ALDA), Cochlear Implant Association, Inc. (CIAI), and Self-Help for Hard of Hearing People (SHHH), which changed its name to Hearing Loss Association of America (www.hearingloss.org) (HLAA). The ALDA (www.alda.org) was formed in 1987 and consists of adults who are **late-deafened**, meaning they lost hearing after the age of 13. ALDA has no membership restrictions and is not tied to any specific mode of communication. ALDA works collaboratively with other organizations around the world serving the needs of late-deafened people and extends a welcome to everyone who supports its goals to join its organization, late-deafened or not (ALDA, 2010).

The CIAI (2005) is a nonprofit organization dedicated to educating and supporting cochlear implant recipients and their families and advocating for and promoting these devices. CIAI has become a part of HLAA, which is the nation's largest organization for people with hearing loss. The HLAA believes that providing information to people with hearing loss, their family and friends, and hearing healthcare professionals is critical. The HLAA has local chapters in the majority of cities in the United States. The National Association of the Deaf (National Association of the Deaf [NAD], 2010a) (www.nad.org) was founded in 1880 in Cincinnati, Ohio, and has had a long history of advocating for the rights of the deaf and hard of hearing.

The establishment of these organizations parallels those of other special interest groups that have been formed by the Deaf, such as Deaf Seniors of America (DSA) or Rainbow Alliance of the Deaf (RAD) for gay and lesbian persons who are also deaf (Andrews, Leigh, & Weiner, 2004). Similarly, individuals who are deaf members of different ethnic backgrounds have formed their own organizations, such as the National Asian Deaf Congress; Deaf Aztlan: Deaf Latino/A Network; National Black Deaf Advocates (NBDA) (Schein, 1989); and Intertribal Deaf Council for American Indians (Andrews et al., 2004).

Physical and Material Well-Being (Health and Living Arrangements)

Hearing loss affects adults' physical and material well-being. The National Academy on an Aging Society (NAOAS) reports that only 39% of people with hearing loss rated their health as "very good" or "excellent" compared with 68% of those with normal hearing (NAOAS, 1999). Moreover, almost one-third of people with hearing loss rated their health as "fair" or "poor" compared with only 9% of those with normal hearing (NAOAS). These findings are consistent with the results of an investigation that found lower subjective health status and higher degrees of physician utilization by adults who were deaf and hard of hearing in comparison to their peers with normal hearing (Zazove et al., 1993).

The communication difficulties of this population may limit their access to healthcare. For example, Iezonni, O'Day, Killeen, and Harker (2004) interviewed adults who believed that their views about their hearing losses and methods of effective communication differed from those of their physicians. They reported difficulties communicating about physical examinations/procedures, medication safety, and using long message menus on telephones. In another study, physicians reported that their most common method of communicating with these patients was through writing, although nearly two-thirds knew that using American Sign Language would be more effective (Ebert & Heckerling, 1995). It is suspected that physicians are ill-trained to work with patients who are deaf (Witte & Kuzel, 2000). At a minimum, medical schools need to teach students not to approach deafness as a pathological condition, but to realize that the Deaf have their own language and cultural traditions (Witte & Kuzel, 2000). In addition, physicians and office staff should use acceptable methods of communication (e.g., telephone-assisted communication, qualified interpreters, and so on) with these patients, including American Sign Language and lipreading (Witte & Kuzel, 2000).

Regarding material well-being, the societal costs of severe-to-profound sensorineural hearing loss are $297,000 per person over the course of a lifetime, with 67% of it attributable to lost work productivity (Mohr et al., 2000). It is assured that these costs have increased during the past decade. In addition, persons aged 51 to 61 years with hearing loss have a median net worth of $65,575 compared with $102,000 for their peers with normal hearing (NAOAS, 1999). Lower achievement of material well-being is a by-product of the effect of hearing loss on educational and professional achievement.

Some occupations have fairly stringent requirements for hearing sensitivity, particularly in jobs that may impact the safety of others. **Auditory fitness for duty (AFD)** has been defined as "possession of hearing abilities sufficient for safe and effective job performance" (Tufts, Vasil, & Briggs, 2009, p. 539). Audiologists may be called upon to perform audiologic evaluations for determining AFD in occupational areas such as air-traffic control, firefighting, law enforcement, public transportation, radio operation, railroad engineering, the military, and the U.S. Coast Guard (Tufts et al., 2009). Audiologic evaluations may determine candidates to be: (1) capable of safely executing the job, (2) able to perform the duties with accommodations, or (3) unsuitable for the position (Begines, 1995; Tufts et al., 2009). Audiologists may play an important role in the selection, evaluation, and fitting of hearing aids and hearing assistive technology (HAT) so that patients may become gainfully employed in their chosen professions. Moreover, audiologists may assist those already in "hearing critical" occupations who develop hearing losses and may need hearing aids and HAT to continue in their present positions.

Adult Role Fulfillment (Education and Employment)

Actress Marlee Maitlin and public speaker and former Miss America Heather Whitestone are examples of women who are deaf and have reached the pinnacles of their professions. Similarly, people who are deaf and hard of hearing can be found in all professions. However, even with acceptance of and excellent accommodations for the members of the Deaf community in Sweden, communication skills were prerequisite to occupational possibilities (DeCaro, Mudgett-DeCaro, & Dowaliby, 2001). MacLeod-Gallinger (1995) found that despite expansion in career awareness and postsecondary educational programs for deaf people, women who are deaf continue to pursue stereotypical female occupations. Furthermore, those women who achieve less than a bachelor's degree often end up among the ranks of the unemployed and underemployed. However, attitudes toward the employability of individuals who are deaf and hard of hearing can change with positive images of strong Deaf role models in the media (Zahn & Kelly, 1995).

Historically, the Deaf have found employment in jobs requiring skilled and unskilled labor. Two popular occupational areas have included printing and employment with the postal service (Andrews et al., 2004). A 15-year follow-up survey indicated that the large majority of 240 college graduates who were deaf or hard of hearing had successfully found employment and reported satisfaction with their lives (Andrews et al., 2004; Schrodel & Geyer, 2000). However, many successfully employed college-educated deaf adults in entry-level positions find a "glass ceiling" and are not provided equal opportunities for advancement (Andrews et al., 2004; Buchanan, 1994; Christiansen, 1994; Schein, 1989).

Although some advances have been made regarding the occupational status of these adults, recent statistics indicate a high school dropout rate of 44% among young adults who are deaf as compared with a 19% rate for their peers with normal hearing (Blanchfield, Feldman, Dunbar, & Gardner, 2001). These poor outcomes may be the result of young adults' low aspirations and lack of awareness of career possibilities. For example, Weisel and Cinamon (2005) asked high school students who were deaf, hard of hearing, and normal hearing to rate the appropriateness of jobs for themselves and for fictitious deaf adults that varied in communication involvement and prestige. All students rated jobs with high communication involvement unsuitable for deaf adults, regardless of the prestige level. Moreover, the young adults with hearing impairment did not perceive prestigious jobs suitable for their own careers, even if communication was irrelevant. Indeed, the students may self-select out of career options due to a lack of awareness of their rights to accommodations under the law (Punch, Creed, & Hyde, 2006). Workers with hearing loss are more likely to be in occupations involving crafts and repair, farming, machine operations, and transportation compared with their hearing peers who are more apt to be in administrative, professional, sales- and/or service-oriented professions (NAOAS, 1999).

These circumstances may change with aggressive career counseling during high school. For example, **school-to-work** (STW) programs are activities, experiences, and opportunities that prepare students for the world of work, including career exploration, integration of academic/vocational curricula, internships, job shadowing, mentoring, and youth apprenticeships (Bonds, 2003). High schools and postsecondary educational institutions have developed STW programs for students due to federal initiatives supporting transition of students who are deaf and hard of hearing into the world of work.

AUDITORY REHABILITATION FOR YOUNG ADULTS WITH HEARING LOSS

Federal laws that ensure children with disabilities a free and appropriate education in the least restrictive environment were covered in the last chapter on the auditory habilitation of school-aged children. We will now consider the transition of two young adults with hearing impairment to the world of work and enrollment at a major university.

Transition to the World of Work

Audiologists and speech-language pathologists must prepare students and their families for the change in laws that affect accommodations received at work or at school. Students and their parents need to know that up until high school graduation, the Individuals With

Disabilities Education Improvement Act (IDEA, 2004) ensures that they are entitled to free and appropriate public education in a least restrictive environment. The IDEA 2004 mandates that each individualized education plan contains information about transition services, beginning no later than age 16, complete with statements about ties to and responsibilities of agencies before the student leaves high school (Hallahan & Kauffman, 2006). Unfortunately, many high school seniors do not benefit from transition planning because many simply give up and quit school. Before discussing transition planning, let's consider some statistics regarding high school graduation rates for this population.

What Does the Evidence Show?

In a recent speech, U.S. Secretary of Education, Arne Duncan, stated that in 2007, nearly 60% of students with disabilities graduated from high school with a regular diploma compared to only 32% twenty years ago. Overall, these statistics suggest improvement. However, what are the graduation rates for students who are deaf and hard of hearing? Communication sciences and disorders professionals should gauge progress on discipline-specific statistics (Hallahan & Kauffman, 2006). Furthermore, a high school diploma does not guarantee success. What are post–high school employment rates for students who are deaf and hard of hearing? What percent of students go on to college or postsecondary training? Evidence has shown that these answers are not always easily and clearly obtained. Factors such as degree of loss, age of onset, and diagnosis impact educational and employment outcomes. Therefore, even discipline-specific statistics must be carefully scrutinized on how estimations are made recording educational and employment achievement of adults with hearing impairment.

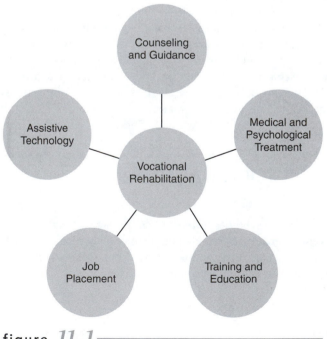

Vocational rehabilitation (VR) has a goal of assisting and empowering persons with disabilities to attain and maintain productive and meaningful employment. Figure 11.1 shows the five major areas of assistance provided through VR.

VR counselors provide counseling, guidance, support, and assistance to adults with disabilities to achieve their job goals. Second, counselors make referrals to physicians and other healthcare professionals to reduce the effects of any conditions related to their clients' disabilities that may interfere with job success. For example, VR counselors may refer their clients to audiologists or speech-language pathologists to limit the effects that hearing impairment have on their clients' employability. Third, VR supports training and education by providing adults with financial assistance to attend postsecondary educational and training institutions. Fourth, VR assists adults with disabilities in obtaining job placement by providing short-term

figure *11.1*

Five major areas of assistance through vocational rehabilitation.

Casebook Reflection

Theresa Calloway: A School-to-Work Student

Theresa Calloway is a 20-year-old enrolled at the Springfield Vocational Technological School that has a Deaf Services Division. Theresa was diagnosed with a bilateral severe sensorineural hearing loss at three years of age. From the time Theresa was a little girl, her mother had her in aural habilitative therapy with a talented speech-language pathologist. The Springfield Public School System had an award-winning program for students who were deaf and hard of hearing. Theresa's parents attended every IEP meeting, parent-teacher conference, and encouraged their daughter to overcome the limitations of her disability. In all of her classes Theresa wore bilateral digital hearing aids and used an FM receiver coupled to her hearing aids via a teleloop. Theresa was an average student and was proud to graduate from high school.

Theresa couldn't wait to enroll in the Springfield Vocational Technological School. She had friends who were hard of hearing who loved the school and Mr. Weber, the VR counselor. She wanted to obtain a certificate in child development through the school's technical division requiring 13 to 24 semester hours. Mr. Weber arranged for her to take classes in the morning and then participate in a school-to-work program in the afternoon. It is common for students in the certificate program to find permanent employment with their in-training placement sites.

Theresa left the campus early to make sure that she arrived on time at Our Little Angels Preschool and Daycare Center. She was nervous, but walked in and greeted the receptionist.

"My name is Theresa Calloway. I'm here to see Mrs. Suarez. I'm the intern from Springfield Tech," explained Theresa.

"Yes, Mrs. Suarez was expecting you," said the receptionist, bending down out of Theresa's view.

"I'm sorry, I didn't hear you," admitted Theresa. "I need to be able to see you to best understand," explained Theresa. "What is your name?"

"Oh," said the receptionist. "My name is Estella. The vans from the schools will be arriving at any

moment. Give me your backpack and I'll lock it up. You can fill out your paperwork later. This is Darcy, one of our lead teachers."

"Hi, Theresa," said Darcy.

"Hi, pleased to meet you," Theresa said, shaking her hand.

"Come outside with me to greet the kids," instructed Darcy. "Here they come."

Theresa and Darcy helped the children off the van from the Springfield Early Education Center.

"I need you to watch the kindergartners play outside," Darcy explained. "You need to be quick on your feet. I'm going to go prepare their snack. If you need me, I'll be right inside."

"Come on, kids! My name is Theresa. Let's go play . . . " said Theresa. "Outside?"

"Yes," Darcy said. "Two girls from high school will be here to help with the older children when their vans arrive. Have fun!"

Theresa couldn't believe that she was actually on the job. The yard was long and narrow. The sandbox was at the far end near the fence. Two boys, Jose and Peter, were eager to play with the earthmoving equipment in the sandbox. Theresa stood by the window with her back to the sandbox talking to the girls who were pretending to walk on a balance beam.

"What's your name?" asked Theresa.

"My name's Madison," said the little girl.

"I'm Courtney," said the other. "I'm going to be a gymnast when I grow up. Theresa, why do you talk funny?"

"I was born with a hearing loss. I had to work very hard to learn how to listen and talk. I have to wear these hearing aids to help me hear," explained Theresa.

"Oh, my grandpa wears those too," Courtney said.

All of a sudden, screams could be heard coming from the sandbox. Courtney and Madison looked at the sandbox in amazement.

"He does?" asked Theresa who wondered why both of the girls were looking beyond her toward the sandbox.

"Theresa! Theresa!" Darcy yelled. "Never take your eyes off the play area! You need to watch all of the children, all the time! Those boys are fighting down there. Can't you hear them?"

"No, I can't. I'm so sorry," Theresa said as she ran with Darcy to break up the fight. She and Darcy pulled the crying boys apart. Jose had a gash in his head from being hit with a dump truck. Peter had sand in his eyes. Two high school girls arrived at the preschool/daycare and came out to help.

"Do you think you can watch these girls while I go clean the boys up?" asked Darcy in a sarcastic tone of voice. "This is Jade and Celeste. They go to Springfield High. You guys get acquainted and watch these kids."

"Hi," Theresa said, a little embarrassed by her mistake.

"Hi," said the girls in unison, talking together in quiet voices about what had happened at school that day and about the dance on Friday night. Gradually, the yard filled with children. Theresa sat on the picnic table carefully watching the children. Soon, she was called in and assisted with snack time. Some of the older children played video games while others did their homework.

"Theresa?" said an older woman. "I'm Mrs. Suarez, the owner of the school. Mr. Weber has talked to me about you. He told me you want to be a preschool teacher."

"Yes," Theresa said. "I'm pleased to meet you, Mrs. Suarez."

"Same here . . . I heard that you had a rough afternoon. Don't worry, that's how we learn," reassured Mrs. Suarez. "Childcare isn't as easy as it looks."

"Tell me about it," said Theresa as they both laughed.

Theresa had a busy afternoon, helping out with snacks and then assisting older students with their homework. Theresa couldn't hear the older students when they tried speaking to her from across the table due to the noise from other children playing board games. Those students became frustrated with Theresa, although she was quite effective in helping with homework when sitting close to a student in a quiet environment. Around 5:30 p.m., Mrs. Suarez asked Theresa if she could take on the role of receptionist for

30 minutes so Estella could go pick her daughter up from dance class.

"Theresa, I need you to answer the phone. Also, please introduce yourself to the parents when they come to pick up their kids," said Mrs. Suarez.

"Sure," Theresa said looking at the multiline phone with concern. She had already had several problems today. She didn't want to tell Mrs. Suarez that she didn't know how to transfer calls. So, she just hoped that no one would call. Then, the phone rang.

"Our Little Angels, Theresa speaking," she said answering the phone.

"Hi, this is Mrs. Pate, I'm afraid I'm going to be very late this evening," said the caller from her cell phone.

"Sorry, I can't hear you. Who is this?" asked Theresa

"Mrs. Pate. Jodie's mom," said the caller.

"Who?" asked Theresa.

"Please let me talk to Estella," asked the caller.

"Estella, is that you?" guessed Theresa.

"No, this is Mrs. PATE!" screamed the caller, who decided to hang up.

Theresa felt way over her head. She didn't know how to transfer calls nor could she understand very well over the telephone. At home, she could hear fine using the equipment that her family got through the phone company. No one else called. Several parents came by to pick up their children. Theresa completed her homework assignment from her morning class. Soon, it was 6:45 p.m. Mrs. Suarez and Theresa were the only ones left besides Jodie Pate.

"I wonder where Ms. Pate is," said Mrs. Suarez looking at her watch. "We close at 6:30 p.m. and charge parents a dollar per minute overtime if they don't phone us. Did Mrs. Pate call?"

"I don't know," Theresa said. "Someone called and hung up."

At that moment a van pulled into the parking lot.

"Mrs. Pate, how are you?" asked Mrs. Suarez. "We were worried because you didn't call."

"I did call, but the young lady answering the phone couldn't understand me. I just gave up," explained Mrs. Pate.

"Mama," Jodie said running to hug her mother.

"Hi, sweetie! Did you have a good day?" asked Mrs. Pate. "Sorry Mommy's late. See you tomorrow."

"Bye, Mrs. Pate," said Mrs. Suarez. "Theresa, if you have difficulty answering telephones, tell me or transfer the call. Everyone who works here must be able to handle the telephone."

"Sorry, Mrs. Suarez," Theresa said, looking down.

Mrs. Suarez liked Theresa from the start. She knew Theresa had a challenging first day, but could recognize someone who loved working with children.

"Are you tired?" asked Mrs. Suarez.

"Yes, ma'am," said Theresa gathering up her belongings.

"Well, we'll see you tomorrow. Have a good evening and thanks for all of your hard work," she complimented. "Bye, Theresa."

"Bye, Mrs. Suarez," said Theresa.

Mrs. Suarez watched her intern walk out to her car. She made a note on her calendar to call Mr. Weber about Theresa's first day.

transitional support for finding and adjusting to regular employment. Fifth, VR assists adults with disabilities to obtain the necessary assistive technology for independent living and employment. The Casebook Reflection shows how these areas of VR dovetail to prepare Theresa Calloway for the world of work.

Mrs. Suarez called Mr. Weber the very next day about Theresa's difficulties. On a positive note, Mrs. Suarez reported that Theresa was punctual, had a good attitude, and easily established rapport with the children. However, Theresa's hearing loss affected her ability to perform required job tasks. For example, she could not understand what was being said across the table when helping children with their homework or during staff meetings in background noise. In addition, she could not operate the multiline phone, understand what was being said, or take messages. Mr. Weber knew that he needed Theresa's permission to talk to her audiologist and the technical school's speech-language pathologist about serving as **job coaches**. Job coaches assist persons with significant disabilities to direct their own support systems and to become successfully employed in careers of their choice. A job coach can be an official employment title (e.g., employment specialist) such as the position that Mr. Weber holds, or it can be a role that a person can serve for a particular client, like the audiologist and speech-language pathologist. For example, the speech-language pathologist and Theresa's audiologist will provide vocational assessment, instruction, overall planning, and interaction assistance with employers, other employees, and the clients of the daycare center. The assessment process is shown in Figure 11.2. For example, the audiologist discovered that Theresa's hearing loss had gotten worse and that she needed new bilateral digital hearing aids equipped with strong telecoils and FM capabilities. The speech-language pathologist confirmed Mr. Weber's reports of Theresa's difficulties with fast paced conversations in background noise and with telephone communication. The third step was obtaining HAT and instruction in communication skills to improve on-the-job performance. Based on their evaluations, the audiologist and speech-language pathologist outlined an Individualized Employment Program for Theresa involving obtaining HAT and setting goals to increase the likelihood of success at Our Little Angels Preschool and Daycare Center. Step four included direct instruction from her audiologist on the multiple uses of the HAT device for classes at the vocational technical school and at work and from the speech-language pathologist on conversational fluency, use of a multiline phone, and the etiquette for taking messages within professional contexts.

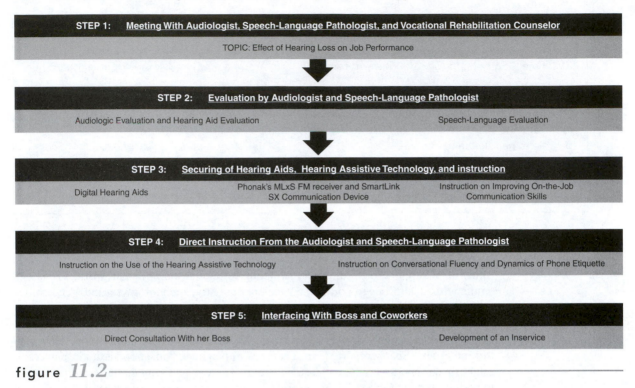

STEP 1: Meeting With Audiologist, Speech-Language Pathologist, and Vocational Rehabilitation Counselor

TOPIC: Effect of Hearing Loss on Job Performance

STEP 2: Evaluation by Audiologist and Speech-Language Pathologist

Audiologic Evaluation and Hearing Aid Evaluation — Speech-Language Evaluation

STEP 3: Securing of Hearing Aids, Hearing Assistive Technology, and instruction

Digital Hearing Aids — Phonak's MLxS FM receiver and SmartLink SX Communication Device — Instruction on Improving On-the-Job Communication Skills

STEP 4: Direct Instruction From the Audiologist and Speech-Language Pathologist

Instruction on the Use of the Hearing Assistive Technology — Instruction on Conversational Fluency and Dynamics of Phone Etiquette

STEP 5: Interfacing With Boss and Coworkers

Direct Consultation With her Boss — Development of an Inservice

figure *11.2*

Vocational rehabilitation assessment process for Theresa Calloway.

The fifth step included interfacing with Theresa's boss and coworkers. For example, Mr. Weber was in direct consultation with Mrs. Suarez regarding Theresa's on-the-job performance. Additionally, the audiologist and speech-language pathologist assisted Theresa in designing an inservice for the preschool/daycare faculty about her hearing loss, her HAT, and how to best communicate with her. In six months, Theresa was a model employee and was hired to work permanently at Our Little Angels Preschool and Daycare. Theresa is an example of successful transition from vocational technical training programs to the world of work. Some students who are deaf or hard of hearing go on to four-year colleges and universities.

Enrollment in Colleges and Universities

Between the years of 1910 and 1965, Quigley, Jenne, and Phillips (1968) conducted a study and found that only 228 deaf or hard of hearing students graduated from a postsecondary school in the United States during that time span. Why do you think that number is so low? Prior to 1965, postsecondary institutions were not equipped to deal with the needs of students with hearing impairment. The only college for students who were deaf and hard of hearing was Gallaudet College, later renamed Gallaudet University, which offered a liberal arts education. Another postsecondary institution emphasizing technical training is the National Technical Institute for the Deaf (NTID). The students at NTID can also take classes with their peers who have normal hearing at the Rochester Institute of Technology (RIT). Students don't have to pay out-of-state tuition at these schools because by law, they must serve students from all 50 states and territories. Postsecondary institutions for the deaf can offer specialized instruction (Berent et al., 2007) for deaf students and may more readily facilitate their psychosocial adjustment than traditional college and universities (Lukomski, 2007).

Most traditional colleges and universities have programs for students with disabilities that provide access to a postsecondary education. Section 504 of the Rehabilitation Act of 1973, as amended, and the Americans With Disabilities Act of 1990 mandated that accommodations must be provided to persons with disabilities to ensure accessibility to programs, services, and activities at postsecondary educational institutions. Section 504 of the Rehabilitation Act of 1973 states, "No otherwise qualified handicapped individual in the United States . . . shall, solely by reason of his handicap, be excluded from participation in, be denied benefits of, or be subjected to discrimination under any program or activity receiving Federal financial assistance." The Americans With Disabilities Act extends civil rights protection for people with disabilities to include public accommodations (stores and businesses), medical treatment, employment, services provided by state and local government, and telecommunication relay services. According to the ADA, a disability is a chronic, long-term, substantially limiting condition that affects one or more major life activities (e.g., walking, sitting, eating, learning, and so on). Title I does not permit discrimination in hiring and terms/conditions of employment based upon disability. It also requires the reasonable accommodation of disabilities and restricts collection and use of medical information from applicants and employees. Title II includes all beneficiaries of programs and services of a public institution, including students and members of the public. Title II requires accessibility of all programs and services, including employment.

In postsecondary schools, students and their parents, not the public agency, must assume responsibility of securing accommodations (Hollins, 2005). Most colleges and universities have programs that work with students with disabilities to ensure that they have an equal opportunity to pursue postsecondary training and/or education. Besides hearing impairment, other examples of disabilities include other health conditions (e.g., asthma, cancer, diabetes, epilepsy or other seizure disorders, kidney disease, lupus, rheumatoid arthritis), mobility impairments (e.g., use of a cane, cart, or wheelchair), psychological disorders (e.g., clinical depression or anxiety), traumatic brain injury, or addictive diseases. Young adults and their parents must assume responsibility to provide appropriate documentation of students' disabilities and to request appropriate accommodations. For example, documentation of hearing impairment should be a letter or report from a physician or audiologist that includes a clearly stated disability (e.g., type, degree, and configuration of hearing loss), the date of evaluation, and how the diagnosis was reached, credentials of the professional, defined level of functioning (e.g., primary mode of communication), and current treatment and medications (e.g., use of hearing aids, cochlear implants, and/or HAT), and how the disability affects academic performance (Hollins, 2005; Laufer, 2000a, 2000b). The report should be current or at least completed within the last calendar year.

Students with disabilities should consider five factors when selecting a college or university. First, like all high school seniors, they should consider universities that offer the best programs in their major field of interest. Second, they should determine if they meet entrance requirements. Third, they should consider the existence and quality of the program for students with disabilities and types of accommodations for those who are deaf and hard of hearing. Fourth, they should self-identify their disabilities on the application form and follow up with a call to the appropriate university officials. Fifth, they should schedule a visit to each school at least six months prior to enrollment because most programs for students with disabilities appreciate at least a semester's notice to secure necessary accommodations.

Most colleges and universities differ in the quality of disability services provided to students. Students and their parents should be sure to ask several key questions. One question that students and their parents should ask is, "What is the school's policy for determining the accommodations for students with disabilities?" (Hollins, 2005; Laufer, 2000a, 2000b). For example, does the school have a "one-size-fits-all" approach so that all students who are deaf and hard of hearing receive the same accommodations? Generally, students with the same disability often require similar accommodations, but individualization of services should be available for each student and tailored to the specific area of study. For example, one student with a hearing loss may need only an FM system, while another student may require an FM system, note-taker services, and extended time on examinations.

Second, how does a student request accommodations and establish eligibility, and what documentation must be provided? A school should have a clearly defined process for requesting and establishing eligibility for accommodations. The requirements should be easily accessible in the information packets for prospective students and on the institution's web page. The process should be described in enough detail with a timeline so that new students have their accommodations in place by the first day of class.

Third, specifically what services can the school provide students having hearing impairment? Schools should have amplified pay phones, TTYs, and HAT in the classroom such as FM, infrared, or induction loop systems that were described in Chapter 7. Schools with adequate services have accessible assistive technology laboratories available for students and faculty. Figure 11.3 shows an assistive technology laboratory at a major university. Accommodations may also include extended time on examinations, quizzes, and note-taker services for students who have poorer than average language skills resulting from their disabilities.

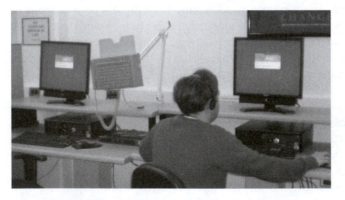

figure *11.3*

An assistive technology laboratory at a major university.

Fourth, are note-taker services available to students with hearing impairment? *Note-taker services* allow students to concentrate on what the professor is saying, rather than struggling to write down everything that is said. Schools that have a variety of note-taker services provide more flexibility than those that have only one option. Note-taker services can range from low- to high-technology options. Low-technology services consist of a peer using carbon paper to make a duplicate copy of class notes for a student with a disability. Alternatively, high-technology note-taking services may include (1) computer-assisted note-taking (CAN), (2) computer-aided speech (C-Print™), and (3) computer-assisted real-time transcription (CART). With **computer-assisted note-taking (CAN)**, note-takers use standard computer keyboards to provide a general summary of what was said, whereas **computer-aided speech (C-Print)** requires the use of regular word-processing systems on computers in addition to special software programs that abbreviate words and use text-condensing strategies that reduce the number of necessary keystrokes. **Computer-assisted real-time transcriptions (CART)** utilizes trained court reporters to record everything that is said in real time. Besides note-taker services, students should inquire about accommodations available in the residence halls. For example, the dormitories should have smoke detectors and fire alarms with lights, and televisions with closed captioning.

Fifth, students who are deaf should ask about the availability of **sign language interpreters**. There are two types of sign language interpreting, those that use American Sign Language (ASL) and those that use **transliteration** or a method used by the majority of sign language interpreters in which the signs maintain the same order as spoken English (Hallahan & Kauffman, 2006). It is advisable to ask for an interpreter, if needed, when students take their initial tour of the campus. If the school cannot provide an interpreter easily, then that may indicate that those services may not always be available when needed due to their cost. It is more cost effective to invest in a single system, such as C-Print, to accommodate all students with hearing impairment than to provide interpreters for each student. Moreover, a recent investigation found no significant difference in the effectiveness of ASL interpreters, C-Print, or simultaneous usage of these accommodations on deaf students' learning (Marschark et al., 2006). However, although students with good reading, writing, and speechreading skills find C-Print acceptable for their needs, programs for students with disabilities should consider providing availability of interpreters for others with special issues (Elliot, Stinson, McKee, Everhart, & Francis, 2001).

Sixth, students should ask about the policies and procedures regarding interaction with faculty members who make accommodations for those with disabilities. At one major southern university, the program for students with disabilities generates an Accommodation Memo for the student for each of their instructor-related accommodations. The memo is given to the student whose responsibility it is to present it to the faculty member for discussion during the first week of class. Ideally, the student should schedule an appointment with the professor to discuss his or her need for accommodations. Some new students may feel uneasy about this process, but they must follow through if accommodations are to be provided in a timely manner. Students are well-advised that accommodations are to be provided from the date of presentation and discussion of the memo, not retroactively. Therefore, students should not expect to take examinations retroactively with accommodations to possibly improve on their performances.

The program for students with disabilities should provide all faculty ample opportunities to learn about aspects of accommodating students with disabilities. Seminars presented in face-to-face or e-learning formats could provide instructors information about what type of accommodations students with certain disabilities need. They should advise that students who have similar disabilities may require different accommodations. Students who are deaf and hard of hearing are no different and although many use HAT, they vary in their need for other accommodations. One student may need an ASL interpreter, while another may need note-taking services and extended time on practical examinations. Faculty may be asked to provide lecture material in advance to ASL interpreters, particularly if the information is technical. In addition, faculty members should ensure that classroom multimedia equipment has captioning capabilities and provides a written text of auditory material from DVDs. Faculty are encouraged to work closely with programs for students with disabilities regarding how best to meet the unique needs of individual students.

Seventh, students should trust their instincts when visiting a university's program for students with disabilities. Students and their parents should be able to meet with the director of the program and should feel at ease in talking with the staff, who should ask them about specific questions about their disabilities and previous accommodations. Alternatively, the director and his or her staff should welcome questions and provide as much information as possible. Students may want to speak candidly with others who are deaf and hard of hearing about their experiences in receiving necessary accommodations. If students do not feel comfortable during their initial visit, they may want to investigate further prior to reaching any conclusions about the quality of the program.

Let's check in on Stacy Sinclair and her visit to State University. In the previous chapter, we looked in on Stacy and her mother during a final meeting with her educational audiologist, Dr. Chow. Following his advice, Stacy and her mother arranged to visit State's program for student with disabilities.

Casebook Reflection

Stacy Sinclair's Visit to State University

"Mom, I don't even want to visit any other schools, I'm going to State!" exclaimed Stacy. "I love the campus and everybody is so friendly! I can't wait to rush and be a Tri-Delt just like you, Mom! I know exactly how I'm going to decorate my dorm room! Can we go shopping for computers when we get home?"

"Young lady, we have one more appointment in 15 minutes at the program for students with disabilities," reminded Mrs. Sinclair.

"OK," agreed Stacy as they walked toward the office. "This must be it. Mom, can you let me do the talking?"

"Sure, sweetie," said Mrs. Sinclair.

"Hi, I'm Stacy Sinclair, and I have an appointment with Dr. Holloway at 2:30 p.m.," Stacy said.

"Hi, I'm Corey, the receptionist. Dr. Holloway will be with you in just one moment," Corey said picking up the telephone. "Dr. Holloway, Stacy Sinclair and her mother are here to see you."

"Thanks, I'll be right out," said Dr. Holloway. "Hi, my name is Dr. Holloway and I'm director of the Program for Students with Disabilities, also known as PSD, at State University."

"I'm Stacy Sinclair, and this is my mother," Stacy said, proudly shaking hands with Dr. Holloway.

"Dr. Holloway, I'm Rose Sinclair," said Mrs. Sinclair, shaking Dr. Holloway's hand.

"I'm pleased to meet you both. Please, have a seat in my office," offered Dr. Holloway. "Corey, no interruptions, please."

"Well, how do you like State so far?" asked Dr. Holloway.

"I love it!" exclaimed Stacy. "I've decided to enroll in the fall."

"That's wonderful," said Dr. Holloway. "I'm so glad that you've made an appointment with us during your visit. Many students with disabilities fail to make proper arrangements for receiving accommodations prior to their enrollment. Stacy, what type of disability do you have?"

"I have a moderately-severe sensorineural hearing loss in both ears and need to wear hearing aids to understand what people are saying, particularly in noise," explained Stacy. "In high school, I used an FM receiver coupled to my hearing aids via direct-audio input for all of my classes."

"Believe it or not, we have over 200 students who are deaf and hard of hearing registered with PSD," reported Dr. Holloway.

"Really?" asked Stacy in amazement. "Wow, that makes me feel better. At West High School, there were only four students that I know of with hearing loss. I felt so different."

"Well, we keep students' disabilities completely confidential and so do the faculty. This is how it works. You must document your disability with our office through a letter or report from a physician or audiologist."

"Yes, Dr. Chow, my educational audiologist, told us about that," recalled Stacy.

"Here is an information sheet about the requirements for documentation with specific instructions for various disabilities," said Dr. Holloway. "Stacy, you said that you used an FM system in most of your classes. We have those available for use, too. State also has an on-campus Speech and Hearing Clinic that works with us."

"Stacy, now you can get your hearing aids serviced at school!" offered Mrs. Sinclair. "How convenient!"

"Examples of other accommodations that students with hearing loss may need include preferential seating for a good view of the instructor's face. Students have also been reassigned if an instructor is difficult to understand due to a foreign accent or facial hair that limits the amount of visual information obtained from speechreading."

"Wow," said Stacy looking at her mom.

"We also offer extended time on examinations, quizzes, and tests for students with weak language skills. We have note-taker services available, too" offered Dr. Holloway.

"Pretty neat," remarked Mrs. Sinclair. "Tell me more about the note-taker service."

"OK," Dr. Holloway said. "Very simply, the student with a disability is given carbon paper and is told to meet with the instructor of the course to identify a note-taker. The instructor may or may not know a good note-taker at the beginning of the class. In that case, a student is asked to volunteer to be a note-taker until someone permanent is found. The instructor may ask students having good grades and neat handwriting to meet with him or her after class and that a notebook and carbon paper will be provided. The instructor maintains the confidentiality of the student having a disability and monitors the quality of the notes taken."

"Wow, that's neat. I wouldn't feel comfortable having other students know that I had an 'extra edge,'" admitted Stacy. "What other accommodations may students with hearing loss need?"

"As I mentioned, they can have extended time on exams, quizzes, and tests," explain Dr. Holloway. "Also, they have access to captioned films and videos and may not have to receive a grade for those without it. For students with more severe hearing loss, interpreter services and use of TTY for phone calls are available."

"How will my teachers know what accommodations I'm allowed?" asked Stacy.

"Good question," said Dr. Holloway. "Each semester, special accommodation memos are generated for you to give to and discuss with your instructors. Please be advised that it is your responsibility to present the memo and talk with your instructors. Accommodations will be provided only from the date of presentation of the memo. We tell professors to maintain students' confidentiality. We expect each student registered with PSD to meet with his or her instructors preferably during the first week of class. Most professors are pleased to make any and all necessary accommodation(s) to ensure the success of their students. Would you like to tour our Assistive Technology Laboratory?"

"Yes," Stacy said, looking at her mother. "Wow, this is really a cool program!"

"This way, it is just down the hall. First, let me introduce you to Jesse. He is our assistive technology specialist and runs the laboratory."

"Pleased to meet you, Jesse," Stacy said, shaking his hand.

"Pleased to meet you, Stacy and Mrs. Sinclair," said Jesse. "I will take you on the tour of the Assistive Technology Laboratory, and then you can meet with Dr. Holloway one last time to answer any remaining questions that you may have."

After Stacy decided she was going to State, she and her parents completed the process, and she was registered to receive accommodations. Stacy soon graduated from high school and had a wonderful summer with a few family trips and working at the local library. In late summer, Stacy and her parents drove to State University so that she could participate in the sorority rush. Hundreds of parents and their children all made a mad rush on the stores to purchase all the must-have amenities, such as mini-refrigerators, DVD players, iPods, bean-bag chairs, etc. Soon, it was time to tell her parents goodbye.

Both Stacy and her roommate pledged Delta Delta Delta sorority. Stacy was so excited when she called home for the first time with the news. Her mother reminded her to go for her follow-up appointment with Dr. Holloway. Stacy agreed, but just wanted to forget about her hearing loss and enjoy all of the orientation week fun. Like Stacy, many college students get a little distracted with all of the free movies, pep rallies, club day, etc. However, Stacy finally got around to making her follow-up appointment with Dr. Holloway. Unfortunately, many students with disabilities follow through with all of the necessary procedures for documentation to receive accommodations, but for whatever reason, decide not to use them. Some college students are embarrassed about receiving accommodations, while others just do not want to go through the hassle. However, students must be counseled that it is no one's fault but theirs if they do not exercise their rights to receive accommodations. They are rudely awakened when they show up at programs for students with disabilities wanting to drop a course or two far past the deadline. Many disability specialists believe that students with disabilities should not be afforded any special privileges, particularly if they did not follow through with securing accommodations. Let's check in on Stacy, who is finally on her own at State University to see how she wrestles with whether to pursue receiving accommodations in the classroom.

Casebook Reflection

Stacy Sinclair's Follow-up Appointment With the Director of the Program for Students With Disabilities

"Hi, Stacy!" said Dr. Holloway. "Are you all settled in?"

"Hi, Dr. Holloway! Yes, all settled in and I love my roommate and my dorm room," Stacy said. "I've got it decorated just the way I like it!"

"Stacy, I'm so glad that you came by to see me. I have a few things that I'd like to ask you," explained Dr. Holloway. "Would you like to be paired with an older student, a senior, who also has a hearing loss? We have a peer-support program here at State University. The peer-counselor I have in mind has done very well. She will be applying to medical school in the fall. We believe that students can relate to other students in ways that PSD staff members can't. Would you like her phone number?"

"Yes, I would," Stacy said.

"Don't feel shy about calling her. She has served as a peer-mentor for two years now. She is so easygoing and enjoys meeting new students," explained Dr. Holloway.

"Thanks, Dr. Holloway," Stacy said, not sure whether she would call the student.

"If you have any difficulties whatsoever, please come to see us," advised Dr. Holloway. "Don't wait until midterm to confront any problems. Catch small problems before they become major ones. . . . Well, Wednesday is the first day of class. Are you ready?"

"Yes, I'm ready," said Stacy, although she wasn't ready at all. "Goodbye, Dr. Holloway."

"Remember, meet with each of your instructors to present and discuss your Accommodation Memo. All of your teachers are requested to use an FM system for you. Don't forget to introduce yourself to each of them," said Dr. Holloway. "Bye, Stacy. Don't be a stranger!"

"I won't," Stacy said.

For the next two nights, Stacy had a difficult time sleeping. She was nervous about her first day of class. During rush, she had time in the evenings to find all of the classrooms so she felt confident that she could find her way to class on time. Finally, Wednesday morning came. Stacy's first class was Biology 101. She was the second person to arrive to class besides the professor. Stacy sat in the back of the lecture hall, which was unusual for her. In high school, she always sat in the front row and all of her teachers knew she had a hearing loss. Stacy sat motionless in her chair, pretending to be reviewing her planner. She watched the professor from the corner of her eye as he prepared the audiovisual equipment. She was relieved when other students started to show up. Stacy felt anxious about introducing herself, presenting her Accommodation Memo, and scheduling an appointment to discuss her instructional needs. She told herself that this was the perfect time. She just couldn't get up from her desk. More and more students arrived and soon the lecture started. Stacy couldn't understand anything that the professor was saying. She doodled in her notebook for the entire 50-minute period. She left the lecture hall almost in tears. She needed to talk to someone, but who? She thought about calling her mother, but Stacy wasn't in the mood for a lecture. Stacy went into her purse to get the number of the peer mentor that Dr. Holloway had given her and punched in the number.

"Hi, I'm Belinda Stephens, I'm sorry I'm unable to come to the phone right now, but if you leave your name, number, and a brief message, I'll get back to you as soon as possible. Thank you for calling," said the student's answering machine.

"Hi, my name is Stacy Sinclair and Dr. Holloway provided your number as a peer mentor. I'm a freshman and I need someone to talk to," Stacy said, on the verge of tears. "My number is 555-4648."

Belinda had just gotten in the door of her apartment when the phone rang, but chose not to answer it because she needed to take her dog out. Belinda listened to Stacy's plea for help and decided to call her immediately.

Stacy was so surprised when her cell phone rang almost as soon as she hung up.

"Hello?" Stacy said, answering the phone.

"Stacy? This is Belinda Stephens. How are you doing?"

"Oh, I'm so glad you called! I really need someone to talk to," Stacy said, feeling somewhat relieved that she was talking to someone who could understand how she was feeling.

"I understand, believe me! Stacy, could you meet me for lunch tomorrow at Mellow Mushroom at 11:45 a.m.?"

"Sure, is that on College Street?"

"Yes, it is, right down from Toomer's Corner. I'll see you then!"

"Sounds like a plan! Bye, Belinda!"

"Bye, Stacy!"

Stacy felt so good after talking to Belinda. Stacy felt like she already had a connection with Belinda, because she had a hearing loss too.

The next day, Stacy arrived at Mellow Mushroom 15 minutes early to be sure not to miss Belinda, who arrived at 11:45 a.m.

"Stacy?" asked Belinda.

"Hi, Belinda. How did you know it was me?" asked Stacy.

"You're the only one waiting," Belinda said with a huge grin.

"Oh yeah," Stacy said, somewhat embarrassed, looking down at her feet.

"Come on, are you hungry?" asked Belinda.

"Starving," admitted Stacy as the waitress took them to their table. As Belinda led the way, Stacy noticed that Belinda had behind-the-ear hearing aids. She could tell from Belinda's speech that she probably had a more severe hearing loss than hers. Stacy wondered if Belinda's first day of college had been as terrifying as hers was. Both students went ahead and ordered their meals.

"Stacy, where are you from?" asked Belinda. "I'm from Mobile."

"I'm from Andalusia," said Stacy.

"What do you want to major in?" asked Belinda.

"I don't know. I want to explore my options for my first year," Stacy explained. "I'd like to be a nurse or a veterinarian. I love animals and I miss my dog."

"Interesting," remarked Belinda. "Vet school is almost as hard to get into as medical school. I'm majoring in biochemistry and am getting my applications to medical school completed. I want to be a pediatrician," explained Belinda.

"Wow," said Stacy.

"How was your first day of class?" asked Belinda. "Did you get to all of your classes?"

"Yes, I did," said Stacy.

"Did you introduce yourself, present your Accommodation Memo, and make an appointment to discuss your accommodations?" asked Belinda, noticing Stacy's face turn red.

"Well, no, I didn't. I was afraid to. I mean, I wanted to, but I just couldn't. I didn't want to bother the professor. He is probably really busy," Stacy explained in a very soft voice. "I sat in the back of the class, glued to my seat. Doesn't that sound stupid?"

"No, Stacy. It doesn't sound stupid. You should have seen me my first day of class," Belinda admitted. "I was pathetic! At least you went to your first day of classes. I decided to pretend I was sick. I wasn't really sick, but it sure felt like I was sick."

"Really?" asked a surprised Stacy. "You are so 'together.' That's hard for me to believe!"

"Well, I realized, though, that if I was going to make it, it was up to me. Sink or swim. I had to become proactive in my own education. My future was in my own hands and I knew it. You've already made a big step by providing documentation of your disability and maintaining contact with PSD. That's half the battle. The rest is just attitude. Who do you have for Biology 101?"

"Dr. Brooster," Stacy answered.

"Dr. B. is awesome!" Belinda confided. "He has always been so helpful to me and always wore the FM transmitter. He encouraged me to come to office hours if I didn't understand something."

"Wow, I feel better. I was afraid that he wouldn't know what an FM system was or why I needed it!" said Stacy.

"Stacy, remember, you are not the first student with a hearing loss who has gone to State,

and you won't be the last either," Belinda said. "Introduce yourself to Dr. B. tomorrow during his office hours and review your accommodations. Professors expect you to do this. Take every advantage that you can. Dr. B. is very accommodating and wants all of his students to do well. Even though he has received notification of your disability and appropriate accommodations, take time to explain how hearing loss affects you and how you learn. Unfortunately, some professors aren't as experienced in accommodating students with hearing loss. Don't assume it's because they don't want to be bothered. Approach them positively and assume it's because of a lack of experience. Most people respond best when approached positively."

"Are there some professors who don't want to be bothered making accommodations?" asked Stacy.

"Yes, I'd being lying if I said there weren't," admitted Belinda. "Thankfully, they are few and far between."

"Have you ever had a teacher who failed to provide you with accommodations?" asked Stacy. "If so, what did you do?"

"Well, a teaching assistant who ran my section of a biology lab would inconsistently use the FM system and often spoke with his back to me. At first, I tried to approach the situation positively. I mentioned to him that I really needed for him to use the FM system during every lab session and to make sure that I saw his face when he spoke. He said he'd try harder. Well, nothing changed."

"What did you do?" asked Stacy.

"Well, I didn't want to be confrontational. I documented the day that I met with him and wrote down exactly what I said. I went to Dr. Holloway to ask for advice. I told her what I did. She said I did the right thing, but I told her that nothing had changed. She suggested that I write a letter to her explaining the problem, with copies to the T.A., the T.A.'s supervisor, my academic advisor, and the Americans with Disabilities compliance officer," explained Belinda. "Needless to say, the T.A. complied with my requests and later apologized. He said that he didn't realize how my hearing loss affects my ability to learn."

"Wow," said Stacy.

"Stacy, most problems are solved without having to file a formal complaint. Most of the time, it is just a case of misunderstanding," said Belinda. "However, State University does have a well-publicized grievance procedure."

"Well, I really appreciate you spending time talking with me, Belinda," thanked Stacy. "I don't feel so alone."

"Hey, any time. Let's plan on getting together once a month. I'm also one of Dr. Brooster's tutors for his section of Biology 101," said Belinda.

"Awesome!" said Stacy. "I'm going to Dr. Brooster's office hours in the morning to introduce myself and talk about my disability and accommodations."

"That's the spirit!" said Belinda.

"One check or two?" asked the waitress.

"Just one. I'll get it," Belinda offered. "You can pay for lunch next time."

"Thanks, Belinda!" Stacy smiled.

"Are you walking back to campus?" asked Belinda.

"Yes," answered Stacy.

"I'll walk with you," Belinda offered.

"Great!" Stacy said as they left the restaurant.

Well, Stacy made a friend and now had a mentor who understood the struggles she faced better than any disability specialist, audiologist, or speech-language pathologist could. Belinda was able to change Stacy's approach to receiving accommodations from being passive to proactive. Stacy realized that federal law mandated her right for accommodations in the classroom and that most of her professors would be more than happy to help her. Stacy also realized that even though noncompliant professors were few and far between, State University had a clearly defined grievance procedure to ensure her rights for accommodations. Sometimes, the advice from audiologists and rehabilitation specialists are not as effective as personal experience relayed through peer mentoring. Belinda will be of great help to Stacy in acclimating to the collegiate life. Just as accommodations for students with disabilities go beyond the confines of the classroom, so do factors relating to enhancing Stacy's quality of life at State University.

AUDITORY REHABILITATION FOR MIDDLE-AGED ADULTS WITH HEARING IMPAIRMENT

Adults who were born with normal hearing may acquire hearing loss during the most productive years of their lives. Hearing loss may develop insidiously or may present suddenly. Both types of hearing losses present with activity limitations, participation restrictions, and reductions in HRQoL, which have been defined in this and other chapters. Before discussing auditory rehabilitation, we will discuss a few issues with both types of hearing losses, insidious and sudden.

Hearing Loss That Develops Gradually

Hearing loss that develops slowly over time may take the young to middle-aged adult by surprise. The person may find that he or she says "huh" or "what" more often or has to turn the television up louder to hear it. Family and friends may complain that the person no longer seems to be listening. When confronted, the person is often in denial because hearing loss is associated with old age, and wearing a hearing aid is stigmatizing. Young to middle-aged adults learn to live with and compensate for hearing losses much to the frustration of their significant others. In fact, it has been found that most people cope with their hearing losses for 10 years or longer before seeking help while the degree of impairment progresses from moderate to severe (Davis, Smith, Ferguson, Stephens & Gianopoulos, 2007; Donahue, Dubno, & Beck, 2009). Some of the other reasons for not getting help may be lack of access to hearing healthcare and affordable hearing aids (Donahue et al., 2009).

Davis, Stephens, Rayment, & Thomas (1992) believed that younger adults with hearing loss who may get help early on may be able to avoid greater disability; social isolation; depression, anxiety, and loneliness; lessened self-efficacy and mastery; and stress in relationships (Andersson & Green, 1995; Bess, Lichtenstein, Logan, Burger, & Nelson, 1989; Campbell, Crews, Moriarty, Zack, & Blackman, 1999; Keller, Morton, Thomas, & Potter, 1999; Kramer, Kapetyn, Kuik, & Deeg, 2002; National Council on the Aging, 1999; Uhlmann, Larson, Rees, Koepsell, & Duckert, 1989; Weinstein & Ventry, 1982). The adult with untreated sensorineural hearing loss may at first experience frustration and impatience followed by anger and pity from family, friends, and coworkers (Andersson & Green, 1995; Bess et al., 1989; Campbell et al., 1999; Keller et al., 1999; Kramer et al., 2002; National Council on the Aging, 1999; Uhlmann et al., 1989; Weinstein & Ventry, 1982).

Sudden Sensorineural Hearing Loss

Sometimes, adults may experience a sudden sensorineural loss of hearing that may occur over a few days or all at once, and 90% of the time it occurs only in one ear (National Institute on Deafness and other Communication Disorders [NIDCD], 2003). The incidence of sudden sensorineural hearing loss is between 5 to 30 cases per 100,000 annually (Nosrati-Zarenoe, Hansson, & Hultcrantz, 2010; Wu, Lin, & Chao, 2006). A variety of conditions may cause sudden sensorineural hearing losses, including infections (e.g., mumps), vascular condition (e.g., atherosclerosis), Meniere's disease, and other miscellaneous causes (Schreiber, Agrup, Haskard, & Luxon, 2010). The average age of patients experiencing sudden sensorineural hearing loss is 50 to 60 years with no specific gender preference (Schreiber et al., 2010). In addition, these patients experience tinnitus and may feel dizzy. It is advised that these patients see a doctor as soon as possible for a complete medical and audiologic evaluation (NIDCD, 2003). In some cases, medical treatment in the form of steroidal therapy can help restore hearing, although some patients recover spontaneously within a few days. If patients do not get better in about two weeks, the damage is probably permanent. Unfortunately, some patients recover only some of their hearing and others' losses get worse. Audiologists play an important role in monitoring and rehabilitating the hearing losses of these patients.

ROLE OF VOCATIONAL REHABILITATION

As covered earlier in this chapter, vocational rehabilitation (VR) is designed to assist people with illnesses or injuries in securing and maintaining suitable employment. VR is funded by the federal government and is provided through state programs, Indian tribes, workers' compensation programs, or private insurance (Trychin & Eckhardt, 2004). Each of these programs has its own subtle nuances, but must comply with applicable federal and state laws. For example, the Alabama Department of Rehabilitative Services has a Vocational Rehabilitation Services unit that has a goal of providing eligible individuals with disabilities opportunities to improve their chances for employment. VR provides educational services; vocational assessment, evaluation, and counseling; job training; assistive technology; orientation and mobility training; and job placement (Alabama Department of Rehabilitative Services [ADRS], 2007). For adults who are deaf and hard of hearing, professionals who are trained in communication, technological, and cultural issues provide the following services (ADRS):

- Vocational counseling and guidance
- Vocational evaluation to determine skills, abilities, and potential to work
- Vocational training
- Purchase of hearing aids and other appropriate communications devices
- Interpreter services for the purpose of obtaining and maintaining employment
- Job placement assistance
- Rehabilitation technology services

Information about clients is kept strictly confidential and is released only to rehabilitation professionals and service providers that are part of an individual's program or of the assessment process to evaluate progress toward goals.

In order to become eligible for VR services, the individual must have a mental or physical disability that keeps him or her from getting and/or keeping a job or requires assistance to secure or maintain a job; or be a recipient of Supplemental Security Income (SSI) or a beneficiary of Social Security Disability Insurance (SSDI) payments and desires to become employed. A rehabilitation counselor is often assigned to an individual's case and must determine within 60 days of application if the person is eligible unless an extension is agreed upon. Trychin and Eckhardt (2004) reported the results of an audit of closed VR cases found that most of the patients who were deaf and hard of hearing had an average age of 45 years compared to other clients whose average age was 30 years and most already had jobs that they needed assistance in keeping. They found that the average cost of providing VR services involved the expenses for the hearing evaluation and hearing aid(s) and involved two visits plus a follow-up appointment.

The role of the rehabilitation counselor is to provide information, resources, counseling and guidance, and possibilities related to the individual's strengths, resources, priorities, concerns, and abilities to assist in preparing for and securing employment. Successful outcomes depend on a close collaboration between the VR counselor and the individual in the development of an individualized plan for employment (IPE) and the attainment of vocational goals. For example, it is up to the individual with a disability to keep scheduled appointments, stay in touch with the VR counselor, and expend sufficient effort toward attaining positive outcomes.

The VR counselor uses existing information about the individual's disability and arranges for further evaluation for eligibility assessment to determine qualification for program eligibility criteria (Trychin & Eckhardt, 2004). If eligible, a Vocational Needs Assessment determines the goals, nature, and scope of the rehabilitation services to be in the IPE. Audiologists can play a key role in providing critical information—not only the results of the hearing evaluation (e.g., type, degree, and configuration of hearing loss), but the vocational impact of the hearing loss including specific on-the-job communication needs listed in Figure 11.4 (Trychin & Eckhardt).

Most of the information is obtained through both observation and interviewing the individual or patient. Audiologists can obtain information about voice quality, auditory and

Communication Requirements
• What type of communication is required of the person on the job on a daily basis?
• Is the person occasionally required to attend meetings or conferences in which important information is presented?
• Does the type of work that the person does require communication while on the telephone or during other activities such as driving or working outside?

Visual Communication
• How skilled and how comfortable is the person with speechreading?
• Does the environment in which the person works facilitate or hinder speechreading?
• Does the person have to communicate while performing other activities, making it difficult to see the speaker?
• Does the person believe that he or she may benefit from speechreading lessons?

Voice Quality
• Is the voice quality of the candidate an issue?
• Does the person appropriately regulate the volume of his or her own speech?
• Is the person's speech clear and easy to understand?

Balance and Vertigo
• Does the patient have balance problems or vertigo?
• If so, is the person's mobility affected?
• Does the job require standing or otherwise maintaining balance?
• Does the job require being in high places or working in the dark or other possibly dangerous locations?

Auditory/Cognitive Processing
• Does the person respond appropriately when asked opened-ended questions?
• Does the person have a (central) auditory processing disorder?

Hearing Technology Maintenance and Usage
• Does the person already own hearing aids? If so, does she know how to:
  ○ Change the batteries?
  ○ Keep the hearing aid clean?
  ○ Use the "T" coil or program controls?
  ○ Manipulate the hearing aid?
• Does the person know how to use, maintain, and troubleshoot HAT?

Independence
• Did the person bring someone else to the appointment?
• If so, was the person dependent on her significant other for answering questions?

Social Interaction
• Does the person interact appropriately with coworkers?

figure *11.4*

Vocational impact of the hearing loss including specific on-the-job communication needs.

Source: Based on *Vocational Rehabilitation and Workers with Hearing Loss,* by S. Trychin and J. Eckhardt, 2004, retrieved from http://www.audiologyonline.com/articles/article_detail.asp?article_id=727.

cognitive processing, independence, and social interaction. For example, the audiologist can assess patients' speech and voice quality during the interview, carefully monitoring its intelligibility, quality, and loudness. At this point, speech-language pathologists may need to provide a diagnostic evaluation to assess patients' strengths and limitations. The patient's job may require communication with coworkers and clients necessitating speech-language therapy or augmentative communication device. In addition, audiologists may use the intake interview to detect the presence of any auditory or cognitive processing difficulties. For example, can the patient not understand audible speech or respond appropriately to open-ended questions? If so, the patient may have difficulty on a job requiring communication in noisy environments. Moreover, patients suspected of having a hearing loss may actually have normal hearing sensitivity, but have a (central) auditory processing disorder. Similarly, audiologists should note if the patient is dependent on a friend or family member to participate in the interview. If so, similar support may be needed on the job. Audiologists can also get a sense of the appropriateness of the patient's social actions during the intake interview. For example, does the patient appropriately respond to questions and keep up with the topic of conversation? If not, the IPE plan may include audiologic rehabilitation for communication tips and strategies.

Information on communication requirements, visual communication, balance and vertigo, and hearing aid technology and its maintenance is obtained through an interview with the patient. The audiologist should ask the patient about the type of on-the-job communication requirements. For example, is the patient required to participate in meetings or conferences in which important information is presented? Is the patient required to communicate on the telephone or when performing various activities in an environment that reduces the visibility or audibility of speech? Some patients may have difficulty understanding what is being said during meetings in noisy rooms, precluding the ability to take minutes for their supervisor. Office assistants who are deaf and hard of hearing may not quite understand enough of what is being said on the telephone in order to write down accurate messages. Similarly, taxi drivers may not understand the desired destination of passengers in a noisy cab. Audiologists' interviews should obtain enough specific information that clearly portrays the on-the-job communication demands of the patient that may indicate the need for accommodations to achieve occupational success.

Audiologists should also ask how dependent, skilled, and comfortable the patient is with **speechreading** or the use of all information available (e.g., lipreading, auditory message, body language, the context, and so on) to understand what is being said. Audiologists may recommend speechreading training for some patients. With only 30% to 40% of the phonemes of the English language being identifiable through vision alone, speechreading may be critical for understanding speech for someone with significant hearing loss. Audiologists should ask these patients when their last comprehensive eye exam was, because poor visual acuity or other ocular problems may adversely affect communication ability. Similarly, the patient should ask if there are any instances at work that make it difficult to speechread, such as excessive glare in a conference room that may be eliminated by closing draperies. The patient may need some coaching in self-advocacy to express communication needs to coworkers, such as letting colleagues know that it is very important to be able to see their faces in order to understand what is being said.

Regarding hearing aid technology and maintenance, it is important to determine if the patient is able to change the batteries, care for, and perform basic hearing instrument troubleshooting. Similarly, it is important to know if the patient knows how to use the telecoil appropriately or different programs on the hearing aids in specific listening situations. Similar questions should be asked of patients who use HAT. Hearing aids and HAT are of no value unless patients understand their use and maintenance. In summary, the purpose of the interview is to provide sufficient information to the VR counselor for the Vocational Needs Assessment in the formulation of the IPE. Let's look in on Mark Ledbetter, a person who is going to need VR services.

Casebook Reflection

Mark Ledbetter: Successful Businessman With a Progressive Sensorineural Hearing Loss

Mark Ledbetter is a 45-year-old executive with a large real estate corporation. He was Executive of the Year three years in a row. He thrived in the business world and was respected by his colleagues. He loved the fast-paced competition, frequently worked 50- to 70-hour weeks, and was constantly on his cell phone, even as he traveled from one appointment to the next. Yet he always found time in his busy schedule to train for competing in triathlons. He took pride in his appearance and his ability to interact with clients, instilling the confidence to close big deals. A few years ago, Mark noticed a change in his ability to understand what was being said to him. He knew that hearing loss ran in his family; his father and grandfather wore hearing aids. Mark's physician referred him to Dr. Goodman for a complete audiologic evaluation. Mark adjusted to the news of his moderate sensorineural hearing loss well and was pleased that he could use completely-in-the-canal (CICs) hearing aids instead of the behind-the-ear (BTE) hearing aid his father wore.

In the last few months, Mark was having extreme difficulty understanding much of anything. He thought that his hearing aids were not functioning properly. Mark struggled at work and started to avoid meetings and directed all calls to his secretary. Mark finally went to see his audiologist, Dr. Goodman.

"Mr. Ledbetter, how nice to see you," said Silvia Delgado. "How are you doing?"

Mark couldn't understand what she was saying, but smiled and nodded as he signed in.

"I don't think my hearing aids are working properly. Can Dr. Goodman check them out and get them repaired?" said Mark, taking his hearing aids out.

"Hi, Mark, come with me to the consult room" said Dr. Goodman. "We haven't seen you for quite some time. What seems to be the trouble?"

Mark couldn't understand much of what Dr. Goodman was saying, but he followed her to the consult room and said, "I think there is something wrong with my hearing aids."

Dr. Goodman took his hearing aids and said that she'd be right back. An electroacoustic analysis revealed that the hearing aids were functioning according to manufacturer's specifications. On her way back to the consultation room, Dr. Goodman looked at Mark's chart and discovered that his last audiologic evaluation was over three years ago!

"Mark, here are your hearing aids," said Dr. Goodman waiting for him to put them in his ears. "And they are functioning properly."

"What?" asked Mark struggling to understand what she said.

"Your hearing aids are OK," said Dr. Goodman in a louder, more deliberate voice. "I noticed that your last audiologic evaluation was over three years ago. I had a cancellation this afternoon. Can you stay an extra hour or so for an audiologic evaluation?"

"Sure," Mark said. "My hearing is not the problem, it is those hearing aids!"

The results of the audiologic evaluation confirmed Dr. Goodman's suspicions of a shift in Mark's hearing from a moderate to a severe sensorineural hearing loss, bilaterally. She suspected that Mark was in denial of the difficulties he was having.

"Mark, I'm afraid that I have some difficult news," Dr. Goodman cautioned. "There has been a significant shift in your hearing sensitivity to the severe range in both ears."

Dr. Goodman could tell that Mark was in shock. "Mark, who is your personal physician?"

"Dr. Patel," Mark said.

"May I call him and explain the situation to get a referral to an **otologist** as soon as possible? An otologist is a physician who specializes in disorders of the ear and hearing."

"Sure," Mark said.

Dr. Goodman quickly called Dr. Patel for a referral to Dr. Rodriguez, an otologist. Dr. Goodman prepared a report for Mark to take to his appointment the next morning. Dr. Rodriguez could find no medical cause for the change in hearing sensitivity and suspected that it was due to hereditary factors.

Dr. Rodriguez referred Mark back to Dr. Goodman for a hearing aid evaluation. Dr. Goodman suspected that Mark's change in hearing sensitivity would have some impact on his job performance and that information for contacting vocational rehabilitation services would be helpful.

Audiologists, like Dr. Goodman, should refer patients to seek vocational rehabilitation services, particularly when their hearing and/or balance problem may affect their ability to seek or maintain employment, as in Mark's case. Audiologists can counsel patients to seek VR services. It may be difficult to convince patients that they are entitled to VR services, because many may believe it is a form of welfare. Although patients do not have to be destitute to receive these services, financial need may be a consideration for some programs. Audiologists may assist patients in preparing for their first appointment by writing a letter detailing how hearing loss affects their employability, securing their last's year's Internal Revenue Service report, and a household report showing expected income and expenditures.

Patients should be counseled that VR counselors may not know much about the needs of clients who are deaf and hard of hearing. Patients must be prepared to explain their disability and its impact on their employability using specific examples. Patients such as Mark may not be able to articulate their needs because of reluctance to get help. Audiologists may need to convince some patients to apply for needed VR services. Let's see how Dr. Goodman counsels Mark on seeking VR services. Audiologists' reports for Vocational Needs Assessment must explain the problem in sufficient detail because most VR counselors may not know the full impact of hearing loss on patients' ability to secure and maintain a job (Trychin & Eckhardt, 2004).

Casebook Reflection

Mark's Follow-up Visit With Dr. Goodman

Dr. Goodman greeted Mark and they went back to her office to talk. She had HAT for him to use during the consultation.

"Well, Mark, it seems that your hearing has shifted into the severe range and will probably not return to the way it was. Did Dr. Rodriguez explain that to you?" asked Dr. Goodman.

"Yes, he did. Is there any possibility that my hearing could get worse?" asked Mark.

"Well, it is difficult to say, but let's concentrate on what we can do now to improve your audibility. You're going to need new hearing aids and CICs are no longer an option," said Dr. Goodman. "I suggest a new style of hearing aid."

"Will I have to wear those behind-the-ear hearing aids?" asked Mark.

"Yes, I think so," advised Dr. Goodman, noting a concerned look on Mark's face. "However, the first thing I'd like to talk with you about is applying for vocational rehabilitation—VR—services. VR is a federal program that assists people with disabilities to seek or maintain employment."

"Is this some sort of public assistance program? I am more than capable of affording any services, hearing aids, and whatever else I may need," Mark stated.

"No, VR services are for everyone and you don't need to be in severe financial need to receive resources," explained Dr. Goodman. "VR services will assist you in getting new hearing aids, HAT, and any other accommodations you may need on the job."

"I don't want to make a big deal out of my hearing loss at work," explained Mark. "I'm one of the leading performers at my firm, and others may perceive my additional hearing loss as a weakness. Before now, no one even knew that I wore hearing aids except for a few close friends."

"Mark, I understand how you feel, but the situation will be far worse if you can't communicate," explained Dr. Goodman.

Mark knew she was right and that he had been avoiding certain responsibilities at work and asked, "What do I need to do?"

"Call this number and request an appointment with a VR counselor. On the basis of this appointment, he or she will decide to pursue an eligibility assessment. The VR counselor may use existing information—for example, your recent audiologic evaluation—or obtain new information to determine eligibility. Additional evaluations may be needed, and I would be happy to continue as your audiologist. My goal now is to help you best prepare for this meeting and then if you qualify for eligibility, carefully describe your communications needs and accommodations."

"How do I best prepare for this appointment?" Mark asked.

"First, make sure that you bring your last year's IRS tax return and a household budget against your income," Dr. Goodman said. "Also, explain in a letter all of the communication situations you're having difficulties with at work, including both visual and auditory communication."

"What do you mean by 'visual communication'?" asked Mark.

"How much difficulty do you have in seeing people's faces when they speak?" asked Dr. Goodman, "You know, for reading lips. . . ."

"Well, it depends," Mark said. "It is very difficult to see people's faces during meetings in the conference room. Usually, a partner is doing a PowerPoint presentation and the lights are dimmed. Also, on very sunny days, I can't see people's faces well who sit with their backs to the window. Too much glare."

"Excellent, this is *exactly* what the VR counselor will need to know," Dr. Goodman said. "In fact, what I would like you to do is use this sheet I've prepared for you to write down typical activities of your job and then the communication problems you're having. Be specific! For example, don't just say, 'Can't understand what people are saying,' but 'I can't understand what people are saying because there is too much background noise.' Take this information sheet with you to your meeting with your VR counselor because it will help you to clearly articulate your problems . . . Also, save it, because it will help in my report to your VR counselor."

"Dr. Goodman," Mark said. "Are these difficulties I encounter just in the office, or could they be difficulties I encounter when traveling for business?"

"Excellent question," Dr. Goodman commented. "Include anything that's job-related. For example, if you have difficulty on your cell phone for business calls, then by all means, write that down. Do you have any other questions?"

"No," Mark answered.

"Fine," said Dr. Goodman. "I'll see you after you've been to your VR counselor. Please use the HAT for as long as you need."

"Thanks!" Mark said.

Mark wasn't too excited about seeking VR services. However, he knew that he needed additional help. His meeting with his VR counselor went well, and she accepted the results from his most recent audiologic evaluation and the medical consultation from Dr. Rodriguez. Mark's VR counselor requested that Dr. Goodman provide a detailed report for his Vocational Needs Assessment.

Hearing loss is just one of several impairments involved in rehabilitative audiology. Another area requiring rehabilitation is tinnitus.

TINNITUS REHABILITATION

Have you ever had ringing in your ears? Maybe you have experienced it every once in a while or after listening to loud music? Ringing in the ears is called *tinnitus*, and it has been defined as the cortical perception of sound in the absence of an actual auditory stimulus (Hazell & Jastreboff, 1990). Another medical definition of **tinnitus** is the perception of sound in one or both ears or in the head when no external sound is present (American Tinnitus Association [ATA], 2009). Some who have tinnitus describe it as "ringing in the ears," although some report hissing, roaring, whistling, chirping, or clicking (ATA). However, experts in the study of tinnitus are in disagreement when trying to establish a single definition of tinnitus.

The American Tinnitus Association (2009) estimates that over 50 million Americans experience tinnitus and that 12 million of those individuals experience it to a degree requiring medical intervention, and 2 million of those experience severe debilitating tinnitus. **Hyperacusis**, a hypersensitivity to the loudness of sounds, can co-occur with tinnitus.

There are several suspected causes of tinnitus including, but not limited to, the following (ATA, 2009):

- Noise-induced hearing loss
- Cerumen, or earwax, buildup in the ear canal
- Certain medications
- Ear or sinus infections
- Jaw misalignment
- Cardiovascular disease
- Tumors
- Head and neck trauma

Children and adults can both experience tinnitus. However, children are less likely to report their experiences because in many cases, children are born with auditory disorders and may have always had a sensation of tinnitus (ATA, 2009). Due to the many causes of this symptom, a multidisciplinary team approach for assessment and management of tinnitus has been advocated (Sandridge et al., 2010). Audiologists are involved in the management of tinnitus and hyperacusis.

Although a variety of treatments of tinnitus have been suggested, no specific treatment is recommended. Frequently, patients with sensorineural hearing loss find relief when they use hearing aids that amplify sounds, which mask their sensation of tinnitus. Some patients with normal hearing are fitted with tinnitus maskers that look like in-the-ear hearing aids and present noise into the ear that masks the tinnitus. Still other patients find relief from a fan or radio noise on their nightstand while sleeping. Other more controversial treatments include drug therapy, biofeedback, and acupuncture. Little evidence has been found that demonstrates the effectiveness of any drug therapies for tinnitus (Patterson & Ballough, 2006), including ginkgo biloba (Hilton & Stuart, 2004). However, a recent randomized controlled clinical trial conducted by Neri et al., (2009) found that melatonin and Sulodexide together were more effective in improving the tinnitus of patients than either melatonin or no treatment at all. Some studies have suggested some psychological benefit of biofeedback in treating patients' reactions to tinnitus (Landis & Landis, 1992; Podashin, Ben-David, Frandis, Gerstel, & Felner, 1991), but these studies have a high risk of bias. For example, neither investigators nor participants were blinded as to the treatments in many of the experiments in this area.

One particularly promising treatment is **tinnitus retraining therapy** (TRT), an approach developed by Pawel Jastreboff and his colleagues that involves educational counseling

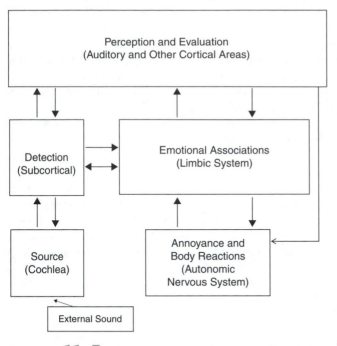

figure 11.5

The neurophysiological model of tinnitus.

Source: Based on "A Neurophysiological Approach to Tinnitus: Clinical Implications," by P. J. Jastreboff and J. W. Hazell, 1993, *British Journal of Audiology, 27,* pp. 7–17.

and sound therapy. The therapy is based on the **neurophysiological model of tinnitus** (Henry, Trune, Robb, & Jastreboff, 2007a; 2007b; Jastreboff & Hazell, 1993) that is shown in Figure 11.5.

According to this model, patients actually perceive and evaluate tinnitus in the auditory and other areas of the cortex. Patients' annoyance with the tinnitus may be due to the dominance of the **limbic** (emotional) and **autonomic nervous** (bodily reactions) **systems**' reaction to the sensation, with the auditory system playing a secondary role (Jastreboff, 2000). The limbic and the autonomic systems provide emotional and physiological responses to sound, respectively. For example, we may be annoyed or even have a "fight or flight" response (i.e., autonomic nervous system) to a loud sound (e.g., siren) that may induce a feeling of fear (i.e., limbic system). These reactions are conditioned reflexes in which an association has been made between a siren and an approaching emergency vehicle racing to an unpleasant event (e.g., fire or crime scene). It may even be after us for exceeding the speed limit! Similarly, many patients have negative conditioned responses to their tinnitus. TRT is based on the premise that the brain has a high degree of plasticity so that sound therapy establishes a positive reaction to a neutral stimulus that retrains these conditioned reflex arcs of the autonomic nervous and limbic systems and, in some cases, secondarily accomplishes **habituation** to the tinnitus (Jastreboff, 2000). Habituation is the reduction of a response to a stimulus after repeated exposure. The end result is that patients are still aware of their tinnitus, but are less bothered by it.

Hazell (2007) suggested that the following TRT exercises could be helpful for patients with tinnitus:

- Read about and be able to explain the neurophysiological model of tinnitus
- Receive counseling to demystify tinnitus
- Experience sound enrichment by the use of pleasant sounds (e.g., fan, sound from an open window)
- Avoid silence
- Conduct self-examination of personal reactions to tinnitus
- Use relaxation techniques when listening to one's own tinnitus

Initially, patients should have a complete audiologic evaluation and an examination by an oto-laryngologist or otologist to determine if there is a medically treatable cause of their tinnitus. The audiologist needs to take a copious case history in order to describe the nature, severity, and precipitating conditions of the tinnitus. One of the first objectives is for the patient to understand and be able to explain the rationale behind Jastreboff's neurophysiological model of tinnitus prior to starting exercises. Patients are more likely to adhere to therapists' recommendations if they understand the scientific reasoning behind the treatment. Educational counseling is aimed at demystifying tinnitus by replacing patients' negative thoughts based on conjecture with positive ones that are based on facts. After all, tinnitus may be a constant reminder to the patient of the possibility of an active disease process, increasing stress level and fear. Assurance that tinnitus is a manageable yet natural phenomenon can empower and change patients' reactions to tinnitus, facilitating the therapeutic process (Hazell, 2007).

Another important component of TRT is sound enrichment that encourages patients to avoid silence by introducing stimuli that are not irritating into their environment (e.g., sound from an open window, the humming of a fan) and do not completely mask the tinnitus. The idea is that the patient should still be able to detect the tinnitus for habituation to occur (Hazell, 2007). Patients with hyperacusis are highly discouraged from wearing earplugs because it increases the sensitivity of the central auditory system to sounds, which is counterproductive to TRT (Hazell, 2007). Other retraining tactics include self-examination of personal reactions to either tinnitus or other unpleasant sounds for very brief periods of time (e.g., 10 seconds). During these brief experiences with their tinnitus, patients practice relaxation techniques designed to reduce both negative feelings and bodily reactions with the assistance of sound enrichment, if necessary (Hazell, 2007). Patients are reminded to have patience because retraining of conditioned reflexes does not happen overnight.

TRT has been shown to be more effective than other types of tinnitus therapy. For example, Henry et al. (2006) investigated the effect of TRT versus tinnitus masking (TM) of patients with clinically significant tinnitus. Investigators alternately assigned participants to treatment groups to avoid selection bias. It was found that patients with more severe tinnitus achieved quicker and more dramatic results with TRT than TM, with similar but less dramatic results obtained for those with moderate tinnitus. Moreover, Davis, Paki, and Hanley (2007) found quick and dramatic reductions in the severity of tinnitus and improvements in quality of life regardless of variations in TRT procedures. In addition, use of only parts of TRT can have benefits for patients. For example, in the following year, Henry, Loovis, et al. (2007) conducted a randomized clinical trial comparing the reduction of symptoms for tinnitus patients who received either TRT–structured counseling, traditional support, or no treatment. Patients who received TRT–structured counseling received greater reduction of symptoms than those who received traditional support or no treatment at all. Hérraiz, Hernandez, Toledano, and Aparicio (2007) conducted a nonrandomized clinical trial to identify factors that may limit the effectiveness of TRT in some patients. The most negative prognostic factor is reticence to use recommended technologies, such as a broadband noise generator. Clearly, evidence supports the use of TRT for improving the quality of life of tinnitus patients. Readers should consult Henry et al. (2007) for more information on TRT.

ADULTS WITH DUAL SENSORY IMPAIRMENT

Dual sensory impairment refers to a patient having both hearing and vision loss. Only about 45,000 people in the United States are **deaf-blind**, or have little or no functional hearing or vision. They have either grown up in the Deaf community using ASL or have acquired deaf-blindness through Usher's syndrome (Spiers & Hammett, 1995). **Usher's syndrome** is a recessive genetic disorder that results in congenital sensorineural hearing loss and progressive visual impairment. Similarly, about 26,000 people in the United States are **deaf and visually impaired**, have little or no functional hearing, but low vision that may be deteriorating due to Usher's syndrome (Spiers & Hammett, 1995). In addition, approximately 366,000 people in the United States are **hard of hearing and blind**, having some hearing impairment but no functional vision (Spiers & Hammett, 1995). They may have gone to schools for the blind or may have been mainstreamed into regular schools and have used their sense of hearing for communication. Last, 312,000 people in the United States are **hard of hearing and visually impaired**, have limited hearing and vision, and may be part of hearing or Deaf communities (Spiers & Hammett, 1995). As can be predicted, adults with dual sensory impairment may receive a wide variety of accommodations based on the status of their disabilities and personal experiences.

Young adults who have dual sensory impairment must transition to the world of work and/or postsecondary educational institutions. They, too, often receive assistance from the Division of Vocational Rehabilitation and programs for students with disabilities at postsecondary educational institutions. Audiologists and speech-language pathologists are part of a team of professionals who may assist these young adults to transition into the world of work and the community. Therefore, it is helpful to know possible referral sources for employment, postsecondary educational, housing, independent living, and legal/advocacy/medical services. Figure 11.6 presents referral sources for young adults with dual sensory impairment in these areas.

Employment Services
Purpose: To assist in finding employment with appropriate accommodations
Examples: Easter Seals, Goodwill Industries, Helen Keller National Center, Lighthouses for the Blind, etc.

Postsecondary Educational Services
Purpose: To provide knowledge and skills to enter the workforce or garner admission to four-year colleges and universities
Examples: Adult education programs, community colleges. correspondence schools, vocational/technical schools, etc.

Housing Services
Purpose: To find safe and affordable places to live
Examples: Centers for independent living, Deaf service centers, private agencies and organizations. state and local housing authorities, etc.

Independent Living Services
Purpose: To provide independent living skills training, counseling, and support
Examples: Assistive technology projects, centers for independent living, departments of social services, etc.

Legal/Advocacy/Medical Services
Purpose: To assist with legal matters, accommodations, and healthcare
Examples: Centers for independent living, community medical referral systems, community mental health services, Deaf service centers, protection and advocacy agencies

figure *11.6*

Referral sources for students with dual sensory impairment.

Audiologists and speech-language pathologists should be aware of the types of accommodations used by students with disabilities such as effective HAT, interpreters, note-takers, tutors, and readers. Students with dual sensory impairment will use HAT similarly to their peers who are deaf and hard of hearing. However, some students who use ASL may require interpreters to sign in a manner that best accommodates their degree of visual impairment. For example, students with low vision may require that the interpreter be very close or use a restricted signing space. Students who are deaf-blind may need to put their hands on those of the interpreter to understand the message through touch (Jordan, 2001b). Other personnel such as note-takers, tutors, and/or readers may be needed for these students to gain access to class notes, textbooks, and other course materials. In addition, programs with students with disabilities should critically evaluate the physical classroom accommodations when scheduling these students (Jordan, 2001b):

- Does the classroom have adequate lighting?
- Are there extensive sources of glare (e.g., fluorescent lights, lots of windows, white walls, or table tops)?
- Is there enough space in the classroom for a guide dog and/or interpreter?
- Are night classes accessible to students with limited night vision who use public transportation?

Some students with dual sensory impairment may require the use of alternate forms of media. It is critical for students' success to meet as early as possible with the instructor regarding receipt of information at the same time as other students (Jordan, 2001b, Senge & Dote-Kwan, 1998). Alternate forms of media include use of large print, Braille, or audiotape (Jordan, 2001b). Other suggestions for accommodations, presented in Figure 11.7, involve audiovisual materials, small-group discussions/activities, oral presentations, examinations, field visits/labs, and teaching style.

VR counselors play an important role in advocating for appropriate on-the-job accommodations for adults who have dual sensory impairment. Moreover, these patients, employers, and healthcare and social services professionals need to be cognizant of the progressive nature of some sensory impairment and the impact on job performance. For example, patients with Usher's syndrome need to be monitored for and counseled about the degenerative nature of the disease and its impact on quality of life (Fishman, Bozbeyoglu, Massof, & Kimberling, 2007). However, the impact of deaf-blindness on job performance may not be quantified accurately with commonly used outcome measures. Möller (2003) assessed the adequacy of the International Classification of Functioning, Disability, and Health (ICF) in describing the on-the-job activity limitations and participation restrictions of adults with deaf-blindness and found that the tool failed to account for all job-related difficulties. The ICF is helpful in describing health impairments in terms of activity and participation.

Dual sensory impairment negatively impacts HRQoL. For example, people with dual sensory impairment who are white or who self-reported to be of an "other" (e.g., not African American) race had an increased risk of mortality compared with their peers with a single or without sensory deficits (Lam, Lee, Gómez-Marin, Zheng, & Caban, 2006). Moreover, women with moderate-to-severe dual sensory impairments were even at greater risk of mortality than those with milder degrees of

Use of Audiovisual Materials
- Use of an interpreter
- Large print or Braille copies of the material
- Use of color overlays to improve contrast vision
- Use of regular lighting
- Verbal description of visual information

Small-Group Discussions/Activities
- Use of an interpreter or HAT
- Communication ground rules (e.g., only one person speaks at a time)
- Conversion of material into alternate form
- Direction of student to alternate meeting place

Oral Presentations by Student
- Use of interpreter to voice what student signs
- Use of oral interpreter if student's speech is unintelligible
- Use of an interpreter to relay information from the class back to the student

Examinations
- Alternate forms of assessment:
  - Oral
  - Interpretation of material into ASL (visually or tactually)
  - Audiotape
  - Extended test-taking time
  - Alternate location with better lighting or with special equipment
- Alternate forms of recording responses:
  - Use of a note-taker
  - Proctor
  - Computer-assisted answers
  - Braille-typed answers
  - Use of writing guides and templates

Field Visits/Labs
- Discussion of location of activity to ensure full participation
- Use of a guide
- Provision for guide dog

Teaching Style
- Stationary lecture style
- Refraining from speaking when writing on the blackboard
- Transfer of class materials into alternate forms (e.g., Braille)
- Lecture speed convenient for interpreter
- Use of communication rules mentioned earlier
- Inclusion of student in classroom activities
- Ensure conversion of materials into alternate forms for class

figure *11.7* ———————————————————————

Accommodations for students with dual sensory impairment.

Source: Based on *Considerations When Teaching Students Who Are Deaf-Blind*, by B. Jordan, 2001, retrieved from http://projects.pepnet.org/downloads/TPSHT_Deaf_Blind.pdf.

impairments (Lee, Gómez-Marin, et al., 2007). The number of employed adults with dual sensory impairment will increase as the population ages, increasing the risk of on-the-job injuries and the need for accommodations (Zwerling, Whitten, Davis, & Sprince, 1998).

Do:
- Speak directly to the person
- Introduce yourself
- Orient to others present and their location
- Include the person in the conversation
- Cue for the appropriate places for conversational turns
- Encourage the person to express himself or herself
- Let the person grab your arm when walking together

Don't:
- Start talking without identifying yourself
- Abandon the person in unfamiliar surroundings
- Ignore the person
- Get frustrated with miscommunications
- Speak for the person
- Push the person to walk ahead of you when walking

figure *11.8*

Do's and don'ts for meeting a person with visual impairments.

Source: Based on "What Do You Do When You Meet a Deaf Blind Person?", 2010, *A to Z Deafblindness*, retrieved from http://www.deafblind.com/whatdbp.html.

Important tips for meeting with persons who are deaf-blind are presented in Figure 11.8. For example, communication partners should speak directly and introduce themselves to the person who is deaf-blind. Whenever needed, it is appropriate to orient the person to others in the communication interaction and indicate their approximate location. Always try to include this person in the conversation and assist in cueing for appropriate places to enter the conversation. Always encourage the person who is deaf-blind to communicate for him- or herself. When walking with these people, partners should allow them to grab their arm and walk side-by-side. Things to avoid are the speaker not identifying him- or herself, and speaking for or ignoring the person in conversations with others. It is also impolite for communication partners to push the person so that he or she walking in front. The most important thing is for people not to get frustrated if misunderstandings occur with people who are deaf-blind.

VESTIBULAR REHABILITATION

It is easy to take our sense of balance for granted. However, if one is unfortunate enough to be one of the 40% of adults who experience balance problems at one time or another, the balance system is something to marvel at and appreciate. The balance system involves several peripheral and central mechanisms. For example, the inner ear has matched pairs of sensory organs for balance located in the **ampulla** of each of the semicircular canals (i.e., **cristaampullaris**), as well as the **otoliths** (i.e., **macula**) in the utricle and the saccule. The utricle is sensitive to horizontal movement; the saccule senses vertical movement. Each of the semicircular canals occupies a separate anatomical plane and is at right angles to the others: (1) superior canal (i.e., coronal plane), (2) posterior canal (i.e., sagittal plane), and (3) horizontal canal (i.e., transverse plane). Alternatively, the utricle and saccule sense gravity and linear acceleration via the macula, which consists of **otoconia**, or calcium carbonate granules located on top of a gelatinous matrix embedded with stereocilia of sensory hair cells. These small granules add mass and increase inertia of the matrix when moving in response to acceleration, bending the stereocilia, indirectly exciting the sensory end organs, for example. With each of the head movements, the inner ear fluid, or endolymph, flows toward or away from the sensory organ and, if the response is the same in the canals in both sides of the head, balance is maintained (Desmond, 2001). These sensory organs send information from the peripheral system to the parts of the nervous system that control eye movement and muscles that maintain our posture. Our visual system has a very important reflex called the **vestibular-ocular reflex**, which is responsible for maintaining a centralized visual image on the retina during head movement. When our head moves in one direction, our eyes move in the opposite direction.

Desmond (2001) stated that the primary function of our balance system is to permit us to interact and maintain contact with our surroundings in a safe and efficient manner. Our sense of balance requires gathering information from the visual, somatosensory, and vestibular senses for integration in the brainstem and for processing in the cortex (Desmond, 2001). Equilibrium is possible if information coming from these sources is predictable and nonconflicting, enabling us to move about the environment with an automatic maintenance of balance (Desmond, 2001). However, when information is in conflict, the brainstem must reflexively adjust, and a sense of imbalance may occur with accompanying vertigo (sensation of spinning) and nausea (Desmond, 2001).

There are many different causes of balance disorders, which many can be classified as peripheral or central. Some causes include (Bauer & Girardi, 2004):

- Benign paroxysmal positional vertigo (BBPV)
- Cerebellar degeneration
- Chemical and pharmacological vestibular toxins
- Head trauma
- Labyrinthitis
- Meniere's disease
- Strokes and vascular problems
- Vestibular neuritis

The prevalence of balance disorders increases with age. For example, an epidemiological study surveying elderly people found that the prevalence of balance disorders was 36% for women and 29% for men at 70 years of age, increasing to 45–50% for those around 90 years of age (Jönsson, Sixt, Landahl, & Rosenhall, 2004). Dizziness in the primary care setting can result from a wide variety of causes in the elderly population (Sloane et al., 1994). We discuss three different balance disorders common in middle-aged adults: benign paroxysmal positional vertigo, vestibular neuritis, and labyrinthitis.

Benign paroxysmal positional vertigo (BPPV) is the most common form of vertigo and results from an asymmetrical fluid movement due to a conflicting response to head movement in one of the semicircular canals. The conflicting response is usually caused from one of the otoconia from the otoliths finding its way to a semicircular canal (most often the posterior), with head movements causing the granule to stimulate the end organs. One treatment for BPPV is **canalith repositioning procedures**, noninvasive, sudden positioning techniques that move the granules back to where they belong. Two successful procedures are the **Epley** and the **Semont** procedures.

The Epley procedure is the most popular in the United States, and its sequence is shown in Figure 11.9 A–E. The patient starts by sitting upright (A). The patient rapidly reclines (while being supported) past the horizontal position toward the side of the head with the problem (e.g., right) at a 45-degree angle, for 30 seconds (B). The patient's head is then turned toward the opposite side (left) and held for 30 seconds (C). Subsequently, the patient is then rolled further in same direction (left), but with his or her chin tilted downward at a 45-degree angle for 30 seconds (D). Finally, the patient sits up (E). A systematic review comparing the efficacy of the Epley maneuver to other treatments or no treatment at all found that it is a safe and effective treatment for posterior canal BPPV, but there was little evidence definitively displaying its superiority over other treatments (Hilton & Pinder, 2004).

The Semont procedure involves a patient rapidly lying on one side, then sitting up, and then rapidly lying on the other. A randomized prospective clinical trial compared

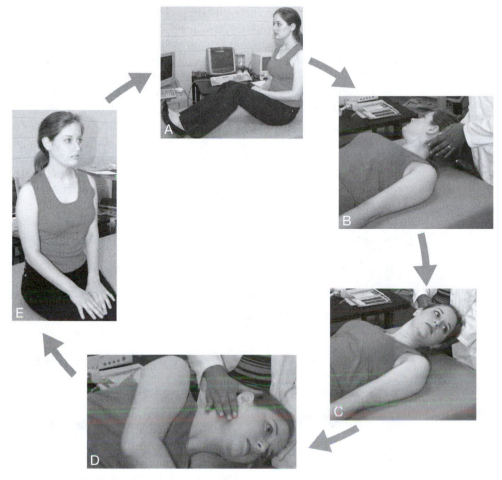

figure *11.9*

The Epley procedure.

the effectiveness of the Semont maneuver, a drug (i.e., flunarizine), and no treatment at all for posterior canal BPPV. The study found that the Semont procedure was the most efficacious and improved patients' quality of life (Salvinelli et al., 2004).

Hearing healthcare professionals who perform canalith repositioning procedures advise patients to wait 10 minutes before leaving the office, to sleep with their head at a 45 degree angle, and to avoid any symptom-provoking head positions (Li & Epley, 2010). Although the vast majority of cases are treated successfully with the preceding procedures, surgeries to cut the ampullary nerve or plug the posterior semicircular canal may be needed to provide relief to some patients (Leveque, Labrousse, Seidermann, & Chays, 2007).

Although some sources say that these two peripheral disorders are the same, vestibular neuronitis and labyrinthitis are different and are the next most two prevalent causes of vertigo. **Vestibular neuritis** is an inflammation of part of the vestibular section of cranial nerve VIII, causing an acute episode of nausea, vomiting, and vertigo (Marill, 2009). **Labyrinthitis** is an inflammatory disorder of the inner ear, or **labyrinth**, a twisting and turning series of osseous spaces set deep within the temporal bone. Co-occurring is a corresponding membranous system that contains the delicate end organs for hearing and balance. Moreover, labyrinthitis presents with a unilateral hearing and loss of vestibular function (Boston, Strasnick, & Steinberg, 2010). The symptoms of both of these peripheral disorders usually subside in a few days to a few weeks. Initial stabilization can be accomplished through bed rest and use of vestibular-depressant medications (e.g., Antivert) (Swartz & Longwell, 2005). Some patients, however, have lingering vertigo, particularly with certain head movements. For many of these patients, **vestibular rehabilitation therapy** (VRT) may be beneficial, which is treatment designed to meet the unique needs of patients with vertigo, dizziness, and/or sense of imbalance. Assessment and treatment of vestibular and balance disorders frequently involve a team of healthcare professionals that may include primary care physicians, otologists, physical therapists, audiologists, and so on. There are many different types of VRT exercises, and they are prescribed based on balance assessments and patients' description of symptoms. Table 11.2 shows some examples for vestibular-ocular reflex stimulation, ocular motor, and gait exercises.

table *11.2*   Examples of Vestibular Rehabilitation Exercises

Exercise	Goal	Description
Vestibulo-ocular Reflex Stimulation (VOR)	Increase the gain of the VOR	• Patient holds a card with printed letters at an arm's length and at a zero-degree azimuth. • Patient fixates eyes on card and then turns his or her head to the right. • Patient turns his or her head back to midline, while still fixated on the card. • Patient repeats the sequence, but turns his or her head to the left. • Patient repeats 20 to 30 times.
Ocular-Motor Exercises	Increase gaze pursuit	• Patient holds a card with printed letters at an arm's length and at a zero-degree azimuth. • Patient fixates eyes on card and moves the card to the right and then back to midline. • Patient repeats the sequence, but the card is moved to the right. • Patient repeats 20 to 30 times.
Gait Exercises	Improve steadiness in walking	• Patient walks beside a wall with hand touching for support, but working toward increasing the number of steps without support with the width of gait reducing until walking heel-to-toe. • Patient walks with the head in motion from left to right, then up and down, but working toward increasing the pace of walk, turning in large circles, turning to the left, then to the right, and then in smaller circles.

Source: Information from *Vestibular Rehabilitation,* by C. A. Bauer and M. Girardi, 2004, retrieved from http://www.fallpreventionclinics.com/docs/Vestibular%20Rehabilitation-Bauer-Girardi.pdf.

The exercises progress from easy to difficult. For example, the gait exercises first begin with walking beside a wall with support, then no support. Later exercises involve walking and moving the head from side to side and then up and down, and so on. The patients who benefit most from VRT are those with stable vestibular symptoms that have not been completely ameliorated through **central compensation**, a reorganization of the processing of information via brain plasticity. Those patients with unstable lesions such as progressively demyelinating diseases or migraine headaches are not good candidates for VRT (Bauer & Girardi, 2004). Migraine headaches, common in young to middle-aged women, can also cause episodic vertigo and represents a new area of investigation (Eggars, 2007). In the next chapter, the vestibular dysfunction and balance disorders in older adults are mentioned in addition to reducing falls risk.

Casebook Reflection

Veterans With Traumatic Brain Injury: A Silent Epidemic

Thus far, we have discussed auditory rehabilitation of young to middle-aged adults including information on managing tinnitus, dual sensory impairment, and vestibular and balance disorders. A "silent epidemic" of veterans with traumatic brain injury are returning from war with profound health issues, many of which include speech, language, and hearing disorders. For some, the struggle is to survive life-threatening injuries. Alternatively, many veterans come home undiagnosed, yet are experiencing unexplained symptoms. Nearly 20% of veterans of Operation Iraqi Freedom and Operation Enduring Freedom have **traumatic brain injury** (TBI), many resulting from blast injuries. TBI has been defined as a physiological disruption of brain functioning resulting from some type of event (Youse, Le, Cannizzaro, & Coelho, 2002). TBI may be classified as **open-** or **closed-head injuries**. Open-head injuries result in penetration of the scalp, skull, and or **meninges** (membranous coverings of the brain) (Youse et al., 2002). Closed-head injuries result from nonpenetrating events resulting from some blow to the head (Youse et al., 2002). A **coup** is the injury resulting directly from a blow; a **contrecoup** is an injury occurring contralaterally to a blow, usually from the brain making impact with the skull. TBI has varying degrees of severity with widespread effects. Mild cases may include a temporary lapse of consciousness or brain dysfunction; severe cases may involve comas and long-term cognitive impairment. Some of the effects of TBI include impairment in the following areas (National Center for Injury Prevention and Control, Centers for Disease Control and Prevention, 2010):

- thinking, including memory and reasoning
- sensation, including taste, touch, smell, hearing, and vision
- language, including receptive and expressive skills
- emotion, causing sadness, depression, or inappropriate action.

In addition, soldiers with TBI have posttraumatic stress syndrome, an anxiety disorder resulting from stressful events of war.

TBI results in hearing loss and tinnitus in a significant proportion of these patients. Moreover, the prevalence of these auditory disorders is greater for those who have TBIs from blast injuries. About 68% of wounded-in-action evacuations are soldiers who are victims of blast injuries (Chandler, 2006). The higher prevalence of blast injuries in these veterans is due to the fact that improvised explosive devices and rocket-propelled grenades are the most common weapons in these wars. Blast injuries can impact the auditory system from the pinna to the auditory cortex, including lacerations to the outer ear, tympanic membrane perforations, ossicular discontinuity, cochlear disturbances, and so on. The types of hearing loss include conductive, sensorineural, and mixed. Interestingly, some evidence suggests that veterans who sustain tympanic membrane perforations are more likely to have concussions and (central) auditory processing difficulties (Lew, Jerger, Guillory, & Henry, 2007). Moreover, these patients frequently have concomitant visual impairments as well as vestibular and balance disorders. These patients have problems that may get worse with age in addition to being at greater risk for dementia.

Many veterans with TBI face a "long road back," requiring an interdisciplinary approach to rehabilitation. Audiologists and speech-language pathologists play key roles on these interdisciplinary teams and provide needed auditory rehabilitation that includes careful collaboration with healthcare professionals in other disciplines. Audiologists conduct the audiologic/vestibular evaluations; select, evaluate, and fit hearing aids and HAT devices; and provide counseling on the care, use, and maintenance of these devices. Patients may attend group hearing aid orientation sessions in addition to individual auditory rehabilitation sessions. Interdisciplinary collaboration may involve working with occupational and physical therapists in facilitating patients' insertion and removal of hearing aids and battery manipulation. Alternatively, speech-language pathologists enhance patients' audiovisual speech recognition abilities and conversational fluency, requiring collaboration with psychiatrists in tailoring sessions conducive to those with anxiety disorders. Indeed, there is a "silent epidemic "of young to middle-aged veterans with TBI and concomitant hearing loss requiring creative and contemporary approaches to auditory rehabilitation for years to come.

HEARING CONSERVATION

Part of auditory rehabilitation of young to middle-aged adults is devoted to the prevention of hearing loss. Exposure to excessive sound levels for extended periods of time can result in **noise-induced hearing loss** (NIHL). The development of NIHL is insidious, in that excessive sound levels have a cumulative effective on the auditory system. Most everyone has experienced tinnitus, a sense of fullness in the ear, and a slight hearing loss after being exposed to excessive sound levels at a concert or visit to a firing range. This phenomenon is known as a **temporary threshold shift** (TTS), or temporary decrease in hearing sensitivity due to exposure to excessive sound levels. Fortunately, TTS is temporary, with hearing threshold levels returning to normal. However, repeated exposures to excessive sound levels lead to **permanent threshold shifts** (PTS), or a nonrecoverable loss of hearing sensitivity. NIHL comes from two sources: occupational and nonoccupational noise exposure. **Occupational noise exposure** is that which occurs in the workplace. The Occupational Safety and Health Administration (OSHA) is a federal agency that was established in 1971 with a mission to prevent work-related injuries, illness, and death (OSHA, 2007). For many years, OSHA has enforced regulations about hearing conservation in the workplace (OSHA, 1983). **Nonoccupational noise exposure** occurs during leisure time and is often sustained while partaking in recreational activities such as listening to music, hunting, and so on.

Occupational Hearing Conservation

Hearing conservation programs are comprehensive efforts aimed at preventing NIHL and frequently involve a team of professionals such as audiologists, data management specialists, engineers (e.g., acoustical, industrial), industrial hygienists, personnel managers, plant managers, physicians (e.g., industrial or otolaryngologists), safety specialists, and supervisors. Audiologists can either direct or provide specific services based on the type of program. Stewart (1994) described three types of hearing conservation programs. An **in-house program** is one in which the entire hearing conservation program is run within a company; this is not too common in the United States. An **out-house program** is one in which the entire hearing conservation program is run by someone external to the company; this, too, is not common in the United States. A **combination program** is run both internally by the company and externally by another party hired to specifically perform some aspect of the program (e.g., audiometric testing). Audiologists' roles in those programs vary in scope and intensity. For example, companies may hire an **industrial audiologist** who specializes in this area of practice to oversee its hearing conservation (e.g., in-house program). Alternatively, an audiologist in private practice may contract to conduct annual audiometric testing of workers for a smaller company (e.g., combination program). Companies in the United States use these types of programs more typically than they use in-house or out-house programs. We will now briefly discuss the major components of a hearing conservation program, including (1) noise monitoring, (2) audiometric testing, (3) hearing protection devices, (4) employee training programs, (5) OSHA accessibility, and (6) recordkeeping.

Noise Monitoring

The purpose of noise monitoring is to determine what workers are at risk for NIHL. Noise monitoring requires the use of instruments called **sound level meters** and/or **noise dosimeters**. Figure 11.10 shows a sound level meter. A sound level meter (SLM) is an instrument that measures sound levels in the environment. It is capable of measuring sound levels via weighting scales (e.g., linear, A, B, C, and so on) that weight different frequency regions based on the sensitivity of human hearing at different intensity levels. Figure 11.11 shows the different weighting scales found on most SLMs. Industrial audiologists measure sound levels on the A-weighting scales, which represent human hearing sensitivity as a function of frequency for moderate intensity levels. Noise dosimeters are special-purpose SLMs that sample the wearer's exposure to sound during a typical work day. SLMs are used in environments that have consistent noise levels. Noise dosimeters monitor noise levels for workers who may be in multiple environments during the workday. Sounds may include those that are **continuous** (i.e., always on), **intermittent** (i.e., on and off), and **impulse** (i.e., short duration and high intensity like a gunshot) and range in levels from 80 to 130 dBA. Specifics on noise measurement are beyond the scope of this textbook; readers are referred to Suter and Berger (2002) for additional information.

Workers who are exposed to 85 dBA for an eight-hour work day should be part of the hearing conservation program. A noise exposure of 85 dBA for an eight-hour work period is called the **action level**, or the threshold for participation in a hearing conservation program. The **permissible exposure level** (PEL) that workers can safely be exposed to is a time-weighted average (TWA) of 90 dBA for an eight-hour period, which is a 100% noise dose or the maximum amount that is considered to be safe for most workers. The PEL depends on the sound level in that there is a **5-dB time-intensity trade-off law**, which states that each time the dB level increases by 5 dB, the permissible duration of exposure decreases by half. Table 11.3 shows the 5-dB time-intensity trade-off rule for various noise levels.

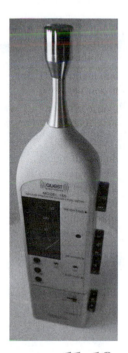

figure *11.10*

A sound level meter.

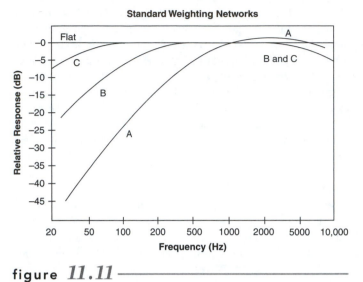

Standard Weighting Networks

figure *11.11*

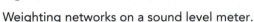

Weighting networks on a sound level meter.

For example, when sound levels increase to 95 dBA, the permissible duration for exposure is four hours. Alternatively, when the level is reduced from 90 dBA to 85 dBA, the allowable duration of exposure doubles from eight to 16 hours. However, sound levels above 115 dBA are not permitted for any duration of time due to the high risk of sustaining NIHL. Noise monitoring is an ongoing process and should be repeated, particularly if a change in sound level is expected from a change in equipment, for example. Workers should be allowed to observe noise monitoring and should be notified if they are at or above the action level.

When workers are found to be exposed to excessive noise levels, there are at least three methods of preventing NIHL. One method is to employ **engineering controls**, which are modifications to equipment or production to reduce noise levels (e.g., replacing a fan belt) to permissible levels. Abating the noise at the source is always the best option. **Administrative controls** are changes in work schedules aimed at reducing workers' exposure to noise. Last, **hearing protection devices** (HPDs) are devices used to attenuate sound at the workers' ear. However, the success of this approach depends on workers' correct and compliant use of HPDs, which are often reported to be uncomfortable.

Audiometric Testing

Audiometric testing should be provided to all workers at or above the action level and should be executed by certified technicians under the supervision of an audiologist, otolaryngologist, or physician and recorded on a standardized audiogram. The Council for Accreditation in Occupational Hearing Conservation (CAOHC), an intersociety council, developed guidelines and standards for occupational hearing conservationists who perform

table *11.3*   5-dB Time-Intensity Trade-off Law for Time-Weighted Averages

Level	Exposure Time Hours
80	32
85	16
90	8
95	4
100	2
105	1

the audiometric testing, among other things (CAOHC, 2007). Each ear should be tested by air conduction at 500, 1000, 2000, 3000, 4000, and 6000 Hz using an audiogram that meets ANSI 33.6-1969 standards in rooms that comply with ambient noise levels for testing.

The audiometer should receive the following calibrations on the following schedule: (1) biological each day, (2) electroacoustic each year, and (3) exhaustive every two years. **Calibration** is the process by which instruments are evaluated for functioning and adjusted to meet manufacturer's specifications. Each worker should have a baseline audiogram within six months of initial employment. Those workers exceeding six months of employment without a baseline audiogram should wear hearing protection. Moreover, workers should have at least 14 hours without workplace noise and are advised to avoid any high sound levels prior to testing establishing the baseline audiogram without a TTS overlay.

After establishment of a baseline audiogram, workers should receive annual audiometric testing. The baseline audiogram is the one against which all others will be compared in assessing existence of a **standard threshold shift** (STS). An STS is an increase of 10 dB or more, taken as an average of the thresholds at 2000, 3000, and 4000 Hz for either ear after the results have been averaged for worker age. Workers with these results are retested within 30 days and are to receive written notification within 21 days if an STS is confirmed. The STS should be reviewed by an audiologist, otolaryngologist, or other physician to determine need for a medical evaluation. If the STS is related to occupational noise exposure, then workers should be fitted, trained, and required to use HPDs and/or told about the need for referral to other health-care professionals. The audiograms with established STSs become the new baseline.

Hearing Protection Devices

Hearing protection devices (HPDs) should be available to workers who are exposed to noise. However, they should be worn by workers who have (1) a TWA of 85 dBA and exceeded six months of employment without a baseline audiogram, (2) a TWA of 90 dBA, or (3) sustained an STS. The company needs to provide a variety of HPDs for workers to choose from. Figure 11.12 shows three types of HPDs: (1) earmuffs, (2) premolded (connected by a string) and (3) formable.

The different types of HPDs differ in sound level attenuation capability, which is indicated by the **noise reduction rating** (NRR). The NRR is a value that indicates the amount of sound attenuation, provided that HPDs are worn properly. The NRR of HPDs is determined in a standardized way, which is beyond the scope of this textbook. Readers are again referred to Suter and Berger (2002) for further explanation.

Earmuff HPDs are considered permanent and have an adjustable spring band for the securing of circumaural cups around users' ears. The band can be worn over the head, behind the head, or sometimes under

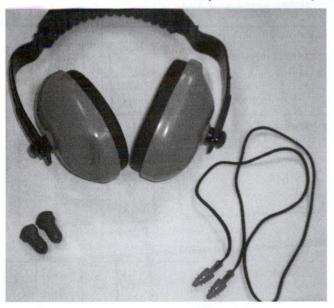

figure *11.12*

Three types of hearing protection devices.

the chin, sometimes resulting in a different NRR for each position. The advantages of these devices are that they are durable, easily verifiable for worker compliance, and somewhat comfortable. Their disadvantages are that they are relatively expensive, hot, and cannot be worn in cramped quarters. Premolded devices are semipermanent flexible HPDs that vary in proportion, consist of a single or triple flange of varying proportions, and must be fitted to workers' ears. The devices for each ear are often adjoined by a string. The advantages of these devices are their low cost and relative durability. Their disadvantages are that they are uncomfortable, and it is difficult to monitor workers' compliance. The formable HPDs are disposable and "one-size-fits-all." Many of these devices are made of foam that is compressed when placed into workers' ear canals and expands to form a sound attenuating seal. The advantages of these devices are their low cost and their relative effectiveness in noise attenuation. Their disadvantages include their discomfort, need for frequent replacements, and difficulty in monitoring for workers' compliance. HPDs can also be custom made, which requires an audiologist to make ear impressions that are sent to a laboratory. The advantages of these devices are their durability, comfort, and noise attenuation abilities. Their greatest disadvantage is their cost.

HPDs must attenuate sound to 90 dBA TWA or 85 dBA for workers who have sustained an STS. The effectiveness of HPDs depends on whether they are worn and, if so, correctly. Therefore, workers must be correctly fit with and trained in the care and use of these devices even though they are often uncomfortable to wear. Workers must understand how noise causes hearing loss and that wearing HPDs is in their best interest. Frequently, management must monitor and enforce their use.

Employee Training Programs, OSHA Accessibility, and Recordkeeping

Employee training should be provided to workers at or above the action level. Training should include instruction on the effects of noise on hearing; purposes, advantages, and disadvantages of various HPDs; and the rationale and procedures for audiometric testing. Regarding OSHA accessibility, all workers should have access to standards, materials for employees, and training materials, upon request. Records for noise exposure should be kept for two years, and those for audiometric testing for three years, with all records transferable to new management. All records should be accessible to OSHA officials and employees.

Efficacy of Hearing Conservation Programs

Despite efforts to develop hearing conservation programs to circumvent NIHL, their effectiveness has been brought into question. Recently, Daniell et al. (2006) assessed the hearing conservation programs at 10 companies in each of 8 industries that have had a high prevalence of workers' compensation cases related to NIHL. They found that hearing conservation programs were incomplete, particularly in maintenance of noise monitoring records, and there was an overreliance on the use of workers' wearing HPDs instead of engineering or administrative controls in the prevention of NIHL. Not only are many companies not following minimal OSHA standards, but some experts believe that those standards are not strict enough. For example, it has been found that changing the 5-dB time-intensity trade-off law to 3-dB (e.g., 100% noise dose = 90 dBA for eight hours, 93 dBA for four hours, and so on) would identify between one-and-a-half to three times as many workers at risk who may avoid NIHL through participation in hearing conservation programs (Daniell et al., 2006).

Nonoccupational Hearing Conservation

From 1970 to 1990, the number of persons 45 to 64 years of age with hearing loss grew 26%; during the same period, hearing loss for persons 18 to 44 years of age grew 19% (Ries, 1994). The prevalence of hearing loss is expected to increase even more due to the numbers of adults at risk for NIHL from nonoccupational noise exposure from listening to music and to the use of firearms (Eisenbeis & Jones, 2007; Morata, 2007). In fact, Shargorodsky, Curhan, Curhan, and Eavey (2010) found that the prevalence of hearing loss in U.S. teenagers is about 20% demonstrating an increase over statistics found in previous studies. Unfortunately, young adults who attend rock concerts producing excessive sound levels report that they are not likely to wear HPDs to circumvent NIHL (Bogoch, House, & Kudla, 2005).

Nonprofessional musicians are also at risk for NIHL. Schmuziger, Patscheke, and Probst (2006) compared audiometric thresholds (e.g., 3000 to 8000 Hz) and existence of other auditory symptoms in nonprofessional musicians who had at least five years of high sound level exposure to their nonmusician peers. The musicians had significantly higher mean high-frequency audiometric thresholds and a greater prevalence of tinnitus and hyperacusis than those in the nonmusician group. However, the musicians who consistently wore HPDs had results similar to the nonmusician group. Therefore, HPDs can be used to protect listeners from excessive sound levels experienced by musicians. The challenge, though, is to convince musicians to wear HPDs that will protect them against NIHL *in the long run.*

Risks of NIHL from loud music to either musicians in a band or to audiences at rock concerts are easily quantifiable. However, potential risks of NIHL from listening to personal listening devices (PLDs) (e.g., Walkmans, iPods, MP3 players, computers with headphones) are difficult to quantify due to individual differences in listening behaviors. In the 1990s, concerns were raised about the risks of NIHL posed by Walkmans. Although nearly four-fifths of young adults listened to them, the listening levels did not seem to pose a risk for NIHL (Wong, Van Hasselt, Tang, & Yiu, 1990). These results were confirmed by Turunen-Rise, Flottorp, and Tvete (1991), who measured the output of personal cassette players and assessed the resulting TTSs in young adults. They concluded that if their sample of young adults was representative of their peer group, most young adults were not at risk for NIHL from normal use of Walkmans.

Increased concern about risks of NIHL from PLDs has resurfaced with the popularity of the iPod, which has become ubiquitous in today's culture. iPods have extended memory capabilities, enabling storage of thousands of songs on a single device. iPod users can simply dictate their play lists for uninterrupted periods of listening, possibly increasing the risks for NIHL. In addition, Fligor and Cox (2004) raised concerns about the output levels of some of the stereo earphones used with some of today's most popular PLDs. They recommended that compact disc users not listen at more than 60% of full volume for any more than 60 minutes per day. They called this the "60-60 rule." In particular, the stock earphones (earbuds) that are provided by Apple with all iPods do not attenuate ambient noise levels, possibly causing users to increase the volume for adequate listening. Fligor and Ives (2006) found that users' preferred listening levels were higher (89 dBA) when listening through the stock earphones in a background of 80 dBA airplane noise than through Etymotic Research ER-6i earphones (78 dBA) that were better able to blockout background noise. However, no significant differences were found when listening in quiet. Portnuff and Fligor (2006) estimated that iPod users could listen through the stock earphones at 70% of full volume for 4.6 hours per day without damaging their hearing.

It is difficult to know exactly how many iPod users are at risk for NIHL. Danhauer et al. (2009) found that approximately two-thirds of university students own iPods. A recent survey completed by Zogby International (2005) found that most adults were not concerned about or aware of possible risks of NIHL from popular electronics. Other dangers include "iPod oblivion" in which users become unaware of their surroundings when listening to these devices (Kuntzman, 2007). iPod oblivion has been blamed on causing several deaths and disabilities. Clearly, public outreach campaigns must be developed about the possible risks of iPod use at high-volume levels. More recently, Portnuff (2010) recommended an "80–90 rule," such that PLDs should not be listened to for more than 90 minutes per day when set at 80% of full volume.

Of all sources of nonoccupational noise exposure, target shooting and hunting pose the greatest risk for NIHL (Clark, 1991). For example, older adults who self-reported using firearms for target shooting and hunting were more likely to have a significantly greater high-frequency sensorineural hearing loss than peers who did not participate in these activities. In addition, the risk for hearing loss increased by 7% for every five years of hunting experience (Nondahl, Cruickshanks, Wiley, Klein, Klein, & Tweed, 2000). The amount of NIHL resulting from use of firearms can compound the damage from occupational noise exposures (Pekkarinen, Iki, Starck, & Pyykkö, 1993; Prosser, Tartari, & Arslan, 1988). Users of firearms for recreational purposes not only sustain NIHL, but experience participation restriction as measured by the *Hearing Handicap Inventory for Adults* (HHIA) (Newman, Weinstein, Jacobson, & Hug, 1990; Stewart, Pankiw, Lehman, & Simpson, 2002). Fortunately, NIHL from use of firearms is 100% preventable through the use of HPDs, if people can be convinced of the benefits of their use (Peck, 2001; Rabinowitz, 2000).

Prevention of Noise-Induced Hearing Loss

Hearing conservation is definitely within the scope of practice of audiologists (ASHA, 2004b). Audiologists' task is to convince various stakeholders that hearing conservation efforts today can circumvent future NIHL. In industry, management must be convinced to abate noise at its sources through engineering and administrative controls so that workers will not be exposed to excessive sound levels. If noise cannot be abated to acceptable levels, then workers must be instructed on the importance of correct usage of HPDs. Management can monitor workers' compliance for wearing HPDs *on the job*, but what they and other adults do to circumvent NIHL in their leisure-time activities is a matter of personal responsibility.

How do audiologists and other medical professionals convince young adults that activities they enjoy can pose a risk of *future* NIHL? It is difficult for young people in their 20s to visualize what life may be like for them at 40, 50, or 60 years of age. Encouraging these individuals to change behaviors in the present to prevent something that may not even happen in the future is difficult. Workers involved in hearing conservation programs frequently receive instruction on the effects of noise on hearing and the importance of wearing HPDs. Educational programs tailored to meet workers' needs have been shown to be effective in increasing workers' compliance (Kerr, Savik, Monsen, & Lusk, 2007; Lusk et al., 2003). Moreover, recently the ASHA, AAA, and other professional organizations have developed public outreach campaigns aimed at promoting the prevention of NIHL from nonoccupational noise exposure.

SUMMARY

In this chapter, we discussed auditory (re)habilitation issues relating to young and middle-aged adults who are deaf and hard of hearing. In particular, the effects of hearing impairment on health-related quality of life (HRQoL) were reviewed. Employment trends of this population were reviewed to highlight the need for transition counseling and VR. Federal legislation mandates that transition programs be in place for high school students with disabilities by the time they reach their 16th birthday or earlier. Two Casebook Reflections illustrated a student in a school-to-work program and a college-bound freshman who were either deaf or hard of hearing. Federal legislation mandating transition programs for this population were reviewed in addition to the role of VR and programs for students with disabilities at colleges and universities. Similarly, VR for middle-aged adults was highlighted in another Casebook Reflection. Dual sensory impairments were defined and issues related to adults were profiled. The chapter also discussed tinnitus rehabilitation, vestibular rehabilitation, and ended with coverage on occupational and nonoccupational hearing conservation.

LEARNING ACTIVITIES

- Visit and interview the director of the program for students with disabilities in your college or university regarding services and accommodations for students who are deaf and hard of hearing. Ask about information for accommodations for students who are deaf and hard of hearing.
- Shadow a VR counselor who works with adults who are deaf and hard of hearing.
- Interview a college student with a hearing loss and ask about the day-to-day challenges both inside and outside the classroom.
- Visit the Internet sites on deaf-blindness to learn more about the obstacles faced by this population.
- Contact an audiologist to observe assessment and remediation of vestibular dysfunction and balance disorders.

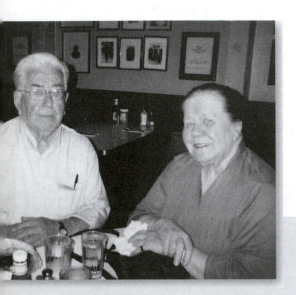

CHAPTER *twelve*

Auditory Rehabilitation for Elderly Adults

LEARNING *objectives*

After reading this chapter, you should be able to:

1. Explain the transdisciplinary and holistic model of auditory rehabilitation for elderly adults.

2. Discuss the characteristics of the elderly population in several domains (communication, physical, sociological, and psychological) and how they may impact auditory rehabilitation.

3. Describe how older adults may enter and progress through the hearing healthcare continuum.

4. Provide and explain the components of a hearing support program in a long-term residential care facility.

5. List and provide details of some home-based auditory training programs.

6. Discuss the efficacy and explain the role of audiologist in fall prevention programs.
7. Recognize the signs of elder abuse.
8. Discuss the impact of dual sensory impairment on the diagnosis and management of older adults.

Improvements in healthcare, nutrition, education, and standards of living have resulted in an increasing proportion of elderly persons living longer. From 1990 to 1997, the number of persons 65 years of age and older increased more than 11 times to 34.1 million with only a threefold increase for the rest of the population (Population Resource Center, 2006).

Approximately 77 million babies were born in the United States during the baby boom experienced from 1946 to 1963 (*Reinventing Aging,* 2005). Persons born during this time period are known as "baby boomers." This segment of the population is expected to increase by 80% to 69 million from 2010 to 2030 when the baby boomer generation retires and accounts for one-fifth of the U.S. population (Population Resource Center, 2006). Most boomers can expect to live to age 83, and many will live into their 90s (*Reinventing Aging,* 2005). According to the National Institutes of Deafness and other Communication Disorders of the National Institutes of Health, hearing loss is now present in approximately 314 of every 1,000 people over 65 years of age, and in about 40–50% of those age 75 and older. Therefore, the number of senior citizens requiring hearing healthcare is expected to dramatically increase.

The baby boomers are expected to challenge the notion of aging in the United States. Our healthcare system has changed from a perspective of living longer to include living well. In the previous chapter, we discussed the impact of sensorineural hearing loss on the health-related quality of life (HRQoL) of young to middle-aged adults. However, the effects on HRQoL of adults over 65 years of age are just as profound with untreated sensorineural hearing loss being associated with isolation, depression, anxiety, and loneliness; lessened self-efficacy and mastery; and stress in relationships when family and friends experience frustration, impatience, anger, pity, and/or guilt toward the older adult with untreated hearing impairment (Campbell, Crews, Moriarty, Zack, & Blackman, 1999; Chisolm et al., 2007; Keller, Martin, Thomas, & Potter, 1999; Kramer, Kapetyn, Kuik, & Deeg, 2002). The purpose of this chapter is to provide readers with the necessary background to provide comprehensive and relevant auditory rehabilitation to older adults.

A TRANSDISCIPLINARY AND HOLISTIC MODEL OF AUDITORY REHABILITATION FOR THE ELDERLY

Several models of auditory rehabilitation have been envisioned for elderly patients. However, meeting the needs of this population with hearing loss in today's complex world requires a holistic approach (Lesner & Kricos, 1995) that is integrated within a transdisciplinary model of hearing healthcare, which breaks down barriers between and among healthcare professionals.

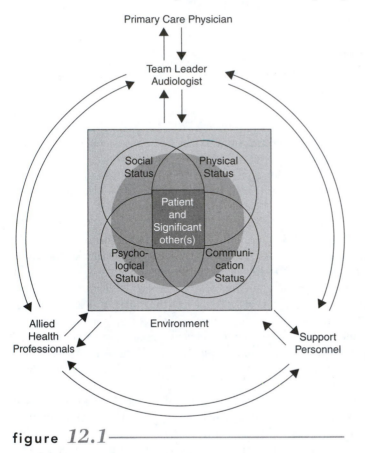

Figure 12.1 shows a holistic and transdisciplinary model of hearing healthcare (Johnson & Danhauer, 2002b).

By integrating a holistic approach (Lesner & Kricos, 1995) within a transdisciplinary framework, the unique characteristics of each patient are taken into consideration for case management in situations requiring complex solutions. At the center of the model are the patients and their significant others. Others in the model include the audiologist (the team leader), the primary care physician, other allied health professionals, and support personnel whose level of participation depends on the individual needs of each patient.

Assessment and treatment of hearing impairment requires consideration of patients' status in multiple domains of functioning (i.e., communication status, physical status, psychological status, and social status) for a holistic approach to auditory rehabilitation (Lesner & Kricos, 1995). The holistic component of the transdisciplinary model of hearing healthcare is reflexive in that strengths and weaknesses in all four areas determine both communication needs and solutions. First, we will discuss common characteristics of the elderly population in each area and then explain important implications for assessment and management of hearing loss.

figure *12.1*

A holistic and transdisciplinary model of hearing healthcare.

Source: Based on "A Transdisciplinary Holistic Approach to Hearing Health Care," by C. E. Johnson and J. L. Danhauer, 2002, *Geriatric Times*, *3*(5), pp. 10–11.

Communication Status

This domain includes considering the types, degrees, and configurations of hearing loss and their effects on activity limitation (i.e., disability) and participation restriction (i.e., handicap); speechreading; audiovisual speech reception, and conversational fluency.

Hearing Loss

Older adults may sustain sensorineural hearing loss due to many etiologies. They may have had a congenital hearing loss or worked in an industry with significant noise exposure, or they may have presbycusis, or hearing loss due to aging. Schuknecht (1964) originally came up with the following four classifications of presbycusis based on the anatomical sites of degeneration, audiometric configurations, and the results of other evaluative tests (Roland, Kutz, & Marcincuk, 2010):

- **Sensory presbycusis** involves loss of sensory and supportive cells at the basal end of the cochlea that progresses toward the apical end and is first manifested by a precipitous high-frequency sensorineural hearing loss usually starting during middle age.

- **Neural presbycusis** results from an atrophy of cochlear neurons throughout the cochlea (basal end more affected than apical) and central auditory pathways with unexpectedly poor speech recognition performance when compared with the patient's pure-tone audiogram.
- **Metabolic presbycusis** results from a degeneration of the stria vascularis (which maintains chemical and bioelectric and metabolic health of the cochlea) that occurs from base to apex in the cochlea, manifesting itself as a relatively flat audiometric configuration.
- **Mechanical presbycusis,** also known as a *cochlear conductive hearing loss*, results from a stiffening of the basilar membrane and a gradually sloping high-frequency hearing loss.

Later, Schuknecht and Gacek (1993) mentioned two additional types of presbycusis: (1) mixed presbycusis and (2) intermediate presbycusis. **Mixed presbycusis** is a combination of two or more different types mentioned previously. **Intermediate presbycusis** is a structural change in the auditory system not significant enough to qualify as any of the other specific types of presbycusis. Figures 12.2 through 12.5 show types of audiometric configurations associated with the four primary classifications of presbycusis.

Some older adults have significantly poorer speech recognition abilities than would be predicted from inspecting their audiograms; these difficulties accelerate with age (Divenyi,

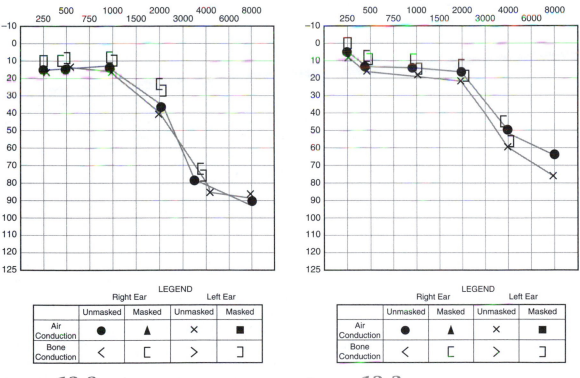

LEGEND

	Right Ear		Left Ear	
	Unmasked	Masked	Unmasked	Masked
Air Conduction	●	▲	×	■
Bone Conduction	<	[	>	]

LEGEND

	Right Ear		Left Ear	
	Unmasked	Masked	Unmasked	Masked
Air Conduction	●	▲	×	■
Bone Conduction	<	[	>	]

figure *12.2*

An audiogram showing sensory presbycusis.

figure *12.3*

An audiogram showing neural presbycusis.

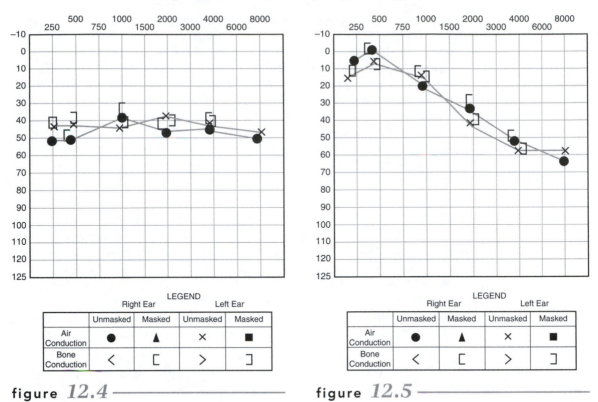

figure *12.4*

An audiogram showing metabolic presbycusis.

figure *12.5*

An audiogram showing mechanical presbycusis.

Stark, & Haupt, 2005). Moreover, evidence suggests the presence of (central) auditory processing dysfunction in the elderly (e.g., Golding, Taylor, Cupples, & Mitchell, 2006). Nabelek and Nabelek (1985) classified elderly adults as "special listeners" who have decreased speech recognition performance in reverberation and noise when compared with younger adults. Recall that *reverberation* is the continuation of acoustic energy due to the reflections of that energy off the room's surfaces although the source of that energy has been terminated. The index of severity for this phenomenon is reverberation time, or the time that it takes for a sound to significantly decay after its termination. Rooms with greater reverberation have longer reverberation times; they tend to be larger in volume and have hard, reflective surfaces. Reverberation tends to prolong vowels such that their energy covers over, or "smears," the energy of the softer consonants that follow. Similarly, noise is any unwanted sound and covers over important cues for speech recognition. Nabelek and Nabelek hypothesized that reverberation and noise reduce the amount of acoustic redundancy necessary for adequate speech recognition in older adults.

Loss of hearing sensitivity and a gradual deterioration of speech recognition abilities may result in activity limitations. For example, older adults may have difficulty understanding their dinner companions in a noisy restaurant or the caller at a bingo game. In addition, they may feel that their hearing loss limits social participation and interaction with their friends and family. As discussed later in this chapter, hearing impairment affects older adults' executing tasks of daily living and restricts their participation with significant others.

Many older adults with hearing loss use other sensory modalities and develop compensatory strategies to assist in understanding in communication situations. Speechreading and audiovisual speech perception are ways in which vision separately and in combination with the auditory system can overcome some of the communication barriers resulting from hearing loss. When most people hear the word *speechreading*, they think of lipreading. However, speechreading is when people use *all* available clues to understand what a person is saying including gestures/body language, facial expressions, situational cues, linguistic cues, and even what is received through the auditory sense (Kaplan, 1996; Lee, 1997).

Audiovisual speech reception occurs when both the auditory and visual senses are used in understanding what is being said, which is affected by age. Cienkowski and Carney (2002) compared the ability of integrating visual and auditory cues in place of articulation and voicing information in three groups of listeners: (1) young adults with normal hearing and vision, (2) older adults with near-normal to normal hearing and vision, and (3) young adults whose hearing was masked by noise to approximate the hearing levels of the older adults. Each of the participants in the study completed a lipreading test and an audiovisual speech reception task using nonsense syllables with conflicting auditory and visual cues (e.g., the visual representation of a syllabic token is /ba/, but is presented auditorily as /da/). They found that although the older adults were as good as the younger adults in integrating auditory and visual information in syllabic identification, they did poorer in lipreading-only conditions (i.e., visual signal only). However, there were qualitative differences in the response choices selected by the various groups, indicating that participants selected the least ambiguous modality. For example, the young adults with normal hearing favored the auditory signal, whereas the older adults and young adults with similarly masked hearing threshold levels frequently used the visual information in selecting responses. The results of this study were consistent with those of Sommers, Tye-Murray, and Spehar (2005), who found that older adults' poorer performance in audiovisual speech reception was due to their reduced speechreading abilities rather than impaired integration abilities.

Conversational fluency is the ability to participate in a discussion with one or more individuals with a minimum of requests for clarification, with an easy conveying of ideas, and with conversational turn-taking resulting in a sharing of speaking time (Erber, 2002). For example, conversations that have many requests for clarification are the result of numerous communication breakdowns. There is an inverse relationship between the number of communication breakdowns and the degree of conversational fluency. Alternatively, an easy exchange of ideas during an interaction means that communication is fluid and the amount of talk-time is shared. The appropriateness of conversational behavior is context-specific and reflects the relationship between the communicative partners. Elderly patients may have difficulty with conversational fluency, especially when they have a hearing loss and must communicate at increased speaker-to-listener distances. For example, Erber, Holland, and Osborn (1998) found that elderly people with hearing loss were rated higher on conversational fluency when wearing amplification and at shorter speaker-to-listener distances than when in unaided conditions at increased speaker-to-listener distances.

Physical Status

The physical status of adults includes general health, visual status, manual dexterity, and fine-motor skills. Readers may be wondering, how can an older person's general health affect auditory rehabilitation? Getting treatment for hearing impairment may not be the top priority for someone who has other chronic health conditions. In addition, patients' visual status may interfere with their ability to speechread; their manual dexterity and fine-motor skills may impact their ability to use hearing aids. The physical status of older adults is discussed in terms of its potential impact on auditory rehabilitation.

General Health

Just because someone is over 65 years of age does not mean that the person has health problems. However, a recent cross-sectional analysis of a national random sample of 1,217,103 Medicare fee-for-service beneficiaries enrolled in either Medicare Part A or Part B found that 82% had one or more chronic health conditions and 65% had multiple afflictions (Wolff, Starfield, & Anderson, 2002). The leading chronic health conditions of this population are arthritis, hypertension, hearing impairment, heart disease, cataracts, deformity/orthopedic impairments, chronic sinusitis, and diabetes (Wolff et al., 2002). During the past two decades, chronic diseases were the leading causes of death for persons 65 years and older with the rank order of prevalence varying among age-race-sex groups. For example, Table 12.1 shows the leading causes of death for persons 65 years of age and older having different ethnic backgrounds. Note that although the leading causes of death are essentially the same across ethnic groups, their prevalence within each group varies. For example, diabetes is not one of the leading causes of death in whites, but ranks third for American Indians. Chronic health conditions can affect elderly persons' HRQoL and auditory rehabilitation.

Arthritis is inflammation of a joint accompanied by symptoms of pain, swelling, and stiffness that can be caused by infection, trauma, degenerative changes, metabolic disturbances, and so on (Arthritis Foundation, 2010). There are more than 100 types of arthritis, but osteoarthritis is the most common type in the United States. It most commonly affects people over 45 years of age and is manifested by joint soreness after overuse or inactivity, stiffness after periods of rest, morning stiffness, or as pain caused by weakening of the muscles surrounding the joint, and joint pain (Arthritis Foundation, 2010). Possible treatments include medications (e.g., analgesics, nonsteroidal anti-inflammatory drugs [NSAIDs], COX-2 inhibitors, and injectable glucocorticoids), physical and occupational therapy, and surgery aimed at controlling pain and other symptoms, improving ability to function in daily activities, and slowing the disease process (Arthritis Foundation, 2010).

table *12.1*   Leading Causes of Death for Persons 65 Years of Age and Older for Different Ethnic Groups

White	Black	American Indian	Asian or Pacific Islander	Hispanic
1. Heart Disease	1. Heart Disease	1. Heart Disease	1. Heart Disease	1. Heart Disease
2. Cancer	2. Cancer	2. Cancer	2. Cancer	2. Cancer
3. Stroke	3. Stroke	3. Diabetes	3. Stroke	3. Stroke
4. COPD*	4. Diabetes	4. Stroke	4. Pneumonia/Flu	4. COPD
5. Flu/Pneumonia	5. Flu/Pneumonia	5. COPD	5. COPD	5. Pneumonia/Flu

*COPD = Chronic Obstructive Pulmonary Disease

Source: Information from *Trends in Aging and Health: Trends in Cause of Death Among the Elderly*, by N. R. Sahyoun, H. Lentzer, D. Hoyert, and K. N. Robinson, 2001, Atlanta, GA: Centers for Disease Control and Prevention: National Center for Health Statistics.

Arthritis can affect patients' **manual dexterity**, which is the skill or ease in using the hands and the arms (Kumar, Hickey, & Shaw, 2000). There are two types of manual dexterity: proximal and distal manual dexterity. **Proximal manual dexterity** involves the ability to raise and lower the arms; **distal manual dexterity** involves use of the hands (Lesner & Kricos, 1995). Arthritis can affect auditory rehabilitation, precluding elderly persons' independence in lifting their arms to ear level for insertion/removal of hearing aids and changing of its batteries (Erber, 2003a). Moreover, a direct and possible correlation between manual dexterity and successful hearing instrument use was found in elderly hearing aid users (Kumar et al., 2000). Parving and Philip (1991) found that 40% of hearing aid users over 90 years of age could not use volume control wheels, 36% could not change their own batteries, and 34% could not clean their earmolds. Therefore, arthritis that impairs manual dexterity may impact elderly persons' use of hearing aids.

Hypertension, defined clinically, is a blood pressure reading of 140/90 mmHg or higher and is estimated to affect 65 million, or 1 in 3, adults in the United States (National Heart, Lung, and Blood Institute, 2010). High blood pressure is also known as "the silent killer" because it does not usually present with any symptoms and, without treatment, can lead to heart failure, kidney failure, aneurysms, stroke, or myocardial infarction (National Heart, Lung, and Blood Institute, 2010). Although there is no cure for hypertension, treatment includes changing one's diet, maintaining a healthy weight, increasing physical activity, quitting smoking, and limiting alcohol intake (National Heart, Lung, and Blood Institute, 2010). Hypertension can affect the hearing status and auditory rehabilitation of elderly patients. For example, Torre, Cruickshanks, Klein, Klein, and Nondahl (2005) found some evidence that women who have had a history of myocardial infarction were twice as likely to have cochlear impairment, although the same history was not significant in men.

Heart disease can be the result of untreated hypertension, and can lead to myocardial infarctions, stroke, and cardiac arrest. Myocardial infarctions can be sudden and intense or start slowly with mild pain and chest discomfort or uneasiness in other areas of the upper body accompanied by shortness of breath, sweating, nausea, or light headedness (American Heart Association, 2006). Signs of stroke include sudden numbness of the face, arm, or leg on one side of the body; confusion or trouble speaking or understanding; impaired vision in one or both eyes; difficulty walking, dizziness, or loss or balance or coordination; or severe headache with no known cause (American Heart Association, 2006). Some risk factors for coronary heart disease factors can be partially or completely ameliorated with a change in lifestyle (e.g., diet and exercise), and others cannot. For example, people cannot change their gender, their age, or hereditary factors, including race. Males are more at risk for heart disease than women, the condition tends to run in families, and over 83% of people who die from heart attacks are over 65 years of age (American Heart Association, 2006). However, people can change their lifestyles to reduce their risks of heart disease by quitting smoking, lowering their cholesterol and blood pressure, adopting an active lifestyle, maintaining a healthy weight, and avoiding stress and excessive alcohol intake (American Heart Association, 2006).

Interestingly, heart disease has been genetically linked to sensorineural hearing loss. Schönberger et al. (2005) have identified a human mutation that causes dilated cardiomyopathy and heart failure preceded by sensorineural hearing loss. In addition, special accommodations might be in order for the auditory rehabilitation of elderly persons who have had strokes, particularly in the management of amplification for those who are paralyzed. For example, patients who are paralyzed on one side need to learn how to insert and remove their hearing aids on the affected side with their nondominant hand (Johnson & Danhauer, 1999).

Diabetes is an endrocrinological disorder in which the body does not produce or efficiently use insulin, a hormone that converts sugar, starches, and other foods into energy (American Diabetes Association, 2010). There are two types of diabetes:

- **Type 1 diabetes** is usually diagnosed in childhood or young adulthood and can result in heart disease (cardiovascular disease), blindness (retinopathy), nerve damage (neuropathy), and kidney damage (nephropathy).
- **Type 2 diabetes** is the most common type and occurs when the body either does not produce enough insulin or the cells in the body do not use the insulin properly to take in sugar directly from the blood.

Some segments of the population are more prone to this condition than others, such as African Americans, Latinos, Native Americans, Asian Americans/Pacific Islanders, and the elderly (American Diabetes Association, 2010). Approximately, 20.8 million children and adults in the United States (7% of the population) have diabetes, 14.6 million of which have been diagnosed and 6.2 million are undiagnosed (American Diabetes Association, 2010). Of those persons 60 years of age and older, 10.3 million, or 20.9% of that segment of the population, has diabetes (American Diabetes Association, 2010). Treatment for diabetes includes diet, exercise, and medication. Compromised blood supply caused by diabetes has been implicated as a contributing etiological factor in the development of sensorineural hearing loss (Vaughan, James, McDermott, Griest, & Fausti, 2006), in addition to loss of sensation in the fingertips, possibly interfering with hearing aid manipulation.

Visual Status

Before discussing common visual disorders in the elderly, we will review the anatomy of the eye.

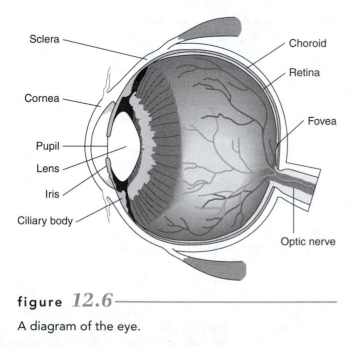

Sclera

Choroid

Retina

Cornea

Fovea

Pupil

Lens

Iris

Ciliary body

Optic nerve

figure *12.6*

A diagram of the eye.

Anatomy of the Eye. The eye and its parts are shown in Figure 12.6.

The **cornea**, a transparent covering, assists in focusing light coming into the eye. The **aqueous humor** is a watery fluid that circulates throughout the front of the eye and maintains a constant pressure. The white part of the eye is the **sclera**, and is made up of a tough and fibrous tissue that provides protection. The **iris** is the part of the eye that denotes its color and dilates to either make the **pupil**, the opening to the eye, larger or smaller to allow more or less light in, respectively. The **lens** is transparent and focuses the light entering the eye by changing shape based on whether objects are close or far away. Light must then pass through the center of the eye, which is filled with a clear, jelly-like substance called the **vitreous humor**. The light focuses on the **retina**, a thin lining of the back of the eye that is sensitive to light and is nourished by the **retinal vessels**.

The retina is composed of several layers. **Photoreceptors** are light-sensitive sensory cells that are of two types: **rods** and **cones**. Rods are used for vision in low light; cones are used for vision in light to see colors and details. These photoreceptors change the visual images on the retina into electrochemical signals. The **retinal pigment epithelium** (RPE) is a dark layer that absorbs excess light, transports oxygen, nutrients, and cellular wastes between the rods and cones and the **choroid**. The choroid is a layer of blood vessels that supply oxygen and nutrients to the outer layers of the retina. **Bruch's membrane** separates the blood vessels of the RPE from the choroids. The macula is the center of the retina and contains a high density of photoreceptor cells that enables sight of fine details. The **fovea** is the center of the macula and is the location of the sharpest visual image. The **optic nerve** consists of a bundle of nerve fibers that sends visual information to the brain.

Visual Disorders in the Elderly.   Like other parts of the body, structural changes within the eye caused by aging result in changes in vision. **Presbyopia** is the aging or the loss of the flexibility of the lens of the eye and the muscles responsible for its shape. Presbyopia commonly occurs after the age of 40 and results in an inability to see things up close. People with presbyopia may report difficulty in reading or a blurriness of objects close by. Presbyopia may also occur with **myopia**, **hyperopia**, or **astigmatism**. Myopia is nearsightedness, meaning that the person can see objects close up very well but has difficulty seeing distant objects that may appear blurry. The prevalence of myopia in the United States is 25.4%, or 30.4 million, of adults over 40 (Eye Diseases Prevalence Research Group, 2004a). Hyperopia, or farsightedness, means that although a person can see distant objects, those that are close may be blurry. The prevalence of hyperopia in the United States is 9.9%, or 11.8 million, of adults over 40 (Eye Diseases Prevalence Research Group, 2004a). An astigmatism is an irregular curvature of the cornea causing problems in how light is focused within the eye and occurs frequently with hyperopia or myopia (University of Michigan Kellogg Eye Center, 2006b). Myopia and hyperopia are often inherited and are diagnosed during childhood. Presbyopia, myopia, and hyperopia are **refractive errors** in which the shape of the eye does not bend light correctly, resulting in a blurred image. They result from a disorder rather than from a disease.

Other common ocular diseases in the elderly include **cataracts**, **glaucoma**, and **age-related macular degeneration**. Cataracts are a clouding of the lens of the eye caused by a combination of factors of increased age resulting in blurry vision, double vision, and sensitivity to light, glare, fading of colors, and frequent changes in eyeglass prescriptions (University of Michigan Kellogg Eye Center, 2007). The clouding of the lens of the eye interferes with the transmission of light to the retina. Cataracts are insidious in that they grow very slowly and most people do not realize that they have them. By age 65, over 90% of people have cataracts, and 50% of those between the ages of 75 and 85 have lost some vision from them (University of Michigan Kellogg Eye Center, 2007). The leading cause of low vision among white, black, and Hispanic people in the United States is cataracts (Eye Diseases Prevalence Research Group, 2004b). Treatment for cataracts is surgical removal and replacement with an artificial lens.

Glaucoma is actually a collection of eye diseases in which abnormal intraocular pressure causes damage to the optic nerve (University of Michigan Kellogg Eye Center, 2007). The most common type of glaucoma is **open-angle glaucoma** in which a constant increase in intraocular eye pressure caused by blockage of the "drainage" angle of the eye reduces visual acuity, contrast sensitivity, and color vision (University of Michigan Kellogg Eye Center, 2007; Weinstein, 2000). Several tests performed by an ophthalmologist can assist in detecting glaucoma by measuring eye pressure (**tonometry**), examining the drainage angle of the eye (**gonioscopy**), evaluating the optic nerve (**ophthalmoscopy**), and assessing the visual field in each eye (**perimetry**) (University of Michigan Kellogg Eye Center, 2007). The treatment for glaucoma depends on the type and severity of each case and may include medication, laser surgery, or operative surgery. Although glaucoma cannot be cured, it can be controlled (University of Michigan Kellogg Eye Center, 2007).

Age-related macular degeneration causes a progressive deterioration of the retina of the eye that may affect vision, particularly in doing close work such as threading a needle, but side or peripheral vision is rarely affected (*Understanding and Coping with Macular Degeneration*, 2006a; University of Michigan Kellogg Eye Center, 2007). The prevalence of this disease in the United States is 1.47%, or 1.75 million people, 40 years of age and older (Eye Diseases Prevalence Research Group, 2004c). The prevalence is expected to increase by 50% (to 2.95 million) by the year 2020 (Eye Diseases Prevalence Research Group, 2004c). In addition, the disease is much more likely to affect Caucasians than African Americans (Eye Diseases Prevalence Research Group, 2004c). Fortunately, many patients have an early form of the disease and experience no loss of vision (*Understanding and Coping with Macular Degeneration*, 2006a). There are two types of macular degeneration: (1) the **dry type**, which is the most common (90% of cases) resulting in the thinning of the macula, and (2) the **wet type**. The wet type accounts for 10% of cases, is the most serious form, and results from an abnormal growth of blood vessels of the macula (*Understanding and Coping with Macular Degeneration*, 2006a; University of Michigan Kellogg Eye Center, 2007). There is no form of treatment for dry macular degeneration, whereas the wet type is treated with laser or photodynamic therapy (*Understanding and Coping with Macular Degeneration*, 2006b).

Vestibular System

Another area of concern is elderly patients' presence of vestibular or balance disorders and risk for falls. The elderly are 10 times more likely to fall than children and 8 times more likely to die from the fall (Runge, 1993). Major causes for falls in the elderly in order of their occurrence are accidents, environmental hazards, falls from bed, gait disturbances, balance disorders or weakness; pain related to arthritis; vertigo due to medications or alcohol; acute illnesses; confusion and cognitive impairment; postural hypotension; visual disorders; central nervous system disorders; syncope; drop attacks; or epilepsy (Rubenstein, 1997). Balance disorders are in the purview of audiologic practice, but require a team approach because of the myriad of etiological factors such as peripheral and central vestibular disorders, age-related multisensory deficits, strokes and vascular insufficiencies, cerebellar degeneration, chemical and drug toxicities, benign paroxysmal positional vertigo, uncompensated Meniere's disease, vestibular neuritis, labyrinthitis, or head trauma (Bauer & Girardi, 2009). For example, audiologists may work with primary care physicians and pharmacists in determining if an elderly patient's prescription medications may be contributing to the sensations of dizziness and vertigo. The following is a listing of drugs that increase the risk of falling:

- Sedative-hypnotic and anxiolytic drugs (especially long-lasting benzodiazepines)
- Tricyclic antidepressants
- Major tranquilizers
- Antihypertensive drugs
- Cardiac medications
- Corticosteroids
- Nonsteroidal anti-inflammatory drugs
- Anticholinergic drugs

- Hypoglycemic agents
- Any medication that is likely to affect balance

Li, Keegan, Sternfeld, Sidney, Quesenberry, and Kelsey (2006) investigated the risk factors among middle-aged and older adults and found that falls occurred outdoors more often than indoors. Moreover, adults who reported more leisure-time physical activities were at higher risk for outdoor falls. Alternatively, they found that adults who had more health issues were at greater risk for indoor falls. Most causes for outdoor falls were uneven surfaces or objects causing trips or stumbles that most often occurred when walking on sidewalks, curbs, or streets. We will discuss fall prevention programs later in the chapter.

Sociological Status

The sociological status of elderly persons includes such factors as the physical environment, social environment, and financial status.

Physical Environment

The physical environment includes where elderly people live and the locations where they spend most of their leisure time.

Place of Residence. Housing for the elderly is a big business, and the market will expand as more boomers reach retirement age. Ideally, most people want to live in their own homes or at least with other family members for as long as possible. However, for some senior citizens, that may not always be possible due to health or financial reasons. For these individuals, considering an out-of-home living arrangement, downsizing, and/or selling the family home may represent a major life transition.

Securing other living arrangements does not mean that the elderly person has to live in a nursing home. Today, there are many residential care options that span a continuum of resident independence, from least restrictive to most restrictive, depending on an individual's needs (Helpguide.org, 2010). Figure 12.7 shows various options along that continuum ranging from independent living to Alzheimer's/dementia care. Independent senior housing includes options such as retirement communities, senior apartment complexes, and congregate living.

Retirement communities are composed of privately owned detached homes, condominiums, and/or apartments that often have scheduled social and recreational activities or other special amenities (e.g., golf memberships) (Helpguide.org, 2010).

Independent Living	Assistance With Activities of Daily Living	Dependent Living
• Retirement Community	• Assisted Living Facilities	• Long-term Residential Care Facility
• Senior Apartment Complexes	• Board and Care Home	• Skilled Nursing Facility
• Congregate Living	• Continuing Care Communities	
• Supported Senior Housing		

figure *12.7*

A continuum of living options for the elderly.

Senior apartment complexes are options used by seniors with low incomes that consist of individual apartments with communal areas for social/recreational activities (Helpguide.org, 2010). **Congregate living** involves senior citizens who have their own apartments in a multiunit building that often has a central kitchen, dining room, and other common areas and other services such as security, on-call staff support, housekeeping, laundry, transportation, and activities (Helpguide.org, 2010). **Supported senior housing** consists of apartments or room/board, as well as meals, social activities, and housekeeping (Helpguide.org, 2010).

Options that include help for seniors' completion of activities of daily living (ADLs) include assisted living facilities, continuing care retirement communities (CCRCs), and assisted living board and care model. **Assisted living facilities** (ALFs) offer a range of accommodations, from shared rooms to upscale private apartments in which residents pay monthly fees based on the services required to meet their level of functioning. A special type of ALF is known as the **board and care model** that has no private apartments, but has residents living in their own rooms in a smaller home-style facility and who may require assistance with ADLs in addition to having mild dementia or memory problems. **Continuing care retirement communities** offer a continuum of care within a single community that offers levels of care so that residents can receive more or less care based on their individual needs (Helpguide.org, 2010).

Long-term residential care is hard to define because the boundaries between primary, acute, and long-term care often overlap (Stone, 2000). **Primary care** is the broad spectrum of care, both preventative and curative, often provided by the elderly person's family physician or internist who serves as the "medical home" (MedicineNet.com, 2006). **Acute care** is treatment provided for immediate healthcare needs by physicians, nurses, and third-party-payer companies (Stone, 2000). A patient having surgery to repair a broken hip receives acute care provided in a hospital. **Long-term care** involves broad-based care aimed at providing services to persons with chronic disabilities to help them complete ADLs (e.g., bathing, dressing, eating, or other personal care) and instrumental activities of daily living (IADLs) (e.g., shopping, meal preparation, money management) involving both **formal** and **informal care providers** (Stone, 2000). Informal care providers, usually friends or family members, are often a spouse or adult child, usually a daughter. Formal care providers are frequently paraprofessionals such as certified nursing assistants, but rehabilitation provided in long-term care facilities is provided by therapists (e.g., physical and occupational). We will discuss later how where an elderly person lives and who provides care are instrumental in planning auditory rehabilitation.

Social Environment

The social environment includes the elderly person's support network (e.g., spouses, family, friends, and acquaintances) and daily activities. Important considerations are: Is the elderly person married? Who does he or she live with? Are family members close by? Who are the elderly person's friends, and how does he or she spend his or her time? Does he or she go to church on a regular basis? Does he or she go out to dinner, to the theatre, or to concerts?

Strong social support networks have positive effects on quality and longevity of life (Giles, Glonek, Luszcz, & Andrews, 2005). Moreover, social engagement is associated with a reduction of depressive symptoms in some older adults (Glass, De Leon, Bassuk, & Berkman, 2006). Therefore, social interaction may assist in improving the HRQoL for older adults.

Many senior citizens find fulfillment in serving others, which may also extend longevity. For example, some evidence has suggested that providing support to others decreases mortality (Brown, Nesse, Vinokur, & Smith, 2003). In addition, volunteering has a protective effect on mortality, particularly for elderly persons who volunteer for one organization or for 40 hours or less a year (Musick, Herzog, & House, 1999). Harris and Thoresen (2005) found that the protective effect of volunteering was stronger for individuals who frequently visited with friends or attended religious services.

Religious activities are important to the elderly and have been found to improve HRQoL. For example, older Mexican American adults who attend church monthly, weekly, and more than weekly show slower rates of cognitive decline than their peers who do not attend religious gatherings (Hill, Burdette, Angel, & Angel, 2006). Moreover, elderly patients who participated in private religious activity (e.g., prayer, meditation, and Bible study) before onset of impairment in completion of ADLs had a significant survival advantage compared with peers who did not (Helm, Hayes, Flint, Koenig, & Blazer, 2000).

Elderly persons' sociological status is highly dependent on their ability to communicate. Therefore, psychosocial problems associated with untreated adult onset sensorineural hearing loss can dramatically impact their HRQoL. Documented problems include social isolation, depression, anxiety; loneliness; lessened self-efficacy and mastery; stress in relationships when family, friends, and coworkers experience frustration, impatience, anger, pity, and/or guilt when interacting with a person having hearing loss; and an increased risk of dementia occurring as function of increasing hearing loss (Andersson & Green, 1995; Bess, Lichtenstein, Logan, Burger, & Nelson, 1989; Campbell, Crews, Moriarty, Zack, & Blackman, 1999; Chisolm et al., 2007; Keller et al., 1999; Kramer et al., 2002; National Council on the Aging [NCOA], 1999; Uhlmann, Larson, Rees, Koepsell, & Duckert, 1989; Weinstein & Ventry, 1982).

Financial Status

Although middle-aged adults look forward to retirement, many elderly adults choose to work or continue employment out of financial necessity. Work later in life has been associated with HRQoL benefits. For example, employment at age 70 years has been correlated with better perceived health, greater independence, and longevity (Hammerman-Rozenberg, Maaravi, Cohen, & Stressman, 2005). Unfortunately, many elderly persons find themselves trying to subsist only on their social security, which, for those with hearing impairment, can preclude the purchase of hearing aids.

Psychological Status

Psychological status includes considerations of mental status, depression, motivation, attitude and expectations.

Mental Status

Some cognitive decline can be expected with aging. Gatehouse, Naylor, and Elberling (2003) found that older adults with poorer cognitive skills had more difficulty understanding speech in noise and received less benefit from hearing aids when compared with seniors without any difficulty. Some elderly persons develop cognitive impairment such as **dementia** and **Alzheimer's disease** (AD). Dementia is a brain disorder that affects an elderly person's ability to carry out his or her daily activities (National Institute on Aging, 2006). AD is the most common form of dementia and initially affects areas of the brain that regulate thought, memory, and language. In the early stages of AD, patients may forget recent events and names of people/objects (National Institute on Aging, 2006). Although some drugs may lessen the severity of symptoms, AD has no cure and ultimately results in death. Two classic physiological signs of AD upon autopsy are (1) plaque deposits of abnormally processed amyloid and precursor protein and (2) neurofibrillary tangles and intracellular accumulations of the cytoskeletal protein tau (Alzheimer's Association, 2010). The following are some key facts about AD (National Institute on Aging, 2006):

- 45 million Americans have it
- Most often starts after age 60 years
- Prevalence increases with age
- Early onset familial AD strikes people between 30 and 60 years of age

Untreated hearing loss is frequently misdiagnosed as a form of dementia (Palmer, Adams, Bourgeois, Durrant, & Rossi, 1999). With the expected increase in the number of persons over 65 years of age, audiologists and speech-language pathologists will play a key role in the identification of older adults at risk for AD and need to know some of the following common characteristics (Cacace, 2007):

- Behavioral and mood changes
- Difficulty performing familiar tasks (e.g., getting dressed, making coffee)
- Disorientation of time and place
- Impaired judgment
- Loss of drive and initiative
- Memory loss
- Misplaced belongings
- Personality changes
- Problems expressing self verbally (e.g., word-finding problems)
- Problems with abstract thinking

Most elderly persons will not develop AD, but may experience problems with the three different types of memory commonly affected by the aging process. Briefly, the three types of memory are (Weinstein, 2000):

- **Sensory memory:** refers to the first, momentary encoding of the incoming information at the input stage.
- **Primary or short-term memory:** lasts longer than sensory memory and has a capacity of five to seven items, permitting the retention of small bits of information over a short period of time.
- **Secondary or long-term memory:** includes information that has been stored for later retrieval and utilization.

Elderly persons are more impaired on tasks that require conscious recollection of things compared with younger adults, but the differences in performance between these groups diminishes when tasks involve automatic activation processes such as the use of mnemonic devices (Light & Singh, 1987). Strategic use of mnemonic devices has been found to aid the memory of elderly persons (O'Hara et al., 2000). In fact, older adults have been known to spontaneously use specific elaborative encoding strategies (Hill, Allen, & Gregory, 1990).

Some evidence suggests that the stability and variability of cognitive abilities in the ninth decade of life and beyond is determined primarily by genetics (McClearn et al., 1997; Plomin, Pedersen, Lichtenstein, & McClearn, 1994). Further, the genetic effect for cognitive functioning in later life is similar for males and females (Read et al., 2006). These findings were based on the investigation of the cognitive abilities of identical twin pairs who were in their 80s and older. Although genetics plays a primary role in later life, maintenance of cognitive skills in later life is supported through consistent participation in mentally stimulating activities such as reading, completing crossword puzzles, taking lifelong learning classes, and so on. We will discuss accommodations for older adults with memory deficits later in this chapter.

Depression

Depression is more than a feeling of being down and lethargic; it is feeling sad all the time without any apparent reason (Helpguide: Depression, 2010). Depression is not a character defect, is treatable, and often can be attributed to physical causes. Being depressed is *not* a normal part of aging, however (Helpguide: Depression, 2010). Depression is the most common mental disorder in later life that presents in community-based primary care (Ell, 2006). The prevalence for major depression among community-dwelling elderly is 1–4% (Mojtabai & Olfson, 2004). Hearing loss can contribute to and even lead to depression and isolation (Campbell et al., 1999, 2006; Keller et al., 1999; Kramer et al., 2002). Communication sciences and disorders professionals should refer elderly patients with suspected depression for further evaluation.

Motivation, Attitude, and Expectations

Motivation to seek help for a hearing loss can be affected by several factors. As people get older, their sense of time left in their lives affects their motivation (Carstensen, 2006). Some seniors may ask, "Why should I get hearing aids at this late stage in my life?" which may mean learning about its care and use. On the other hand, some elderly patients may feel that hearing aids will enhance their relationships and time left with family. Patients can be classified into four categories based on their attitudes toward hearing aids and auditory rehabilitation (Goldstein & Stephens, 1981). **Type I attitude** is strongly positive toward hearing aids and auditory rehabilitation. **Type II attitude** is essentially positive toward hearing aids and auditory rehabilitation, but the patient presents with some complicating factor such as previous unsuccessful use of amplification, difficult-to-fit loss, and so on. **Type III attitude** is essentially negative toward hearing aids and auditory rehabilitation, but the patient is at least willing to consider receiving an audiologic evaluation. Frequently, these patients are in denial of their problem. **Type IV attitude** is strongly negative toward hearing aids and auditory rehabilitation. These patients typically do not want any assistance for their hearing loss, may be members of the Deaf community, and may harbor great resentment toward communication sciences and disorders professionals. Insight into patients' attitude types may assist the audiologists in tailoring counseling approaches to address unique patient needs.

Patients' attitudes can ultimately affect clinical outcomes. Wilson and Stephens (2003) investigated whether the reason for referral and attitudes toward amplification affected patients' satisfaction and use of hearing aids. Although they found that the reason for referral had no impact, attitudes toward hearing aids did affect patient outcomes. In addition, Brooks and Hallam (1998) found that patients who were less distressed by their hearing losses did not want hearing aids and used them for fewer hours per day than patients more affected by their hearing impairment. Similarly, patients who felt that they did not need hearing aids rated their effectiveness lower in listening situations as compared with those patients with a greater self-perceived need for amplification. Last, patients who felt stigmatized by the visual presence of hearing aids reported greater difficulty in the care and handling of their hearing instruments than other patients. Therefore, auditory rehabilitation should be tailored to meet the unique needs and attitudes of patients.

THE ELDERLY AND THE HEARING HEALTHCARE CONTINUUM

It is important to understand how elderly patients may enter into and progress through the **hearing healthcare continuum**. They may enter the system via a hearing screening at their physician's office that results in a referral to an audiologist for assessment and rehabilitation of a hearing loss. We will now discuss each part and the continuum of the hearing healthcare system, which includes the following steps:

- Screening
- Audiologic evaluation
- Auditory rehabilitation evaluation
- Hearing aid treatment and rehabilitation

Screening for Hearing Loss

As mentioned in an earlier chapter, one elderly person in three has hearing loss, and it is the third most common chronic healthcare condition for the elderly (Campbell et al., 2002). Only 20% of the 28 million who have hearing loss pursue amplification (NCOA, 1999). With the number of elderly citizens expected to increase dramatically over the next 30 years, communication sciences and disorders professionals must explore ways of increasing senior citizens' accessibility to hearing healthcare.

As with diabetes, the elderly patient may go undiagnosed with hearing loss for many years, possibly resulting in significant activity limitation and participation restriction. However, as of January 1, 2005, the Centers for Medicare and Medicaid Services (CMS) added a new benefit, an initial preventative physical examination (IPPE) only during Medicare Part B beneficiaries' first six months of enrollment (Solodar & Chapell, 2005). This is where primary care physicians (PCPs) are invaluable in identifying senior citizens who may have hearing loss and referring them for further audiologic evaluation. The new **Welcome to Medicare Examination** must include a review of the beneficiary's medical and social history, potential for depression, functional ability and level of safety, including screening for hearing impairment and falls risk, and examination of height, weight, blood pressure, visual acuity, and an electrocardiogram (Card, 2005). Based on the results of the examination, beneficiaries are educated, counseled, and referred for any health problems. Unfortunately, the length and focus of PCPs' consultations with patients vary and are often mediated by several factors that may preclude screening certain chronic health conditions like hearing loss and balance system disorders (Wilson & Childs, 2006). For example, Cohen, Labadie, and Haynes (2005) surveyed 260 physicians (85 responded = 32.7% response rate) and found that although 97.6% of the respondents felt that hearing loss affected patients' HRQoL, only 60% performed any hearing screenings. Maybe more physicians would screen for these problems if they knew that self-report screening tools were available for use that could be completed during patients' intake case histories.

The most frequently used hearing screening questionnaire for the elderly is the *Hearing Handicap Inventory for the Elderly–Screening Version* (HHIE–S) (Ventry & Weinstein,

1982). The HHIE–S is easily administered, with only 10 items that probe social and emotional impact of hearing loss (see Appendix 12.1). Patients respond to each item (e.g., "Does a hearing problem cause you to feel embarrassed when you meet new people?") by answering "yes," "no," or "sometimes." "Yes" responses earn 4 points, "no" responses earn 0 points, and "sometimes" responses earn 2 points. The higher the HHIE–S score, the greater is the perceived hearing handicap of the patients. The HHIE–S has a sensitivity of 72% and a specificity of 77% (Bess et al., 1995). The HHIE–S final score can range from 0 to 40 points. Moreover, patients who score from 0 to 8 points have a 13% probability of actually having a hearing loss (Bess et al., 1995). Alternatively, patients who score between 26 and 40 points on the HHIE have an 84% probability of having significant hearing loss.

To screen for prevalent problems such as vestibular and balance disorders in the elderly, a paper-and-pencil test should also be considered by healthcare professionals. One tool is the *Dizziness Handicap Inventory* (DHI) (Jacobson & Newman, 1990), which is a 25-item self-report questionnaire that has a shorter screening version. The DHI was designed to measure the handicapping effects of vestibular dysfunction. The 25 items are grouped into three content domains of functional, emotional, and physical aspects of dizziness and unsteadiness. Patients respond to each item (e.g., "Does looking up increase your problem?") by answering "yes," "no," or "sometimes." "Yes" responses earn 4 points, "no" responses earn 0 points, and "sometimes" responses earn 2 points. The higher the DHI score, the greater is the self-perceived handicap effects of the vestibular or balance problem. The final DHI scores can range from 0 (i.e., no perceived handicap) to 100 (i.e., significant perceived handicap). Therefore, the higher the score, the greater is the perceived handicap of the patients. The DHI was found to have high internal consistency and high test-retest reliability. Jacobson, Newman, Hunter, & Balzer (1991) administered the DHI to 367 patients and found that greater perceived handicap (higher scores on the DHI) was highly related to abnormal findings on balance function testing.

Besides having their hearing screened by a physician, elderly patients may enter the hearing healthcare continuum through hearing screenings in the community. For example, community agencies for the elderly commonly arrange senior health fairs providing screening for a variety of conditions such as osteoporosis, diabetes, obesity, and, frequently, hearing loss. Both audiologists and speech-language pathologists attend such fairs and conduct pure-tone screening tests and provide basic information about referral sources and hearing healthcare. The elderly may also respond to newspaper ads placed by local audiologists who are conducting "open houses" in which participants receive hearing screenings and demonstration of the latest product lines in amplification.

Various methods are used by audiologists in screening for hearing loss in the elderly. The best screening methods are those that identify patients with a particular condition for further testing and excuse those individuals without a condition. In one example, Scudder, Culbertson, Waldron, and Stewart (2003) evaluated the effectiveness of various screening tools for older adults. The predictive validity for hearing loss in the elderly was assessed when using a **distortion product otoacoustic emissions** (DPOAEs) handheld screener, pure-tone screening, screening otoscopy, self-assessment of communication (e.g., the HHIE), and case-history screening. DPOAEs are an objective method of assessing outer hair cell integrity by delivering stimuli via a probe and measuring the emissions from sensory cells. Predictive validity is the degree with which the results of a screening test correlate to those of a criterion measure, and in this case, an audiogram. They found that pure-tone screening had good predictive validity for actual hearing loss in this population when a 25-dB HL pass-fail criterion was used. In addition, screening otoscopy ratings were reliable over time and screeners. However, the DPOAE handheld screener was reliable for pass-refer outcome, but it did not have good predictive validity for hearing loss in the elderly. Moreover, self-assessment scores did not predict compliance with referral recommendations. Therefore, even though the elderly may report significant hearing handicap on a self-report questionnaire such as the HHIE–S, it does not mean that they will follow through with recommendations for further audiologic evaluation after failing a hearing screening. The use of valid screening methods in identifying older adults with hearing loss is useless unless patients comply with recommendations for audiologic evaluation. More recently, Jupiter (2009) suggested that using DPOAEs is effective for screening elderly patients who cannot respond on other screening vehicles.

Audiologic Evaluation

Audiologic evaluation of elderly patients may require some accommodations. At minimum, a complete diagnostic evaluation of elderly patients should include the following (ASHA, 1997):

- Assessment of most comfortable listening levels (MCLs) and loudness discomfort levels (LDLs)
- Functional status on an annual basis to identify any significant changes
- Immittance testing
- Otoacoustic emissions testing
- Pure-tone air-conduction testing at 250, 500, 1000, 2000, 3000, 4000, and 8000 Hz
- Reliable functional communication assessment scales
- Speech-recognition or speech-detection thresholds
- Suprathreshold word recognition testing

Figure 12.8 shows some accommodations that can be made when testing elderly patients who may have poor memory, movement deficits, disorientation, fading attention/distractibility, slower response time, and/or speech-language difficulties (based on Weinstein, 1995). For example, simplifying instructions, using repetition, checking comprehension, using frequent conditioning/reconditioning trials, providing extensive opportunities for practice, and offering verbal reinforcement and reassurances can modify testing procedures for older adults with memory problems.

At the completion of the diagnostic evaluation, the audiologist determines the need for a medical referral to a licensed physician and determines if the patient is a candidate for amplification. Audiologists should carefully and clearly present the audiometric results and possible treatment options, which will most likely involve the use of amplification. Use of tips for informational counseling mentioned by Margolis (2004) that were described in Chapter 2 may be particularly useful for elderly patients. General considerations for the determination of hearing aid candidacy are covered in Chapter 6 on amplification.

Counseling at this stage in the rehabilitation process is critical because even an elderly person who knows that he or she has a hearing loss may not choose to pursue amplification. Kricos (2006a, 2006b) believes that audiologists may not be cognizant of the elderly adults' degree of problem awareness and level of readiness for hearing aids. Smith and Kricos (2003) surmised that there are three levels of acknowledgment of hearing problems in elderly patients: **complete acknowledgment** (e.g., I definitely have a hearing impairment), **partial acknowledgment** (e.g., I may have a problem, but I don't need to get treatment for it yet),

Poor memory	**Fading attention/distractable**
• Simplify instructions	• Reduce length of test sessions
• Use repetition	• Limit sessions to a maximum of 20 to
• Check comprehension	30 minutes
• Use frequent conditioning/reconditioning trials	• Schedule 2 to 3 sessions, if necessary, to
• Offer extensive opportunities for practice	complete the test battery
• Offer verbal reinforcement and reassurances	

Poor memory
- Simplify instructions
- Use repetition
- Check comprehension
- Use frequent conditioning/reconditioning trials
- Offer extensive opportunities for practice
- Offer verbal reinforcement and reassurances

Movement deficits
- Evaluate different strategies before initiating testing
- Select natural and easy responses
- Select responses in patient's behavioral repertoire (e.g., hand raising, tissue use, waving)
- Be consistent in selection of response behavior

Disorientation
- Allow patient to listen to spoken voice prior to initiation of test

Fading attention/distractable
- Reduce length of test sessions
- Limit sessions to a maximum of 20 to 30 minutes
- Schedule 2 to 3 sessions, if necessary, to complete the test battery

Slower response time
- Slow down rate of tonal presentation
- Allow patient's behavior to dictate the pace

Speech and language
- Evaluate speech reception and word recognition using relevant materials
- Use simple commands and common questions
- Consider eliminating speech perception testing for patients with severe word-finding difficulties, failing memory of recent events, or reduction of vocabulary

figure *12.8*

Suggestions for modifications in audiologic evaluations for elderly patients.

Source: Based on "Auditory Testing and Rehabilitation of the Hearing-Impaired," by B. E. Weinstein, 1995. In R. Lubinski (Ed.), *Communication and Dementia* (pp. 223–237), San Diego, CA: Singular.

and **nonacknowledgment** (e.g., I don't have a problem; people around me mumble). Partial acknowledgment or nonacknowledgment may result in a failure to pursue amplification because their perceived problem "may not be that bad." Therefore, audiologists should be sensitive to the degree of acknowledgment in their elderly patients so that appropriate counseling can be provided prior to commencement of auditory rehabilitation. Otherwise, elderly patients who do not or only partially acknowledge the hearing loss may return their hearing aids for lack of perceived benefit (Kricos, 2006b).

Differential counseling should be implemented for older adults in the different stages of acknowledgment (Kricos, 2006b). Kricos (2006b) provided some techniques to explore with patients who only partially or do not acknowledge their hearing losses. First, they suggested providing information about hearing loss and its affect on communication. For example, some patients may not recognize that they are showing signs of a hearing loss. Second, they suggest having patients return in three to six months after having monitored their hearing abilities in a variety of situations using self-awareness materials as shown in Figures 12.9, 12.10, and 12.11. After careful reflection, partial acknowledgers or nonacknowledgers might just realize the extent of their communication problems. Further acknowledgment of hearing loss may occur during the next stage of self-perception of communication needs, performance, and selection of goals for treatment.

Auditory Rehabilitation Evaluation

The audiologic evaluation may not obtain all of the information that may be beneficial in planning auditory rehabilitation. Once the audiologic evaluation has determined the presence of a hearing loss, the auditory rehabilitation evaluation begins. For some patients, assessment of

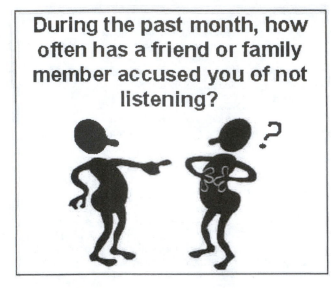

figure *12.9* ──────────────────────

Materials for self-reflection about hearing loss.

Source: From *Audiologic Rehabilitation with the Geriatric Population*, P. B. Kricos, 2006, retrieved from www.audiologyonline.com/articles/ article_detail.asp?article_id=1673. Reprinted with permission.

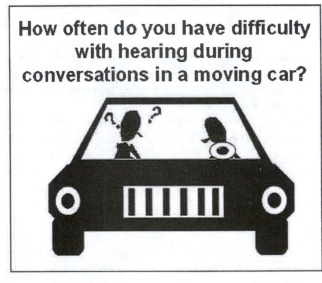

figure *12.10* ──────────────────────

Materials for self-reflection about hearing loss.

Source: From *Audiologic Rehabilitation with the Geriatric Population*, P. B. Kricos, 2006, retrieved from www.audiologyonline.com/ articles/article_detail.asp?article_id=1673. Reprinted with permission.

activity limitations and participation restriction may be satisfactory for selecting hearing aids and the need for HAT. For other patients, audiologists may detect a need for additional counseling regarding realistic benefits to be derived from the use of amplification. Alternatively, other patients may need evaluation of how nonauditory factors may influence the rehabilitative process. Moreover, patients with more severe hearing losses may need one-on-one auditory rehabilitation necessitating assessment of audiovisual speech reception abilities and conversational fluency. Therefore, the patients' needs determine the extent of the auditory rehabilitation evaluation.

Assessment of Activity Limitation, Participation Restriction, and Nonauditory Factors

As discussed in Chapter 6, on hearing aids, audiologists together with patients should establish goals for auditory rehabilitation. As with all patients, some measurement of the contribution of the older adult's hearing loss on activity limitations, participation restrictions, and effect on general health should be made. The self-report instruments mentioned in that chapter may be useful. The *Client-Oriented Scale of Improvement* (COSI) (Dillon, James, & Gillis, 1997) is frequently used to select and prioritize difficult communication situations to target for improvement through the use of amplification. However, it is important to use tools that have been normed on the elderly population. For example, it is inappropriate to use the *Hearing Handicap Inventory for Adults* (HHIA) (Newman, Weinstein, Jacobson, & Hug, 1991) on elderly adults instead of the HHIE (Ventry & Weinstein, 1982). Furthermore, Kricos (2006b) suggested asking elderly patients the following questions:

- What types of situations do you find most troubling?
- Do you have difficulty separating out and attending to voices from multiple talkers?

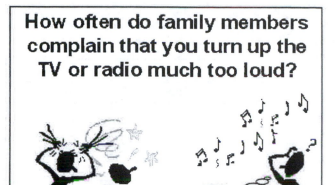

figure *12.11* ——————————————

Materials for self-reflection about hearing loss.

Source: From *Audiologic Rehabilitation with the Geriatric Population,* P. B. Kricos, 2006, retrieved from www.audiologyonline.com/articles/article_detail.asp?article_id=1673. Reprinted with permission.

- How much effort does it take to communicate in difficult versus easy listening situations? And how does it affect you?
- Do you have difficulties attending to one talker and then having to shift your attention to other talkers?
- Do you think that your hearing loss is affecting you psychologically or socially?

Information gleaned from this process can assist in setting goals for auditory rehabilitation and in selecting the right type of hearing aid, features, and assistive listening technology.

Serious consideration should be given to assessment of the nonauditory factors discussed earlier in the chapter and how they affect the auditory rehabilitation process for elderly patients. Table 12.2 shows a checklist of potentially important variables for consideration prior to beginning auditory rehabilitation with elderly patients.

For example, knowledge of the patients' general health may indicate the need for referrals to other healthcare professionals or special scheduling of appointments. Patients who have very poor corrected vision may require specialized features on their hearing aids or use of handheld magnifiers during the hearing aid delivery (see the section "Dual Sensory Impairment" later in the chapter). Furthermore, patients' manual dexterity, finger sensitivity, and fine-motor skills may be important factors in the selection of their hearing aids. Patients with poor fine-motor skills and finger sensitivity may require hearing aids that use larger batteries and have larger controls. In addition, patients who have poor proximal manual dexterity and are unable to lift their arms and hands to ear level may require a spouse, family member, or caregiver to insert and remove hearing aids.

Assessment of the elderly patient's psychological status may reveal that some of the problems in communication may be due to a cognitive decline. Audiologists might consider using simple mental status screening questionnaires such as the *Mini-mental States Examination* (MMSE) (Folstein, Folstein, & McHugh, 1975), particularly for patients over 80 years of age (Kricos, 2006a). Some patients may have some form of dementia and/or be in the early stages of AD. For these patients, Kricos (2006a) suggested careful counseling of the individuals and their family using a collaborative problem-solving approach. She suggested that solutions beyond hearing aids should be considered such as hearing assistive technology (HAT), controlling the communication environment to reduce listening difficulties, formal listening training, attention to the patient's self-efficacy for managing communication challenges, and clear speech training for frequent communication partners.

Hearing impairment may be the most undetected chronic healthcare condition in Alzheimer's patients because they may be able to communicate in quiet settings; additional signs of hearing loss may be masked by other behavioral manifestations of the disease

table *12.2*   Checklist of Potentially Important Variables for Consideration Prior to Beginning Auditory Rehabilitation With Elderly Patients

Physical Status

	Good	Fair	Poor
• General health	____	____	____
• Visual status (close vision with glasses)	____	____	____
• Manual dexterity	____	____	____
• Finger sensitivity	____	____	____
• Fine motor skills	____	____	____

Notes:

Psychological Status

	Good	Fair	Poor
• Mental status	____	____	____
• Motivation/Attitude	____	____	____
• Outlook	____	____	____

Notes:

Social Status

	Yes	No
• Participates in community activities	____	____
• Communicates in noisy environments	____	____
• Goes to worship services	____	____
• Lives independently	____	____
• Lives with spouse	____	____
• Has supportive, extended family nearby	____	____

Notes:

Communication Status

	Good	Fair	Poor
• Has good communication skills	____	____	____
• Has good conversational fluency	____	____	____
• Has good audiovisual communication skills	____	____	____

Notes:

Financial Status

	Yes	No
• Resources for purchasing hearing aids?	____	____

Source: Information from *Guidebook for Support Programs in Aural Rehabilitation*, by C. E. Johnson and J. L. Danhauer, 1999, San Diego, CA: Singular.

(Palmer, Adams, Bourgeois, Durrant, & Rossi, 1999). Palmer et al. found a reduction of caregiver-identified problem behaviors and an increase in appropriate social behaviors in patients with AD after being fitted with hearing aids. Therefore, a diagnosis of AD should not preclude the consideration of hearing aids, provided an adequate support system is in place for safe and consistent use of the device. Other psychological considerations may include poor patient motivation and/or a bleak outlook on life, necessitating a referral to a mental health professional.

Consideration of sociological status may reveal the types and amount of social activities enjoyed by patients, indicating a need for further probing for problematic listening situations or for considering special hearing aid features such as the use of directional microphones. The use of the *Client Oriented Scale of Improvement* (COSI) (Dillon, James, & Ginis, 1997) is useful for collaborating with patients in nominating problematic listening situations. For example, understanding communication partners in a noisy restaurant may indicate a need for a digital hearing aid with digital noise reduction and use of adaptive directional microphones. In addition, consideration of the older adult's living arrangements may indicate who should be present during the hearing aid delivery and who may assist the patient with hearing aid care and use, if needed.

Assessment of Audiovisual Speech Reception

Besides determining the type, degree, and configuration of hearing loss, assessment of communication status involves assessing elderly patients' speechreading abilities, audiovisual speech reception, and conversational fluency. Speechreading tests have been used over the past century and consist of syllables, words, and/or sentences that the examiner presents without voice and the patient repeats what was said. Patients' responses are scored on the number of words or sentences correctly identified. Appendix 12.2 contains List A of the sentence subtest of the *Utley Test of Lipreading Ability* (Utley, 1946). The Utley has three subtests: sentences (Lists A and B), words (Lists A and B), and stories that require the answering of questions (Hipskind, 2007). The sentence subtest is the most frequently administered part of the tests, with each form containing 125 words to score. Examiners present each sentence twice at a distance of 3 to 5 feet from the patient. The normative data for List A are on the scoresheet. The problems with these tests are a high degree of variability in the test situation due to the sentences, the speechreader, the talker, and the interaction of the talker and the sentence (e.g., Demorest & Bernstein, 1992; Yakel, Rosenblum, & Fortier, 2000). A survey found that although a group of rehabilitative audiologists felt that speechreading was important, the majority were concerned about the lack of validity in test results. Speechreading can also be assessed using some of the instruments for assessing audiovisual speech reception.

One effective means of evaluating audiovisual speech reception includes use of techniques and technologies used in training. For example, speech tracking is a procedure requiring a partner to read materials to the patient who repeats *exactly* what has been said (De Filippo & Scott, 1978). The dependent variable is the rate of understanding, or the number of words from the text that are understood, per second. If a word or phrase is not repeated back verbatim, then the clinician acknowledges the error and provides clues so that the patient can figure out what the word or phrase was. The clues should not be gestural, but verbal. For example, the clinician should provide words that are opposite of the word missed or use a similar sounding word (e.g., "Sounds like _____"). The reading material may be from books, newspaper articles, and/or magazines. The assessment may involve different conditions (Spitzer, Leder, & Giolas, 1993):

- Without the hearing aid (lipreading)
- With lipreading and the hearing aid together
- With the hearing aid only and no other visual cues

A major problem with speech tracking is that it is highly individualistic due to inter-speaker differences and variations in how patients respond to these variations (Levitt, 2006).

A relatively new software program, Computer-Assisted Tracking, maintains the interactive nature of the technique, but reduces the sources of variation (Levitt, 2006). The program was also designed for patients to self-train at home. Adults are busy and cannot always take time off from work to go to therapy. Over the past 20 years, three computerized audiovisual speech perception training programs have been developed for both adults and children: (1) *Computer-Assisted Speech Perception Evaluation and Training* (CASPER) developed by Boothroyd and colleagues at the City University of New York (Boothroyd, 1987), (2) *Computer-Aided Speechreading Training* (CAST) by Pichora-Fuller and colleagues (Benguerel & Pichora-Fuller, 1988; Pichora-Fuller & Benguerel, 1991) and (3) a computerized videodisc system (Tye-Murray, Tyler, Bong, & Nares, 1988). More recently, Boothroyd (2008) and his colleagues at San Diego State University have developed *Computer-Assisted Speech Perception Evaluation and Training of Sentences* (CasperSent), a multimedia program with an aim to evaluate and train sentence-level speech perception.

Assessment of Conversational Fluency

Earlier in the chapter when defining conversational fluency, it was stated that some characteristics of conversational fluency are a sharing of speaking time, with a minimum of requests for clarification, and an easy conveying of ideas. Tye-Murray (2008) recommended the use of two indices in measuring the amount of speaking time per conversational partner: (1) mean length of turn, in words (MLT); and (2) mean length of turn ratio (MLT ratio). The **mean length of turn** (MLT) is defined as the average number of words used by a person during a conversational turn. It is computed by counting the number of words used by a speaker within a conversation and then dividing by the number of speaking turns. The **mean length of turn ratio** (MLT ratio) is simply the ratio of the patient's MLT per the conversational partner's MLT. In order to calculate these values, a representative sample of conversation must be obtained involving the patient on a familiar topic or at least one that provides an opportunity for a collection of a representative sample to determine his or her level of conversational skill. The conversation should be tape recorded and written down, word-for-word. It is best to select a segment for analysis from the middle of the conversation exchange rather than the beginning or ending of the tape when communication is either starting up or winding down. Let's calculate these measures using the following conversation exchange.

CONVERSATION EXAMPLE 1

Audiologist: "Where did you go on vacation this summer?"

Patient: "We went to Scottsdale, Arizona, and stayed at a resort."

Audiologist: "Are you and your wife golfers?"

Patient: "She isn't, but I am. She likes to lie out by the pool."

Audiologist: "I can imagine that it gets pretty warm there during the summer."

Patient: "Oh yes! It averages about ninety degrees Fahrenheit, but very low humidity."

Audiologist: "With the low humidity, you probably don't feel the heat as much."

Patient: "Oh yes, my wife and I don't even feel the heat."

The first step in computing MLT is to count the total number of words used by each conversational partner. The second step is to count the number of conversational turns had by each partner. The third step is to divide the total number of words by the number of conversational turns to compute the MLT for each speaker. Let's do the computations.

Computations for Example 1

	Audiologist	Patient
Step 1: Count the number of words	38	46
Step 2: Count the number of turns	4	4
Step 3: Divide number of words by the number of turns	9.5	11.5

Therefore, the MLT for the audiologist is 9.5 words per turn versus 11.5 words per turn for the patient. The MLT ratio is computed by dividing the MLT of the patient by the MLT of the audiologist, which is 1.2. What does the MLT ratio mean? An MLT ratio of 1.0 signifies that the mean length of turn, in words, of the patient and the audiologist are approximately the same, exemplifying equal conversational turn time. The MLT of 1.2 from the first conversation indicates that the patient uses more words per turn than the audiologist. A number less than one indicates that the MLT of the patient is, on average, less than the audiologist and represents a comparative proportion of MLT of the patient to the audiologist. For example, an MLT ratio of 0.8 means that, on the average, the patient's MLT is 80% of the audiologist's. Conversely, if the number is greater than 1, it represents that, on the average, the patient's MLT is greater than the audiologist's. For example, an MLT ratio of 2.0 means that, on the average, the patient uses twice as many words per turn than the audiologist.

Readers might be wondering, what does MLT and MLT ratio have to do with conversational fluency? Well, before answering that question, let's look at a conversational exchange between an audiologist and a patient who clearly has poor conversational fluency due to hearing loss.

CONVERSATIONAL EXAMPLE 2

Audiologist: "Where did you go on vacation this summer?"

Patient: "What?"

Audiologist: "Where did you go on vacation this summer?"

Patient: "Where did I go?"

Audiologist: "Yes, where did you and your wife go on vacation this summer?"

Patient: "We went to Scottsdale and stayed at a resort."

Audiologist: "Are you and your wife golfers?"

Patient: "Are we . . . what?"

Audiologist: "Are you and your wife golfers?"

Patient: "Is my wife what?"

Clearly the patient in this example has a difficult time in conversational fluency. Again, let's do the computations.

Computations for Example 2

		Audiologist	Patient
Step 1:	Count the number of words	40	21
Step 2:	Count the number of turns	5	5
Step 3:	Divide number of words by the number of turns	8	4.2

The MLT is 8 for the audiologist and 4.2 for the patient. Therefore, the MLT ratio is 0.525, meaning that the patient only uses 52% of the number of words per utterance compared to the audiologist, indicating reduced turn time.

With the patient only using about half the number of words that the audiologist does, it could mean that the conversation may be one sided, with the audiologist doing most of the talking and moving the interaction along. The low MLT ratio signifies poor conversational fluency, particularly due to the patient. However, this might not always be the case, because some communication situations lend themselves to lower MLT ratios than others. For example, a person probably would have a low MLT and MLT ratio when being interrogated by a policeman who had just pulled him or her over for speeding. Therefore, the context of the conversation has a lot to do with whether the MLT and MLT ratio denotes low or high conversational fluency. If we look at the last example and apply other criteria, we can determine that the patient has poor conversational fluency. For example, the number of requests for clarification was high and the exchange of ideas was low. So, other criteria should also be used in assessing conversational fluency.

Tye-Murray (2008) suggested different methods of measuring conversational fluency: (1) interview, (2) questionnaire, (3) daily log, (4) group discussion, (5) structured communication interaction, and (6) unstructured communication interaction. The **interview method** involves directly asking patients their subjective impressions of conversational fluency in various communication situations. For example, patients are asked about who (e.g., common communication partners), what (e.g., topic, vocabulary used), where (e.g., at the bingo hall, at church), when (e.g., how long conversations last), and why (e.g., to order at a restaurant, to catch up with friends) of their typical, day-to-day conversations. In addition, patients can also indicate if they have difficulty with conversations with certain people or settings by saying "yes," "no," or "sometimes." The interview method solicits information that can be used to seek unique solutions to patients' problems.

The **questionnaire method** uses the traditional income/outcome measures mentioned in this and other chapters to get an idea of conversational fluency. Many of these scales have items that directly ask about conversational difficulties. For example, one of the items on the *Self-Assessment of Communication* (Schow & Nerbonne, 1982) asks, "Do you experience communication difficulties in situations when conversing with a small group of several persons? (for example, with friends or families, co-workers, in meetings or casual conversations, over dinner or while playing cards, etc.)," to which patients respond: "1, almost never (or never)," "2, occasionally (about $\frac{1}{4}$ of the time)," "3, about half of the time," "4, frequently (about $\frac{3}{4}$ of the time)," or "5, practically always (or always)." The questionnaire method can be done quickly, but may not probe deep enough into the specifics of patients' conversational difficulties.

The **daily log method** asks patients to answer the same questions about conversational behaviors encountered each day. The daily log has a page(s) for each day for patients to write their names and the date. Questions such as "Did you tell a conversational partner that you did not understand what was said?" are asked of the patient, to which they circle "yes" or "no." Audiologists can examine the daily logs from a week or so to determine patterns of difficulties frequently encountered with specific communication partners or settings.

The **group discussion method** involves having a group of patients with hearing loss and their significant others discuss potentially difficult listening situations. This strategy might be particularly effective for orientation groups of new hearing aid users. For example, group members may elect to discuss conversational problems encountered on the telephone, in the car, at the movies, in a restaurant, and so on. The group discussion method can elicit peer support and suggestions in seeking solutions to problems. Unfortunately, not everyone may feel comfortable participating; therefore, audiologists and other group members may not gain much information about the communication difficulties of reluctant patients.

The **structured communication interaction method** involves using mock situations to simulate realistic conversational interactions. For example, the patient and a communicative partner select a topic to talk about for a period of up to five minutes while the audiologist uses a sheet to rate conversational fluency. Topics can include current events, common hobbies, vacation sites, sports, and so on. Figure 12.12 shows the TOPICON rating sheet that the audiologist uses to describe conversational skills of the patient.

The sheet has spaces for the recording of the patient's name, date, and the topic of conversation. Because partners' familiarity with the topic can influence conversational fluency, the audiologist rates the familiarity of the topic for the patient and the communicative partner as either high or low. The audiologist also rates conversational skills (e.g., presuppositions, receptive ability [audio, visual, audio + visual], expressive abilities, motivation/attention, turn-taking, specificity/accuracy, and so on) of the patient as either "1, excellent," "2, good," "3, fair," or "4, poor." In addition, a space is provided to record qualitative comments about the interaction.

Two other structured tools developed by Erber (1988, 1996) are: (1) *Questions for Aural Rehabilitation: Quest? AR,* and

---

Topic: _Fishing_   Topic: _Familiarity_

		Clinician	
		Low	High
	Low	☐	☒
Client			
	High	☐	☐

Rating Scale
1. Excellent
2. Good
3. Fair
4. Poor

	Rating			
	1	2	3	4
Overall fluency of discourse:			X	

Factors related to conversational fluency:

	1	2	3	4
a. presupposition				X
b. receptive abilities (A, V, A-V)	X			
c. expressive abilities				X
d. motivation, attention				X
e. turn-taking			X	
f. specificity/accuracy			X	
g. new vs old information			X	
h. nonverbal communication			X	
i. topic maintenance				X
j. cooperation				X
k. time-sharing			X	
l. verification			X	
m. independent repair		X		
n. meta-communication		X		
o. other				

Comments:

Poor topic maintenance (even though on a familiar topic): client frequently asks for clarification.

figure *12.12*

TOPICON rating sheet.

(2) *ASQUE*. Quest? AR is actually a therapy technique that can be used to assess conversational fluency. Quest? AR provides question-and-answer practice using a predetermined set of questions on a specific topic. ASQUE categorizes questions into five different categories: (1) yes-no questions (YQ) (e.g., Did you go to the store last night?), (2) choice questions (CQ) (e.g., Do you want the red car, white car, or blue car?), (3) information-eliciting (wh-) questions (IQ) (e.g., Where are you going on your vacation?), (4) opinion-eliciting (how-why) questions (OQ) (e.g., Why do you think he feels that way?), and (5) assertions (AS) (e.g., She baked that apple pie?).

The **unstructured communication interaction method** uses "real-life" communication situations to assess conversational fluency. The major advantage of this approach is high external validity in the measurement of behavior. However, the disadvantage of this approach is that the audiologist has very little control over the topic and other conversational parameters. For example, if one communicative partner knows little about the topic, measures of conversational fluency may be a reflection of the partner's lack of knowledge rather than the performance of the patient. With this method, conversational fluency can be assessed through the computation of MLT/ MLT ratio, use of the TOPICON rating sheet, or specialized software.

Flynn (2003) stated that *Dyalog,* a computer software program, can assist audiologists in objectively measuring conversational fluency. Dyalog was developed by Norman P. Erber and records conversational breakdowns with the pressing of spacebar on a computer keyboard. Dyalog can measure the following parameters: total duration of the conversation (in seconds), time taken by clarification, the proportion of clarification time, the number of clarifications, and the average time taken by a clarification (Flynn, 2003). Audiologists can use Dyalog in real-time or by using a videotape recording procedure (Caissie & Rockwell, 1993).

Hearing Aid Treatment

Dr. James Jerger (2007) has called hearing aids "the cornerstone of auditory rehabilitation." Desirable characteristics of hearing aids change as patients age. Meister, Lausberg, Kiessling, von Wedel, and Walger (2002) found that although younger adults' top attribute for hearing aids is to hear speech in noise, elderly patients most value speech recognition in quiet situations, followed by understanding in noisy environments and ease of manipulation. The details of the hearing aid selection, evaluation, and fitting process are discussed and exemplified in the Casebook Reflection involving Bill and Dottie Roberts in Chapter 6. It is important that elderly patients should not be stereotyped, and some seniors may need more assistance than others in managing their hearing aids. Therefore, the structuring and the content of the hearing aid delivery may be a critical factor in some elderly patients' compliance and successful use of amplification. There are so many things to do in adjusting to amplification for older adults that many seniors may believe that they cannot gain self-mastery in this domain and may return their hearing aids to the provider or manufacturer.

Audiologists may need to work on building elderly patients' self-confidence in mastering the use of amplification. **Self-efficacy** has been defined as the confidence a person has in completing a set of skills requisite for success in achieving a particular goal (Bandura, 1986). Smith and her colleagues have applied this concept to auditory rehabilitation, particularly toward the hearing aid delivery and orientation process (Smith & West, 2006). If older adults with hearing impairment have high self-efficacy toward amplification, they are more likely to keep and use their hearing aids, rather than return the devices. Smith and West suggest incorporating the following principles into the hearing aid delivery to increase patients' self-efficacy:

- Starting with simple skills and progressing toward more difficult tasks
- Offering extensive practice during the initial delivery, follow-up appointments, and hearing aid orientation groups
- Suggesting practice of skills at home
- Engaging in role play
- Setting clear and specific goals

We will further discuss Smith and West's suggestions for increasing hearing aid self-efficacy during hearing aid orientation groups.

Regarding scheduling appointments, extra time may be needed for the hearing aid delivery appointment because the elderly may need more time processing new information, have more questions, or require additional practice of basic skills. Whenever possible, spouses, adult children, hired companions, or significant others who will assist in the hearing aid adjustment process should attend the delivery. These patients and their significant others should be encouraged to be active learners by asking questions. Periodically, audiologists should check patients' comprehension because sometimes patients will just nod their heads that they understand when they actually do not. Patients should also be required to demonstrate basic skills such as insertion/removal of the device, changing of a battery, and so on.

Some patients may require extra time and additional practice in basic hearing aid manipulation. For example, even though most hearing aids do not have volume control wheels, it was not unusual for elderly patients to sometimes get confused on how they worked and benefited from additional cueing. For example, cueing might take the form of a diagram showing a side view of hearing aid wearer with arrows going toward the eyes and the word "louder" in large font and arrows going backward (i.e., away from the eyes) with the word "softer" in smaller font. Some patients may benefit from mnemonic devices with this task such as, "If you want to hear more (i.e., louder), roll the wheel toward your nose to be 'nosy.'" Similar strategies may be developed for seniors to get use to switching between programs on digital hearing aids. Additionally, a "cheat-sheet" printed in large font may be all that is needed for an elderly hearing aid wearer to learn the sequence of steps in using the telephone. Audiologists can be creative in devising strategies for the elderly in self-mastery of hearing aid use and care.

As mentioned in Chapter 6, a lot of information is presented and several skills are demonstrated during a typical hearing aid delivery. No patient, regardless of age, can be expected to absorb every detail or be proficient at every single skill without real-life experience with the hearing aids and additional exposure to the information and practice. In fact, elderly hearing aid wearers who participated in a hearing aid manipulation training protocol (HATP) performed better than their peers who did not on a questionnaire focusing on handling hearing aids, volume control adjustment, and controlling the listening environment (Chartrand, 2005). The HATP training was administered to the elderly hearing aid wearers over two 30-to-45-minute visits. Chartrand explained that the HATP was designed and tested to expand the elderly hearing aid users' understanding about psychoacoustics, his or her own voice dynamics, and utilization of hearing aids as a coping strategy to improve speech understanding in noise. During each HATP session, participants were given practice on each exercise until they demonstrated some mastery of the new skills. They practiced each exercise on their own for a minimum of 15 minutes per day or until they felt more confident in accomplishing the task. Therefore, elderly patients and their significant other(s) should seek out additional training and practice with their hearing aids. In addition to HATPs, elderly hearing aid wearers and their significant others should attend group hearing aid orientation programs to assist in the adjustment process.

Hearing Aid Orientation Groups

Hearing aid orientation groups are composed of new and experienced hearing aid wearers and their significant others attending sessions geared toward promoting successful use of amplification. Hearing aid orientation groups were first introduced when servicemen started returning home from World War II with significant hearing loss (Ross, 2009). The government assembled a variety of specialists to develop auditory rehabilitation programs at military hospitals such as Borden, Deshon, and Walter Reed as well as the United States Naval Hospital in Philadelphia (Ross, 2009). In those early days, veterans with hearing loss sat through classes for as long as eight hours a day for eight weeks on topics such as speechreading.

Andragogy and the Development of Hearing Aid Self-Efficacy

Andragogy involves learning strategies that engage the adult learner (Bruegemann, 2005; Knowles, Holton, & Swanson, 2005). Bruegemann (2005) has drawn parallels between andragogy Malcolm Knowles's theories of adult learning, and effective hearing aid orientation groups. Figure 12.13 shows five principles of adult learning.

The first principle of adult learning theory is that self-concept promotes self-direction. Effective hearing aid orientation groups do not consist of didactic teaching (e.g., audiologists' lectures), but should be highly interactive and directed by participants' needs. A second principle of adult learning theory is that learner experience is used as a powerful teaching tool. For example, participants learn vicariously from each other's experiences in adjusting to amplification. Third, adult learning is oriented for immediate application, consisting of information and skills that new hearing aid users can apply and use *now* to improve communication. Fourth, adults are eager to learn what is important in the fulfillment of their roles in their day-to-day activities such as a member of their community organization, a communicative spouse, a bridge partner, and so on. Fifth, adult learners are internally motivated to learn information and skills that are relevant to their personal goals. To maximally benefit from hearing aid orientation group experiences, new hearing aid wearers require a strong locus of control

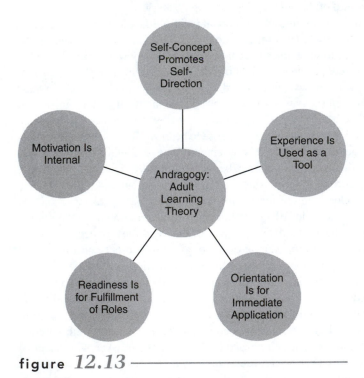

figure 12.13

Five principles of adult learning.

Sources: Based on *Andragogy and Aural Rehabilitation*, by P. M. Bruegemann, 2005, retrieved from http://www.audiologyonline.com/articles/pf_article_detail.asp?article_id=1445; *The Adult Learner*, Sixth Edition, by M. Knowles, E. E. Holton, and R. A. Swanson, 1984, Burlington, MA: Elsvier.

and a high degree of self-efficacy toward adjustment to amplification. Smith and West (2006) suggest a framework for fostering hearing aid self-efficacy beliefs through four major sources: (1) mastery experience, (2) vicarious experiences, (3) verbal persuasion, and (4) physiological and affective states.

Mastery experience is achieved through the reviewing of information and using the practice of skills to increase patients' hearing aid self-mastery (Smith & West, 2006). Wayner (2005) suggested a group hearing aid orientation program consisting of three sessions whose overall goals and specific objectives are depicted in Figure 12.14. For example, session 1 reviews important knowledge already covered during the hearing aid delivery such as hearing aid components, switches, and controls; characteristics of batteries; and listening strategies with amplification. The first session also demonstrates basic skills and provides opportunities for practice such as removal/insertion of the earmold/hearing aid, cleaning and care of hearing aids, and use of hearing aids with the telephone. Moreover, the session progresses from the simple to more complex and difficult information and skills. For example, listening experiences and steps of hearing aid use are presented in a hierarchy, from easy to difficult, to foster self-mastery. In addition, subsequent sessions not only review old information and have opportunities for practicing mastered skills, but also contain more advanced aspects of hearing aid use and communication strategies. Sometimes, experienced hearing aid users who obtain new devices may benefit from hearing aid refresher (HAR) courses (Wayner, 2005) with a curriculum shown in Figure 12.15.

Vicarious experiences can promote hearing aid self-efficacy through participants' observation of each other's successes (Smith & West, 2006). For example, patients' difficulties in using the telephone may be eased when observing others achieve success. In addition, members of hearing aid orientation groups can develop an *esprit de corps* and can gain confidence and learn as much from each other as from hearing healthcare professionals. Other types of vicarious experiences may include the use of skits to practice newly learned communication strategies. For example, patients who typically bluff their way through conversations may feel more confident in executing requests for clarification in the real world if first practiced in group therapy.

Verbal persuasion enhances hearing aid self-efficacy through the use of positive statements about a person's ability to succeed (Smith & West, 2006). Participants can be effective sources of support for each other. For example, not only can participants offer solutions to each other's problems, but they can provide verbal and nonverbal encouragement, instilling a sense of confidence of mastery over a particularly difficult communication situation. In addition, positive reinforcement from hearing healthcare providers can enhance participants' belief in their abilities to become effective communicators through the use of amplification.

Physiological and affective states influence patients' degree of self-efficacy in the performance of certain tasks (Smith & West, 2006). A supportive hearing aid orientation group in quiet and pleasant surroundings may reduce patients' anxiety about their hearing loss and use of amplification. Audiologists should be particularly sensitive to participants' frustration levels in learning new information or skills. The rate of presentation of new information can be slowed down for easier comprehension by older or less educated patients (Smith & West, 2006). It is not uncommon for patients to verbalize with great emotional distress the aggravation in trying to communicate with significant others who refuse to modify their conversational style to facilitate comprehension. Audiologists should listen for "hot button" topics and have participants relax and calmly explain sources of anxiety. Approaching problems with a sense of calmness may generalize to patients' belief in their abilities to master difficult listening situations and partners.

CLASS I

Overall Goals: To inform the patient about the insertion, care, operations, and gradual adjustment schedule regarding hearing aid use. Further, to acquaint the patient with practical use of the telephone and assistive devices.

Specific Objectives:
  (1) Administration of the Communication Performance Assessment
  (2) Review of hearing aid components, switches, and controls
  (3) Review of removal and insertion of the earmold/hearing aid
  (4) Review of cleaning and care of the earmold and the hearing aid
  (5) Maintenance and care of the hearing aid
  (6) Review of the characteristics of the batteries
  (7) Hierarchy of listening experiences and steps in hearing aid use
  (8) Review of listening strategies with amplification
  (9) Practice use of the telephone (demonstration and training)
 (10) Introduction of additional assistive listening devices
 (11) Reschedule for HAO Class II

CLASS II

Overall Goals: To utilize visual cues and supplementary listening skills to facilitate effective communication.

Specific Objectives:
  (1) Review questions from previous class
  (2) Inquire if there are any questions or problems
  (3) Perform a battery check
  (4) Review removal and insertion of earmold or hearing aid
  (5) Review and discuss patient's audiogram
  (6) Perform visual awareness exercises
  (7) Introduce the importance of visual cues
  (8) Introduce speechreading
  (9) Review listening attentiveness activities
 (10) Exercises in situational cues and association techniques
 (11) Exercises in gestures and facial expressions
 (12) Schedule 30-day check and HAO Class III

CLASS III

Overall Goals: To simulate various listening conditions and teach the patient coping strategies. Further, to provide troubleshooting methods for maintenance of hearing aids.

Specific Objectives:
  (1) Review questions from previous class
  (2) Perform a battery check
  (3) Review the importance of visual cues
  (4) Further speechreading practice
  (5) Exercises in identifying contextual cues
  (6) Review keys to effective listening
  (7) Communication strategies
  (8) Tips for communicating with persons with hearing impairment
  (9) Troubleshooting the hearing aid
 (10) Practical speechreading and auditory training in various settings (e.g., hospital cafeteria, auditorium, or use of background party noise tape)
 (11) Re-administration of the Communication Performance Assessment
 (12) Hearing Aid Use and Satisfaction measure
 (13) Present information about hearing aid insurance, the Patient Information Center, and self-help groups
 (14) 30-day check with audiologist

figure *12.14* ————————————————————————

Hearing aid orientation (HAO) curriculum.

Source: Reprinted from *The Hearing Journal,* December 2005, Vol. 58, No. 12, pp. 32–35, by permission of *The Hearing Journal* and its publisher, Lippincott/Williams & Wilkins.

Overall Goals:
- To offer patients who have used hearing instruments in the past and accompanying persons a review about insertion, care, operations, and a gradual schedule of adjustment for new hearing aid use
- To review and practice the use of the telephone, assistive devices, visual cues, and supplementary listening strategies to facilitate effective communication
- To review coping strategies
- To provide troubleshooting methods for maintaining hearing aids

Specific Objectives:
(1)   Provide description of session including goals and objectives
(2)   Complete Hearing Aid Use and Satisfaction Measure for experienced hearing aid users
(3)   Determine each participant's past experience with amplification to include:
    (a)   Type/style
    (b)   How long worn
    (c)   How much worn
    (d)   How amplification has helped
    (e)   Problems experienced
    (f)   Special concerns and questions
(4)   Review hearing aid care, wearing schedule, maintenance, and troubleshooting
(5)   Provide overview of assistive listening devices and systems (ALDs)
(6)   Review communication strategies to include:
    (a)   Listening strategies
    (b)   Visual strategies
    (c)   Contextual and situational cues
(7)   Discuss factors that can control the communication environment to include:
    (a)   Background noise
    (b)   Lighting
    (c)   Distance
    (d)   Preferential seating
    (e)   Restaurant/meeting place exercise
    (f)   Implications for home
(8)   Telephone tips and practice
(9)   Distribute information about:
    (a)   Equipment available for hearing aid maintenance
    (b)   Battery order form
    (c)   Self-Help for Hard-of-Hearing People (SHHH), (Hearing Loss Association of America [HLAA])
    (d)   Local chapter of SHHH
    (e)   Warranty information
    (f)   Insurance information

figure *12.15* —————————————————————————

Suggested hearing aid refresher (HAR) curriculum.

Source: Reprinted from *The Hearing Journal*, December 2005, Vol. 58, No. 12, pp. 32–35, by permission of *The Hearing Journal* and its publisher, Lippincott/Williams & Wilkins.

Outcome Measures for Hearing Aid Orientation Groups

We have discussed the use of outcome measures for patients in Chapter 6 on amplification. However, outcome measurement of hearing aid orientation groups warrants some discussion. Kricos and Lesner (2000) suggested using the following methods for evaluating these programs:

- Observations by professional staff
- Attendance patterns
- Knowledge area tests

- Measures of hearing aid use
- Measures of hearing aid benefit
- Measures of hearing aid satisfaction

Audiologists and speech-language pathologists can observe participants' application of skills learned in the group during the social interaction portion of the hearing aid orientation group. For example, staff may use the TOPICON rating sheet to assess generalization of communication strategies to general conversations. Moreover, Johnson and Danhauer (1999) adapted additional information provided by Kricos and Lesner (1997) into development of the *Hearing Aid Orientation Group Interaction Checklist* that assesses characteristics of interactive portions of hearing aid orientation groups (see Appendix 12.3). For example, clinicians should occupy no more than 30% talk time during interactive portions of these sessions (Kricos & Lesner, 1997). Other outcome measures are the attendance records of participants and their significant others. If the hearing aid orientation group is enjoyable and useful, patients usually attend. However, attendance may decline if the group fails to meet participants' expectations and needs.

Knowledge area tests can also be excellent formative outcome measures for the instructional portion of hearing aid orientation groups by quizzing participants' recall of the information covered during the previous week's session. For example, audiologists and/or speech-language pathologists may devise skits showing appropriate and inappropriate conversational behaviors. Participants can problem-solve, offering suggestions for improvement in a nonthreatening atmosphere. Assessment can also be more formal through administration of written quizzes and demonstration of new skills.

Measures of hearing aid use, benefit, and satisfaction can also be useful outcome measures for hearing aid orientation groups. For example, Kricos and Lesner (1997) developed a series of questions adapted by Johnson and Danhauer (1999) into a *Hearing Aid Skills Checklist* that professional staff can use when unobtrusively observing participants' use of amplification (see Appendix 12.4). Audiologists can also choose to administer traditional outcome measures after completion of the hearing aid orientation group to measure benefit (e.g., *Abbreviated Profile of Hearing Aid Benefit* [Cox & Alexander, 1998]) or satisfaction (e.g., *Satisfaction with Amplification in Daily Life* [Cox & Alexander, 1999]) from amplification.

What Does the Evidence Show?

Hawkins (2005) conducted a systematic review on the efficacy of counseling-based group auditory rehabilitation programs. His search focused on studies that (1) had adult participants with hearing impairment; (2) involved group auditory rehabilitation programs; (3) used a randomized, controlled clinical trial, quasi-experimental, or pre- and post-intervention design; (4) utilized outcome measures for HRQoL, hearing aid benefit and satisfaction; and (5) were published in peer-reviewed journals. The strategy involved using relevant search strings in three search engines and inspecting references in articles and textbooks. Twelve studies were identified and were included in the systematic review, although some had risk of bias. The author concluded that there was good evidence to support the contention that group auditory rehabilitation based on counseling resulted in improved HRQoL (e.g., reduction in self-perceived hearing handicap) and better use of communication strategies and hearing aids.

Additional Auditory Rehabilitation

The communication problems of elderly patients are often successfully addressed through the placement of hearing aids and through the use of HAT. Some seniors, however, require additional auditory rehabilitation to reap the full benefits of amplification. In particular, some adults fitted with frequency transposition hearing aids or cochlear implants may need individual therapy to restructure listening strategies (Abrahamson, 2001). Audiologists and speech-language pathologists provide one-on-one auditory rehabilitation with seniors and may work on audiovisual speech reception and conversational fluency. Baseline performances obtained during the auditory rehabilitation evaluation establish the need for and starting points for therapy, which is usually provided on a short-term basis. Clinicians may use their own or commercially available materials that have been compiled by Abrahamson (2001) and are shown in the following lists.

Complete Curricula

- *Learning to Hear Again: An Audiologic Rehabilitation Guide, Second Edition* (Wayner & Abrahamson, 2000)
- *Learning to Hear Again with a Cochlear Implant; An Audiologic Rehabilitation Curriculum Guide* (Wayner, Abrahamson, Casterton, 1998)

Auditory and Auditory/Visual Perceptual Training and Speechreading

- *Hear Again at Home: A Home Training Program for Adults with Hearing Loss: Receiver's Manual* (Plant, 2000a)
- *Hear Again at Home: A Home Training Program for Adults with Hearing Loss: Talker's Manual* (2000b)
- *Communication Training for Older Teenagers and Adults: Listening, Speechreading, and Using Conversational Strategies* (Tye-Murray, 1998)
- *Quest?AR: Communication Practice* (Erber 1996)
- *Analytica: Analytical Testing and Training Lists* (Plant, 1998)

Complete curricula contain activities and materials for all aspects of group and individual auditory rehabilitation. Wayner and Abrahamson (2001) developed a complete curriculum, *Learning to Hear Again, Second Edition*, which is replete with specific activities, instructions, and ready-to-use materials that may be duplicated for patients and their families. The program addresses many topics regarding hearing aids, HAT, communication strategies, and organized into a three-ring binder. The authors also developed *Learning to Hear Again with a Cochlear Implant: An Audiologic Rehabilitation Curriculum Guide* composed of activities and materials for telephone use, communication strategies, speechreading, and auditory training for cochlear implant users and their families. Purchase of these curricula provides clinicians with everything they need in providing auditory rehabilitation.

As mentioned in Chapter 6, speechreading is a process by which listeners put together information from a variety of sources (e.g., lipreading; facial expressions; gesture, posture, and movement; situational cues; the topic of conversation; rules of the language; news of the day; motivation to understand; and residual hearing) to derive meaning (Cherry & Rubenstein, 1988). A general orientation to speechreading is to explain to patients that it is a lot more than lipreading, or watching the speaker and deriving meaning from recognition of the visible aspects of articulation. Speechreading is using the mind to make a good guess in understanding what someone is trying to say by using the following (Cherry & Rubenstein, 1988):

- lipreading: What sounds are identifiable from the visible aspects of phoneme production?
- facial expressions: How do facial expressions provide insight into what is being said?
- gesture, posture, and movement: How does body language provide clues as to what is being said?
- situational cues: How can situational cues assist in figuring out what people are saying?
- knowing the topic: How can knowing the topic assist in understanding what is said during a conversation?
- knowledge of the language: How can knowledge of the language help to fill in gaps in a message?
- keeping informed: How can keeping informed on current events assist in understanding what people are talking about?
- emotional factors: How can motivation and self-confidence aid in understanding what is being said?
- residual hearing: How can residual hearing be used to understand what is being said?

Therapy may include creating scenarios in which patients are provided some information, but must use cues to figure out the complete message. For example, clinicians may present a sentence without context, such as "My name is Barbara and I will be taking care of you tonight. What would you like to drink?" and ask patients to repeat what was said. Patients may have difficulty even getting a few words correct. However, if they are told that they have just been seated at a restaurant, patients will quickly understand the importance of contextual cues and how knowledge of typical situations can assist in decoding messages.

Patients need to be made aware of how they, their communicative partners, the environment, and the message affect communication. Patients need to be aware that their vision affects their ability to speechread and that their visual acvity needs to be at least 20/40 to be able to access all of the visible aspects of speech (Hipskind, 2007). They must understand that they need to keep motivated and that some people are better at speechreading than others. Similarly, they need to realize that some communicative partners may be easier to speechread than others. Those who speak clearly and naturally and are clean shaven are easier to speechread than those who are not. It is more difficult to speechread someone who is smoking or chewing when speaking. Moreover, communicative partners who are aware of the communicative needs of those with hearing loss will naturally try to provide the necessary visual cues. Patients need to be made cognizant of the importance of seeking environmental conditions conducive for optimal speechreading such as speaker-to-listener distances of 3 to 5 feet and viewing angles of 0 to 45 degrees. Also, adequate lighting and an avoidance of glare aid in creating an environment that facilitates communication. In addition, patients can be shown how some aspects of the message are easier to speechread than others. Certain sounds that look the same on the mouth, causing listeners the most confusion, are called **visemes.** The following table shows eight different viseme groups, their visible characteristics, and the phonemes, both voiced (v) and voiceless (vs), appearing in real words (adapted from Cherry & Rubenstein, 1988). The consonants /p/, /b/, and /m/ are all in the same viseme group and are **homophones** and **homophonous** with each other. Homophones are phonemes in the same viseme group (e.g., /p/, /b/, and /m/); homophonous means that sounds look the same on the mouth such as /p/, /b/, and /m/ all being made with the lips closed.

Viseme Groups	Visible Characteristics	Example Words
p (vs), b (v), m (v)	Lips closed	pat, bat, mat
f (vs), v (v)	Upper teeth touch lower lip	fat, vat
th (vs), th (v)	Tongue between teeth	thistle, though
wh (v), r (v)	Lips rounded	why, rye
sh (vs), zh (v), tsh (vs), dzh (v)	Teeth together; lips rounded	shop, azure, chat, gym
s (vs), z (v)	Teeth closed; lips in a smile	side, zoom
t (vs). d (v), n (v), l (v)	Tongue tip up	tide, died, nine, line
k (vs), g (v), ng (v)	Back of tongue tip up	riK, riG, ring

Two different approaches to speechreading training have emerged over the years: **analytic** and **synthetic**. Analytic approaches are based on the premise that the individual parts (e.g., syllables) of the message must be identified before the whole message can be understood. Synthetic approaches are based on the notion that a basic understanding of the entire message is important regardless of which individual parts are identified. The following table compares and contrasts the analytic versus synthetic approach to speechreading (Hipskind, 2007).

	Analytic	Synthetic
Definition	An approach to speechreading based on the premise that individual parts (e.g., syllables) must be identified prior to the understanding of the entire message	An approach to speechreading built on the notion that a general understanding of the entire message is most important, regardless of which of the individual parts are identified
Basic Unit	Syllable	Sentence
Strategy	Start with highly contrastive phonemic elements, progressing to finer discriminations	Start with highly contextually dependent materials and work toward more novel content
Example of Behavioral Objectives	• Patient will correctly discriminate among words with /i/ versus /u/ (e.g., "beet" versus "boot") • Patient will discriminate consonant pairs that differ in place of production and share either voice or manner (e.g., "kite" versus "tight")	Patient will speechread a narrative and then answer questions about its content
Example Materials	Lists of words with specific phonemic contrasts	Sentences, paragraphs, stories that have appropriate content and provide context for the development of speechreading abilities

Clinicians can make or use preexisting curricula; most of the materials mentioned previously offer activities and materials for speechreading. Creating materials for analytic speechreading training may be extremely time consuming. Therefore, Abrahamson (2001) recommended Plant's (1994) *ANALYTICA: Analytic Testing and Training Lists*, which contains 379 lists of monosyllabic words that differ by a single phoneme.

Conversational fluency was defined earlier in the chapter as the ability to participate in a discussion with one or more individuals with a minimum of requests for clarification, an easy conveying of ideas, and turn-taking that results in a sharing of speaking time (Erber, 1993; Tye-Murray, 2008). Older adults with hearing loss need to realize that everyone has breakdowns in communication. The major task is to teach them about ways of detecting breakdowns and unobtrusive strategies for repair shown in the following table with examples of their use (Tye-Murray, 2008).

Strategy	Example of Use
Repetition	"Could you please repeat the beginning of the sentence?"
Rephrasing	"Could you please say that in another way? I'm not following you."
Elaboration	"Could you tell me a little more?"
Simplification	"Could you say that again using fewer words?"
Indication of the Topic	"What are you talking about now? I'm not following you."
Confirmation of the Message	"Your phone number is 555-2453?"
Provision of Feedback	"You are talking loud enough, but could you slow down just a little?"
Writing the Message Down	"Could you please write that down for me?"
Fingerspelling	"Could you fingerspell that name for me?"

Clinicians can demonstrate these skills to patients and their family first in therapy, then with guided practice, and then they can use them in their day-to-day interactions with others. Progress can be measured post-intervention using the same techniques for assessment in the auditory rehabilitation evaluation.

Home-Based Auditory Rehabilitation

In today's fast-paced world, adults who are deaf and hard of hearing may find it difficult to find either the time or the availability of individual auditory rehabilitation therapy in their communities. Similarly, audiologists and speech-language pathologists may find it difficult to get reimbursed for these services. Fortunately, technological advancements have enabled the delivery of auditory rehabilitative training via computers allowing for a consistent, cost-effective, and convenient way of bringing therapy into patients' homes (Sweetow & Sabes, 2007). Moreover, few audiologists offer these as part of their services, and there is no insurance coverage for these programs (Ross, 2005).

Ross (2005) reviewed four home-based auditory training programs available via the computer and the Internet. One program is the *Listening and Communication Enhancement*

(LACE), which focuses on auditory training in addition to a few communication tips. LACE was developed by Robert Sweetow, Ph.D., an audiologist at the University of California at San Francisco. The program is four weeks long and requires the completion of 30-minute sessions five days a week. The types of listening tasks with specific purposes in the program include:

- recognizing speech in babble to prepare for listening in noise
- understanding rapid speech to keep up with fast talkers
- discerning speech in competition with a single speaker to zero in on specific talkers
- repeating words that appear before a target word in a sentence to improve memory
- selecting the correct word that was completely masked when presented in a sentence to improve processing and use of contextual cues

Recent evidence suggests that LACE training demonstrates significant improvements. For example, using a between-group, within-subject design with pre- and post-training objective and subjective outcome measures, Sweetow and Sabes (2006) randomly assigned 65 participants to two groups. One group received LACE training immediately following baseline testing, and another group received training as a cross-over group. Participants receiving LACE training demonstrated statistically significant improvements in all but one outcome measure. Sweetow and Sabes stated that a possible limitation in the widespread application of LACE is that not everyone is a computer user. In a larger study, Henderson-Sabes and Sweetow (2007) found that patients who had the poorest baseline scores, greatest degree of loss, and highest hearing handicap scores achieved the greatest amount of benefit from LACE training, although there was great variability among participants. They also reported that some patients with modest amounts of objective improvement reported subjective impressions with LACE training. Some contraindications for using LACE include having:

- less than an eighth-grade reading level
- a poor command of the English language
- a serious cognitive impairment
- insufficient manual dexterity to use a computer mouse, keyboard, or DVD remote
- significant vision problems

LACE may be purchased through Neurotone (www.neurotone.com).

A second program, *Sound and Beyond,* developed by the House Ear Institute, consists of eight modules. This program focuses on auditory training and communication tips for cochlear implant users, or hearing aid users with severe to profound hearing loss. *Sound and Beyond* consists of a variety of listening tasks of varying difficulty. Patients' starting points are determined through an assessment process. The listening modules provide users with immediate feedback. Users can stop, rewind, and replay stimuli as often as desired. Some of the specific tasks include (1) same/different pure-tone recognition, (2) identification of environmental sounds in quiet and in noise, (3) male versus female voice identification, (4) vowel and consonant recognition, (5) word discrimination, and (6) music appreciation: identification of musical instruments and melodies. Each task builds in complexity, depending on the accuracy of patients' responses. For example, for the stimuli in the same/different pure-tone recognition task, the difference in pitch separation for the target tone are distinct at first but are quite similar in more advanced training tasks. *Sound and Beyond* is available through the Cochlear Corporation.

Another home-based auditory training program is *Seeing and Hearing Speech* distributed by the Sensimetrics Corporation in Somerville, Massachusetts. The program consists of four training modules: (1) vowels; (2) consonants; (3) stress, intonation, and length; and (4) everyday communication. Each training module is preceded by an explanation of the content (e.g., articulatory movements and communication tips), and training stimuli can be presented auditory-only, visually-only, or audiovisually based on patients' training needs. The training stimuli can be presented via a variety of talkers, at different loudness levels, and in the presence of six different types of noise based on patients' needs. The idea is for the patient to select a challenging stimulus, but not one that is impossible. The program has both practice and test conditions. The practice conditions require that the patient select the particular stimulus. However, the test conditions present the stimuli in a random order. Patients are provided immediate feedback regarding their performance and, if unsuccessful, may opt to try again or go on to the next item.

Another home-based auditory training program is *Conversation Made Easy* by Nancy Tye-Murray, available from the Central Institute of the Deaf in St. Louis, Missouri. The program consists of three training modules accessible on five CDs: (1) Sounds (one CD), (2) Sentences (two CDs), and (3) Everyday Situations (two CDs). The Sounds program consists of a speaker producing a syllable that a patient must identify by selecting from a series of 3 to 12 foils. Patients receive immediate feedback because when an error is made, the stimulus is repeated and the correct answer is presented. The Sounds program was designed to help patients distinguish between sounds that look or sound the same during production. All consonants of the English language are utilized and are presented in varying vowel context. The Sentences program consists of 160 sentences that are divided into 8 exercises with 20 sentences each. A speaker presents a sentence, and patients select a picture that best represents the meaning of the stimulus. In this way, patients have to understand just the meaning of the sentence rather than recall it verbatim. If an incorrect picture is selected, the patient selects from five different repair strategies that present the primary sentence in a variety of ways: (1) repetition, (2) simplification, (3) rephrasing, (4) use of key words, and (5) modification into two shorter sentences. The goal of this program is to train patients to be assertive communicators by use of appropriate conversational repair strategies. The Everyday Situations program consists of a number of video clips of typical communication situations (e.g., party, restaurant). Each video ends with a speaker saying an utterance that patients must understand by selecting a picture from four foils presented on the screen that best matches the meaning of the message. This program trains conversational repair strategies in the same way as the Sentences program and includes additional conversational repair strategies such as having the patient inform the speaker how to remedy the communication situation (e.g., to look at the listener when talking).

COCHLEAR IMPLANTS AND THE ELDERLY

Cochlear implants have been shown to be a viable treatment for adults with severe to profound hearing loss who do not receive much benefit from amplification. However, cochlear implant surgery has risks that some may feel are too great to consider this treatment option for the elderly. As described in Chapter 8, cochlear implantation requires general surgery. For patients over 70 years old, the risks of dying are 5 to 10 times greater than for younger patients undergoing the same surgical procedure (Kozak, 1993). Elderly patients should have a presurgical assessment to detect the presence of any cardiopulmonary diseases and other related risk

Flap Wound	Temporal Bone/ Central
• Flap necrosis	Nervous System
• Wound separation	• Facial paresis or palsy
• Wound infection	• Facial nerve stimulation
	• Perilymphatic fistula
Device-Related	• Tympanic membrane perforation
• Intrinsic device failure	• Meningitis
• Extracochlear insertion	• Dizziness or vertigo
• Compressed electrode	• Taste disturbance
• Device migration	• Tinnitus alterations

figure *12.16* —————————————————

Otologic complications from cochlear implant surgery.

Source: Based on "Cochlear Implants in the Geriatric Population: Benefits Outweigh Risks," by C. A. Buchman, M. J. Fucci, and W. M. Luxford, 1999, *Ear, Nose, and Throat Journal, 78*, p. 492.

factors (e.g., diabetes mellitus, coronary artery disease, stroke) (Buchman, Fucci, & Luxford, 1999).

In addition to the inherent risks of general surgery, cochlear implantation presents some otologic complications. For example, Figure 12.16 shows possible otologic complications from cochlear implant surgery with the elderly being more susceptible to flap problems due to a compromised blood supply that might be caused by chronic hypertension, diabetes mellitus, or atherosclerotic vaso-occlusive disease, or because of thinning skin (Buchman et al., 1999, p. 492). Recall that the surgeon must peel back a flap of skin and muscle to expose the bone during surgery. The skin tissue can die due to compromised blood supply, or the surgical wound could become separated and infected. However, Buchman et al. (1999) stated that most flap/wound and device-related risks can be avoided with proper preparations.

Buchman et al. (1999) stated that of all the possible temporal bone or central nervous system complications, dizziness and vertigo are of most concern for the elderly who often have multisensory (e.g., visual, vestibular, or proprioceptive) balance disturbance or vertigo. Cochlear implantation may further disturb an already impaired vestibular system (Brey et al., 1995). Therefore, Buchman and colleagues (1999) recommended that elderly patients with uncompensated vestibulopathy or significant imbalance should have a preoperative vestibular evaluation to determine the risk-benefit ratio when considering cochlear implants.

Research has shown that the elderly benefit as much as younger adults from cochlear implantation. For example, Chan and colleagues (2007) conducted a retrospective chart review and found that older adults between the ages of 56 and 77 performed comparably to a group of younger adults who were primarily under 50 years of age, but were matched for duration of profound sensorineural hearing loss. Similarly, Labadie, Carrasco, Gilmer, and Pillsbury (2000) did a retrospective analysis of postlingually deafened individuals and found no significant difference between operative time, anesthesia time, length of hospitalization, or word recognition scores between younger (mean age = 46.9 years) and older adults (mean age = 71.5 years). The results of these studies suggest that elderly adults should not be discriminated against when considering candidacy for cochlear implantation. See Chapter 8 for further discussion of older adults and cochlear implantation.

HEARING HEALTHCARE IN LONG-TERM RESIDENTIAL CARE FACILITIES FOR THE ELDERLY

Increasingly, communication sciences and disorders professionals will find themselves providing services to elderly persons in long-term residential care facilities. Before we consider the realities of this service delivery site, let's consider an all-too-common scenario for the elderly in long-term care.

Casebook Reflection

Beatrice and Long-Term Care

Beatrice, an 86-year-old stroke survivor with a bilaterally severe sensorineural hearing loss, had recently recovered from a broken hip and was well cared for by her husband, Duke. They had just celebrated their 60th wedding anniversary. Duke had been the picture of health until he had a massive heart attack and passed away. Beatrice was all alone in the world. She felt overwhelmed in her big house all by herself.

Beatrice was so glad to see her daughter, Vivian, her son, Vick, and their families who had traveled all the way from California to attend Duke's funeral. Vivian and Vick realized that their mother could no longer live by herself in that huge house. Vick's family and Vivian and her family returned to California after the funeral. Vick stayed behind to help his mother with the estate.

Beatrice could understand everything when wearing her hearing aids, although she had difficulty keeping up with a fast-paced conversation. Due to her stroke, Beatrice had a difficult time expressing herself and was partially paralyzed on one side, precluding independent use of hearing aids. She was able to use a walker, but felt safest in a wheelchair. Duke had recently purchased a motorized chair so she could zip around the house and garden. Beatrice enjoyed going to church, friends' houses, and playing bingo at the Elks Club. Beatrice no longer drove and had relied on her husband to communicate for her and to assist her with the activities of daily living, but now he was gone.

Vick and Vivian recommended putting the family house up for sale and placing their mother in a long-term care facility. Beatrice did not like the idea, but there were few alternatives. Vick visited the facility to discuss his mother's move. Although he stated that she had a hearing loss, he did not mention that she had hearing aids. Vick had already missed two weeks of work. He told Beatrice that he, Vivian, and their families would

be back at Christmastime to visit. Beatrice hugged her son as she was taken to her room in a wheelchair. In the evening, the nurse's assistant helped Beatrice undress and get ready for bed and removed her hearing aids and placed them in the dresser drawer.

The next morning, another nurse's assistant introduced herself and helped Beatrice with bathing and dressing, placed her into a wheelchair, and took her to the cafeteria. Beatrice kept pointing to the dresser drawer and her ears while vocalizing, but the nurse's assistant did not pay any attention to her. Beatrice ate and then another nurse's assistant took her to the television room. Beatrice tried to get the attention of staff by pointing to her ears and yelling hearing aids, but her speech was unintelligible and the nurse's assistants just shook their heads. Soon it was time for lunch, more television, then dinner, and then bedtime. The next morning, Beatrice was able to get the nurse's assistant to open the dresser drawer and take out her hearing aids. She tried to put them in Beatrice's ears, but with no success. She and Beatrice became frustrated, but the nurse's assistant had to get Beatrice to the cafeteria so she wouldn't miss breakfast. The nurse's assistant left the hearing aids on Beatrice's bed with the intention of bringing them to the attention of the head nurse. She got involved with another resident and forgot about Beatrice's hearing aids, which were scooped up with the laundry. Beatrice never knew what happened to her hearing aids. She soon just gave up.

By Christmastime, Beatrice was withdrawn and noncommunicative. The staff physician became increasingly concerned about her because she was lying in bed all day and eating very little. Vick and Vivian flew out early and were shocked to see how their mom had deteriorated in only a few months. Vick asked about his mother's hearing aids and the nursing staff said they did not know she had any.

Scenarios such as Beatrice's are all too common. The prevalence of hearing loss is high in residents of these facilities; few receive the adequate auditory rehabilitation for their problems (Ferguson & Nerbonne, 2003; Garahan, Waller, Houghton, Tisdale, & Runge, 1992; Schow, 1982; Thibodeau & Schmitt, 1988). For example, Cohen-Mansfield and Taylor (2004a, 2004b) estimated that 70–90% of elderly residents in long-term care facilities have some degree of hearing impairment. These investigators assessed the rates of hearing impairment and hearing aid use among residents of a large long-term care facility in the mid-Atlantic region of the United States; they estimated that this condition went undetected in over half of the residents. Some of the reasons for hearing aid nonuse in these facilities were lack of knowledge of staff members, inappropriate delegation and care procedures, hearing instrument design and fit issues, and difficulty in residents' handling of devices (Cohen-Mansfield & Taylor, 2004b).

Service provision in these facilities is challenging, but should be comprehensive in its scope and function. Audiologists rarely provide consistent services in these facilities due to logistical complications and lack of reimbursement for their efforts. Johnson and Danhauer (1999) initiated the concept of developing auditory rehabilitation support programs in long-term residential care facilities to ensure that residents who are deaf and hard of hearing may meet the communication needs of their environments. Support programs are necessary when traditional auditory rehabilitation service provision may be difficult and require the participation of audiologists, speech-language pathologists, other allied-health personnel, physicians, family members, and residents. Support programs may provide a "safety net" in ensuring communication accessibility for these residents. Figure 12.17 shows the possible components of a support program in the area of patient, facility, and special services.

Patient Services

Within two weeks of admission to a long-term residential care facility for the elderly, patients should have their hearing screened and necessary referrals made (ASHA, 1997). The Omnibus Reconciliation Act (OBRA, 1987) determined the nature and care provided to residents in long-term care facilities. For example, all nursing-home residents receiving federal support must be assessed using a form called the Minimum Data Set for Nursing Home Resident Assessment and Care Screening (MDS) (OBRA, 1987). Section C of the MDS, "Communication/Hearing Patterns," contains two questions pertaining to residents' adequacy of hearing for everyday functioning with hearing aids.

Otoscopy and pure-tone hearing screening should be conducted whenever possible. Valid audiometric screenings and diagnostic hearing evaluations may be difficult to obtain due to the high ambient noise levels within the environment. Lankford and Hopkins (2000) assessed ambient noise levels in 10 different nursing-home settings and compared the results to the American National Standards Institute S3.1 1999 criteria for maximum permissible noise levels and suggested the use of insert earphones when sound-treated booths are not available.

An otoscopic examination should be completed to inspect for the presence of cerumen impaction and collapsing ear canals and to assess the integrity of the tympanic membrane (Schultz & Mowry, 1995). Following otoscopy, residents should undergo pure-tone air-conduction screening at 500, 1000, 2000, and 4000 Hz at 30 dB HL (Schultz & Mowry, 1995). Valid pure-tone hearing screening sometimes is not possible at 500 Hz due to

Patients Services
- Audiometric and receptive-communication screening
- Cerumen management program
- Diagnostic hearing evaluations
- Hearing aid fitting
- Hearing aid evaluation
- Hearing aid repair
- Hearing aid maintenance program
- Hearing assistive technology: selection, fitting, and orientation
- Direct consultation with residents, physicians, families, social workers, nursing staff, and significant others
- Weekly in-house visits
- Emergency services

Facility Services
- Ombudsman Reconciliation Act: Receptive Communication Classification of All New Admissions—Minimum Data Set (MDS)
- Patient-specific screening report for medical records
- Inservice training
- Americans with Disabilities Act (ADA): Review and Recommendations for Compliance
- Fall prevention

Special Services
- Hospice-patient care
- Fundraising
- Hearing aid safety cords

figure *12.17* ————————————————————————————

Components of auditory rehabilitation support programs in long-term residential care facilities for the elderly.

Source: Based on "Older Adults in Long-term Care Facilities," by D. Schultz and R. B. Mowry, 1995, in P. B. Kricos and S. A. Lesner (Eds.), *Hearing Care for the Older Adult: Audiologic Rehabilitation*, pp. 167–184, Boston: Butterworth-Heinemann.

ambient noise levels. If pure-tone hearing screening is not possible, then the following questions should be asked of residents (ASHA, 1997):

- Does the person require repetition of verbal questions, instructions, or messages?
- Has a family member or caregiver voiced concerns about the adequacy of the individual's hearing?
- Does the person complain of current or past difficulty hearing or understanding?
- Does the person complain of current or past history of head noise, ear pain, or ear discharge?

If the answer to any of these questions is "yes," then appropriate referrals should be made to PCPs and/or for audiologic services. The results of any screening procedures should be documented in a report for placement into patients' files.

Patients failing hearing screenings should be referred for either cerumen management and/or audiologic evaluation. The prevalence for impacted cerumen among nursing-home residents has been found to be as high as 34% (Mahoney, 1993). Moore, Voytas, Kowalski, and Maddens (2002) found that 65% of residents in a skilled nursing facility had impacted cerumen in at least one ear and that hearing and cognitive status improved after management of the problem as compared with a control group of peers. Risk factors for cerumen impaction include ear canal hairs, use of hearing aids, bony growths resulting from osteophytes or osteomas, and past history of ear wax impaction (Meador, 1995). Although cerumen management can be performed by a variety of healthcare professionals, it is within the audiologist's scope of practice to do so (ASHA, 2004; Ballachanda, 1995). Audiologic evaluations on-site in long-term care facilities are difficult due to ambient noise levels and transportation of equipment. Ideally, arrangements for transportation from the facility to an audiology clinic would make audiologic evaluations and hearing aid evaluation and fitting appointments possible for residents.

Evaluating and fitting residents of long-term care facilities with hearing aids does not guarantee success. Cohen-Mansfield and Taylor (2004b) found that 69% of residents in a large, not-for-profit long-term care facility had problems with their hearing aids. Moreover, the vast majority (86%) of those residents needed assistance in managing the devices. Unfortunately, less than half of the staff had any training on the care and use of hearing aids. In addition, for almost one-third of the hearing aid users, no responsibility for assisting the resident had been assigned within the facility. Cohen-Mansfield and Taylor (2004b) state that increasing hearing aid use in this population requires change at multiple levels, including at the institutional level, establishing policy by mandating staff training and, at the individual unit level, by developing care/follow-up procedures. For example, facility administrators must make a commitment to promote the successful use of hearing aids by residents. At the unit level, the nursing staff should organize a hearing aid maintenance program based on the needs of each resident regarding his or her level of care. Long-term care facilities have multiple levels of independence. Therefore, a hearing aid monitoring program should reflect multiple levels according to patients' ability to use and care for their devices. The *Guidelines for Audiology Service Delivery in Nursing Homes* (ASHA, 1997) has four levels of care: independent, partial assistance, full assistance, and supervised use.

At the **independent level**, patients are completely responsible for their hearing aids. For example, these patients can insert/remove their own hearing aids, work the controls, and test/change their own hearing aid batteries. Patients who live in assisted living facilities may benefit from installation of a Hearing Aid Check station in a common area equipped with hearing aid stethoscopes, battery checkers, forced-air bulbs, wax picks, alcohol pads, and so on. Patients should be instructed to report any problems with loss of, or damage to, their hearing aids either to family members, nursing staff, or an audiologist.

The **partial assistance level** is also for patients who are primarily responsible for the care and maintenance of their hearing aids, but they may need assistance with these tasks. For example, patients may have limited ability to lift their arms high enough to insert or remove their hearing aids.

The **full assistance level** is appropriate for patients who do not have the ability to care for their hearing aids. Most often, the nursing staff holds the hearing aids and puts them on patients in the morning and retrieves them at night. At this time, nurses should remove the batteries and place the hearing aids into dehumidifiers to remove excess moisture. The dehumidifiers should be labeled with each patient's name and room number. The nursing staff is also responsible for completing daily visual and listening inspections on patients' hearing instruments and performing basic troubleshooting requiring hearing aid check kits at nurses' stations.

The **supervised-use level** is one in which the nursing staff assumes complete responsibility for patients' hearing aids. In fact, patients can use hearing aids only with one-on-one supervision of staff members. Patients requiring supervised use usually have some sort of cognitive impairment such as AD. As in other levels of hearing aid assistance, the nursing staff is required to maintain care of hearing aids and report any significant problems to audiologists. Audiologists can make weekly visits to provide on-site care to residents with hearing aids. Furthermore, audiologists can be in direct consultation with residents, physicians, families, social workers, and so on regarding hearing healthcare and hearing aids. Provisions can be made for emergency services that could include express delivery of hearing aids needing repair and use of loaner hearing aids.

Facility Services

Auditory rehabilitation support programs also include services to facilities. One important service audiologists can provide is the receptive communication screening for all new admissions in addition to generating the screening records for residents' files. Other services include inservices for nursing, administrative, and ancillary staff; Americans With Disabilities Act (1990) compliance review and audit; and a fall prevention program.

Inservice Training. Inservices are classes offered to healthcare professionals and paraprofessionals that teach knowledge and skills to assist in the execution of their on-the-job duties. Some healthcare professionals must earn a specified amount of **continuing education units** to meet state licensure and national board certification requirements. Inservices can be informational, skill-based, or a combination of informational and skill-based. Informational inservices are didactic and are presented in a lecture format. Skill-based formats teach participants skills via learning laboratories. Informational and skill-based inservices use both formats for conveying knowledge and teaching new skills. Different inservice formats require different learning environments. For example, informational inservices can be conducted in meeting rooms. However, skill-based inservices require rooms with moveable furniture and ample space for necessary equipment and practice.

An inservice program is critical for development of auditory rehabilitation support programs. Audiologists and speech-language pathologists have the expertise to provide inservices to staff on topics such as how to communicate with seniors who have hearing loss; assist residents with the use and care of their hearing aids, hearing assistive technology, and cochlear implants; basic principles of the Americans With Disabilities Act (1990); and so on. Audiologists and speech-language pathologists need to know the characteristics of effective inservice programs.

Effective inservice programs have six defining characteristics. First, inservices should be taught by licensed audiologists and speech-language pathologists. Second, inservices should be competency-based, specifically addressing what participants will know and be able to do. Skill-based inservices on the care and use of hearing aids should have specific learning objectives such as, "By attending this inservice, participants will be able to check the voltage of any size battery, determine its adequacy, and then replace it, if necessary." Third, inservices should be well-equipped and staffed such that there should be enough battery checkers, batteries, and hearing aids for each participant to have ample practice with the devices. In addition, for skill-based inservices, the instructor-to-participant ratio should be no more than 1 to 4. Fourth, inservice programming should be ongoing and current. Because these facilities experience frequent staff turnover, the same sequence of inservices should be presented throughout the year for new hires and to refresh the knowledge and skills of others. Moreover, inservices should include the latest technology such as teaching competencies with new styles of hearing aids. Fifth, inservices should be well-documented in that upcoming events should be advertised using appropriate signage indicating topic, time, and place, and certificates of completion should be placed in participants' personnel files. Sixth, inservices should be rigorously evaluated in terms of participants' knowledge/skills and impressions of the learning experience. Although knowledge gleaned from informational inservices can be assessed via paper-and-pencil tests, participants should be expected to demonstrate new skills (e.g., insertion and removal of hearing aids from residents' ears). Instructors should routinely solicit participants' evaluations of the inservices so that improvements can be made. Knowledgeable staff are essential for successful auditory rehabilitation support programs in long-term care facilities. For example, all staff should know about the Americans With Disabilities Act (ADA, 1990) and follow any facility rules about compliance with this law.

Americans With Disabilities Act (ADA: 1990) Compliance Review and Audit.   The ADA (1990), discussed in Chapters 10 and 11, is a federal law passed in 1990 (Public Law 101-336) to provide protection from discrimination based on an individual's disability. The law has five major sections: (1) Employment, (2) Public Services and Transportation, (3) Public Accommodations and Commercial Facilities, (4) Telecommunications, and (5) Miscellaneous Provisions. Hearing loss is but one of a myriad of disabilities to consider. Communication sciences and disorders professionals should be aware of what is required under the law and ways to improve communication accessibility when providing services to the elderly. Effective communication under the ADA means that reasonable measures are taken to ensure that people with hearing impairment have access to goods, services, and facilities; are not excluded, denied services, segregated, or treated differently from others; and that information is accessible and useable (ASHA, 1991). Providing necessary auxiliary communication aids and services and making auditory information available to persons who are deaf and hard of hearing is required to achieve effective communication under the ADA. The following is a list of ways in which long-term residential care facilities may comply with the ADA (ASHA, 1991):

- Establishing appropriate attitudes and behaviors
- Modifying the communication setting
- Providing auxiliary aids and services
- Responding to auxiliary aids and services requests
- Providing materials in accessible formats
- Keeping written materials simple and direct
- Providing visual as well as auditory information
- Providing a means for written exchange of information
- Informing the public of available accommodations
- Maintaining devices in good working condition
- Consulting communication sciences and disorders professionals

Fall Prevention.   Thirty percent to 40% per year of elderly adults who live independently experience a fall, and the frequency of falling increases with age (Rao, 2005). Falls result in injuries, such as hip fractures, and reduced HRQoL (Cranney et al., 2005). As discussed earlier, falls in the elderly can result from a myriad of causes. However, approximately one-third of falls may be attributable to accidents and environmental hazards and another third due to gait issues, balance disorders, or weakness (Rubenstein & Josephson, 2002).

Falls are a problem in long-term residential care facilities, too. Each year, a typical 100-bed nursing home reports 100 to 200 falls, but many falls go unreported (Rubenstein, 1997). Of those falls, 1,800 are fatal, while 10% to 20% result in serious injuries with 2% to 6% of those causing fractures (Rubenstein, Robbins, Schulman, Rosado, & Osterweil, 1988). Figure 12.18 lists possible causes for falls in nursing homes, and Figure 12.19 describes how to assess a patient after a fall.

What Does the Evidence Show?

Gillespie and colleagues (2009) conducted a systematic review of randomized controlled clinical trials assessing the effectiveness of various interventions for preventing the risk and rate of falls of elderly persons living in the community. The risk of falls is the likelihood of taking a spill; the rate of falls is the actual number that occurs during a period of time. The investigators searched multiple databases and ultimately included 111 trials involving 55,203 participants. They found that the following interventions reduced the risk (rif) and/or rate (raf) of falls:

- Exercise programs including tai chi (rif, raf)
- Assessment and multifactorial interventions (raf)
- Home-safety improvements for persons with visual problems or who were at greater risk for falling (raf)
- Reduction in the use of certain medications (raf)
- Primary-care administered home programs (rif)

The results of the systematic review indicated that a variety of interventions have had effectiveness in reducing the risk and/or rate of falls of elderly people.

- Weakness
- Walking or gait problems
- Environmental hazards
  - Wet floors
  - Poor lighting
  - Lack of bed rails
  - Clutter
  - Incorrect bed height
- Improperly maintained or fitted wheelchairs
- Medications (psychoactive drugs such as sedatives)
- Difficulty in transferring (e.g., from a bed to a chair)
- Poor foot care
- Poorly fitting shoes
- Inappropriate use of walking aids such as canes

figure *12.18*

Causes of falls in nursing homes.

Source: Based on "Preventing Falls in the Nursing Home," by L. Z. Rubenstein, 1997, *Journal of the American Medical Association, 278*, pp. 595–596.

Audiologists can team up with other healthcare providers in developing fall prevention programs. Fall prevention, therefore, requires a team approach that may include audiologists, nurses, otolaryngologists, otologists, PCPs, physical therapists, and so on. Audiologists assess for vestibular dysfunction and balance disorders in addition to providing treatment for BPPV and stable but symptomatic and uncompensated deficits (see Chapter 11). **Formal fall prevention programs** may be documented efforts within specific facilities that employ healthcare professionals full-time or on a consultative basis who serve a role on the fall prevention team. Alternatively, **informal teaming for balance issues** may occur on a case-by-case basis whereby audiologists may consult with PCPs regarding patients' prescription medication that may be contributing to dizziness and vertigo. Suggestions can be made to assess patients who have fallen to identify a cause or address risk factors in

- Assess patients after a fall to identify and address risk factors
- Offer physical conditioning and/or rehabilitation classes to:
  - Improve strength and endurance
  - Physical therapy
  - Gait training
  - Walking programs
- Monitor usage of medication that may affect the balance system
- Provide hip pads to those most at risk to prevent hip fractures
- Consider use of alarm systems alerting staff to residents needing help (e.g., getting out of bed)
- Reduce falls in living spaces
  - Keep the floor clear of clutter
  - Safely tuck telephone and electrical cords out of walkways
  - Keep the floor clean
    - Clean up grease, water, and other liquids immediately
    - Don't wax floors
  - Use non-skid throw rugs
  - Install hand rails in stairways
  - Have grab bars in the bathroom by toilets and in showers
  - Use elevated toilet seats
  - Move frequently used objects from high places
  - Use sturdy step stools with hand rails

figure *12.19* —————————————————————————

Assessing patients after they fall.

Source: Based on "Prevention of Falls in Older Patients," by S. S. Rao, 2005, *American Family Physician, 72,* pp. 81–88.

their environments. Inquiries into the types and dosages of drugs may reveal medications affecting the balancing system. Audits of residents' living spaces may indicate hazards such as cluttered surfaces, exposed electrical cords, slippery surfaces, or placement of frequently used objects on shelves requiring the use of stools, increasing the risk of falls. Strategic placement of handrails in stairways, grab bars in the bathrooms, and elevated toilet seats may also prevent falls. Development of physical conditioning and/or rehabilitation classes may assist residents in increasing their strength and endurance. Moreover, injuries may be prevented through use of alerting systems by residents at risk for falls that may need assistance in walking. Some administrators may feel that the use of restraints may reduce the number of falls in long-term residential care facilities for the elderly. However, the use of restraints does not reduce the likelihood of falls or other injuries (Capezuti, 2004).

Special Services

Special services in long-term facilities for the elderly may include participating in hospice-patient care, residential care fundraising, and provision of hearing aid safety cords.

Hospice-Patient Care. Long-term care facilities frequently deal with end-of-life issues. **Hospice** is care designed to provide comfort and support to patients and their families when a life-limiting illness no longer responds to cure-oriented treatments (Hospice Foundation of America, 2006). Hospice does not administer care that extends life or quickens death for those who are suffering. However, hospice provides **palliative care**, which has been defined by the World Health Organization as the active total care of patients whose disease is not responsive to curative treatment (Center for Advancement of Palliative Care, 2006). For example, customarily hospice services would involve minimization of pain for a patient with a terminal disease rather than chemotherapy aimed at shrinking a tumor. Audiologists can be of great assistance to hospice care by loaning HAT and providing other hearing healthcare services for facilitating end-of-life interactions involving elderly patients and their family and friends.

Fundraising. Audiologists may participate in resource seeking/fundraising activities for the auditory rehabilitation support programs and for residents needing resources to pursue hearing aids. For example, local philanthropic groups may provide funds for development of a HAT lending library or start-up funds for a residents' hearing club. Moreover, audiologists may assist residents in securing funding for hearing aids through organizations such as Hear Now sponsored through the Starkey Hearing Foundation. Hear Now is a national nonprofit program committed to assisting persons who are deaf and hard of hearing with limited financial resources who permanently reside within the United States. The organization salvages used hearing aids that are donated by persons who no longer need them. Audiologists may apply to be Hear Now providers who volunteer fitting and follow-up services to qualified patients.

Hearing Aid Safety Cords. Audiologists can also provide hearing aid safety cords for residents so that their hearing aids will not get lost. Hearing aids have a knack for getting lost under the bed, being left in the cafeteria, or tumbling through the laundry. Use of hearing aid retention and protection devices such as Ear Gear from Oticon for children ages birth to 3 years may be useful for protecting residents' hearing aids from damage and loss.

Another critical issue that long-term healthcare facilities need to be concerned with is elder abuse, which is discussed in the next section.

ELDER ABUSE

Communication sciences and disorders professionals must be able to recognize elder abuse, which is defined as any knowing, intentional, or negligent act by a caregiver or any other person that harms or risks the well-being of a vulnerable adult (National Center on Elder Abuse, 2007). Elder abuse can occur in many forms, such as physical, emotional, sexual, exploitive, neglect, and/or abandonment, and it affects people of all ethnic backgrounds and all socioeconomic levels. Some of the signs of elder abuse include any visible injuries (e.g., bruises, broken bones, and abrasions), sudden changes in behavior, bedsores, unattended medical needs, verbal abuse, strained relationships, and sudden changes in financial situations. Table 12.3 shows the types, definitions, and symptoms of elder abuse (National Center on Elder Abuse, 2007).

The elderly are not only abused by others, but also neglect their own care. Some signs of self-neglect include hoarding, discontinuation of medication, self-endangerment

table *12.3*   Types, Definitions, and Symptoms of Elder Abuse

Type of Abuse	Definition	Symptoms
Physical	The use of physical force that may result in bodily injury, physical pain, or impairment.	• Bruises, black eyes, welts, lacerations, rope marks • Bone fractures, broken bones, and skull fractures • Sprains, dislocations, and internal injuries/bleeding • Broken eyeglasses/frames, physical signs of being subjected to punishment, and signs of being restrained • Laboratory findings of medication overdoses or under utilization of prescribed drugs • An elder's report of being hit, slapped, kicked, or mistreated • An elder's sudden change in behavior • The caregiver's refusal to allow visitors to see an elder alone

(Continued)

table *12.3* (*Continued*)

Type of Abuse	Definition	Symptoms
Sexual	Nonconsensual sexual contact of any kind with an elderly person	• Bruises around the breasts or genital area • Unexplained venereal disease or genital infections • Unexplained vaginal or rectal bleeding • Torn, stained, or bloody underclothing • An elder's report of being sexually assaulted or raped
Emotional or Psychological	The infliction of anguish, pain, or distress through verbal or nonverbal acts	• Being emotionally upset or agitated • Being extremely withdrawn and noncommunicative or nonresponsive • Unusual behavior usually attributed to dementia (e.g., sucking, biting, rocking) • An elder's report of being verbally or emotionally mistreated
Neglect	The refusal or failure to fulfill any part of a person's obligations or duties to an elder	• Dehydration, malnutrition, untreated bed sores, and poor personal hygiene • Unattended or untreated health problems • Hazardous or unsafe living conditions/arrangements • Unsanitary and unclean living conditions (e.g., dirt, fleas, lice on person, soiled bedding, fecal/urine smell, inadequate clothing) • An elder's own report of being abandoned
Abandonment	The desertion of an elderly person by an individual who has assumed responsibility for providing care for an elder, or by a person with physical custody of an elder	• The desertion of an elder at a hospital, a nursing facility, or other similar institution • The desertion of an elder at a shopping center or other public location • An elder's own report of being abandoned
Financial or Material Exploitation	The illegal or improper use of an elder's funds, property, or assets	• Cashing an elderly person's checks without authorization or permission • Forging an older person's signature • Misusing or stealing an older person's money or possessions • Coercing or deceiving an older person into signing any document (e.g., contracts or will) • The improper use of conservatorship, guardianship, or power of attorney
Self-neglect	The behavior of an elderly person that threatens his/her own safety	• Dehydration, malnutrition, untreated, or improperly attended medical conditions, and poor personal hygiene • Hazardous or unsafe living conditions/arrangements • Unsanitary or unclean living quarters • Inappropriate and/or inadequate clothing or lack of the necessary medical aids (e.g., eyeglasses, hearing aids, and dentures) • Grossly inadequate housing or homelessness

Source: Information from the National Center for Elder Abuse, 2007, retrieved from www.elderabusecenter.org.

(e.g., leaving a stove burning), poor personal hygiene, inappropriate clothing (e.g., no coat in the winter), confusion, poor housekeeping, and/or dehydration. The National Center on Elder Abuse estimated that in 1996, more than 500,000 people over 60 years of age were victims of elder abuse and that only 16% of cases were actually reported, while 84% cases were hidden. If elder abuse is suspected and a patient is in a life-threatening situation, 9-1-1 should be called. Otherwise, Eldercare Locator may be called at 1 (800) 677-1116 Monday through Friday from 9:00 a.m. to 5:00 p.m. Eastern time.

DUAL SENSORY IMPAIRMENT

Dual sensory impairment is present when a person has concurrent visual and hearing impairment. Visual impairment, like hearing impairment, varies by degree. **Low vision** is a term used for situations in which visual acuity is 20/70 or worse and cannot be corrected by conventional eyeglasses (University of Michigan Kellogg Eye Center, 2007), which is different than **blindness**. Blindness is a visual acuity of no less than 20/200 in the better eye with correction or a visual field no greater than 20 degrees (American Federation for the Blind, 2007). Although these definitions provide classifications based on visual testing, they do not provide information on patients' functional visual abilities. Great caution must be used in labeling patients based on visual testing.

Berry, Mascia, and Steinman (2004) estimated that by age 70, 21% of those living in the United States will have dual sensory impairment. In addition, 70% of elderly persons with severe vision impairment will also have significant hearing loss (Heine & Browning, 2002). A recent retrospective review of 400 randomly selected charts of 1,472 veterans who presented to audiology and optometry outpatient clinics over a single year had a prevalence of hearing impairment ranging from 41.6% to 74.6%, 7.4% for vision impairment including blindness, and 5.0% to 7.4% for dual sensory impairment (Smith, Bennett, & Wilson, 2008). In addition, the prevalence of dual sensory impairment increased with age with 0% <65 years of age, rising to >20% for those older than 85 years (Smith et al., 2008). The prevalence of dual sensory impairment is expected to rise as the number of elderly people increases.

Effect of Dual Sensory Impairment on the Elderly

Older adults with dual sensory impairment not only have problems associated with their sensory impairments, but many have additional conditions from aging alone, such as arthritis and memory impairment (Saunders & Echt, 2007). Brennan, Horowitz, and Su (2005) investigated the relation of dual and single sensory impairments on everyday competence of elderly persons in completing ADLs and **instrumental activities of daily living** (IADLs). Recall that ADLs are tasks such as getting dressed, brushing one's teeth, and so on; IADLs are tasks such as preparing dinner, going grocery shopping, planning a budget, and so on. The Longitudinal Study on Aging, which followed 5,151 individuals age 70 and older in 1984, provided data for this investigation. One-fifth of the older adults reported dual sensory impairment, which resulted in greater difficulty completing ADLs and IADLs than for the elderly reporting single sensory impairment. In addition, a high degree of dual impairment was associated with difficulty in performing three (preparing meals, shopping, and using the telephone) out of six IADL tasks when compared to those with visual impairments only. The researchers also found that the cognitive status of the elderly was a good predictor of the difficulty encountered in completion of ADLs and IADLs. Dual sensory impairment affects HRQoL or older adults' abilities to socialize, communicate with others, and live independently (Berry et al., 2004). For example, depression, anxiety, lethargy, and social dissatisfaction have been reported by elderly persons with dual sensory impairment. Visual difficulties can also affect the balance of the elderly (Anand, Buckley, Scally, & Elliott, 2003a, 2003b).

Implications for Audiologic Assessment and Auditory Rehabilitation

The prevalence and resulting effects of dual sensory impairment warrant periodic vision and hearing screening of the elderly. In addition, audiologists should always ask about vision on the case history form because visual impairment may be present but not noticeable (Blumsack, 2003). Some of the difficulties these patients may have are being able to detect, identify, and locate (1) warning sounds, (2) familiar stationary sound sources, (3) obstacles, (4) moving sound sources in the environment, and (5) sounds from auditory alerting devices (e.g., signals for when it is safe to cross the street) (Blumsack, 2003). Clinical environments should be enhanced for optimal auditory and visual transmission of information including quiet environments, use of sound absorptive materials to reduce reverberation, and good lighting with a minimization of glare (Saunders & Echt, 2007).

Figure 12.20 presents suggestions for how to communicate with and perform audiologic assessments and auditory rehabilitation on patients with dual sensory impairment (Blumsack, 2003; Saunders & Echt, 2007; Weinstein, 2000). Saunders and Echt (2007) suggest using clear speech with seniors with dual sensory impairment, including slowing the rate of speech to facilitate information processing. Weinstein presents several recommendations regarding how to improve verbal communication with adults with dual sensory impairment. First, it is important to introduce yourself by name to the person with dual sensory impairment. Second, for patients with very low vision or who are blind, it is important to alert them when you are entering or leaving the room. Third, speak to the patient before touching him or her, particularly before performing any audiologic procedure such as otoscopy, placement of earphones, inserting probe for otoacoustic emissions testing, and so on. Fourth, always approach the patient from the side of his or her better eye. Fifth, communication sciences and disorders professionals should speak directly to the patient rather than to significant others. Patients with dual sensory impairment usually present to appointments with significant others, but this does not mean that they speak for the patient.

Similarly, Blumsack (2003) recommended several considerations for audiologic assessment of these patients. As mentioned earlier, audiologists should include items on their case history form regarding patients' visual history, visual acuity, visual field impairments, problems related to glare, use of special devices (e.g., hand magnifiers), and whether the patients are under the care of a vision specialist. Blumsack (2003) also recommended facilitation of the patients' mobility into the test booth by marking steps with bright contrasting tape, reducing the likelihood of stumbling, in addition to using furniture that is in contrast with the background color of the booth. Moreover, care must be taken to avoid glare, to ensure adequate lighting in the test booth, and to modify written materials so that they can be read by patients with low vision (Blumsack, 2003). For example, she suggested that glare can be avoided by illuminating the booth with multiple, evenly spaced incandescent lights and using dimmer switches to control the intensity of lighting for each patient. However, she cautioned against adjusting the intensity of light within the booth to be

Considerations for Communication (Weinstein, 2000)
- Introduction by name
- Alerting the patient when you enter or leave the room
- Approaching the patient on the side of his or her better eye
- Allowing the patient to speak for him- or herself
- Speaking directly to the patient

Considerations for the Audiologic Assessment (Blumsack, 2003)
- Vision screening and monitoring
- Detailed inquiry regarding:
  - Visual acuity
  - Visual field impairments
  - Problems related to glare
  - Use of special devices (e.g., magnifiers or special lenses)
  - Collaboration of a visual specialist
- Use of appropriate lighting inside and outside the audiometric booth
- Use of high contrast furniture and threshold markings
- Use of appropriate written materials (Weinstein, 2000)
  - Print text promoting the highest possible contrast between light and dark, preferably using black and white
  - Space letters widely
  - Use extra-wide margins, especially for bound materials, such that the materials can be read on a flat surface
  - Use large fonts (e.g., 16- to 18-point)
  - Use ordinary typeface, upper and lower case lettering, and/or boldface print
  - Do not use paper that has a glossy finish

Considerations for Auditory Rehabilitation (Blumsack, 2003; Saunders & Echt, 2007; Weinstein, 2000)
- Services provided in conjunction with a certified vision rehabilitation therapist
- Assessment of visual acuity for speechreading
- Considerations for Selecting, Fitting, and Delivery of Hearing Aids and Hearing Assistive Technology (HAT)
  - Provisions for appropriate accommodations
    - Lighting
    - Visual aids (e.g., hand magnifiers)
    - Scheduling of longer appointment times
  - Special features for hearing aids
  - Special features for HAT: Telephone Features for Patients with Dual Sensory Impairment
    - Make sure the keypad has:
      - Large buttons
      - Good color contrasts
    - Make sure the telephone has:
      - A paging feature
      - Memory and redial features

figure *12.20* ─────────────────────────────

Suggestions for working with patients with dual sensory impairment.

Sources: Based on "Audiological Assessment, Rehabilitation, and Spatial Hearing Considerations Associated with Visual Impairments in Adults: An Overview," by J. T. Blumsack, 2003, *American Journal of Audiology, 12,* pp. 76–83; "An Overview of Dual Sensory Impairment in Older Adults: Perspectives for Rehabilitation," by G. H. Saunders and K. V. Echt, 2007, *Trends in Amplification, 11,* pp. 243–258; *Geriatric Audiology,* by B. E. Weinstein, 2000, New York: Thieme.

significantly brighter or dimmer than the light in the examination room in order to avoid problems for patients who have difficulties adapting to changes in ambient lighting. Similarly, provisions should also be made for optimally conveying information via printed material: (1) the highest possible contrast between the colors (e.g., black and white), (2) widely spaced letters, and (3) large fonts (e.g., 16 to 18 point) with ordinary typeface using upper and lower case (Blumsack, 2003). Messages in all uppercase lettering are difficult for anyone to read! Weinstein (2000) also suggested using wide margins so that books and booklets can be read on a flat surface.

Regarding auditory rehabilitation, Blumsack (2003) recommended service provision in conjunction with a certified vision rehabilitation therapist. Unfortunately, joint rehabilitation efforts between audiologists and optometrists/ophthalmologists are rare (Smith et al., 2008). Vision specialists can determine if patients' visual acuity is less than 20/80 at a distance of 5 feet, which is critical for determining the effectiveness of speechreading. Visual impairment should also be a consideration for the selection, fitting, and delivery of hearing aids and HAT through the use of visual aids (Blumsack, 2003; Saunders & Echt, 2007; *Understanding and Coping with Macular Degeneration,* 2006b):

- Strong reading lenses are good to use because the patient's hands are free to manipulate hearing aids, for example.
- Hand magnifiers provide greater magnification than strong reading glasses and may have a built-in light source that provides increased contrast for reading.
- Stand magnifiers provide greater magnification than the hand magnifiers and have legs that sit directly on a flat surface so that patients may view and/or manipulate their hearing aids.

Electronic magnifiers provide the greatest magnification for reading and/or near-vision tasks. Saunders and Echt (2007) suggest using a closed-circuit video magnifier that can show hearing aids up close or other objects on a television monitor.

Several features are important to consider when selecting amplification for patients with dual sensory impairment. Blumsack (2003) recommended that patients with low vision select their own case color, use a magnetic tool for battery manipulation, request a large-print instruction manual, investigate which wax guards are easiest to use, and order large-font "R" and "L" stamped onto the hearing aids for easy identification. In addition, she suggested that patients be told to manipulate their hearing aids over a high-contrast color towel. Seniors with dual sensory impairment may find Duracel Easytabs and Energizer EZ Change particularly useful in changing hearing aid batteries (Saunders & Echt, 2007). Blumsack (2003) and Saunders and Echt (2007) suggested that audiologists use tactile cues for teaching blind patients how to use hearing aids and that they schedule longer appointments. Saunders and Echt (2007) said that having patients touch and experiment with the control mechanisms may be key in successful manipulation of their hearing aids. Weinstein (2000) stated that these patients should be encouraged to practice new skills during the hearing aid delivery to instill confidence and a sense of mastery over amplification. Saunders and Echt (2007) advocated facilitating mastery of amplification using the **patient teach-back method** by having older adults repeat and show their new hearing aid knowledge and skills.

Regarding selection of appropriate HAT, special considerations should be made for patients with dual sensory impairment. For example, Weinstein (2000) suggested using phones with keypads with large buttons and a good contrast in colors. In addition, telephones that have memory and redial features reduce the need for these patients to punch in frequently called numbers, minimizing the chance for errors. Further, a paging feature allows these patients to find the handsets for cordless telephones that have been misplaced. The same suggestions for hearing aid delivery also apply in the delivery of HAT to patients with dual sensory impairment.

SUMMARY

This chapter began with discussing a transdisciplinary model of hearing healthcare focusing on older patients and their families. Primary consideration should be given to patients' unique characteristics regarding their communication status, physical status, psychological status, and social status for a holistic approach to hearing healthcare. Audiologists must learn to break down barriers between and among healthcare providers in providing auditory rehabilitation to elderly patients, especially in long-term, residential care facilities. Service provision is discussed as patients progress through the hearing healthcare continuum. The chapter concluded with coverage of elder abuse and dual sensory perception in the elderly.

LEARNING ACTIVITIES

- Contact someone who is 85 years of age or older and interview him or her about what life is like for them, their daily joys and struggles. How closely does this person match the characteristics of elderly persons discussed in the chapter?
- Shadow an audiologist whose clientele consists mostly of older adults and, if you can, observe service delivery in a long-term care facility.
- Interview a speech-language pathologist who provides auditory rehabilitation to older adults, and ask this person what specialized skills and knowledge they believe are required to provide these services.
- With a classmate, administer as well as take the *Utley, A Test of Lipreading Ability* (Utley, 1946) and/or the *Denver Quick Test of Lipreading Ability* (Alpiner, 1982).
- Observe an audiologist performing balance testing and vestibular rehabilitation training.

APPENDIX 12.1

Hearing Handicap Inventory
for the Elderly–Screening Version (HHIE–S)

Name: _____   Date: _____

INSTRUCTIONS: *Answer "Yes," "No," or "Sometimes" for each questions by placing an "X" in the appropriate box. Do not skip a question if you avoid a situation because of a hearing problem. If you use a hearing aid, please answer according to the way you hear with the aid.*

Question	Yes	No	Sometimes
1. Does a hearing problem cause you to feel embarrassed when you meet new people?			
2. Does a hearing problem cause you to feel frustrated when talking to members of your family?			
3. Do you have difficulty when someone speaks in a whisper?			
4. Do you feel handicapped by a hearing problem?			
5. Does a hearing problem cause you difficulty when visiting friends, relatives, or neighbors?			
6. Does a hearing problem cause you to attend religious services less often than you would like?			
7. Does a hearing problem cause you to have arguments with family members?			
8. Does a hearing problem cause you difficulty when listening to TV or radio?			
9. Do you feel that any difficulty with your hearing limits or hampers your personal or social life?			
10. Does a hearing problem cause you difficulty when in a restaurant with relatives or friends?			
SCORING: 1. Count the number of "X" marks in the "yes" and "sometimes" categories. 2. Multiply that sum by the indicated value (e.g., # of "Yeses" × 4 = ____). 3. Write the product in the space provided. 4. Add the products together to obtain a total score.	____ × 4 ____		____ × 2 ____

Total Score Interpretation:

Score _____

   0–8 = No handicap

10–24 = Mild to moderate handicap

26–40 = Severe handicap

Source: Based on "Identification of Elderly People with Hearing Problems," by I. M. Ventry and B. E. Weinstein, 1983, *ASHA, 25,* pp. 37–42.

APPENDIX 12.2
Utley Test of Lipreading Ability

Practice List

1. Good morning.
2. Thank you.
3. Hello.
4. How are you?
5. Goodbye.

Form A

1. All right.
2. Where have you been?
3. I have forgotten.
4. I have nothing.
5. That is right.
6. Look out.
7. How have you been?
8. I don't know if I can.
9. How tall are you?
10. It is awfully cold.
11. My folks are home.
12. How much was it?
13. Good night.
14. Where are you going?
15. Excuse me.
16. Did you have a good time?
17. What did you want?
18. How much do you weigh?
19. I cannot stand him.
20. She was home last week.
21. Keep your eye on the ball.
22. I cannot remember.
23. Of course.
24. I flew to Washington.
25. You look well.
26. The train runs every hour.
27. You had better go slow.
28. It says that in the book.
29. We got home last night at six o'clock.
30. We drove to the country.
31. How much rain fell?

Source: Based on "A Test of Lipreading Ability," by J. Utley, 1946, *Journal of Speech Disorders, 11,* pp. 109–116.

APPENDIX 12.3

Hearing Aid Orientation Group Interaction Checklist

INSTRUCTIONS: *Use this form when observing patients interacting in hearing aid orientation group. Answer each question by checking the appropriate box. Space has been provided at the bottom of this form for notes.*

Question	Yes	No
Is/are the instructor(s) talking no more than 30% of the time?	☐	☐
Are group members actively participating in sessions?	☐	☐
Are family members/significant others participating in sessions?	☐	☐
Do patients make use of visual cues and watch speakers' faces?	☐	☐
Do patients use effective repair strategies?	☐	☐
Are patients assertive communicators?	☐	☐
Do patients offer suggestions to speakers in order to improve communication?	☐	☐
Are patients comfortable in stating publicly that they have hearing losses?	☐	☐
Do patients attempt to modify the environment to maximize communication?	☐	☐
Do patients come to the sessions wearing their hearing aids?	☐	☐
Do patients use assistive technology?	☐	☐
Are patients' nonverbal signals indicative of their comprehension of and interest in group topics?	☐	☐
NOTES:		

Source: Based on "Evaluating the Success of Adult Audiologic Rehabilitation Support Programs," by P. B. Kricos and S. A. Lesner, 2000, *Seminars in Hearing, 21,* pp. 267–279.

APPENDIX 12.4

Hearing Aid Skills Checklist

INSTRUCTIONS: *Use this form when observing patients when they come in for their first appointment after hearing aid delivery. Answer each question by checking the appropriate box. Space has been provided at the bottom of this form for notes.*

Question	Yes	No
Is the hearing aid being worn?	☐	☐
Is the hearing aid inserted into the ear correctly?	☐	☐
Is the battery inserted correctly?	☐	☐
Is the battery adequately charged?	☐	☐
Is the volume adjusted appropriately?	☐	☐
Is the remote control used appropriately?	☐	☐
Are the programs appropriately used?	☐	☐
Is the hearing aid functioning properly?	☐	☐
Can the patient remove/insert the hearing aid properly?	☐	☐
Are the earmold and hearing aid clean?	☐	☐
Can the patient use the aid properly on the telephone?	☐	☐
NOTES:		

Source: Based on "Evaluating the Success of Adult Audiologic Rehabilitation Support Programs," by P. B. Kricos and S. A. Lesner, 2000, *Seminars in Hearing, 21,* pp. 267–279.

Glossary

2-cc coupler: A hollow, hard-walled chamber that simulates a human ear for the purposes of standardized assessments of hearing instrument functioning

5-dB time-intensity trade-off law: States that each time the dB level increases by 5 dB, the permissible duration of exposure decreases by half

abnormal refractive errors: Visual disorders including astigmatisms, hyperopia, and myopia

Academy of Rehabilitative Audiology (ARA): A professional organization composed of communication sciences and disorders professionals dedicated to the excellence in hearing care through the provision of comprehensive rehabilitative and habilitative services (ARA, 2006)

acclimatization: Accommodations the brain must make due to the changes of acoustic information coming from the periphery due to amplification

accommodations: Adjustments in procedures or rules that permit students with disabilities access to an education

acknowledging and reflecting feelings: A counseling skill involving reflecting on what the patient may be feeling about a particular issue

acoustic dampers: Material placed in the tubing of an earmold or earhook (e.g., tone hook) of a BTE hearing aid with a net result of smoothing out any acoustical peaks in the output of the hearing aid that may be painful to patients

acoustic highlighting: Emphasizing certain words that are difficult to hear through the use of suprasegmentals (e.g., rhythm and intonation)

acquired hearing loss: Hearing loss that develops after the development of spoken language or after the completion of formal schooling

action level: A noise exposure of 85 dBA for an eight-hour work period and serves the threshold for participation in a hearing conservation program (50% noise dose)

activities of daily living (ADLs): Such activities as getting dressed, brushing one's teeth, and so on

activity: The execution of a task or action of an individual; has to do with what the patient can do

activity limitations: Difficulties that an individual may have in executing tasks, particularly those involving speech, speech understanding, and communication

acute care: Physicians', nurses', and third-party payers' companies choose and provide treatment usually for immediate medical needs (Stone, 2000)

adaptive procedures: Tests in which the difficulty of the assessment condition is based on the accuracy of patients' previous responses

administrative controls: Changes in work schedules aimed at reducing workers' exposure to noise

affective goals: Goals set on the psychosocial implications of hearing loss such as, "I don't want to feel embarrassed anymore because of not hearing," or "I don't want to feel isolated because of my hearing loss" (Valente, Abrams, et al., 2006)

affective statements: Statements of social and emotional concerns regarding hearing loss

affirmations: Statements of appreciation, understanding, as well as compliments that validate patients

age of onset: The chronological age of a patient when a hearing loss develops

ageism: Discrimination of people on the basis of their age, usually involving the elderly

Agency for Healthcare Research and Quality (AHRQ): Part of the Department of Health and Human Services that is concerned with health services research and supports efforts to improve the quality, safety, efficiency, and effectiveness of healthcare (AHRQ, 2007)

age-related macular degeneration: A progressive deterioration of the retina of the eye that may affect vision particularly in doing close work such as threading a needle, but side or peripheral vision is rarely affected (*Understanding and Coping with Macular Degeneration,* 2006a; University of Michigan Kellogg Eye Center, 2007)

air-bone gap: A difference of more than 10 dB between bone- and air-conduction thresholds at the same frequency and in the same ear

air-conduction hearing aids: Hearing aids with output transducers that convert the amplified signal that is heard via air conduction through the outer, middle, and the inner ears

air-conduction stimuli: Sounds that travel through the outer ear, middle ear, and inner ear

Alzheimer's disease (AD): The most common form of dementia; initially affects areas of the brain that regulate thought, memory, and language

amblyopia: A visual disorder known as "lazy eye" and is the result of one eye failing to develop normally, but can be corrected during infancy or early childhood (University of Michigan Kellogg Eye Center, 2006a)

American Sign Language: The language of the Deaf community with its own syntax; semantics is used extensively within and among the Deaf community within the United States

ampulla: The dilated portions of the semi-circular canals in the inner ear

analog hearing aids: Hearing instruments based on a technology in which sound pressure is turned into an analogous waveform represented by variations in electrical voltage for processing (Dillon, 2001)

analytic approach to speechreading: Based on the premise that the individual parts (e.g., syllables) of the message must be identified before the whole message can be understood (Hipskind, 2007)

andragogy: Learning strategies to engage adult learners (Bruegemann, 2005; Knowles, Holton, & Swanson, 2005)

anotia: The absence of a pinna

Anti-kickback Statute: Prohibits healthcare professionals from receiving remunerations for referrals to providers for services reimbursable through federal programs

appliances: Devices that provide benefits to patients irrespective of their individual skill level

Appraisal of Guidelines for Research and Evaluation Instrument (AGREE): An evaluative tool for assessing the thoroughness of the process for developing a clinical practice guideline

aqueous humor: A watery fluid that circulates throughout the front of the eye and maintains a constant pressure

arthritis: Inflammation of a joint accompanied by symptoms of pain, swelling, and stiffness that can be caused by infection, trauma, degenerative changes, metabolic disturbances, and so on (Arthritis Foundation, 2010)

Articulation Index: An estimation of the availability of speech energy expressed in percent ranging from 0%, no audibility, to 100%, complete audibility

assessing: Determining the nature of a patient's complaint hearing loss or balance disorder (Stockman et al., 2004)

assisted living facilities (ALFs): Residences that offer a range of accommodations, from shared rooms to upscale private apartments, in which residents pay monthly fees based on the services required to meet their level of functioning (Helpguide.org, 2010)

assistive listening devices (ALDs): Devices that are conceived and applied to ameliorate the auditory problems faced by individuals with hearing loss

assistive listening technology system: An assistive device, a human operator of the device, and an environment in which a functional activity involving hearing is to take place (Cook & Hussey, 2002)

assistive technology: A "broad range of devices, services, strategies, and practices that are conceived and applied to ameliorate the problems faced by individuals who have disabilities" (Cook & Hussey, 2002; p. 5)

assistive technology system: An assistive device, a human operator of the device, and an environment in which a functional activity is to take place (Cook & Hussey, 2002)

associations: Connections or relationships between variables, such as between risk factors and certain diseases

astigmatism: An irregular curvature of the cornea causing problems in how light is focused within the eye; occurs frequently with hyperopia or myopia (University of Michigan Kellogg Eye Center, 2006b)

asymmetric audiometric results: Audiometric results in each ear are different

attack time: The length of time, in milliseconds, that it takes for the compression circuit to activate after onset of a loud sound

Audibility Index: An estimation of the audible speech energy available calculated from the patient's air-conduction thresholds superimposed on the Count-the-Dot Audiogram

audiogram: A graph used to record the results of an audiologic evaluation

audiologic rehabilitation: Includes services provided by audiologists to minimize the effects of hearing loss, balance problems, or other auditory disorders on patients' lives

audiometer: An instrument used to measure hearing sensitivity

audiovisual speech reception: The use of both auditory and visual senses to understand what is being said

audism: A term that describes how the hearing establishment is perceived as imposing its values onto Deaf culture by defining its members as a group of individuals who have the same affliction needing treatment (Harlan, 1999)

auditory brainstem response testing (ABR): A non-behavioral test that measures how the auditory nerve conducts impulses from the periphery to the auditory brainstem pathways in response to auditory stimuli

auditory deprivation: Loss of some integrity of the sensory system due to a lack of external auditory stimulation (Kochkin, 2000)

auditory discrimination: The ability to differentiate between types of auditory stimuli (e.g., "Are /pa/ or /ba/ the same syllables or different?")

auditory fitness for duty: "Possession of hearing abilities sufficient for safe and effective job performance" (Tufts, Vasil, & Briggs, 2009; p. 539)

auditory habilitation: Providing services to children with congenital hearing loss or hearing loss present at birth or acquired before the acquisition of speech and language

auditory habilitative approach: A particular methodology used to develop the auditory, speech, and language skills through a child's use of his or her residual hearing

auditory neuropathy/dyssynchrony (AN/AD): Dysfunction of cranial nerve VIII that impedes the transmission of neural impulses generated in the periphery that go to the central auditory nervous system, resulting in a neural hearing loss

auditory pattern recognition: The ability to recognize patterns in acoustic stimuli (e.g., "Can you recognize patterns in sequences of low- and high-pitched tones?")

auditory performance decrements with competing acoustic signals: The tendency for the ability to understand speech to decrease with increasing distortion (e.g., "Can speech continue to be understood even though the signal-to-noise ratio decreases and reverberation time increases?")

auditory performance decrements with degraded acoustic signals: The tendency for the ability to understand speech to decrease when some of its redundancy is reduced, such as when the message has some of its energy removed through filtering (e.g., "Can you understand these words that have most of their spectral energy above 600 Hz filtered out?")

auditory rehabilitation: An "ecological, interactive process that facilitates one's ability to minimize or prevent the limitations and restrictions that auditory dysfunctions can impose on well-being and communication, including interpersonal, psychosocial, educational, and vocational functioning" (ASHA, 2001)

auditory steady state response: Electrophysiological examination that provides an accurate estimation of patients' pure-tone audiograms

Auditory-Oral: A communication option that encourages the use of the child's residual hearing with the aid of amplification, but also stresses the use of speechreading

Auditory-Verbal approach: An approach to facilitating oral language development in children with hearing impairment that strongly emphasizes the development of listening skills through the use of residual hearing with amplification and discourages the use of visual cues in training (Med-El, 2005)

aural rehabilitation: Services and procedures for facilitating adequate receptive and expressive communication in individuals with hearing impairment (ASHA, 1984)

Aural-Oral: See *Auditory-Oral*

automatic gain control (AGC) hearing aids: Control the gain automatically based on the level of the signal being amplified (ANSI S3.22.2003, Section 3.16)

autonomic nervous system: Part of the nervous system that controls involuntary reactions of the body (e.g., smooth muscles and glands)

autosomal dominant disorders: An inheritance pattern in which one parent has the genetic mutation, expresses the disorder, and has a 50% chance of passing it on to his or her children

autosomal recessive disorders: An inheritance pattern in which both parents are carriers of the genetic mutation, but usually do not express it and have a 25% chance of having a child with the disorder, 50% chance that their child will be a carrier, and 25% chance that their child will be normal

being comfortable with silence: A listening skill that incorporates the realization that periods of quiet can assist conversational partners to reflect on what has been said

behavioral tests: Assess patients' conscious response to auditory stimuli

behind-the-ear hearing aid (BTE): A style of hearing aid with its electrical components built in a case that is situated behind the pinna and is coupled to patients' ears via earmolds using tubing

benchmarking: Comparing an individual performance to evidence-based, normative outcomes

benchmarks: Evidence-based projected performance levels after cochlear implant activation

benign paroxysmal positional vertigo (BPPV): The most common form of vertigo; results from an asymmetrical fluid movement due to a conflicting response to head movement in one of the semicircular canals

best evidence: Evidence at the highest levels of evidence with minimal experimental bias

bias: The measurable influence on a dependent variable that is not attributable to the independent (e.g., treatment) variable

bilateral contralateral routing of the signal (BICROS): A hearing aid arrangement for patients who have asymmetrical losses, with the better ear having a significant but aidable loss and a nonfunctional ear

bimodal stimulation: Occurs when a hearing aid is worn in the ear opposite to the cochlear implant

biopsychosocial model: Perspective that combines the medical and social models of disability

blends: Two consonants produced in combination (e.g., /sk/)

blindness: A visual acuity of no less than 20/200 in the better eye with correction or a visual field no greater than 20 degrees (American Federation for the Blind, 2007)

block diagram: A graph that shows how energy flows through the components of an electronic device

Bluetooth technology: An industrial specification for wireless personal area networks (PANs) that provides a means for wireless communication between devices (e.g., mobile phones, laptop computers, digital cameras, and so on) via an unsecure short-range radio frequency

board and care model: A type of assisted living facility that has no private apartments, but has residents living in their own rooms in a smaller home-style facility; residents may require assistance with activities of daily living in addition to having mild dementia or memory problems (Helpguide.org, 2010)

body functions: Physiological functions of body systems (including psychological functions)

body hearing aid: A style of hearing aid worn on the body (e.g., in a pocket) that has a cord connecting it to a receiver coupled to patients' ears by means of snap ring earmolds

body structures: Anatomical parts of the body such as organs, limbs, and their components

bone-anchored hearing aids: An osseointegrated bone-conduction hearing aid combining a sound processor with a small titanium fixture that is surgically implanted behind the ear

bone-conduction hearing aids: Hearing aids with output transducers that convert the amplified signals to vibrations that are delivered by an oscillator pressed firmly against the skin of the skull via a steel spring coupled to a band

bone-conduction stimuli: Sounds that bypass the outer and middle ears (i.e., conductive mechanism) to stimulate directly the inner ear (i.e., sensorineural mechanism) through vibration of the bones of the skull

"bottom up" strategies: Attempts to enhance the signal being heard and assist patients overcome processing problems by developing their perceptual skills through auditory training (ASHA, 2005a, 2005b)

brain plasticity: Ability of the cortex to reorganize as a result of repeated experiences, such as auditory training

breathiness: The perception that too much air is being expended during speech

Bruch's membrane: A membrane that separates the blood vessels of the retinal pigment epithelium from the choroid

bullying: Demeaning, threatening, intimidating, physically harming, or abusing someone in any way (Smith & Monks, 2008)

calibration: The process by which instruments are evaluated for functioning and adjusted to meet manufacturer's specifications

Campbell Collaboration: An independent nonprofit organization that provides evidence-based information for making decisions regarding social, behavioral, and educational sciences

canalith repositioning procedures: Noninvasive, sudden positioning techniques that attempt to move granules (i.e., otoconia) back to where they belong

canonical babbling: An advanced form of babbling consisting of consonant-vowel (e.g., CV like /ba/) or consonant-vowel-consonant-vowel (e.g., CVCV like /baba/) utterances

case history: A form used for collecting relevant patient information in an organized fashion

case studies: Studies involving specific individuals described in detail with results compared to historical controls

case-control studies: Research in which participants are recruited after they have developed some type of pathology along with a disease-free control group, are measured on some type of predictor variable, and then statistically compared for significant differences on predictor variables suggesting possible causes or associative variables for developing a pathology

cataracts: A clouding of the lens of the eye caused by a combination of factors of aging; results in blurry vision, double vision, sensitivity to light, glare, fading of colors, and frequent changes in eyeglass prescriptions (University of Michigan Kellogg Eye Center, 2007)

Center for Evidence-Based Medicine (CEBM): A center in England with an aim "to promote evidence-based healthcare and provide support and resources to anyone who wants to make use of them" (www.cebm.net) (CEBM, 2010)

(central) auditory processing disorders ([C]APD): Patients with normal hearing sensitivity, but who have difficulty with certain auditory skills due to problems in the central auditory nervous system

central compensation: A reorganization of the processing of information via brain plasticity

central hearing losses: Congenital or acquired damage to the auditory nerve, pathways, or cortex that may cause hearing loss or other processing problems

CHARGE syndrome: A recognizable and often life-threatening birth defect that occurs in approximately 1 in every 9,000 to 10,000 births and may cause craniofacial anomalies, complex heart and breathing problems, as well as vision, hearing, and balance impairments (The CHARGE Syndrome Foundation, 2010)

choroid: A layer of blood vessels that supply oxygen and nutrients to the outer layers of the retina

circular questioning: An interviewing technique to find out the role of the relevant significant others in the patient's life (Palazzoli, Boscalo, Cecchin, & Prata, 1977)

classic ITE hearing aid: A style of in-the-ear hearing aid that fills all or part of the concha portion of the pinna

classroom noise: Unwanted sound that comes from inside the classroom (e.g., children talking and computer noise)

classroom types: Instruction areas that may be (1) closed classrooms, (2) open area concepts, (3) split grades, or (4) portable classrooms

client-centered approach: A counseling approach characterized by empathetic listening, unconditional positive regard, counselor congruence, and listening with concern (Sweetow, 1999)

clinical expertise: Knowledge, skills, and experiences of a practitioner in addition to recommendations from clinical practice guidelines

Clinical Practice Development Process: A document developed by the American Academy of Audiology stating the process by which clinical practice guidelines should be developed

clinical practice guidelines (CPG): A systematically defined set of recommended procedures based on scientific evidence and/or expert opinion that have been designed to yield specific, well-defined outcomes (American Academy of Audiology, 2009b)

clinical practice standards: An explicitly and systematically defined set of required procedures and practices based on scientific evidence and/or expert opinion that have been designed to yield specific, well-defined outcomes outcomes (American Academy of Audiology, 2009b)

closed captioning: The process of converting a television program or home video's dialogue, sound effects, and narration into words that appear on the screen (National Captioning Institute, 2005)

closed classrooms: Traditional classrooms in which teachers and students are in a completely enclosed space

closed-head injuries: An injury resulting from nonpenetrating blows to the head (Youse, Le, Cannizzaro, & Coelho, 2002)

clusters: Three consonants produced in combination (e.g., /skr/)

cochlear implant mapping: The process of setting or adjusting the speech processor for a cochlear implant based on the patient's dynamic range of each electrode and electrode pair

cochlear implant team: A group of healthcare professionals involved in the cochlear implantation of patients, from candidacy to rehabilitation

cochlear implant team coordinator: A professional that is the main contact for patients and their families interested in cochlear implants and organizes the pre-implant evaluation

cochlear implants: Surgically implanted cochlear prostheses that bypass the damaged peripheral auditory system to directly stimulate nerve VIII for hearing

cochlear ossification: Build-up of new bone in response to bacterial meningitis that may have caused an infection in the cochlea

cochleostomy: A surgical procedure in which a hole is drilled into the basal turn of the cochlea for the purpose of inserting a cochlear implant electrode into the scala tympani

Cochrane Collaboration: An international organization devoted to assisting users in making informed healthcare decisions via systematic reviews

Cochrane Library: A source published by Wiley that contains several databases to be used in evidence-based practice

cognitive goals: Goals based on objective statements of the ability to hear during certain activities such as "to be able to hear my grandchildren on the telephone" or "to be able to hear the doorbell when I'm in my bedroom" (Valente, Abrams, et al., 2006)

combination program: A hearing conservation program run both internally by the company and externally by another party hired to specifically perform some aspect of the program (e.g., audiometric testing)

comment: A language facilitation technique in which something is said that keeps the conversation going or encourages a child (DesJardin & Eisenberg, 2007; Tye-Murray, 2008)

communication match: Patients' expressed needs in a professional interaction are heard and met by clinicians

communication mismatch: Replying to patients' affective statements (i.e., from the heart) with informational statements (i.e., from the brain)

compensatory strategies: Efforts made to overcome (central) auditory processing disorders and obtain information when the comprehension of auditory information is compromised due to factors internal or external to the child (e.g., use of a study buddy, note-taker service, etc.)

complete acknowledgment: Total recognition of a problem (e.g., I definitely have a hearing impairment)

completely-in-the-canal (CIC): A style of in-the-ear hearing aid, also known as a *deep-canal fitting* because the instrument is lodged out of sight, around the first bend of the ear canal, frequently requiring use of an extraction string for removal

comprehension: The ability to derive meaning of an auditory stimulus

compression hearing aids: Hearing aids with circuits that compress the wide range of input levels found in everyday sounds into a smaller range in the output signal that ultimately goes into patients' ears

computer-aided speech (C-Print™): Technology for note-taking requiring the use of regular word-processing systems in computers in addition to special software that abbreviate words and use text condensing strategies that reduce the number of necessary keystrokes

computer-assisted note-taking (CAN): Note-taking system in which note-takers use standard keyboards to provide a general summary of what was said

computer-assisted real-time transcriptions (CART): Technology for note-taking utilizing trained court reporters to record everything that is said in real time

conditioned oriented response audiometry (COR): A testing paradigm to be used with infants as young as 6 months that is similar to visual reinforcement audiometry, but differs in that responses are rewarded only with visual reinforcement (e.g., animated toys behind smoked-Plexiglass) if the head turn is made toward the loudspeaker (or earphones) actually presenting the auditory stimulus

conductive hearing loss: Loss of hearing sensitivity due to a problem in the outer ear (e.g., impacted ear wax [i.e., cerumen], growths, or infections that may obstruct the ear canal) or middle ear (e.g., a perforation in the tympanic membrane, a presence of fluid in the middle ear space, otitis media, a cholesteatoma) that prevents transmission of sound energy into the inner ear

cones: Photoreceptors used for vision in light to see colors and details

Conference on Guidelines Standardization Statement (COGS): A list and explanation of 18 desirable characteristics of evidence-based clinical practice guidelines that promote their appropriate implementation (Shiffman et al,, 2003)

confidence intervals (CI): A range within which the effect size may fall based on a specific probability level; a 95% CI means that the same results are to be expected 95 times out of every 100 times the study is replicated (Cox, 2005)

configuration: Describes the shape or direction the air-conduction threshold symbols assumes in either the right and/or left ear when placed on an audiogram

conflict of interest: A situation in which a person's personal and professional interest may be, or may give the appearance of being, in conflict with appropriate patient care that could possibly impede professional judgment

congenital aural atresia: The absence or failure of the development of the external auditory canal apparent at birth

congenital hearing loss: Hearing loss present at birth

congregate living: A living arrangement for senior citizens who have their own apartments in a multiunit building that often has a central kitchen, dining room, and other common areas and other services such as security, on-call staff support, housekeeping, laundry, transportation, and activities (Helpguide.org, 2010)

consensus: Reaching agreement regarding important issues facing the professions

CONSORT Statement: A document designed to improve the quality of reporting clinical trials particularly in medicine

contemplation: The stage in which patients are ambivalent in that they acknowledge the problem but are resistant to change

continuing care retirement communities: A model of residential care that offers a continuum of services within a single community by offering various levels of care so that residents can move from one level to another based on their individual needs

continuing education: Formal acquisition of knowledge and skills beyond those obtained in professional training programs

continuing education units (CEUs): Credits awarded upon completion of courses, seminars, or other training that meet professional education requirements

continuous interleaved stimulation (CIS): A speech coding strategy that estimates the envelope of the acoustic wave by coding the amplitude of the signal in six to eight bandpass filters at > 800 pps

continuous sound: Sound that is always on

contract grading: Establishing a contract between teacher and students about what criteria are used for evaluation

contract-for-service model: An educational audiology service delivery model in which audiologists are hired by school systems to perform duties as specified in a contract

contralateral routing of the signal: A hearing aid arrangement for patients with a unilateral hearing loss in which a microphone and FM transmitter are placed at the poorer or unaidable ear for transmission of sound to an FM receiver at the better ear

contrecoup: An injury occurring contralaterally to a blow, usually from the brain making impact with the skull

conversational fluency: The ability to participate in a discussion with one or more individuals with a minimum of requests for clarification, with an easy conveying of ideas, and with conversational turn-taking resulting in a sharing of speaking time (Erber, 1993)

cornea: A transparent covering, assists in focusing light coming into the eye

cost-effectiveness question: Compares the relative costs versus benefits of clinical procedures and treatments

co-teaching: Regular and special education teachers teaming up to teach specific subjects to students with and without disabilities

counseling: "The gathering of information through careful listening, the conveying of information, and the making of adjustments in one's strategies based on that knowledge" (Sweetow, 1999, p. 3)

counselor congruence: Occurs when the verbal statements of the counselor matches his or her body language

Count-the-Dot Audiogram: A graph that has 100 dots superimposed onto an audiogram for the purpose of calculating an Articulation or Audibility Index for a patient

coup: An injury resulting directly from a blow to the head

Crista ampullaris: A sensory organ for balance located in the semi-circular canals

criterion-referenced measures: Compare a student's performance against his or her own performance

cross-check principle: To confirm behavioral assessments with non-behavioral results

cross-cultural competence: The ability to understand the origin of one's bias (e.g., personal history), but yet establish a common ground with patients from diverse backgrounds

cross-professional competence: The ability to competently execute services within one's scope of practice to a diverse patient population toward positive outcomes in a wide variety of service delivery sites in collaboration with other professionals

cross-sectional studies: Also known as prevalence studies, cross-sectional studies determine the number of individuals that have a particular disorder or disease at one point in time per the number of people at risk

Cued Speech: A visual communication system that incorporates eight handshapes and four hand positions (cues) that represent how sounds are said while talking, providing help to the child in distinguishing sounds that look the same on the mouth

cued speech transliterater: A professional who cues what is said in a classroom or other venue to a person with hearing impairment

cul-de-sac resonance: The nasalization of speech sounds during vowel production

cultural sensitivity: A willingness to learn about and address needs of *every* patient

culturally and linguistically diverse patient: Every patient who has a culture and who is influenced by gender, geographic location, age, language ability, sexual orientation, and gender identification (ASHA, 2003)

culture: A group of people who share a common characteristic (e.g., race, ethnicity, gender, age, sexual preference, religion, or geographic regions) in addition to shared beliefs, behaviors, traditions, and mores

"culture shock": A series of disorienting encounters when a person's basic values, beliefs, and patterns of behavior are challenged by another culture (Lynch, 1997)

cytomegalovirus: A member of the herpes virus family; the most common congenital infection and one of the leading causes of hearing loss present at birth

daily log method: A method of assessing conversational fluency that asks patients to answer the same questions about their interactive behaviors encountered each day (Tye-Murray, 2008)

deaf: Having PTAs or SRTs in excess of 80 to 90 dB HL and not being able to use residual hearing to understand speech without the use of visual cues even when wearing hearing aids

deaf and visually impaired: Having no functional hearing and limited visual acuity

deaf-blind: Having little or no functional hearing or vision

deafness: "A hearing impairment that is so severe that the person is impaired in processing linguistic information through hearing, with or without amplification, [and] that adversely affects a child's educational performance" (300.7[c][3] of the Individuals with Disabilities Education Act)

decisional balance sheet: A chart that assists audiologists and patients to sort out ambivalent feeling toward change

decreased penetrance: When a genetic trait is expressed in a mild form (e.g., mild hearing loss)

degree of hearing loss: The severity of hearing impairment based on predefined categories that may vary among course instructors, clinical supervisors, and textbooks

dementia: A brain disorder that affects an elderly person's ability to carry out his or her daily activities (National Institute on Aging, 2010)

dependent variable: In a research study, a variable that is caused, influenced, or measured according to the change influenced by a treatment on it

depression: More than a feeling of being down and lethargic; it is feeling sad all the time without any apparent reason (*Helpguide: Mental Health Issues,* 2006)

detection: The ability to tell the presence or absence of an auditory stimulus

determination: The stage in which patients are more open to change than they are resistant to change

diabetes: An endrocrinological disorder in which the body does not produce or efficiently use insulin, a hormone that converts sugar, starches, and other foods into energy (American Diabetes Association, 2010)

diagnostic evaluation: A thorough assessment process; for example, a process that uses a recognized "gold standard" test to confirm the existence and extent of a hearing loss

diagnostic questions: Seeks to compare the relative efficacy, effectiveness, or efficiency of two assessment tools

diaphragm: A large muscle in the chest that contracts and moves downward to create negative air pressure in the lungs relative to the outside of the body

didactic teaching approaches: A teaching style involving teachers relaying material to students, such as in traditional lectures

digital feedback suppression scheme: An internal feature in a hearing aid that eliminates feedback before it is noticeable to the patient

digital hearing aids: Hearing instruments that change acoustic energy to electrical voltages that are converted to a binary number code by the analog-to-digital (A/D) converter, which in turn is processed by a computer chip, then sent to the digital-to-analog (D/A) converter that changes the binary number code back into electrical voltage that will be transduced by the receiver into acoustic energy

digitally programmable analog or hybrid hearing aids: Hearing instruments that transform acoustic energy into electrical voltage for processing that is accomplished by digitally controlled circuits inside the hearing aid that are

manipulated externally by the audiologist using a computer or by the user via a remote control (Dillon, 2001)

diphthong distortion: An error in vowel production such that a diphthong is substituted for by a single vowel or monothong

diphthongalization: Changing a regular, single vowel or monothong into a diphthong (e.g., /e/ into /eI/)

diphthongs: A vowel that is a combination of two vowels, resulting in movement of the second formant during its production (e.g., /a/ + /I/ = /aI/)

diplophonia: The perception that a voice has two fundamental frequencies

direct-audio input (DAI): A series of electrical contacts that connects an external signal source via a plug or external shoe to the input of a hearing aid, bypassing the microphone (Ross, 2006)

direct service delivery: Therapy directly provided by audiologists and speech-language pathologists in the schools

directional (microphone): An input transducer that picks up sounds from in front of the hearing aid wearer

directional hearing aids: Have microphones that change their output as a function of the direction from which sound waves arrive at the input of a hearing aid (Frye, 2005)

disability: An umbrella term for impairments, activity limitations, and participation restrictions

discipline specific sources: Sources of information used by audiologists and speech-language pathologists

discrimination: Differential treatment of members of a group based on prejudice

discrimination: The ability to tell whether two auditory stimuli are the same or different

distal manual dexterity: The ability to use the hands (Lesner & Kricos, 1995)

distortion product otoacoustic emissions (DPOAEs): An objective method of assessing outer hair cell integrity by delivering two tones (f_1 and f_2) via a probe and measuring the emissions from sensory cells in the form of a distortion product ($2f_1$-f_2)

dizziness: A general feeling of imbalance

domestic sources: Sources of evidence originating within the United States

dominant transmission: An inheritance pattern in which only one gene is needed for the trait to be passed on

double-blinded prospective randomized, controlled clinical trials (DBPRCTs): Clinical trials that meet the following criteria: (1) data are collected *after* enrollment of participants, (2) participants are randomly assigned to treatment and control groups, and (3) neither participants nor researchers have knowledge of those assignments

double-blinding: Occurs when neither the experimenter nor the participant has knowledge of administration of the treatment/intervention or placebo

dropouts: Participants who are recruited, but fail to complete an experimental protocol

dry type of macular degeneration: The most common (90% of cases) type of macular degeneration resulting in the thinning of the macula in the eye

dual sensory impairment: The existence of both hearing loss and vision loss in the same patient

dynamic range: Decibel range between threshold (e.g., 10 dB HL) and sounds that are uncomfortably loud (e.g., 90 dB HL)

earhook: Part of a BTE hearing aid that rests on top of the pinna, securing the device in place on the ear

earmold: Custom-made earpieces that couple hearing aids to patients' ears

eclectic approach (to auditory habilitation): Use of a conglomeration of techniques from aural habilitative approaches in order to meet the needs of the patient

educational audiologists: Hearing healthcare professionals that provide services to children in schools

effect sizes: "A metric that expresses the magnitude of a result, such as the differences in mean scores for two different hearing aids, within the context of the individual variation in scores" (Cox, 2005; p. 432)

effectiveness: The extent to which treatments provide positive patient outcomes in real world settings (ASHA, 2004c; 2005c)

efficacy: The degree to which intervention results in positive outcomes in ideal settings such as laboratory settings (ASHA, 2004c; 2005c)

efficiency: The extent to which one treatment provides relatively better outcomes than other treatments (ASHA, 2004c; 2005c)

egocentrism: Negative attitudes toward other people when comparing their cultures against one's own

electric auditory brainstem response (EABR): An auditory brainstem response test using an electric stimulus (Voll, 2005)

electrical threshold level (T-level): The amount of current provided by a cochlear implant electrode that results in the patient just being able to detect the sensation of hearing

electroacoustic analysis: A process completed by a hearing aid analyzer that determines if a hearing aid is functioning according to manufacturer's specifications

electroacoustics: The process of how acoustic energy enters a hearing aid, is changed to electrical energy, is processed, and then changed back to acoustic energy for delivery to a patient's ear

electrode array: Consists of electrodes that are paired and aligned along on a wire that is inserted into the cochlea (e.g., round window) during surgery for cochlear implantation

electromagnetic devices: Types of partially implantable hearing aids necessitating use of an external processor that turns acoustic energy to electromagnetic energy that is sent across the skin to a coil on a vibrating ossicular prosthesis (VORP) setting the stapes into vibration (Shohet, 2010)

empathetic listening: A technique used in client-centered therapy; involves not only hearing what patients are saying, but being able to relate to their feelings

engineering controls: Modifications to equipment or production to reduce noise levels (e.g., replacing a fan belt) to permissible levels in the workplace

enlarged vestibular aqueduct syndrome (EVAS): A disorder in which the vestibular aqueduct is larger than usual that causes fluctuating sensorineural hearing losses in some patients

environmental factors: What make up the physical, social, and attitudinal environment in which people live and conduct their lives

Epley procedure: A canalith repositioning procedure

equivalent input noise (EIN) level: An electroacoustic parameter that evaluates if the hearing aid is producing noise on its own

ethical practice board: A group of members of the American Academy of Audiology appointed to investigate and adjudicate peers who have reportedly violated the AAA's Code of Ethics

etiologic questions: Investigates the relative risk of certain exposures (e.g., noise) for developing a certain disease or disorder (e.g., noise-induced hearing loss)

evidence-based practice (EBP): Integrates high-quality research evidence, practitioner expertise, and patient preferences and values into the process of making clinical decisions (ASHA, 2004c)

expansion and modeling: Language facilitation techniques of repeating what the child says and adding more to it (DesJardin & Eisenberg, 2007; Tye-Murray, 2008)

expectation bias: Anything that may be done by experimenters or participants who expect certain results that influence the outcomes of the study

experimenter bias: Anything that the experimenter does that has measurable influence on the dependent variable that is not attributable to the independent variable

expert clinical opinion: The knowledge and skills of recognized leaders in the field who have established themselves through clinical work and/or scholarly activity

external noise: Unwanted noise that comes from outside of a building (e.g., playground noise and traffic noise)

extra corporeal membrane oxygenation (ECMO): A medical procedure in which a machine outside the body delivers oxygen to a patient's blood, much like the heart and lungs are supposed to do

eyeglass hearing aid: A style of hearing aid that has its electronic components housed in the temple of the glasses and is coupled to patients' ears by means of earmolds using tubing

facial recess approach: A method of surgically accessing the middle ear through the mastoid through a niche lateral to the facial nerve canal

facilitative language techniques: Things caregivers can do to enhance children's communication

Familiar Sounds on the Audiogram: A tool consisting of an audiogram that has speech and other familiar sounds superimposed at the frequency and hearing level of their approximate spectral energy

Federal Anti-kickback Statute: Law that prohibits healthcare professionals from receiving payments for referrals to providers for services reimbursable through federal programs such as Medicaid or Medicare

feedback: A whistling sound that comes out of the hearing aid receiver that is picked up again by the microphone, or reamplification of previously amplified sound

first-fit programming: Manufacturers' fitting programs that set hearing aids so that patients are allowed to get accustomed to their new hearing instruments

flutter echo: The ricocheting of reflected sound bouncing between two parallel structures

forest plots: Graphs of effect sizes and corresponding confidence intervals for studies

formal care providers: Paraprofessionals such as certified nursing assistants who care for the elderly

formal fall prevention programs: Documented efforts within specific facilities that employ healthcare professionals full-time or on a consultant basis who serve a role on the fall prevention team

fovea: The center of the macula that is the location of the sharpest visual image

free and appropriate public education (FAPE): A principle of the IDEA (2004) stating that children with disabilities should be provided with an appropriate education at no cost to their families

frequency modulation (FM) systems: Systems that transmit the signal via radio waves to a receiver

frequency response curve / frequency range (f_1 and f_2): An electroacoustic parameter that assesses whether the hearing aid is amplifying a range of frequencies specified by the manufacturer

frequency shaping: Differential amplification of certain frequency regions or the "sculpting" of the frequency response of a hearing aid to accommodate various configurations of hearing loss via the use of more than one channel or frequency band

full assistance level: A level of hearing aid care in a residential facility for patients who do not have the ability to care for their hearing instruments

full-on gain curve: An electroacoustic parameter that with an input to the microphone being a tone, sweeping from low to high frequency at 50 or 60 dB SPL, and the controls set for maximum levels, it is the *gain* of the hearing aid as a function of frequency

functional gain: The difference in unaided and aided thresholds for warbled tones presented through loudspeakers in an audiometric test booth

functioning: All body functions, activities, and participation

fundamental frequency (Fo): The number of times the vocal folds open and close per second

gain processing: How hearing aid circuitry amplifies sounds in certain frequency regions

gathering information: Obtaining a patient's pertinent background information (Stockman et al., 2004)

generic sources: Sources of information used across disciplines

genetics consultation: An appointment with a qualified healthcare professional (e.g., clinical geneticist, genetics counselor, or clinical molecular geneticist) that includes genetic testing and counseling

genotype: What is in a person's genes

glaucoma: A collection of eye diseases in which abnormal intra-ocular eye pressure causes damage to the optic nerve (University of Michigan Kellogg Eye Center, 2007)

gold standard: A test considered to be the most valid and reliable measure that diagnoses a disease or disorder against which all other methods are to be compared (e.g., audiogram is the gold standard of measure for hearing sensitivity)

gonioscopy: Examining the drainage angle of the eye

group discussion method: A method of assessing conversational fluency involving a group of patients with hearing loss and their significant others discussing potentially difficult listening situations (Tye-Murray, 2008)

group-amplification systems: Devices used to transmit a speaker's voice (either live or via multimedia) to an audience of listeners and are classified by how the signal travels to the listener(s)

Guidelines for the Audiologic Management of Adult Hearing Impairment: One of the first clinical practice guidelines in auditory rehabilitation using an evidence-based process for its development (Valente, Abrams, et al., 2006)

habituation: The reduction of a response to a stimulus after repeated exposure

hand cue: Clinicians and parents cover their mouths with their hands while speaking, eliminating visual cues and encouraging children to rely and develop their auditory skills. It has a secondary function when placed near children's mouths indicating that it is their turn to speak (Pollack, 1997)

hand-searching: Searching for evidence in journals or unpublished studies

hard of hearing: Typically having PTAs or SRTs that are less than about 80 dB HL and functionally being able to understand speech without the use of visual cues with assistance from hearing aids

hard of hearing and blind: Having some hearing impairment, but no functional vision (Spiers & Hammett, 1995)

hard of hearing and visually impaired: Having limited hearing and vision and may be part of hearing or Deaf communities (Spiers & Hammett, 1995)

hard technologies: Devices or parts that can be easily purchased by the consumer, assembled, and used (Cook & Hussey, 2002)

hardwired systems: An assistive listening device in which the speaker, or sound source, is physically tethered to the listener via a wire

HAT system: See *assistive listening technology system*

Hawthorne effect: The tendency for participants to act differently when they know they are part of a research experiment

"head shadow effect": Occurs when the head casts a shadow for high frequency sounds

health: A state of complete physical, mental, and social well-being; not merely the absence of disease or infirmity (World Health Organization, 2001)

health-related quality of life (HRQoL): The impact of an illness or a disease on an individual's physical, mental, and social well-being (Abrams, Chisolm, & McArdle, 2005)

hearing aid analyzer: A device that is used to determine if a hearing aid is functioning according to manufacturer's specifications

hearing aid dependent systems: An amplification system that requires use of a hearing aid that is coupled or attached to the jack or microphone

hearing aid effect: Negative public impressions of persons who wear hearing aids

hearing aid independent systems: An amplification system that requires use of a receiver or hardwire amplifier that has an input jack, volume control wheel, and earphone jack

hearing aid orientation groups: New and experienced hearing aid wearers and their significant others attending sessions geared toward promoting successful use of amplification

hearing assistive technology (HAT): A range of devices, services, strategies, and practices that are conceived and applied to ameliorate the auditory problems faced by individuals with hearing loss

hearing assistive technology system: See *assistive listening technology system*

hearing conservation programs: Comprehensive efforts aimed at preventing noise-induced hearing loss (NIHL); frequently involves a team of professionals such as audiologists, data management specialists, engineers (e.g., acoustical, industrial, and so on), industrial hygienists, personnel managers, plant managers, physicians (e.g., industrial or otolaryngologists), safety specialists, and supervisors

hearing impairment: An impairment in hearing, whether permanent or fluctuating, that adversely affects a child's educational performance but that is not included under the definition of deafness in section [(300.7(c)(5)) of the Individuals with Disabilities Education Act]

hearing protection devices (HPDs): Devices (e.g., earplugs) used to attenuate sound at workers' ears

heterosexism: The belief that love relationships between a man and a woman are superior to homosexual partnerships

high-frequency average OSPL-90: An electroacoustic parameter for hearing aids that with an input to the microphone being a tone, sweeping from low to high frequency at 90 dB SPL, and the controls set for maximum levels, is the average output taken at 1000, 1600, and 2500 Hz from the OSPL90 curve and must be within + or − 4 dB of manufacturer's specifications

high-frequency full-on average gain: An electroacoustic parameter for hearing aids that, with an input to the microphone being a tone, sweeping from low to high frequency at 50 or 60 dB SPL, and the controls set for maximum levels, is the average gain (i.e., output minus input) taken at 1000, 1600, and 2500 Hz full-on gain curve and must be within + or − 5 dB of manufacturer's specifications

high-risk register: A collection of conditions that increases the likelihood for presence or development of hearing loss

homophones: Phonemes in the same viseme group (e.g., /p/, /b/, and /m/)

homophonous: Sounds that look the same on the mouth such as /p/, /b/, and m/ all being made with the lips closed

hook-up: The initial delivery and fitting of the cochlear implant, which usually takes about two hours

hospice: Care designed to provide comfort and support to patients and their families when a life-limiting illness no longer responds to cure-oriented treatments (Hospice Foundation of America, 2006)

Huggies: Hearing aid accessories that consist of a plastic loop that is attached to the hearing aid case, surrounds the ear, and snugly holds the behind-the-ear device in place

hybrid cochlear implant: Devices that simultaneously provide acoustic input through a hearing aid for the lower frequencies and electrical stimulation of afferent auditory nerve fibers tuned to the higher frequencies via a cochlear implant in the same ear

hyperacusis: Hypersensitivity to the loudness of sounds; can co-occur with tinnitus

hyperopia: Farsightedness, meaning that although a person can see distant objects, those that are close may look blurry (University of Michigan Kellogg Eye Center, 2006d)

hypertension: A blood pressure reading of 140/90 mmHg or higher that is estimated to affect 65 million or 1 in 3 adults in the United States (National Heart, Lung, and Blood Institute, 2010)

incidental learning: Unplanned learning or the natural acquisition of information (Moeller, 2010)

identification: The ability to label an auditory stimulus

IEP grading: Using IEP long-term goals and short-term objectives for criteria in assessment

impairments: Problems in body function or structure or of a physiological or psychological function such as a significant deviation or loss

impedance: The opposition to the flow of energy (e.g., electricity)

impulse sound: A short duration, high-intensity sound like a gunshot

inadequate sampling: Occurs when the participants in a sample do not represent the population of patients from which the results are to be generalized

incidence: The number of new cases of a particular disease during a specified time period

incidental learning: Unplanned learning or the natural acquisition of information (Moeller, 2010)

incidental learning methods: Language instruction methods that use incidental learning

independent level: A level of hearing aid care in a residential facility at which patients are completely responsible for their hearing instruments

independent variables: What is manipulated by the experimenter in trying to test a hypothesis

independent work periods: Students concentrate on assignments during class time

individual family services plan (IFSP): A written document developed by a team of professionals that states the programs, services, and equipment that the public agency must provide to the 0- to 2-year-old child and his or her family

individualized education plan (IEP): A written document that stipulates the special education programs and services, long-term goals and short-term objectives, any accommodations and related services provided by the public agency to a child with a disability

Individuals with Disabilities Education Act (IDEA): A federal law that ensures that all children with disabilities are entitled to a free and appropriate public education in the least restricted environment

induction loop system: System that consists of a microphone, an amplifier, and a large loop that turns the signal into electromagnetic energy

industrial audiologist: A hearing healthcare professional who specializes in this area of practice to oversee hearing conservation programs (e.g., in-house program)

informal care providers: Usually friends or family members (e.g., often a spouse or adult child, usually a daughter) of elderly people

informal teaming for balance issues: Occurs on a case-by-case basis whereby audiologists may consult with other healthcare professionals about balance (e.g., primary care physicians regarding patients' prescription medication that may be contributing to dizziness and vertigo)

information literacy: The knowledge and skills for effectively and efficiently finding relevant high-quality evidence for clinical decision-making

informational counseling: Providing information related to hearing loss, its diagnosis, and management to patients and their family members (English, 2002)

infrared systems: Systems that transmit a signal via infrared light rays

in-house program: A hearing conservation program run completely within a company; this is not too common in the United States

input: How information gets into the brain

input compression: Reduces the gain of the hearing aid based on the input level in order to match the range of intensities that are audible, yet comfortable for patients, also known as dynamic range compression (Frye, 2005)

input/output function: An electroacoustic parameter that shows the output of a hearing aid as a function of the input stimulus

inservices: Continuing education opportunities to teach knowledge and skills on selected topics

instrumental activities of daily living (IADLs): Tasks such as preparing dinner, going grocery shopping, planning a budget, and so on

intention-to-treat analysis: A procedure that compares the results of patients in groups to which they were originally assigned; requires obtaining their data, regardless of whether or not they completed the experimental protocol (Hollis & Campbell, 1999)

interactive teaching: Teaching styles including teacher-to-student and student-to-student interactions that may involve small or large groups

interdisciplinary teams: Involves professionals from different disciplines who possess discipline-specific skills, plus the ability to contribute to a team effort in accomplishing goals (ASHA, 1996)

intermediate presbycusis: Subclinical structural changes in the auditory system due to aging that are not significant enough to qualify as a specific type of presbycusis

intermittent sound: Sound that goes on and off

internal noise: Unwanted sound that comes from inside the school but outside the classroom (e.g., hallway noise and noise from the cafeteria)

internal validity: The degree of certainty that any measureable treatment effects on the dependent variable were due to the independent variable and not to other factors (Haynes & Johnson, 2009)

International Classification of Functioning, Disability, and Health (ICFDH): A classification system and model that provides a standard language and framework for use in describing health and health-related states

international sources: Sources of evidence originating outside the United States

interpreters: Professionals who translate what is said into another language, such as American Sign Language

interprofessional documents: Documents generated by groups of individuals who represent different professional organizations usually involving multidisciplinary issues

intervention question: Focuses on the relative efficacy, effectiveness, or efficiency of two treatments for a specific patient or population

interview method: A method for determining conversational fluency by directly asking patients about their subjective impressions of their abilities in various communication situations (Tye-Murray, 2008)

in-the-canal (ITC) hearing aid: A style of in-the-ear hearing aid that fits into the external ear canal, leaving most, if not all, of the concha free and its acoustic properties unaffected

in-the-ear (ITE) hearing aids: A category of hearing aid style that (1) includes classic in-the-ear, in-the-canal, and completely-in-the-ear model; (2) does not require earmolds; and (3) has its electronic components housed completely within a custom-made shell or earpiece

intonation: The variation of fundamental frequency over time

intraprofessional documents: Documents generated by professional organizations (e.g., ASHA or AAA) to guide their members (e.g., audiologists and speech-language pathologists)

inverse square law: Describes how the sound pressure level of a signal changes as a function of distance from the source (e.g., a reduction of 6 dB SPL with each doubling of distance)

iris: The part of the eye that denotes its color, which dilates making the opening of the eye larger or smaller to let either more or less light in, respectively

itinerant: Traveling from school-to-school providing services to students

labyrinth: A twisting and turning series of osseous spaces set deep within the temporal bone

labyrinthitis: An inflammatory disorder of the inner ear or labyrinth

language sample: An exact transcription of a patient's use of language including what is communicated by all participants along with notation of relevant context

late-deafened: Losing hearing after the age of 13 years

least restrictive environment (LRE): A principle in special education that to the greatest extent possible, children with hearing loss should be educated with their peers who are nondisabled (IDEA, 2004; Johnson, 2000)

lens: A transparent structure that focuses the light entering the eye by changing shape based on whether objects are close or far away

level grading: Providing letter grades (e.g., A, B, C, and so on) and level of difficulty (e.g., 1, 2, and 3)

levels of evidence: A hierarchy of rigor used in evaluating research methodology

libby horn: A type of tubing in which the diameter of the tubing gets larger from the earhook to its connection to the earmold; can increase the amount of high-frequency amplification

limbic systems: Part of the brain that deals with emotions

linear hearing aids: Have a direct and predictable output as a function of input level of the signal and gain of the hearing aid

linguistic mapping: A language facilitation technique of saying what you think the child is trying to say by identifying what is around you (or context) to convey meaning (DesJardin & Eisenberg, 2007; Tye-Murray, 2008)

lipreading: Watching the speaker and deriving meaning from recognition of the visible aspects of articulation

listening bubbles: Proximities for communication, or distances at which children consistently respond to quiet, typical, and loud sounds (Anderson, 2007)

listening through filters: A pitfall in counseling involving identifying so closely with patients, particularly children, that listening is colored by personal experiences of the professional

listening with the third ear: Involves listening with the heart for patients' affective statements that indicate unmet social or emotional issues regarding hearing loss

localization: The ability to identify the origin of a sound

long-term average speech spectrum (LASS): The intensity of speech as a function of frequency

long-term care: Broad-based care aimed at providing services to persons with chronic disabilities to function in completing activities of daily living (ADLs) (e.g., bathing, dressing, eating, or other personal care) and instrumental activities of daily living (IADLs) (e.g., shopping, meal preparation, money management)

loudness discomfort levels (LDLs): Levels of sound that are judged to be uncomfortable by the patient

low vision: Visual acuity less than 20/70 that cannot be corrected by conventional eyeglasses (University of Michigan Kellogg Eye Center, 2007)

macro search strategies: The order in which databases are searched for evidence-based practice

macromovements: Body movements used by Verbotonal therapists for facilitating the auditory perception of children with hearing impairment

macula: Sensory end organs for balance located in the utricle and saccule of the inner ear

macula: The center of the retina; contains a high density of photoreceptor cells that enables sight of fine details

macular degeneration: See *age-related macular degeneration*

magnetic resonance imaging: A diagnostic procedure in which radio waves are applied to the body so that the nuclear magnetic resonance of atoms produces images of internal organs and tissues on a computer (Merriam-Webster's Medical Dictionary Online, 2008)

mainstreaming: Educating children with disabilities with their nondisabled peers

maintenance: The stage when patients must sustain their efforts to change

maladaptive behaviors: Those actions that interfere with or sabotage the auditory (re)habilitation process (e.g., nonadherence to recommendations and denial)

manual dexterity: The skill or ease in using the hands and the arms (Kumar, Hickey, & Shaw, 2000)

mapping: See *cochlear implant mapping*

masking: A procedure used by an audiologist that ensures that the non-test ear does not participate or interferes with audiometric testing

mastery experience: The reviewing of information and the practice of skills to increase patients' hearing aid self-mastery (Smith & West, 2006)

mastoidectomy: Partial or complete removal of the mastoid process and bone

maximal technology: HAT devices that replace the sense of hearing with other senses, such as visual or tactile

maximum comfort level (C-level): The highest current level of sensation that a cochlear implant patient can tolerate for an extended period of time without causing discomfort

maximum OSPL-90: An electroacoustic parameter for hearing aids that with the input to the microphone being a tone, sweeping from low to high frequencies at 90 dB SPL, and the controls set for maximum levels, is the highest point on the OSPL-90 curve and must be no higher than 3 dB of manufacturer's specifications

mean length of turn (MLT): A measure of conversational fluency defined as the average number of words used by a person during a conversational turn

mean length of turn ratio (MLT ratio): The ratio of the patient's MLT per the conversational partner's MLT

mean length of utterance (MLU): The average number of morphemes used per utterance

mechanical presbycusis: A cochlear conductive hearing loss, resulting in a stiffening of the basilar membrane due to aging resulting in a gradually sloping high-frequency hearing loss

medical home: A high-quality and cost-effective approach to providing accessible, family-centered, ongoing, comprehensive, coordinated, and compassionate care to children through assignment of a primary healthcare provider who knows the child on an individual basis, acknowledging any special needs and cultural background for achievement of maximum potential

medical model: Perspective that disability is a characteristic of a person or patient directly caused by disease, trauma, or other health condition requiring medical care provided by a professional

medical model of deafness: Classifies those with hearing loss as "sick" individuals trying to get well (Lane et al., 1996)

memories: Different settings on the hearing aid that listeners may use for different listening situations

meninges: Membranous coverings of the brain

meta-analysis: The use of special statistical procedures that combine the results of more than one investigation in order to measure the magnitude of a treatment effect

metabolic presbycusis: A degeneration of the stria vascularis (which maintains chemical, bioelectric, and metabolic health of the cochlea) due to aging that occurs from base to apex in the cochlea, manifesting itself as a relatively flat audiometric configuration

method of explicit categorization: Defining and presenting information to patients with topics presented in the following order: recommendations, diagnosis, results, and prognosis

micro search strategies: Specific techniques for searching within a database for evidence-based practice

micromovements: Movements of the speech musculature, according to those using the Verbotonal Method

microphone: An input transducer that changes sound pressure into variations in electrical voltage

microtia: Deformity of the pinna, which is usually smaller than normal

minimal technology: HAT devices that augment patients' listening abilities

mitochondrial disorders: Hereditary disorders resulting from abnormalities in the mitochondria of the cells of the body

mixed hearing losses: A loss of hearing sensitivity resulting from problems in both the conductive and sensorineural mechanism

mixed presbycusis: A combination of two or more different types of presbycusis

modified live voice presentation: The audiologist presents the speech stimuli on a speech perception test via the microphone on the audiometer while monitoring his or her voice on a volume meter

motivational interviewing protocol: Elicits self-motivational statements from ambivalent patients to become motivated for change (Miller & Rollnick, 2002)

multiculturalism: The acknowledgment that society is composed of many different groups or cultures

multidisciplinary screening for central auditory processing disorders: Screening tests administered by professionals in more than one field to identify those who need a comprehensive central auditory processing evaluation

multidisciplinary teams: Utilizing discipline-specific skills and viewing rehabilitation efforts as the combined efforts of each discipline involved (ASHA, 1996)

multiple disabilities: Presence of more than one disability in a patient

multiple grading: Dividing a unit into sections for specific grading (e.g., participation, achievement, progress)

multisensory approach: A method for facilitating oral spoken language in children with hearing loss that provides input via other senses besides audition such as vision or vibrotactile

mutations: Genetic abnormalities

myopia: Nearsightedness, meaning that the person can see objects close up very well, but has difficulty seeing distant objects that may appear blurry (University of Michigan Kellogg Eye Center, 2006e)

narrative grading: Writing a descriptive evaluation of a student's work

neonatal intensive care unit (NICU): The nursery where the most fragile and sickest babies go after birth including, but not limited to those who are premature, have multiple birth defects, or severe medical issues (e.g., heart, lung, gastrointestinal, or other life-threatening conditions)

neural hearing loss: A hearing impairment that occurs due to difficulties that cranial nerve VIII (i.e., statocoustic nerve) has in transmitting electrical impulses from the peripheral to the central auditory nervous system

neural losses: A hearing impairment that occurs due to difficulties that cranial nerve VIII (i.e., statoacoustic nerve) has in transmitting electrical impulses from the peripheral to the central auditory nervous system

neural plasticity: The ability of the brain to form new connections and reorganize itself through the processing of sensory information from auditory experiences (Tremblay & Kraus, 2002)

neural presbycusis: An atrophy of cochlear neurons throughout the cochlea (basal end more affected than apical) and central auditory pathways due to aging with an unexpectedly poor speech recognition performance when compared with the patient's pure-tone audiogram

neurofibromatosis: A group of three genetically distinct hereditary conditions that results in tumors arising from the cells of the supportive tissue of neurons

neuromaturation: Development of the nervous system

Neurophysiological Model of Tinnitus: A model that explains how patients neurologically and physiologically respond to the sensation of tinnitus

neutralization: Vowels are substituted for the neutral vowel *schwa*

noise: Any unwanted sound

noise dosimeters: Special purpose sound level meters that sample the wearer's exposure to sound during a typical work day

noise reduction rating (NRR): A value that indicates the amount of sound attenuation, provided that HPDs are worn properly

noise-induced hearing loss (NIHL): Hearing loss resulting from exposure to excessive sound levels

nonacknowledgment: Failure to recognize a problem (e.g., I don't have a problem; people around me mumble)

nonbehavioral tests: Tests that measure physiological responses to sound

nonoccupational noise exposure: Noise encountered in recreational or leisure activities

nonprofessional counseling: Providing information and support for emotional crises that involve discipline-specific issues (English, 2002)

nonrandomized intervention studies: Types of experimental designs that do not use random assignment (e.g., participants to treatment and control groups)

nonsyndromic: When hearing loss usually occurs without other disabilities

norm-referenced measures: Compare children's performances against those of a peer group

occlusion: The degree to which an earmold or hearing aid blocks the ear canal

occlusion effect: Patient-generated sounds (e.g., vocalizations) vibrate the mandible, which in turn does the same thing to the cartilaginous walls of the outer ear canal, which increase the sound pressure level of low-frequency sounds in an occluded ear (Mackenzie, Mueller, Ricketts, & Konkle, 2004)

occupational noise exposure: Noise encountered in the workplace

omnidirectional (microphone): An input transducer that picks up sound from all around the hearing aid wearer

open area concepts: Eight or more classes located in the same space without any walls, permitting team teaching and cross-grouping of children who can move easily from class to class

open-angle glaucoma: A type of glaucoma caused by constant increase in intraocular eye pressure resulting in a blockage of the "drainage" angle of the eye that reduces visual acuity, contrast sensitivity, and color vision (University of Michigan Kellogg Eye Center, 2007; Weinstein, 2000)

open-ear fitting hearing aids: A relatively new style of hearing aid that is similar to a behind-the-ear hearing aid, but whose electrical components fit into a smaller case that fits high on the pinna and couples to the ear via a thin wire and receiver

open-head injuries: An injury resulting from a penetrating blow to the head involving the scalp, skull, and/or meninges (Youse, Le, Cannizzaro, & Coelho, 2002)

open-set speech recognition: A response format in which patients write down or repeat test stimuli instead of selecting a response from a group of options

opthalmoscopy: Evaluating the optic nerve

optic nerve: A bundle of nerve fibers that sends visual information to the brain

osseointegration: The process by which the small titanium implant of the bone-anchored hearing aid adheres to the surrounding tissue in the mastoid bone (Cochlear Americas, 2006)

otoacoustic emissions testing: An objective, noninvasive test of outer hair cell integrity involving presenting stimuli into the ear canal (acoustic energy) that travel through the middle ear (mechanical energy), and then into the inner ear (bioelectric energy) to which the sensory cells emit a response that travels in the reverse direction and is measured in the ear canal

otoacoustic emissions: Responses emitted by the outer hair cells that are either spontaneous or evoked

otoconia: Calcium carbonate granules located on top of a gelatinous matrix embedded with stereocilia of sensory hair cells in the macula in the vestibular system

otoliths: A sensory end organ for balance located in the utricle or saccule of the inner ear

otosclerosis: A disease in which a bony growth forms on the otic capsule and particularly on the stapes footplate

otoscope: An illuminated, magnifying scope for looking into the ears

outcome measures: Data collected to determine the benefit of treatment and frequently involve the use of self-assessment scales

out-house program: A hearing conservation program run by someone external to the company

output: The sound pressure level coming out of the receiver of a hearing aid (i.e., input + gain)

output compression: Output-limiting that compresses or reduces gain in order to limit the maximum output so that it is not uncomfortable to patients (Frye, 2005)

output of information: How a child expresses what he or she has learned in the classroom in the form of performance on tests, class assignments, and contributions to class discussions

output sound pressure level-90 (OSPL-90): An electroacoustic parameter for hearing aids with an input to the microphone being a tone, sweeping from low to high frequencies at 90 dB SPL with the settings set for maximum output capabilities, it is the output as a function of frequency

palliative care: The active total care of patients whose disease is not responsive to curative treatment defined by the World Health Organization (Center for Advancement of Palliative Care, 2006)

parallel talk: A language facilitation technique which is simply using words to describe what the child is attending to or doing (DesJardin & Eisenberg, 2007; Tye-Murray, 2008)

paraphrasing: A counseling technique involving repeating back what the patient has said

paraprofessionals: Teachers' aides who provide valuable support in the classroom

parent-initiated model: Diagnosis of hearing loss is a direct result of parents taking the initiative of scheduling an appointment with their pediatrician because of their concerns about their child's auditory behavior

partial acknowledgment: Limited recognition of a problem (e.g., I may have a problem, but I don't need to get treatment for it yet)

partial assistance level: A level of hearing aid care in a residential facility in which patients are responsible for the care and maintenance of their hearing instruments, but they may need assistance with these tasks

participant bias: Anything that a participant does that has a measurable influence on the dependent variable that is not attributable to the independent variable

participation: Involvement in life situations

participation restrictions: Problems an individual may experience, restricting involvement in life situations, particularly in communicating with specific partners in specific situations

patient selection criteria: General characteristics that individuals must have to be considered for cochlear implant candidacy

patient teach-back method: New hearing aid users repeat and show knowledge and skills they have learned (Saunders & Echt, 2007)

patient-safety questions: Evaluates the relative risks versus benefits of clinical procedures for specific patients or populations

peak clipping: Occurs when linear hearing aids reach their maximum output limit; successive increases in input do not result in complementary increases in the output of the signal whose amplitude is trimmed

peer-reviewed publications: Those publications that are reviewed by experts in the field and must meet certain criteria for publication

percent total harmonic distortion: An electroacoustic parameter that determines if the hearing aid is adding extra energy at frequencies that are whole-number multiples of input stimuli that could compromise the quality of the output signal, particularly if it is speech

perilingual hearing loss: A hearing loss that develops between 3 and 5 years of age or during the period of rapid speech and language acquisition

perimetry: Assessing the visual field in each eye

permanent conductive hearing loss: A loss of hearing sensitivity resulting from problems in the outer or middle ear that may not be completely ameliorated through medical management (e.g., congenital aural atresia)

permanent threshold shifts (PTS): Permanent and nonrecoverable loss of hearing sensitivity due to exposure to excessive sound levels

permissible exposure level (PEL): Time-weighted average (TWA) of 90 dBA for an eight-hour period, a 100% noise dose, and the maximum amount that is considered to be safe for most workers

personal adjustment counseling: Efforts to assist patients and their families cope with and solve problems caused by the secondary social and emotional effects of hearing loss

personal listening devices (PLDs): iPods, compact disc players, and MP3 players used by individuals to listen to music or other forms of entertainment

persuasion: A pitfall in counseling involving audiologists and speech-language pathologists convincing patients, particularly children, to see things their way

phenotype: Genetic traits that are actually expressed by the person (e.g., hair or eye color)

phonation: Vibration of the vocal folds

phonology: How speech sounds come together to form words

photoreceptors: Light-sensitive sensory cells

physiological and affective states: Conditions that influence patients' degree of self-efficacy in the performance of certain tasks (Smith & West, 2006)

Pidgin Sign: A combination of American Sign Language (ASL) and Signing Exact English (SEE)

piezoelectric devices: Types of implantable hearing aids that send electrical current through components containing piezoelectric crystals that result in increased vibration of the stapes ossicle (Shohet, 2010)

placebos: Inactive (i.e., sugar pill) conventional medications or procedures that are administered in the exact same way as the experimental treatment and serve as a comparison for experimental interventions

play audiometry: A testing paradigm for which children complete a motoric task (e.g., dropping blocks in a bucket, putting pegs in a board, etc.) for their response indicating detection of an auditory stimulus

portable classrooms: Moveable educational enclosures often utilized when the number of students exceeds the physical capabilities of a school

position statements: Documents supported by available scientific evidence and/or expert opinion put forth by professional organizations consistent with their intrinsic and/or extrinsic goals and objectives (AAA, 2009b)

postlingual hearing loss: A hearing loss that develops after the age of 5 or after speech and language development

potentiometers: Adjustable controls on analog hearing aids that audiologists manipulate to set electroacoustic parameters

power analysis: A statistical procedure conducted at the beginning of the experiment that determines the sample size needed to detect a significant difference when, in fact, it does exist

practice guidelines: A systematically defined set of recommended procedures based on scientific evidence and/or expert opinion that has been designed to yield specific, well-defined outcomes (AAA, 2009b)

pragmatics: The use of language in context

preferred practice patterns: Statements that define universally applicable characteristics of specific clinical activities, including definitions, regarding which professionals perform the procedures, expected outcomes, clinical indications, clinical processes, setting and equipment specifications, and documentation (ASHA, 2006b)

prejudice: Negatively judging someone without adequate knowledge or reason

prelingual hearing loss: A hearing loss that develops before the acquisition of speech and language

pre-literacy activities: Things that caregivers can do to prepare children for reading (e.g., reading books together)

presbycusis: Hearing impairment due to aging

presbyopia: The aging or the loss of the flexibility of the lens of the eye and the muscles responsible for its shape

prescriptive methods: Formulas that estimate the amount of hearing aid gain and output based on patients' audiometric thresholds

prevalence: The number of persons afflicted per a segment of the population

prevalence studies: Studies that determine the number of individuals that have a particular disorder or disease at one point in time per the number of people at risk (Newman, Browner, Cummings, & Hulley, 2001)

primary care: The broad spectrum of care, both preventative and curative, often provided by elderly persons' family physicians or internists who serve as their "medical home" (MedicineNet.com, 2006)

primary measurement methods: The investigator collecting and analyzing his or her own data for an experiment

primary or short-term memory: A type of memory that lasts longer than sensory memory and has a capacity of 5 to 7 items, permitting the retention of small bits of information over a short period of time (Weinstein, 2000)

procedural safeguards: Procedures ensuring that the rights of children with disabilities and their families are protected and each state must develop a system guaranteeing those rights (Johnson, 2000)

professional counseling: Mental health professionals (e.g., psychiatrists, psychologists, social workers) use their training to help people solve pervasive life problems (English, 2002)

professional-centered approach: A counseling approach in which the clinician asks the questions; is in control; has the role of diagnosing, reaching conclusions, and reporting; makes professional decisions regarding the needs of the patient and family; and is responsible for all decisions (Sweetow, 1999)

programs: See *memories*

promontory stimulation test: A needle electrode is inserted through the tympanic membrane and placed on the promontory with a surface electrode placed on the opposite cheek to measure for patients' sensation when the auditory nerve is stimulated

proportional frequency compression hearing aids: A hearing aid option for patients who have hearing losses greater than 60 dB HL in the higher frequencies with circuitry that actually moves critical "high-frequency" speech information into the lower frequency regions where patients usually have better hearing sensitivity (Davis, 2001)

prospective studies: Participants are recruited prior to the collection of data

prospective cohort studies: Investigations in which participants are recruited in the present before an outbreak of a disease or disorder to assess who does and does not develop a particular condition in the future (Frattali, 1998)

providing feedback: A counseling skill that involves making descriptive and specific statements to the patient to ensure accurate communication

proximal manual dexterity: The ability to raise and lower the arms (Lesner & Kricos, 1995)

pulsatile tinnitus: A noise in the head that pulsates, similar to a heartbeat and is usually vascular in nature

pupil: The opening to the eye

pure-tone average 1 (PTA1): The arithmetic average of the air-conduction thresholds for 500, 1000, and 2000 Hz

pure-tone average 2 (PTA2): The arithmetic average of the air-conduction thresholds taken at 1000, 2000, and 4000 Hz

pure-tone stimuli: Used for audiometric testing; have energy at discrete frequencies presented at various hearing levels

pure-tone threshold: The softest pure tone, measured in dB HL, that a patient can detect 50% of the time and is plotted on the audiogram with special symbols

quasi-experimental studies: See *nonrandomized intervention studies*

quasi-transcranial contralateral routing of the signal (CROS): Another name for the transcranial CROS that acknowledges that the signal is delivered by more than one way to the better ear (Valente, Valente, & Mispagel, 2006)

questionnaire method: A method of determining conversational fluency using traditional income/outcome measures (Tye-Murray, 2008)

racism: The belief that one race is superior to another

random assignment: Participants are assigned to treatment groups based purely on chance (e.g., each has a 50-50 chance of being assigned to receive a placebo or a treatment)

real-ear probe-tube microphone measurement system: Measures what the hearing aid is doing *inside* the patient's ear and if it is amplifying sound at the appropriate frequencies

real-ear-to-coupler difference: The difference between sound pressure level as a function of frequency measured at a specific point in the ear canal to that when measured in a 2-cc coupler

real-time captioning: The use of captions that are created and displayed simultaneously for lectures/presentations such as training seminars, corporate meetings, sporting, or other "live" events (Robson, 2008)

reassurance: A pitfall in counseling involving telling patients, particularly children, that they should not feel the way that they do and that the situation is not as bad as it seems

recasting: A language facilitation technique of simply restating a child's statement as a question, or vice-versa (DesJardin & Eisenberg, 2007; Tye-Murray, 2008)

receiver: An output transducer that changes variations in electric voltage back out into sound pressure or acoustic energy

recessive transmission: An inheritance pattern that requires two copies of a gene for a trait to be passed on

recommending: Advising and/or counseling a patient about potential treatment plans (Stockman et al., 2004)

recruitment: Abnormal growth in the sensation of loudness of sounds

red flags: Indications that patients are not making average progress with their implants (Robbins, 2005)

redundancy: Meaning that is coded in multiple ways in the speech signal

reference test gain: An electroacoustic parameter of hearing aids obtained with an input to the microphone being a tone, sweeping from low to high frequency at 60 dB SPL, and the volume control set at a specific level or at a level that yields an output that is 17 dB below the high-frequency average OSPL-90

referring: Providing a patient access to clinical services (Stockman et al., 2004)

reflective listening: A strategy by which professionals take a guess at what the patient means by using a statement that contains the word "you" and rephrasing what the patient has already said

refractive errors: Errors caused by the shape of the eye not bending light correctly, resulting in a blurred image

relapse: The stage in which the patient chooses not to continue the effort to change and returns to the original state

related services: Supportive services that are needed for a child to benefit from special education and may be provided by a variety of school personnel (e.g., audiologists, educational interpreter, school counselors, school nurses, school psychologists, school social workers, speech-language pathologists) (IDEA, 2004)

release time: The length of time, in milliseconds, that it takes for a compression circuit to deactivate after a decrease in sound level

remote microphone hearing assistive technology (RMHAT): Technology in which the microphone is not located on the body of the person who has a hearing impairment, such as personal FM systems, group/individual sound-field systems, and induction loop systems

reports: Testimonies or accounts of factual information related to professional issues identified by a professional organization (AAA, 2009b)

resonance: A tendency for objects to vibrate when energy at its natural frequency is applied resulting in amplification

retina: A thin lining of the back of the eye that is sensitive to light

retinal pigment epithelium: A dark layer that absorbs excess light, transports oxygen, nutrients, and cellular wastes between the rods and cones and the choroid

retinal vessels: The blood vessels that nourish the retina

retirement communities: Common living arrangements for the elderly consisting of privately owned detached homes, condominiums, and/or apartments that often have scheduled social and recreational activities or other special amenities (e.g., golf memberships) (Helpguide.org, 2010)

retrocochlear (hearing loss): Hearing losses caused by congenital or acquired damage or disease (e.g., tumors) to the auditory nerve and its pathways and reception and processing areas in the cortex

retrospective cohort study: Studies that identify a sample of individuals who already have a disorder and then measures predictor variables (Cummings et al., 2001)

retrospective studies: Data are collected after some sort of event or occurrence

reverberation: The continuation of acoustic energy due to the reflections of that energy off of the floor, ceiling, and walls of a room after the source of the sound has been terminated (Crandell & Smaldino, 2005)

reverberation time: The time it takes for the sound to decrease 60 dB after the source of the sound has been terminated

reverse mainstreaming: The inclusion of nondisabled children from regular education into special education programs

rods: Photoreceptors used for vision in low light

safety-net metaphor: All of the services (protections, professionals, and accommodations) provided to a child who is deaf or hard of hearing in the classroom

sampling bias: The measurable influence on the dependent variable that assignment of participants to treatment or control groups that is directly not attributable to the independent variable

sarcasm: When words convey one meaning, but the way the message is said signifies another

scheduling: Selecting the time for a patient to receive clinical services (Stockman et al., 2004)

school-based model: An educational audiology service delivery model in which audiologists are full-time employees of the school district or educational agency

school-to-work programs (STW): Activities, experiences, and opportunities that prepare students for the world of work, including career exploration, integration of academic/vocational curricula, internships, job shadowing, mentoring, and youth apprenticeships (Bonds, 2003)

schwannomas: Tumors arising from the sheaths of cranial and spinal nerves and often invade the internal auditory canal or cerebellopontine angle in over 90% of gene carriers with NF2 (Kanowitz et al., 2004; Wagner, 2006)

sclera: The white part of the eye that is made up of a tough and fibrous tissue that protects the eye

scope of practice: An official document of a professional organization that specifies appropriate areas of practices for its members

Scottish Intercollegiate Guidelines Network: A group devoted to improving the quality and consistency of healthcare for the citizens of Scotland

screening: A short process that serves to identify persons who may have a condition (e.g., hearing loss) needing further evaluation from those who do not

search strings: Words and/or phrases input into databases in order to retrieve the most relevant information on a topic

secondary measurement methods: Experimenters or clinicians considering or analyzing data collected from other investigators

secondary or long-term memory: A memory that includes information that has been stored for later retrieval and utilization

segmentals: Phonemes of the language

self-assessment scales: Questionnaires filled out by patients and significant others that are designed to measure the impact of hearing loss in various areas of life

self-efficacy: The confidence a person has in completing a set of skills requisite for success in achieving a particular goal (Bandura, 1986)

self-talk: A language facilitation technique of simply talking about what you're doing (DesJardin & Eisenberg, 2007; Tye-Murray, 2008)

semantics: The meaning of words

Semont procedure: A canalith repositioning procedure

senior apartment complexes: Housing options used by seniors with low incomes that consist of individual apartments with communal areas for social/recreational activities (Helpguide.org, 2010)

sensation level (SL): The number of decibels above a certain reference threshold

sensitivity: The accuracy with which screening protocols identify those who have a disorder

sensitivity levels: Determines the softest sound to be picked up by the microphone of a cochlear implant

sensorineural hearing losses: A loss of hearing sensitivity resulting from a problem in the inner ear, usually the result of hair cell damage as a result of noise exposure, ototoxic drugs, aging, and so on

sensory hearing loss: A loss of hearing sensitivity resulting from damage to the ear's inner or outer hair cells

sensory losses: A loss of hearing sensitivity resulting from damage to the ear's inner or outer hair cells

sensory memory: The first, momentary encoding of the incoming information at the input stage (Weinstein, 2000)

sensory presbycusis: Loss of sensory and supportive cells at the basal end of the cochlea due to age that progresses toward the apical end and is first manifested by a precipitous high-frequency sensorineural hearing loss usually starting during middle age

sentence recognition threshold: The lowest signal-to-noise ratio resulting in 50% sentence recognition

sequential implantation: Having one ear implanted first, and then the other ear during a second surgery

service delivery site: A place where auditory rehabilitative services are provided

sexism: A belief that one gender is superior to the other

signal expectation/time delay: Language facilitation technique of showing the child that you are waiting for their response (DesJardin & Eisenberg, 2007; Tye-Murray, 2008)

signal-to-noise ratio (S/N): The index of severity for noise; defined as the relative level of signal, in decibels (dB), in relation to that of the background noise

Signing Exact English: A manual communication system that aims to represent spoken English on the hands as accurately as possible

sign language interpreter: Professionals who serve to translate spoken language into sign language

silhouette inductor: An ear-level device worn behind the ear, much like a hearing aid, that provides a stable signal to the telecoil from a particular device (e.g., a type of receiver)

silicagel: A desiccant material that pulls moisture out of the hearing aid

simultaneous implantation: Both ears receiving cochlear implants during the same surgery

single-sided deafness: A normal ear on one side and a deaf or nonfunctional ear on the other

situational teaching: Teaching within meaningful contexts, according to those using the Verbotonal Method

Sixty/Sixty (60/60) rule: An advisory that says that people should limit their listening to their personal listening devices (e.g., iPods) to no more than 60% of full volume for 60 minutes per day (Fligor & Cox, 2004)

small-group instruction: One instructor teaching 10 students or less

social model: Perspective that views disability as a socially-created problem, not as an attribute of the person

soft technologies: Human components such as decision-making, strategies, and training

somatosensory senses: Senses that provide information about the body's position using skin and muscle receptors

sound-field amplification systems: FM transmitter that sends the speaker's voice to strategically placed loudspeakers in a classroom in order to improve the signal-to-noise ratio (S/N)

sound lateralization: Place of sound perception in the head (e.g., "Where does the sound seem to be coming from in your head? Do you hear it in the left ear, right ear, or in the center of your head?")

sound level meter: Instruments that measure sound levels, in decibels, in the environment

sound localization: Locating the origin of a sound in space

sound surveys: Sound measurement in noisy areas

sound transmission loss: The number of decibels that are attenuated from one side of a partition to another

Sounds on the Audiogram Chart: A figure consisting of common every day sounds and phonemes of the English language superimposed on an audiogram according to their spectral energy (e.g., approximate frequency and hearing level)

SPEAK: Cochlear implant processing scheme that breaks the signal into many (e.g., 20) bandpass filters, scans for those having the greatest amplitude, and then conveys that information via low pulse rates

special interest divisions: Groups of members of American Speech-Language-Hearing Association who share professional areas of interest and expertise

special purpose hearing aids: Amplification at frequency regions outside of that which would be considered conventional, also known as low-frequency- or high-frequency-emphasis hearing aids

specific auditory habilitation approach: The exclusive use of one approach to develop the auditory, speech, and language skills through children's use of their residual hearing (e.g., Auditory-Verbal Approach, the Ling Method, and Verbotonal Method)

specificity: The accuracy with which screening protocols accurately dismiss those individuals who do not have a particular disorder

spectrographic analysis: Use of computers in digitizing and analyzing the duration, frequency, and intensity of speech in addition to other parameters

speech awareness threshold (SAT): The softest hearing level at which the patient can detect the presence of speech

speech coding strategy: The methods that designate how acoustic signals (frequency, intensity, and timing) are modified by the cochlear implant speech processor and turned into electrical impulses that are sent to the electrodes that stimulate the auditory nerve

speech recognition score: The percent of words correctly repeated back when presented at suprasthreshold level

speech recognition threshold (SRT): The softest hearing-threshold level that the patient can repeat back or point to pictures on a board representing *spondee words* with 50% accuracy

speech tracking: An auditory training procedure requiring a partner to read materials to the patient who repeats *exactly* what has been said (De Filippo & Scott, 1978)

speech-language pathology assistants: Paraprofessionals who assist and are supervised by licensed speech-language pathologists

speechreading: A process by which listeners put together information from a variety of sources (e.g., lipreading; facial expressions; gesture, posture, and movement; situational cues, the topic of conversation; rules of the language; news of the day; motivation to understand; and residual hearing) to derive meaning (Cherry & Rubenstein, 1988)

spill over: When the electromagnetic signal from one room interferes with that of another

spiral ganglion: A collection of nerve cells that have fibers that send signals from the cochlea up the auditory pathway toward the brain

split-grade classrooms: One teacher responsible for instructing children from two different grade levels necessitating two or more activities occurring in the same enclosure

SPL-O-GRAM: Output targets for hearing aids that ensure that the long-term average speech spectrum is audible

spondee words: Compound words consisting of two syllables that are of equal stress (e.g., baseball, hot dog, armchair)

square-foot-to-student ratios: The number of square feet allotted to each child in a classroom setting

standard threshold shift (STS): An increase of thresholds of 10 dB or more taken as an average for 2000, 3000, and 4000 Hz for either ear after the results have been corrected for worker age

Stark Law: A civil law that prohibits physician "self-referral" in that they cannot refer patients to entities in which they or their family members have financial holdings

statistical power: The degree with which a significant difference between groups or conditions may be found if, in fact, it exists

stay-put principle: Mandates that children remain in their current educational placement during mediation processes

stereotype: A collection of characteristics attributed to a particular group

stimulable: The child is primed to respond when presented with a particular stimulus

stimulus-response paradigm: The basic unit of aural habilitative therapy in which the clinician presents a stimulus for the patient to respond to that is subsequently reinforced

strabismus: A visual disorder known as "cross eye" or wall eye; patients cannot align their eyes at the same time under normal conditions without one of the eyes turning in, up, or out (Kellogg Eye Center, 2006c)

structured communication method: A method of assessing conversational fluency involving mock situations to simulate realistic communication interactions (Tye-Murray, 2008)

subject bias: See *participant bias*

subject self-selection bias: A source of bias in an experiment when patients who volunteer for an experiment differ in some way from those who opt not to, possibly affecting results

supervised-use level: A level of hearing aid care in a residential facility in which the nursing staff assumes complete responsibility for patients' hearing instruments

supplementary aids and services: Those things that support a child with disabilities in general education such as assistive technology

supported senior housing: A living arrangement for senior citizens consisting of apartments or room/board, as well as meals, social activities, and housekeeping (Helpguide.org, 2010)

suprasegmentals: The prosodic aspects of language such as rhythm and intonation

suprathreshold levels: Levels that are above threshold and are usually presented at a comfortable level

surprise model of diagnosis: Diagnosis of hearing loss as a result of newborn hearing screening programs that surprise parents when their child is referred to an audiologist for an audiologic evaluation that confirms presence of hearing impairment

surrendering the role of expert: A counseling technique allowing patients, particularly children, to find their own answers instead of telling them what to do (English, 2001)

surrogate endpoints: Dependent variables measured in experimental studies that may indicate immediate outcomes, but that may not be representative of long-term status

syndromic hearing loss: When hearing loss presents with other disabilities that result from a recognized genetic condition

syntax: How words come together to form sentences

synthetic approach to speechreading: This approach to speechreading is based on the notion that a basic understanding of the message is important regardless of which individual parts are identified (Hipskind, 2007)

systematic review: Studies that involve asking research questions; searching for evidence; evaluating investigations; and analyzing results of several studies together; and making overall conclusions regarding the consistency of findings supporting the use of a clinical procedure or effectiveness of a particular treatment

Tadoma method: A means of communicating with deaf-blind individuals who place his or her thumb on the speaker's lips and other three fingers along the jaw line to understand what someone is saying through the tactile sense

task forces: Teams of professionals recruited by professional organizations to assess and/or determine appropriate strategies for issues affecting professional practice and pertaining to the recognized areas of audiology and speech-language pathology (AAA, 2009b)

team approach: A group of healthcare professionals collaborate to provide auditory rehabilitation to lessen the effects of hearing impairment on patients and their families

team teaching: Two or more teachers combining their classes together in one classroom

telecoil (t-coil): An induction coil (i.e., metal rod surrounded by many turns of a copper wire) that produces a voltage that can be amplified by the hearing aid when in close proximity to an alternating magnetic field that flows through it (Dillon, 2001)

Telecommunications Relay Service (TRS): A service that provides special operators available 24 hours a day,

seven days a week, who can type whatever is said so that it appears on the TTY user's screen

teleloop: A loop worn around the neck that attaches to a receiver of some sort that creates an electromagnetic field so that the user may access the signal via the telecoil program in his or her hearing aid or cochlear implant

telemetry: A procedure that measures the impedances and voltages when current is passed through a cochlear implant to determine if the electrodes are functioning in compliance with manufacturer's specifications

temporal integration: The ability of the auditory system to integrate acoustic energy over time (e.g., "Can you still detect the tone presented at the same sound pressure level even though it is only half of its previous duration?")

temporal masking: The ability to detect or recognize acoustic signals that have been masked by sounds that either come before or after them in time (e.g., "Can you still identify the consonant that is being masked by a noise that comes before it?")

temporal ordering: The ability to sequence the order of items presented auditorily (e.g., "Can you repeat the sequence of numbers in the order in which they were presented?")

temporal resolution: The ability to detect very fine temporal aspects of an auditory stimulus (e.g., "Can you detect the tiny gaps in the burst of noise you are about to hear?")

temporary threshold shift (TTS): Temporary and reversible decrease in hearing sensitivity due to exposure to excessive sound levels

third-party payers: An entity other than the healthcare provider or patient who reimburses for procedures performed, diagnoses made, and certain devices, supplies, and/or other equipment for patients (ASHA, 1996)

tinnitus: Noises, and more specifically "ringing", in the head

tinnitus retraining therapy (TRT): An approach developed by Pawel Jastreboff and his colleagues to treat patients' reaction to tinnitus that involves educational counseling and sound therapy

tolerance values: Determination of how accurately a hearing aid must perform on each parameter to be considered to be in line with the manufacturer's specifications

tonality: The spectral pitch of phonemes, according to those using the Verbotonal Method

tone hook: See *earhook*

tonometry: Measuring eye pressure

tools: Devices that provide benefit to patients that require some skill to use

"top down" strategies: Focus on the development of compensatory strategies to overcome processing problems relying on central resources of language, memory, and attention (ASHA, 2005a, 2005b)

Total Communication: A philosophy supporting the use of every and all means to communicate with children who are deaf; uses simultaneous exposure of a formal sign-language system (based on English), finger spelling (manual alphabet), natural gestures, speechreading, body language, oral speech, and the use of amplification

transcranial CROS: A fitting for patients with a unilateral hearing loss consisting of a high gain or output in-the-ear or behind-the-ear hearing aid to the unaidable ear such that sound from that side is amplified and then transferred to the cochlea of the better or normal ear by bone conduction through the cranium (Valente, Abrams, et al., 1995)

transdisciplinary teaming: Breaking down boundaries between and among professional disciplines so that members of one profession may assist in providing cross-disciplinary services to patient populations who may be unserved or underserved

transducer: A device that changes one form of energy to another and is classified by the transformation that takes place (e.g., acoustic-to-electric)

transient evoked otoacoustic emissions (TEOAEs): An objective method of assessing outer hair cell integrity by delivering click stimuli via a probe and measuring the emissions from sensory cells

transition services: Efforts made to assist children with disabilities and their families with changes in educational programming or status

transliteration: Method used by sign language interpreters

traumatic brain injury (TBI): A physiological disruption of brain functioning resulting from some type of event (Youse, Le, Cannizzaro, & Coelho, 2002)

treating: Ameliorating or lessening the impact of a hearing loss and/or balance disorder, modifying a patient's hearing and/or communication status (Stockman et al., 2004)

treatments/interventions: Procedures administered to lessen the effects of, or cures for, a disease or a disorder

TTY: An abbreviation for text telephone permitting hard-of-hearing individuals to communicate by telephone; also called a telecommunications device for the deaf or TDD

two-frequency pure-tone average: The average of the two best air-conduction thresholds at 500, 1000, and 2000 Hz and is used when one of the thresholds is significantly below the other two (e.g., 20 dB HL at 500 Hz, 25 dB HL at 1000 Hz, and 70 dB HL at 2000 Hz)

type I attitude: A strongly positive attitude toward hearing aids and auditory rehabilitation (Goldstein & Stephens, 1981)

type I diabetes: An endrocrinological disorder that is diagnosed in childhood or young adulthood in which the body does not produce or efficiently use insulin, frequently resulting in heart disease (cardiovascular disease), blindness (retinopathy), nerve damage (neuropathy), and kidney damage (nephropathy)

type II attitude: An essentially positive attitude toward hearing aids and auditory rehabilitation, but the patient presents with some complicating factor such as previous unsuccessful use of amplification, difficult-to-fit loss, and so on (Goldstein & Stephens, 1981)

type II diabetes: An endrocrinological disorder usually diagnosed in adulthood in which the body does not produce or efficiently use insulin; the most common type of diabetes

type III attitude: An essentially negative attitude toward hearing aids and auditory rehabilitation, but the patient is at least willing to consider receiving an audiologic evaluation (Goldstein & Stephens, 1981)

type IV attitude: A strongly negative attitude toward hearing aids and auditory rehabilitation (Goldstein & Stephens, 1981)

unconditional positive regard: Accepting patients, their values, and decisions regardless of the clinician's background

unisensory approaches: Auditory habilitation approaches that emphasize the use of audition for the development of spoken language while discouraging the reliance on speechreading

United States Preventive Services Task Force (USPSTF): A group that analyzes scientific evidence and then grades the clinical recommendations regarding health practices

unstructured communication method: A method of assessing conversational fluency that uses real-life communication situations (Tye-Murray, 2008)

use of minimal encouragers and verbal followings: A counseling technique involving simply saying short phrases (e.g., "Uh-huh," "Go on," and so on) to show patients that their communication partner is listening and that they should continue talking

Usher syndrome: An autosomal recessive genetic disorder that results in congenital sensorineural hearing loss and progressive visual impairment

variation in expressivity: When a genetic trait may express itself in variable degrees (e.g., slight to profound hearing loss)

velopharyngeal port: An opening between the oral and nasal cavities

vents: Tunnels in earmolds or in-the-ear styles of hearing aids that connect the outside environment to the inside of the ear canal, which can taper the amount of low-frequency amplification through use of little plugs with holes of different diameters

verbal persuasion: The enhancement of hearing aid self-efficacy through the use of positive statements about a person's ability to succeed (Smith & West, 2006)

Verbotonal Method: An approach for facilitating oral spoken language in children with hearing loss developed by Petar Guberina

vernix caseosa: A fatty lipid material that is left over from the amniotic fluid on the baby's skin that can be present in the ear canal and may interfere with newborn hearing screening

vertigo: Sensation of spinning

vestibular aqueduct: A small opening in the temporal bone that serves as a passageway for part of the membranous labyrinth, the endolymphatic duct, to travel outside of the inner ear to terminate at the endolymphatic sac at the level of the dura mater

vestibular neuritis: An inflammation of part of the vestibular section of cranial nerve VIII, causing an acute episode of nausea, vomiting, and vertigo (Marill, 2009)

vestibular rehabilitation therapy (VRT): Treatment designed to meet the unique needs of patients with vertigo, dizziness, and/or a sense of imbalance

vestibular-ocular reflex: A reflex responsible for maintaining a centralized visual image on the retina during head movement

vicarious experiences: The promotion of hearing aid self-efficacy through new hearing aid wearers' observation of other patients' successes

video otoscopes: An illuminated, magnifying scope for looking into the ears that contains a camera within a probe that is placed at the outer opening of the external auditory canal

viseme: Groups of phonemes that look the same on the mouth when articulated, like /f/ and /v/

visual acuity examination: An examination performed by a pediatric ophthalmologist because children with hearing loss may also have visual problems

visual reinforcement audiometry (VRA): A testing paradigm to be used with infants as young as 6 months old and rewards their head-turn responses to auditory stimuli presented through loudspeakers (or earphones) using visual reinforcers (e.g., animated toys behind smoked Plexiglas)

visually impaired: Having visual acuity less than 20/70 that cannot be corrected by conventional eyeglasses (University of Michigan Kellogg Eye Center, 2007)

vitreous humor: The center of the eye, which is filled with a clear, jelly-like substance

vocational rehabilitation (VR): Professional activities with a goal of assisting and empowering persons with disabilities attain and maintain productive and meaningful employment

voice quality: The degree of breathiness, roughness, strain, and overall noise during speech production (Monsen, 1979)

vowel neutralization: A type of vowel substitution in which vowels may be substituted for the neutral vowel *schwa* or a lax vowel may be used in place of a tense one (e.g., /I/ for /i/), or vice-versa (e.g., /i/ for /I/)

vowel substitution: Using one vowel in place of another

Welcome to Medical Examination: A one-time preventative examination for patients turning 65 years old conducted by a primary care physician to include a review of the beneficiary's medical and social history, potential for depression, functional ability and level of safety, including screening for hearing impairment and falls risk, and examination of height, weight, blood pressure, visual acuity, and an electrocardiogram (Card, 2005)

well-baby nursery: A nursery for babies who do not need any specialized services

wellness model of deafness: Views deafness not as an impairment to be treated, but as a different culture, rather than a group with a disability (Lane et al., 1996)

wet type of macular degeneration: Accounts for 10% of macular degeneration cases and is the most serious form; results from an abnormal growth of blood vessels of the macula (*Understanding and Coping with Macular Degeneration,* 2006a; University of Michigan Kellogg Eye Center, 2007)

wired systems: Hardwired systems in which the speaker, or sound source, is physically tethered to the listener via a wire

wireless systems: Listening systems that do not tie or connect the speaker, or sound source, to the listener with a wire

World Health Organization (WHO): The United Nations specialized agency for health

x-linked disorders: Mutation found on genes located on the sex chromosome

zero reject: A policy that the public agency must provide an educational program for all children, regardless of the child's disability

References

Abel, D., & Hahn, R. (2006). Relationships with hearing aid manufacturers. In T. A. Hamill (Ed.), *Ethics in audiology* (pp. 61–74). Reston, VA: American Academy of Audiology.

Abrahamson, J. (2001). *Materials for audiologic rehabilitation: Help getting started.* Retrieved from http://www.hearingreview.com/issues/articles/2001–08_02.asp

Abrams, H. B. (2000). *Outcome measures in audiology: Knowing we've made a difference.* Retrieved from http://www.audiologyonline.com/articles/article_detail.asp?article_id=236

Abrams, H. B., & Chisolm, T. H. (2007). *Audiology and quality of life: Is there a connection?* Retrieved from http://www.audiologyonline.com/articles/article_detail.asp?article_id=1816

Abrams, H. B., Chisolm, T. & McArdle, R. (2002). A cost-utility analysis of group audiologic rehabilitation: Are the benefits worth the cost? *Journal of Rehabilitation Research and Development, 39,* 549–558.

Abrams, H. B., Chisolm, T. H., & McArdle, R. (2005). Health-related quality of life and hearing aids: A tutorial. *Trends in Amplification, 9,* 99–109.

Abrams, H. B., Hnath-Chisolm, T., Guerreiro, S. M., & Ritterman, S. I. (1992). The effects of intervention strategy on self-perception of hearing handicap. *Ear and Hearing, 13,* 371–377.

Academy of Doctors of Audiology. (2010). *Au.D. history and timeline.* Retrieved from http://www.audiologist.org/aud-history.html

Academy of Rehabilitative Audiology. (2010). *ARA Statement of Purpose.* Retrieved from http://www.audrehab.org

Advanced Bionics. (2009). *Candidacy criteria.* Retrieved from http://www.advancedbionics.com/For_Professionals/Audiology_Support/Candidacy_Criteria.cfm?langid=1

Agency for Healthcare Research and Quality (AHRQ). (2010). *About AHRQ.* Retrieved from http://www.ahrq.gov/about/

AGREE Collaboration. (2007). Retrieved from http://www.agreecollaboration.org

Alabama Board of Examiners in Speech-Language Pathology and Audiology. (2010). *Alabama Board of Examiners in Speech-Language Pathology and Audiology (ABESPA).* Retrieved from http://www.abespa.org

Alabama Department of Vocational Rehabilitation. (2007). *Deaf/hard of hearing services.* Retrieved from http://www.rehab.state.al.us/Home/default.aspx?url=/Home/Services/VRS/Blind+and+Deaf+Services/Deaf+Services

Alexander Graham Bell Academy for Listening and Spoken Language (AGBALSL). (2010). *Auditory-Verbal therapy.* Retrieved from http://nc.agbell.org/NetCommunity/Page.aspx?pid=360

Allen, R., (2002). *Hearing aids: Reasonable expectations for the consumer.* Retrieved from http://www.audiologyonline.com/articles/article_detail.asp?article_id=347

Alpiner, J. B. (1982). *Handbook of adult rehabilitative audiology.* Baltimore, MD: Williams & Wilkins.

Altman, E. (1996). Meeting the needs of adolescents with impaired hearing. In F. N. Martin & J. G. Clark (Eds.), *Hearing care for children* (pp. 197–210). Boston: Allyn & Bacon.

Alzheimer's Association. (2010). *Alzheimer's disease.* Retrieved from http://www.alz.org/alzheimers_disease_alzheimers_disease.asp

American Academy of Audiology. (1993). *Auditory integration training.* Retrieved from http://www.audiology.org/resources/documentlibrary/Pages/AuditoryIntegrationTraining.aspx

American Academy of Audiology. (2003). *Pediatric amplification protocol.* Retrieved from http://www.audiology.org/resources/documentlibrary/Documents/pedamp.pdf

American Academy of Audiology. (2004a). *Scope of practice.* Retrieved from http://www.audiology.org/resources/documentlibrary/Pages/ScopeofPractice.aspx

American Academy of Audiology. (2004b). *Ethical practice guidelines on financial incentives from hearing instrument manufacturers.* Retrieved from http://www.audiology.org/resources/documentlibrary/Documents/financialincentives.pdf

American Academy of Audiology. (2006a). *American Academy of Audiology Political Action Committee.* Retrieved from http://www.audiology.org/advocacy/pac/Pages/default.aspx

American Academy of Audiology. (2006b). *The clinical practice guidelines developmental process.* Retrieved from http://www.audiology.org/resources/documentlibrary/Documents/financialincentives.pdf

American Academy of Audiology. (2009a). *Code of ethics.* Retrieved from http://www.audiology.org/resources/documentlibrary/Pages/codeofethics.aspx

American Academy of Audiology. (2009b). *Academy documents glossary.* Retrieved from http://www.audiology.org/resources/documentlibrary/Pages/AcademyDocumentsGlossary.aspx

American Academy of Audiology. (2009c). *Coding.* Retrieved from http://www.audiology.org/practice/coding/Pages/default.aspx

American Academy of Audiology. (2009d). *Clinical practice guideline: Remote microphone hearing assistance technology for children and youth from 0 to 21 years.* Retrieved from http://www.audiology.org/resources/documentlibrary/Documents/HATGuideline.pdf

American Academy of Otolaryngology, Head, and Neck Surgery. (2006). *Hearing aid timeline.* Retrieved from http://www.entlink.net/museum/exhibits/HearingAid-Timeline.cfm

American Academy of Otolaryngology, Head, and Neck Surgery. (2010). *Fact sheet: When your child has tinnitus.* Retrieved from http://www.entnet.org/HealthInformation/Child-Tinnitus.cfm

American Academy of Pediatrics. (1997). *Children's health topics: Medical home.* Retrieved from http://www.aap.org/healthtopics/medicalhome.cfm

American Academy of Pediatrics. (2003). *Eye examination in infants, children, and young adults.* Retrieved from http://aappolicy.aappublications.org/cgi/reprint/pediatrics:111/4/902.pdf

American Academy of Pediatrics, Joint Committee on Infant Hearing. (2007). Year 2007 position statement: Principles and guidelines for early hearing detection and intervention programs. *Pediatrics, 120,* 898–921.

American Academy of Pediatrics, Task Force on Newborn and Infant Hearing. (1999). Newborn and infant hearing loss: Detection and intervention. *Pediatrics. 103,* 527–530

American Board of Audiology. (2005). *Application handbook.* Reston, VA: American Board of Audiology.

American Board of Audiology. (2007). *Board certification in audiology with a specialty in cochlear implants candidate application handbook.* Reston, VA: American Board of Audiology.

American Board of Audiology. (2010). *Cochlear implant specialty certification.* Retrieved from: http://www.americanboardofaudiology.org/specialty/ci.html

American Diabetes Association. (2010). *Diabetes basics.* http://www.diabetes.org/diabetes-basics/?utm_source=WWW&utm_medium=GlobalNavDB&utm_campaign=CON

American Federation for the Blind. (2007). *Understanding vision loss.* Retrieved from http://www.afb.org/seniorsite.asp? SectionID=63

American Heart Association. (2006). *Diseases and conditions.* Retrieved from http://www.heart.org/HEARTORG/Conditions/Conditions_UCM_001087_SubHomePage.jsp

American National Standards Institute. (2002). *ANSI S12.60-2002, Acoustical performance criteria, design requirements and guidelines for schools.* Melville, NY: Author.

American National Standards Institute. (2003). *Standards for specifications of hearing aid characteristics. S 3.22.* New York: Author.

American Speech-Language-Hearing Association. (1984). *Definition of and competencies for aural rehabilitation* [Relevant paper]. Retrieved from http://www.asha.org/policy

American Speech-Language-Hearing Association. (1990). *Audiometric symbols* [Guidelines]. Retrieved from http://www.asha.org/policy

American Speech-Language-Hearing Association. (1991). *Communication and the Americans with Disabilities Act.* Rockville, MD: Author.

American Speech-Language-Hearing Association. (1996). *Curriculum guide to managed care.* Rockville, MD: Author.

American Speech-Language-Hearing Association. (1997). *Guidelines for audiology service delivery in nursing homes* [Guidelines]. Retrieved from http://www.asha.org/policy Date Accessed: August 17, 2007.

American Speech-Language-Hearing Association. (2001). *Knowledge and skills required for the practice of audiologic/aural rehabilitation [knowledge and skills]* (Revised 2001). Retrieved from http://www.asha.org/policy

American Speech-Language-Hearing Association. (2002). *Guidelines for audiology service provision in and for schools.* Retrieved from http://www.asha.org/policy

American Speech-Language-Hearing Association. (2004a). *Knowledge and skills needed by speech-language pathologists and audiologists to provide culturally and linguistically appropriate services* [knowledge and skills]. Retrieved from http://www.asha.org/policy

American Speech-Language-Hearing Association. (2004b). *Scope of practice in audiology [scope of practice].* Retrieved from http://www.asha.org/policy

American Speech-Language-Hearing Association. (2004c). *Evidence-based practice in communication disorders: An introduction* [Technical report]. Retrieved from http://www.asha.org/policy

American Speech-Language-Hearing Association. (2004d). *Roles of speech-language pathologists and teachers of children who are deaf and hard of hearing in the development of communicative and linguistic competence* [Guidelines]. Retrieved from http://www.asha.org/policy

American Speech-Language-Hearing Association. (2005a). *(Central) auditory processing disorders* [Technical report]. Retrieved from http://www.asha.org/policy

American Speech-Language-Hearing Association. (2005b). *(Central) auditory processing disorders—The role of the audiologist* [Position statement]. Retrieved from http://www.asha.org/policy

American Speech-Language-Hearing Association. (2005c). *Evidence-based practice in communication disorders* [Position statement]. Retrieved from http://www.asha.org/policy

American Speech-Language-Hearing Association. (2005d). *Acoustics in educational settings* [Position statement]. Retrieved from http://www.asha.org/policy

American Speech-Language-Hearing Association. (2006a). *Tips for working with interpreters.* Retrieved from http://www.asha.org/practice/multicultural/issues/interpret.htm

American Speech-Language-Hearing Association. (2006b). *Preferred practice patterns for the profession of audiology* [preferred practice patterns]. Retrieved from http://www.asha.org/policy

American Speech-Language-Hearing Association. (2006c). *Special interest division 7, aural rehabilitation and its instrumentation.* Retrieved from http://www.asha.org/members/divs/div_7.htm

American Speech-Language-Hearing Association. (2007). *Scope of practice in speech-language pathology* [scope of practice]. Retrieved from http://www.asha.org/policy

American Speech-Language-Hearing Association. (2009a). *Division 7, aural rehabilitation and its instrumentation.* Retrieved from http://www.asha.org/members/divs/div_7.htm#miss

American Speech-Language-Hearing Association. (2009b). *Steps in the Process of Evidence-Based Practice: Step 2: Finding the Evidence.* Retrieved from http://www.asha.org/members/ebp/finding.htm

American Speech-Language-Hearing Association. (2010). *Code of ethics.* Retrieved from http://www.asha.org/policy

American Tinnitus Association. (2009). *ATA's top 10 most frequently asked questions.* Retrieved from http://www.ata.org/for-patients/faqs

Americans with Disabilities Act of 1990, Public Law 101–336, 42 U.S.C. 12101 *et seq.: U.S. Statutes at Large, 104,* 327–378 (1991).

Anand, V., Buckley, J. G., Scally, A., & Elliott, D. B. (2003a). Postural stability in the elderly during sensory perturbations and dual tasking: The influence of refractive blur. *Investigative Ophthalmology and Visual Science, 44,* 2285–2291.

Anand, V., Buckley, J. G., Scally, A., & Elliott, D. B. (2003b). Postural stability changes in the elderly with cataract simulation and refractive blur. *Investigations in Ophthalmology and Visual Science, 44,* 4670–4675.

Anderson, I., Schmidt, M., Buchreiter, T., & Bisanar, K. (2004). Handling of the MED-EL TEMPO + ear-level speech processor by paediatric cochlear implant users and their parents. *International Journal of Audiology, 43,* 579–584.

Anderson, K. (1989). *Screening Instrument for Targeting Educational Risk (SIFTER) in Children with Identified Hearing Loss.* Tampa, FL: Educational Audiology Association (previously by Pro-Ed and Interstate Publishers and Printers).

Anderson, K., & Matkin, N. (1996). *Preschool Screening Instrument for Targeting Educational Risk (SIFTER) in Children age 3–Kindergarten.* Tampa, FL: Educational Audiology Association.

Anderson, K., & Matkin, N. (1998). *Hearing loss counseling pads.* Tampa, FL: Educational Audiology Association.

Anderson, K. A. (2007). *ELF–Early listening function–Discovery tool for parents and caregivers of infants and toddlers (4 months to 3 years).* Retrieved from http://kandersonaudconsulting.com/uploads/ELF_Questionnaire.pdf

Anderson, K. A., Goldstein, H., Colodzin, L., & Iglehart, F. (2005). Benefit of S/N enhancing devices to speech perception of children listening in typical classrooms with hearing aids or a cochlear implant. *Journal of Educational Audiology, 12,* 14–28.

Anderson, K. A., & Smaldino, J. J. (1998). *Listening inventory for education: An efficacy tool (LIFE).* Westminster, CO: Educational Audiology Association.

Anderson, K. A., & Smaldino, J. J. (2000). *Children's Home Inventory for Listening Difficulty (CHILD).* Retrieved from http://www.oticonusa.com/eprise/main/SiteGen/Uploads/Public/Downloads_Oticon/Pediatrics/CHILD_Questionnaire.pdf

Anderson, T., Weichbold, V., D'Haese, P. S. C., Szuchnik, J., Quevedo, M. S., Martin, J., . . . Phillips, L. (2004). Cochlear implantation in children under the age of two—What do the outcomes show us? *International Journal of Pediatric Otorhinolaryngology, 68,* 425–431.

Andersson, G., & Green, M. (1995). Anxiety in older hearing-impaired persons. *Perceptual Motor Skills, 81,* 552–554.

Andrews, J. F., Leigh, I. W., & Weiner, M. T. (2004). *Deaf people: Evolving perspectives from psychology, education, and sociology.* Boston: Allyn & Bacon.

Angelocci, A. A., Kopp, G. A., & Holbrook, A. (1964). The vowel formants of deaf and normal-hearing eleven-to-fourteen-year-old boys. *Journal of Speech and Hearing Disorders, 29,* 156–160.

Apple, Incorporated. (2010). *iPod sales per quarter.* Retrieved from http://www.apple.com/pr/library/2009/01/21results.html.

Archbold, S. M., Nikolopoulos, T. P., & Lloyd-Richmond, H. (2009). Long-term use of cochlear implant systems in paediatric recipients and factors contributing to non-use. *Cochlear Implants International, 10,* 25–40.

Arizona Commission for the Deaf and the Hard of Hearing. (2003). *TTY etiquette.* Retrieved from http://www.acdhh.org/assets/user_upload/TTY_etiquette12-09.pdf

Arlinger, S. (2000). Can we establish internationally equivalent outcome measures in audiological rehabilitation? *Ear and Hearing, 21,* 97S–99S.

Arthritis Foundation. (2010). *Disease center.* Retrieved from http://www.arthritis.org/disease-center.php?disease

Association of Late-Deafened Adults. (2010). Retrieved from http://www.alda.org

A to Z to Deafblindness. (2010). *What do you do when you meet a deafblind person?* Retrieved from http://www.deafblind.com/whatdbp.html

Babbidge, H. (1965). *Education of the deaf in the United States: A report to the Secretary of Health, Education, and Welfare by his advisory committee of education of the deaf.* Washington, DC: United States Government Printing Office.

Babeu, L., Kricos, P., & Lesner, S. (2004). Application of the Stages-of-Change Model in audiology. *Journal of the American of Rehabilitative Audiology, 37,* 41–56.

Baguley, D. M., Bird, J., Humphriss, R. L., & Prevost, A. T. (2006). The evidence base for the application of contralateral bone-anchored hearing aids in acquired unilateral sensorineural hearing loss in adults. *Clinical Otolaryngology, 31,* 6–14.

Ballachanda, B. P. (1995). *The human ear canal.* San Diego, CA: Singular/Delmar Cengage Learning.

Bance, M., Abel, S. M., Papsin, B. C., Wade, P., & Vendramini, J. (2002). A comparison of the audiometric performance of bone-anchored hearing aids and air-conduction hearing aids. *Otology and Neurotology, 23,* 912–919.

Bandura, A. (1986). *Social foundations of thought and action. A social cognitive theory.* Englewood Cliffs, NJ: Prentice Hall.

Barringer, D. G., Mauk, G. W., Jensen, S., & Woods-Kerschner, N. (1997). Clinical report I: Survey of parents' perceptions regarding hospital-based newborn hearing screening. *Audiology Today, 9*(1), 18–19.

Basura, G. J., Eapen, R., & Buchman, C. A. (2009). Bilateral cochlear implantation: Current concepts, indications, and results. *Laryngoscope, 119,* 2395–2401.

Battat, B., Berger, S., Killion, M., & Kozma-Spytek, L. (2003). *Hearing aids and digital cell phones: Providing intelligent answers to your patients' questions.* Virtual seminar provided by the American Academy of Audiology, September 19, 2003.

Bauer, C. A., & Girardi, M. (2004). *Vestibular rehabilitation.* Retrieved from http://www.fallpreventionclinics.com/docs/Vestibular%20Rehabilitation-Bauer-Girardi.pdf

Bauer, P. W., Wippold, F. J. II, Goldin, J., & Lusk, R. P. (2002). Cochlear implantation in children with CHARGE association. *Archives of Otolaryngology—Head and Neck Surgery, 128,* 1013–1017.

Beauchaine, K. L. (2001). An amplification protocol for infants. In R. C. Seewald & J. S. Gravel (Eds.), *A Sound Foundation Through Early Amplification* (pp. 105–112). Warrenville, IL: Phonak Hearing Systems.

Beck, L. (1999). *The NIDCD/VA hearing aid clinical trial and evidence-based decision-making in the VA.* Paper presented at the Annual Convention of the American Speech-Language-Hearing Association, San Francisco, CA.

Beebe, H. (1953). *A guide to help the severely-hard-of-hearing hearing child: Testing their hearing/ways to develop normal speech.* Basel, Switzerland: S. Karger.

Begines, T. (1995). Fitness and risk evaluation. *Spectrum, 21*(1), 9–11.

Behar, A., MacDonald, E., Lee, J., Cui, J., Kunov, H., & Wong, W. (2004). Noise exposure of music teachers. *Journal of Occupational and Environmental Hygiene, 1,* 243–247.

Bellis, T. J. (2003). *Assessment and management of central auditory processing disorders: Disorders in the educational setting from science to practice* (2nd ed.). Clifton Park, NY: Delmar Thomson Learning.

Bellis, T. J., & Ferre, J. M. (1999). Multidimensional approach to the differential diagnosis of central auditory processing disorders in children. *Journal of the American Academy of Audiology, 10,* 319–328.

Bell-Krotoski, J., & Tomancik, E. (1987). The repeatability of testing with the Semmes-Weinstein Monofilaments. *The Journal of Hand Surgery, 12,* 155–161.

Benguerel, A.-P., & Pichora-Fuller, M. K. (1988). Design of a computer-assisted speechreading training system. *Annual Bulletin of the Research Institute of Logopedics and Phoniatrics, 22,* 105–116.

Bentler, R., & Chiou, L. K. (2006). Digital noise reduction: An overview. *Trends in Amplification, 10,* 67–82.

Bentler, R. A. (2005). Effectiveness of directional microphones and noise reduction schemes in hearing aids: A systematic review of the evidence. *Journal of the American Academy of Audiology, 16,* 473–484.

Bentler, R. A., Niebuhr, D. P., Johnson, T. A., & Flamme, G. A. (2003). Impact of digital labeling on outcome measures. *Ear and Hearing, 24,* 215–224.

Berent, G. P., Kelly, R. R., Aldersley, S., Schmitz, K. L., Khalsa, B. K., Panara, J., & Keenan. S. (2007). Focus-on-form instructional methods promote deaf college students' improvement in English grammar. *Journal of Deaf Studies and Deaf Education, 12,* 8–24.

Berlin, C. I., Hood, L., Morlet, T., Rose, K., & Brashears, S. (2003). Auditory neuropathy/dys-synchrony: Diagnosis and management. *Mental Retardation and Developmental Disabilities Research Review, 9,* 225–231.

Berry, P., Mascia, J., & Steinman, B. A. (2004). Vision and hearing loss in older adults: "Double trouble." *Care Management Journals, 5,* 35–40.

Bess, F. H. (2000). The role of generic health-related quality of life measures in establishing audiological rehabilitation outcomes. *Ear and Hearing, 21,* 74S–79S.

Bess, F. H., Dodd-Murphy, J., & Parker, R. A. (1998). Children with minimal sensorineural hearing loss: Prevalence, educational performance, and functional status. *Ear and Hearing, 19,* 339–354.

Bess, F. H., Lichtenstein, M. J., Logan, S. A., Burger, M. C., & Nelson, E. (1989). Hearing impairment as a determinant of function in the elderly. *Journal of the American Geriatrics Society, 37,* 123–128.

Beyer, C. M., & Northern, J. L. (2000). Audiologic rehabilitation support programs: A network model. *Seminars in Hearing, 21,* 257–265.

Bishop, D. V. (1983). Comprehension of English syntax by profoundly deaf children. *Journal of Child Psychology and Psychiatry and Allied Disciplines, 24,* 415–434.

Blamey, P., Arndt, P., Bergeron, F., Bredberg, G., Brimacombe, J., Facer, G., . . . Whitford, L. (1996). Factors affecting auditory performance of postlinguistically deaf adults using cochlear implants. *Otology and Neuro-otology, 1,* 293–306.

Blanchfield, B. B., Feldman, J. J., Dunbar, J. L, & Gardner, E. N. (2001). The severely to profoundly hearing-impaired population in the United States: Prevalence estimates and demographics. *Journal of the American Academy of Audiology, 12,* 183–189.

Blood, G. W., Blood, I., & Danhauer, J. L. (1977). The hearing aid effect. *Hearing Instruments, 28*(6), 12.

Blood, G. W., Blood, I., & Danhauer, J. L. (1978). Listeners' impressions of normal-hearing and hearing-impaired children. *Journal of Communication Disorders, 11,* 513–518.

Blood, I. M., & Blood, G. W. (1999). Effects of acknowledging a hearing loss on social interactions. *Journal of Communication Disorders, 32*(2), 109–120.

Blumsack, J. T. (2003). Audiological assessment, rehabilitation, and spatial hearing considerations associated with visual impairments in adults: An overview. *American Journal of Audiology, 12,* 76–83.

Boehm, A. E. (1971). *Boehm test of basic concepts.* Austin, TX: Pro-Ed.

Bogoch, I. I., House, R. A., & Kudla, I. (2005). Perceptions about hearing protection and noise induced hearing loss of attendees at rock concerts. *Canadian Journal of Public Health, 96,* 69–72.

Bonds, B. G. (2003). School-to-work experiences: Curriculum as a bridge. *American Annals of the Deaf, 148,* 38–48.

Boothroyd, A. (1987). CASPER: A computer-assisted program for speech-perception testing and training. *Proceedings of the 10th Annual Conference of the Rehabilitation Society of North America,* 734–736.

Boothroyd, A. (2006a). Opening comments. Paper presented at the State-of-the-Science (SOS) Conference on Hearing Enhancement, Gallaudet University, September 18–20, 2006.

Boothroyd, A. (2006b). *CasperSent: An example of computer-assisted speech perception testing and training at the sentence level.* Paper presented at the State-of-the-Science (SOS) Conference on Hearing Enhancement, Gallaudet University, September 18–20, 2006.

Bossuyt, P. M., Reitsma, J. B., Bruns, D. E., Gatsonis, C. A., Glasziou, P. P., Irwig, L. M., . . . de Vet H. C. W., for the STARD Group. (2003). Toward complete and accurate reporting of studies of diagnostic accuracy. The STARD initiative. *Annals of Internal Medicine, 138,* 40–44.

Boston, M. E., Strasnick, B., & Steinberg, A. R. (2010). *Inner ear labyrinthitis.* Retrieved from http://emedicine.medscape.com/article/856215-overview

Boswell, S. (2005, Feb. 8). New IDEA law brings relief, worry for school clinicians. *The ASHA Leader.*

Boughman, J. A., Vernon, M., & Shaver, K. A. (1983). Usher syndrome: Definition and estimate of prevalence from two high-risk populations. *Journal of Chronic Diseases, 36,* 595–603.

Bowe, F. G. (2004). *Birth to eight: Early childhood special education* (3rd ed.). Clifton Park, NY: Thomson Delmar Learning.

Bowen, S. K. (2008). Coenrollment for students who are deaf or hard of hearing: Friendship patterns and social interactions. *American Annals of the Deaf, 153,* 285–293.

Boyd, P. J. (2006). Effects of programming thresholds and maplaw settings on acoustic thresholds and speech discrimination with the MED-EL COMBI 40+ cochlear implant. *Ear and Hearing, 27,* 608–618.

Boys Town National Research Hospital. (2010). *Making the decision.* Retrieved from http://www.boystown hospital.org/hearingLoss/cochlearImplant/Pediatric CochlearImplantProgram/Pages/MakingtheDecision .aspx

Brackett, D. (2002). Management options for children with hearing loss. In J. Katz (Ed.), *Handbook of clinical audiology* (5th ed., pp. 758–766). Baltimore, MD: Lippincott Williams & Wilkins.

Bratt, G. W. (1999). *Electroacoustic assessment of hearing aid performance in NIDCD/ VA clinical trial.* Paper presented at the Annual Convention of the American Speech-Language-Hearing Association, San Francisco, CA.

Brennan, M., Horowitz, A., & Su, Y. P. (2005). Dual sensory loss and its impact on everyday competence. *Gerontologist, 45,* 337–346.

Brennan, M., Su, Y. P., & Horowitz, A. (2006). Longitudinal associations between dual sensory impairment and everyday competence among older adults. *Journal of Rehabilitation Research and Development, 43,* 777–792.

Brenza, B. A., Kricos, P. B., & Lasky, E. Z. (1981). Comprehension and production of basic semantic concepts by older hearing impaired children. *Journal of Speech, Language, and Hearing Research, 24,* 414–419.

Brey, R. H., Facer, G. W., Trine, M. B., Lynn, S. G., Peterson, A. M., & Suman, V. J. (1995). Vestibular effects associated with implantation of a multiple channel cochlear prosthesis. *American Journal of Otology, 16,* 424–430.

Brookhouser, P. E. (1987). Ensuring safety of deaf children in residential schools. *Otolaryngology, Head, and Neck Surgery, 97,* 361–368.

Brooks, D. N., & Hallam, R. S. (1998). Attitudes to hearing difficulty and hearing aids and the outcome of audiological rehabilitation. *British Journal of Audiology, 32,* 217–226.

Brown, N. C., James, K., Liu, J., Hatcher, P. A., & Li, Y. (2006). Newborn hearing screening. An assessment of knowledge, attitudes, and practice among Minnesota physicians. *Minnesota Medicine, 89*(12), 50–54.

Brown, P. M., & Foster, S. B. (1991). Integrating hearing and deaf students on a college campus. Successes and barriers as perceived by hearing students. *American Annals of the Deaf, 136,* 21–27.

Brown, S. L., Nesse, R. M., Vinokur, A. D., & Smith, D. M. (2003). Providing social support may be more beneficial than receiving it: Results from a prospective study of mortality. *Psychological Science, 14,* 320–327.

Browning, G. G., & Gatehouse, S. (1994). Estimation of the benefit of bone-anchored hearing aids. *Annals of Otology, Rhinology, and Laryngology, 103,* 872–878.

Bruegemann, P. M. (2005). *Andragogy and aural rehabilitation.* Retrieved from http://www.audiologyonline .com/articles/pf_article_detail.asp?article_id=1445

Brunnberg, E., Bostrom, M. L., & Berglund, M. (2008). Self-rated mental health, school adjustment, and substance use in hearing-impaired children. *Journal of Deaf Studies and Deaf Education, 13,* 324–335.

Buchanan, R. (1994). Building a silent colony: Life and work in the deaf community of Akron, Ohio from 1910 to 1950. In C. J. Erting, R. C. Johnson, D. L. Smith, & B. D. Snider (Eds.), *The deaf way* (pp. 250–259). Washington, DC: Gallaudet University.

Buchino, M. A. (1993). Perceptions of the oldest hearing child of deaf parents: On interpreting, communication, feelings, and role reversal. *American Annals of the Deaf, 138,* 40–45.

Buchman, C. A., Fucci, M. J., & Luxford, W. M. (1999). Cochlear implants in the geriatric population: Benefits outweigh risks. *Ear, Nose, and Throat Journal, 78,* 489–494.

Burton, S. E., Pandya, A., & Arnos, K. S. (2006, January 17). Genetics and hearing loss: An overview. *The ASHA Leader.*

Bush, P. J., & Robin, D. L. (1980). Racial differences in encounter rates for otitis media. *Pediatric Research, 14,* 1115–1117.

Byrne, D., Dillon, H., Ching, T., Katsch, R., & Keidser, G. (2001). The NAL-NL1 procedure for fitting nonlinear hearing aids: Characteristics and comparisons with other procedures. *Journal of the American Academy of Audiology, 12,* 37–51.

Bzoch, K. R., League, R., & Brown, V. L. (2003). Receptive-expressive emergent language test, third edition (REEL-3). Austin, TX: Pro-Ed.

Caban, A. J., Lee, D. J., Gómez-Marin, O., Lam, B. L., & Zheng, D. (2005). Prevalence of concurrent hearing and visual impairment in U.S. adults: The National Health Interview Survey, 1997–2002. *American Journal of Public Health, 95,* 1940–1942.

Cacace, A. T. (2007). Aging, Alzheimer's disease, and hearing impairment: Highlighting relevant issues and calling for additional research. *American Journal of Audiology, 16,* 2–3.

Caissie, R., & Rockwell, E. (1993). A videotape analysis procedure for assessing conversational fluency in hearing-impaired adults. *Ear and Hearing, 14,* 202–209.

Calderon, R. (2000). Parental involvement in deaf children's education programs as a predictor of child's language, early reading, and social emotional development. *Journal of Deaf Studies and Deaf Education, 5,* 140–155.

Caleffe-Schenck, N. (2005). *Auditory-verbal therapy: Developing spoken language through listening with children who are deaf.* Retrieved from http://www.thecni .org/reviews/16-spring05-p12-caleffe-schenck.pdf

Calvert, D., & Silverman, S. (1975). *Speech and deafness.* Washington, DC: Alexander Graham Bell Association for the Deaf.

Cambra, C. (2002). Acceptance of deaf students by hearing students in a regular classroom. *American Annals of the Deaf, 147,* 38–45.

Campbell, V. A., Crews, J. E., Moriarty, D. G., Zack, M. M., & Blackman, D. K. (1999). Surveillance for sensory impairment, activity limitation, and health-related quality of life among older adults – United States, 1993–1997. *Mortality and Morbidity Weekly Report Centers for Disease Control Surveillance Summary, 48,* 131–156.

Capezuti, E. (2004). Minimizing the use of restrictive devices in dementia patients at risk for falling. *Nursing Clinics of North America, 39,* 625–647.

Cappelli, M., Daniels, T., Durieux-Smith, A., McGrath, P. J., & Neuss, D. (1995). Social development of children with hearing impairments who are integrated into general education classes. *Volta Review, 97,* 197–208.

Card, R. O. (2005). How to conduct a "Welcome to Medicare" visit. *Family Practice Management, 12,* 27–29, 31–32.

Carmen, R. (2009). *When a loved one resists help for their hearing loss.* Retrieved from http://www .betterhearing.org/aural_education_and_counseling/ articles_tip_sheets_and_guides/hearing_loss_and_a_ loved_one_detail.cfm

Carron, J. D., Moore, R. B., & Dhaliwal, A. S. (2006). Perceptions of pediatric primary care physicians on congenital hearing loss and cochlear implantation. *Journal of the Mississippi State Medical Association, 47(2),* 35–41.

Carrow-Woolfolk, E. (1995). *The oral and written language scales.* Los Angeles, CA: Western Psychological Services.

Carstensen, L. L. (2006). The influence of a sense of time on human development. *Science, 312,* 1913–1915.

Cellular Telecommunications and Internet Association (2005). Retrieved from http://www.ctia.org/

Center for Advancement of Palliative Care. (2006). *Center for Advancement of Palliative Care Manual: World Health Organization Definition of Palliative Care.* Retrieved from http://64.85.16.230/educate/content/ elements/whodefinition.html

Center for Evidence-Based Medicine. (2010). *Center for evidenced-based medicine.* Retrieved from http://www .cebm.net/

Centers for Disease Control and Prevention. (2008). *Early hearing detection and intervention program. Summary of 2006 national EHDI data* (version 3). Retrieved from http://www.cdc.gov/ncbddd/ehdi/documents/EHDI_ Summ_2006_Web.pdf

Centers for Disease Control and Prevention. (2009). *Historical moments in newborn hearing screening.* Retrieved from http://www.cdc.gov/ncbddd/hearingloss/ ehdi-history.html

Centers for Disease Control and Prevention. (2010). *Use of vaccines to prevent meningitis in persons with cochlear implants.* Retrieved from http://www.cdc.gov/vaccines/ vpd-vac/mening/cochlear/dis-cochlear-gen.htm

Chadha, N. K., Gordon, K. A., James, A. L., & Papsin, B. C. (2009). Tinnitus is prevalent in children with cochlear implants. *International Journal of Pediatric Otorhinolaryngology,73,* 671–675.

Chan, S. (1997). Families with Asian roots. In E. W. Lynch & M. J. Hanson (Eds.), *Developing cross-cultural competence: A guide for working with children and their families* (2nd ed., pp. 251–354). Baltimore, MD: Brookes.

Chan, S. (1997). Families with Pilipino roots. In E. W. Lynch & M. J. Hanson (Eds.), *Developing cross-cultural competence: A guide for working with children and their families* (2nd ed., pp. 355–408). Baltimore, MD: Brookes.

Chan, V., Tong, M., Yue, V., Wong, T., Leung, E., Yuen, K., & van Hasselt, A. (2007). Performance of older adult cochlear implant users in Hong Kong. *Ear and Hearing, 28,* 52S–55S.

Chandler, C. (2006, July 11). Blast related ear injury in current U.S. military operations. *The ASHA Leader.*

Chang, D. T., Ko, A. B., Murray, G. S., Arnold, J. E., & Megerian, C. A. (2010). Lack of financial barriers to pediatric cochlear implantation: Impact of socioeconomic factors on access and outcomes. *Archives of Otolaryngology Head and Neck Surgery, 136,* 648–657.

Chang, J. T., Morton, S. C., Rubenstein, L. Z., Mojica, W. A., Maglione, M., Suttorp, M. J., . . . Shekelle, P. G. (2004). Interventions for the prevention of falls in older adults: Systematic review and meta-analysis of randomized clinical trials. *British Medical Journal, 328,* 680.

CHARGE Syndrome Association. (2010). *About CHARGE.* Retrieved from http://www.chargesyndrome.org/about- charge.asp

Chartrand, M. S. (2005). *Effectiveness of hearing aid manipulation training for elderly hearing aid users.* Retrieved from http://www.audiologyonline.com/articles/article_detail.asp?article_id=1400

Chatelin, V., Kim, E. J., Driscoll, C., Larky, J., Polite, C., Price, L., & Lalwani, A. K. (2004). Cochlear implant outcomes in the elderly. *Otology and Neurotology, 25,* 298–301.

Chen, D. A., Backous, D. D., Arriaga, M. A., Garvin, R., Kobylek, D., Littman, T., . . . Lura, D. (2004). Phase I clinical trial results of the Envoy System: A totally implantable middle ear device for sensorineural hearing loss. *Otolaryngology, Head, and Neck Surgery, 131,* 904–916.

Chermak, G. D., & Musiek, F. E. (2007). *Handbook of (central) auditory processing Disorders: comprehensive intervention – volume II.* San Diego, CA: Plural.

Cherry, R., & Rubenstein, A. (1988). Speechreading instruction for adults: Issues and approaches. *Volta review 90*(5), 289–306.

Ching, T. Y., Dillon, H., & Byrne, D. (1998). Speech recognition of hearing-impaired listeners: Predictions from audibility and the limited role of high-frequency amplification. *Journal of the Acoustical Society of America 103,* 1128–1140.

Ching, T. Y., Psarros, C., Hill, M., Dillon, H., & Incerti, P. (2001). Should children who use cochlear implants wear hearing aids in the opposite ear? *Ear and Hearing, 22,* 365–380.

Ching, T. Y., Scollie, S. D., Dillon, H., & Seewald, R. (2010). A cross-over, double-blind comparison of the NAL-N1 and the DSL v4.1 prescriptions for children with mild to moderately severe hearing loss. *International Journal of Audiology, 49*(Suppl. 1), S4–S15.

Ching, T. Y. C., & Hill, M. (2005). *The Teacher's Evaluation of Aural/Oral Performance of Children (TEACH).* Retrieved from http://www.outcomes.nal.gov.au/LOCHI%20assessments-teach.html

Ching, T. Y. C., & Hill, M. (2007). The Parent's Evaluation of Aural/Oral Performance of Children (PEACH) Scale: Normative data. *Journal of the American Academy of Audiology, 18,* 220–235.

Ching, T. Y. C., Incerti, P., & Hill, M. (2004). Binaural benefits for adults who use hearing aids and cochlear implants in opposite ears. *Ear and Hearing, 25,* 9–21.

Chisolm, H., Abrams, H. B., & McArdle, R. (2004). Short- and long-term outcomes of adult audiological rehabilitation. *Ear and Hearing, 25,* 464–477.

Chisolm, T. H., Johnson, C. E., Danhauer, J. L., Portz, L. J. P., Abrams, H. B., Lesner, S., . . . Newman, C. W. (2007). A systematic review of health-related quality of life and hearing aids: Final Report of the American Academy of Audiology Task Force on the Health-Related Quality of Life Benefits of Amplification in Adults. *Journal of the American Academy of Audiology, 18,* 151–183.

Christiansen, J. (1994). Deaf people and the world of work: A case study of deaf printers in Washington, DC. In C. J. Erting, R. C. Johnson, D. L. Smith, & B. D. Snider (Eds.), *The deaf way* (pp. 260–267). Washington, DC: Gallaudet University.

Cienkowski, K. M., & Carney, A. E. (2002). Audio-visual speech perception and aging. *Ear and Hearing, 23,* 439–449.

Cienkowski, K. M., & Pimental, V. (2001). The hearing aid 'effect' revisited in young adults. *British Journal of Audiology, 35,* 289–295.

Clark, J. G., & English, K. (2003). *Counseling in audiologic practice: Helping patients and families adjust to hearing loss.* Boston: Allyn & Bacon.

Clark, W. W. (1991). Noise exposure from leisure activities: A review. *Journal of the Acoustical Society of America, 90,* 175–181.

Clarke Schools for Hearing and Speech. (2010a). *Clarke campuses.* Retrieved from http://www.clarkeschool.org/programs-and-schools/clarke-campuses

Clarke Schools for Hearing and Speech. (2010b). *Philadelphia campus.* Retrieved from http://www.clarkeschools.org/programs-and-schools/clarke-campuses/philadelphia/philadelphia-about

Cochlear Americas. (2009). *Baba support materials.* Retrieved from http://www.professionals.cochlearamericas.com/cochlear-products/baha/baha-support-materials

Cochlear Americas. (2010). *Cochlear implant candidate criteria.* Retrieved from http://www.professionals.cochlearamericas.com/sites/default/files/resources/criteria%20card.pdf

Cochrane Collaboration. (2009). *Cochrane handbook for systematic reviews of interventions, version 5.0.2.* Retrieved from http://www.cochrane-handbook.org/

Cohen, S. M., Labadie, R. F., & Haynes, D. S. (2005). Primary care approach to hearing loss: The hidden disability. *Ear, Nose, and Throat Journal, 84,* 26, 29–31, 44.

Cohen-Mansfield, J., & Taylor, J. W. (2004a). Hearing aid use in nursing homes. Part 1: Prevalence rates of hearing impairment and hearing aid use. *Journal of the American Medical Directors Association, 5,* 283–288.

Cohen-Mansfield, J., & Taylor, J. W. (2004b). Hearing aid use in nursing homes. Part 2: Barriers to effective utilization of hearing aids. *Journal of the American Medical Directors Association, 5,* 289–296.

Colletti, V. (2006). Auditory outcomes in tumor and non-tumor patients fitted with auditory brainstem implants. *Advances in Otorhinolaryngology, 64,* 167–185.

Colletti, V., Carner, M., Miorelli, V., Guida, M., Colletti, L., & Fiorino, F. (2004). Cochlear implant failure: Is an auditory brainstem implant the answer? *Acta Otolaryngologica, 124,* 353–357.

Colletti, V., & Shannon, R. V. (2005). Open set speech perception with the auditory brainstem implant? *Laryngoscope, 115,* 1974–1978.

Colorado Department of Education. (2008). *(Central) auditory processing deficits: A team approach to screening, assessment, and intervention process.* Retrieved from http://www.cde.state.co.us/cdesped/download/pdf/APDGuidelines2008.pdf

Commission on Education of the Deaf. (1988). *Toward equality: Education of the deaf.* Washington, DC: United States Government Printing Office.

Compton, C. (1999). Assistive technology for deaf and hard of hearing people. In J. G. Alpiner, & P. A. McCarthy (Eds.), *Rehabilitative audiology* (3rd ed., pp. 441–469). Baltimore, MD: Lippincott Williams & Wilkins.

Compton, C., Lewis, D., Palmer, C., & Thelen, M. (1994). *Assistive technology: Too legit to quit.* Pittsburgh, PA: Support Syndicate for Audiology.

Cone-Wesson, B., Rance, G., & Sininger, Y. (2001). Amplification and rehabilitation strategies for patients with auditory neuropathy. In Y. Sininger & A. Starr (Eds.), *Auditory neuropathy: A new perspective on hearing disorders* (pp. 233–249). San Diego, CA: Singular/ Delmar Cengage Learning.

Cook, S. M., & Hussey, S. M. (2002). *Assistive technologies: Principles and practice* (2nd ed.). St. Louis, MO: Mosby.

Cosetti, M., & Roland, J.T., Jr. (2010). Cochlear implantation in the very young child: Issues unique to the under-1 population. *Trends in Amplification, 14,* 46–57.

Council for Accreditation in Occupational Hearing Conservation (CAOHC). (2007). *What is CAOHC?* Retrieved from http://www.caohc.org/what_is_caohc/

Courtois, J., Johansen, P. A., Larsen, B. V., & Beilin, J. (1988). Hearing aid fitting in asymmetrical hearing loss. In J. H. Jensen (Ed.), *Hearing aid fitting: Theoretical and practical views* (pp. 243–255). 13th Danavox Symposium, Copenhagen: Stougaard Jenson.

Cox, R., & Alexander, G. (1995). The abbreviated profile of hearing aid benefit. *Ear and Hearing, 16,* 176–183.

Cox, R., & Alexander, G. (1999). Measuring satisfaction with amplification in daily life: The SADL scale. *Ear and Hearing, 20,* 306–320.

Cox, R., & Alexander, G. (2000). Expectations about hearing aids and their relationship to fitting outcome. *Journal of the American Academy of Audiology, 11,* 368–382.

Cox, R., & Alexander, G. (2001). Validation of the SADL. *Ear and Hearing, 22,* 151–160.

Cox, R., Hyde, M., Gatehouse, S., Noble, W., Dillon, H., Bentler, R., . . . Hallberg, L. (2000). Optimal outcome measures, research priorities, and international cooperation. *Ear and Hearing, 21*(4 Suppl.), 106S–115S.

Cox, R. M. (2004). Page 10: Waiting for evidence-based practice for your hearing aid fittings? *The Hearing Journal, 57*(8), 10, 12, 14, 16, 17.

Cox, R. M. (2005). Evidence-based practice in provision of amplification. *Journal of the American Academy of Audiology, 16,* 419–438.

Cox, R. M., & Alexander, G. C. (2002). The International Outcome Inventory for Hearing Aids (IOI-HA): The psychometric properties of the English version. *International Journal of Audiology, 41,* 30–35.

Cox, R. M., Alexander, G. C., & Beyer, C. M. (2003). Norms for the International Outcome Inventory for Hearing Aids. *Journal of the American Academy of Audiology, 14,* 404–413.

Cox, R. M., Stephens, D., & Kramer, S. E. (2002). Translations of the International Outcome Inventory for Hearing Aids (IOI-HA). *International Journal of Audiology, 41,* 3–26.

Crandell, C. C., & Smaldino, J. J. (2002). Room acoustics and auditory rehabilitation technology. In J. Katz (Ed.), *Handbook of clinical audiology* (5th ed., pp. 607–630). Baltimore, MD: Lippincott Williams & Wilkins.

Crandell, C. C., & Smaldino, J. J. (2005). Acoustical modifications in classrooms. In C. C. Crandell, J. J. Smaldino, & C. Flexer (Eds.). *Sound field amplification: Application to speech perception and classroom acoustics* (2nd ed., pp. 132–141). Clifton Park, NY: Thomson Delmar Learning.

Cranney, A. B., Coyle, D., Hopman, W. M., Hum, V., Power, B., & Tugwell, P. S. (2005). Prospective evaluation of preferences and quality of life in women with hip fractures. *Journal of Rheumatology, 32,* 2393–2399.

Crockett, R., Wright, A. J., Uus, K., Bamford, J., & Marteau, T. M. (2006). Maternal anxiety following newborn hearing screening: The moderating role of parents' knowledge. *Journal of Medical Screening, 13,* 20–25.

Croog, S. H. (1993). Current issues in conceptualizing and measuring quality of life. In *Quality of life assessment: Practice, problems, and promise* [Proceedings of a workshop]. Washington, DC: U.S. Department of Health and Human Services.

Cross, T. G., Nienhuys, T. G., & Kirkman, M. (1985). Parent-children interaction with receptively disabled children: Some determinants of material speech style. In K. E. Nelson (Ed.), *Children's language* (pp. 247–290). Hillsdale, NJ: Lawrence Erlbaum.

Cunningham, R. F. (2007). *Protocols for fitting infants and young children with amplification.* Retrieved from http://www.audiologyonline.com/articles/article_detail.asp?article_id=1829

Cummings, S. R., Newman, T. B., & Hulley, S. B. (2007). Designing an observational study: Cohort studies. In S. B. Hulley, S. R. Cummings, W. S. Browner, D. G. Grady, N. Hearst, & T. B. Newman (Eds.), *Designing clinical research* (3rd ed., pp. 97–126). Baltimore, MD: Lippincott William & Wilkins.

Curtiss, S., Prutting, C. A., & Lowell, E. L. (1979). Pragmatics and semantic development in young children with impaired hearing. *Journal of Speech, Language, and Hearing Research, 22,* 534–552.

Danhauer, J. L., Blood, G. W., Blood, I., & Gomez, N. (1980). Professional and lay observers' impressions of preschoolers wearing hearing aids. *Journal of Speech and Hearing Disorders, 45,* 415–422.

Danhauer, J. L., Johnson, C. E., Byrd, A. E., DeGood, L., Meuel, C., Pecile, A., & Koch, L. (2009). Survey of college students on iPod use and hearing health. *Journal of the American Academy of Audiology, 20,* 5–27.

Danhauer, J. L., Johnson, C. E., Finnegan, D., Hansen, K., Lamb, M., Lopez, I. P., . . . Williams, V. (2006). A case study of an emerging community-based early hearing detection and intervention program: Part II. Team building with otolaryngologists and pediatricians using a survey approach. *American Journal of Audiology, 15,* 33–45.

Danhauer, J. L., Johnson, C. E., Finnegan, D., Lamb, M., Lopez, I. P., Meuel, C., . . . Latiolais, L. N. (2006). A national survey of pediatric otolaryngologists and early hearing detection and intervention programs. *Journal of the American Academy of Audiology, 17,* 708–721.

Danhauer, J. L., Pecile, A. F., Johnson, C. E., Mixon, M., & Sharp, S. (2008). Parents' compliance and impressions of a maturing community-based early hearing detection and intervention program: An update. *Journal of the American Academy of Audiology, 19,* 612–629.

Daniel, E. (2007). Noise and hearing loss: A review. *Journal of School Health, 77,* 225–231.

Daniell, W. E., Swan, S. S., McDaniel, M. M., Camp, J. E., Cohen, M. A., & Stebbins, J. G. (2006). Noise exposure and hearing loss programmes after 20 years of regulations in the United States. *Occupational and Environmental Medicine, 63,* 343–351.

Davis, A., & Rafaie, E. A. (2000). Epidemiology of tinnitus. In R. S. Tyler (Ed.), *Tinnitus handbook* (pp. 1–23). San Diego, CA: Singular/Delmar Cengage Learning.

Davis, A., Smith, P., Ferguson, M., Stephens, D., & Gianopoulos, I. (2007). Acceptability, benefit, and costs of early screening for hearing disability: A study of potential screening tests and models. *Health Technology Assessment, 11,* 1–294.

Davis, A., Stephens, D., Rayment, A., & Thomas, K. (1992). Hearing impairment in middle age: The acceptability, benefit, and cost of detection (ABCD). *British Journal of Audiology, 26,* 1–14.

Davis, J. M., Elfenbein, J., Schum, R., & Bentler, R. A. (1986). Effects of mild and moderate hearing impairments on language, educational, and psychosocial behavior of children. *Journal of Speech and Hearing Disorders, 51,* 53–62.

Davis, M., Jackson, R., Smith, T., & Cooper, W. (1999). The hearing aid effect in African-American and Caucasian males as perceived by female judges of the same race. *Language, Speech, and Hearing Services in the Schools, 30,* 165–172.

Davis, P. B., Paki, B., & Hanley, P. J. (2007). Neuromonics tinnitus treatment: Third clinical trial. *Ear and Hearing, 28,* 242–259.

Davis, W. E. (2001). *Proportional frequency compression in hearing instruments.* Retrieved from http://www.hearingreview.com/issues/articles/2001-02_04.asp

Day, P. S. (1986). Deaf children's expression of communicative intentions. *Journal of Communication Disorders, 19,* 367–385.

Deafblindinfo.org. (2010). Retrieved from http://www.deafblindinfo.org/

Deaf Mentor (2006). *Deaf Mentor.* Retrieved from http://www.skihi.org/DeafMent.html

De Boysson-Bardies, B., Halle, P., Sagart, L., & Durand, C. (1989). A cross-lingustic investigation of vowel formants in babbling. *Journal of Child Language, 16,* 1–17.

DeCaro, J. J., Mudgett-DeCaro, P. A., & Dowaliby, F. (2001). Attitudes toward occupations for deaf youth in Sweden. *American Annals of the Deaf, 146,* 51–59.

De Filippo, C., & Scott, B. L. (1978). A method for training and evaluating the reception of ongoing speech. *Journal of the Acoustical Society of America, 63,* 1186–1192.

Demorest, M. E., & Bernstein, L. E. (1992). Sources of variability in speechreading sentences: A generalizability analysis. *Journal of Speech, Language, and Hearing Research, 35,* 876–891.

Demorest, M. E., & Erdman, S. A. (1987). Development of the communication profile for the hearing impaired.

Journal of Speech and Hearing Disorders, 52, 129–143.

Dengerink, J. E., & Porter, J. B. (1984). Children's attitudes towards peers wearing hearing aids. *Language, Speech, and Hearing Services in the Schools, 15,* 205–209.

Des Jardin, J. L., & Eisenberg, L. S. (2007). Maternal contributions: Supporting language development in young children with cochlear implants. *Ear and Hearing, 28,* 456–469.

Desmond, A. (2001). *Dizziness and balance disorders: Evaluation and treatment.* Chatham, IL: Micromedical Technologies.

de Villiers, J., de Villiers, P., & Hoban, E. (1994). The central problem of functional categories in English syntax of oral deaf children. In H. Tager-Flusberg (Ed.), *Constraints on language acquisition: Studies of atypical children* (pp. 9–47). Hillsdale, NJ: Lawrence Erlbaum.

de Villiers, P. A. (1988). Assessing English syntax in hearing-impaired children: Elicited production in pragmatically motivated situations. In R. R. Kretchmer & L. W. Kretchmer (Eds.), *Communication assessment of hearing impaired children: From conversation to classroom* [Monograph supplement]. *The Journal of the Academy of Rehabilitative Audiology, 21,* 41–71.

Dillon, H. (2001). *Hearing aids.* Sydney, Australia: Boomerang Press.

Dillon, H., James, A., & Ginis, J. (1997). Client oriented scale of improvement (COSI) and its relationship to several other measures of benefit and satisfaction provided by hearing aids. *Journal of the American Academy of Audiology, 8,* 27–43.

Divenyi, P. L., Stark, P. B., & Haupt, K. M. (2005). Decline of speech understanding and auditory thresholds in the elderly. *Journal of the Acoustical Society of America, 118,* 1089–1100.

Dobie, R. (1999). A review of randomized clinical trials in tinnitus. *Laryngoscope, 109,* 1202–1211.

Dodd, M. C., Nikolopoulos, T. P., Totten, C., Cope, Y., & O'Donoghue, G. M. (2005). Cochlear implants: 100 pediatric conversions from the body worn to the Nucleus Esprit 22 ear level processor. *Otology and Neurotology, 26,* 635–638.

Doggett, S., Stein, R. L., & Gans, D. (1998). Hearing aid effect in older females. *Journal of the American Academy of Audiology, 9,* 361–366.

Donahue, A., Dubno, J. R., & Beck, L. (2009). Guest editorial: Accessible and affordable hearing health care for adults with mild to moderate hearing loss. *Ear and Hearing, 31,* 2–6.

Dorros, C., Kurtzer-White, E., Ahlgren, M., Simon, P., & Vohr, B. (2007). Medical home for children with hearing loss: Physician perspectives and practices. *Pediatrics, 120,* 288–294.

Duncan, A. (2010). *Keeping the promise to all America's children: Secretary Arne Duncan's remarks to the Council of Exceptional Children on April 21, 2010.* Retrieved from http://www2.ed.gov/news/speeches/2010/04/04212010.html

Dunn, C. C., & Marciniak, K. (2009). *Options for preserving residual hearing with a cochlear implant.* Retrieved from http://www.audiologyonline.com/articles/article_detail.asp?article_id=2167

Dunn, L. M., & Dunn, D. M. (2007). *Peabody picture vocabulary test–fourth edition (PPVT-4).* Boston, MA: Pearson.

Dunn, L. M., Robertson, G. J., & Eisenberg, J. L. (1979). *Peabody picture vocabulary test – revised.* Circle Pines, MA: American Guidance Service.

Earobics. (2010). *Earobics.* Retrieved from http://www.earobics.com

Ebert, D. A., & Heckerling, P. S. (1995). Communication with deaf patients. Knowledge, beliefs, and practices of physicians. *Journal of the American Medical Association, 273,* 227–229.

Educational Audiology Association. (2005). *Sounds on the audiogram chart.* Tampa, FL: Author.

Educational Audiology Association. (2009). *School-based audiology advocacy series.* Retrieved from http://www.edaud.org/displaycommon.cfm?an=1&subarticlenbr=86

Edwards, C. (2005). From system selection to enhancement of listening skills: Considerations for the classroom. In C. C. Crandell, J. J. Smaldino, & C. Flexer (Eds.), *Sound field amplification: Application to speech perception and classroom acoustics* (2nd ed., pp. 166–191). Clifton Park, NY: Thomson Delmar Learning.

Egan, K. (1998). *The skilled helper: A problem management approach to helping* (6th ed.). Pacific Grove, CA: Brooks/Cole.

Eggars, S. D. (2007). Migraine-related vertigo: Diagnosis and treatment. *Current Pain Headache Reports, 11,* 217–226.

Eisenbeis, J. F., & Jones, S. C. (2007). What did you say? Pump up the volume: Noise-induced hearing loss in the young. *Modern Medicine, 104,* 112–113.

El-Hakim, H., Papsin, B., Mount, R. J., Levasseur, J., Panesar, J., Stevens, D., & Harrison, R. V. (2001). Vocabulary acquisition rate after pediatric cochlear implantation and the impact of age at implantation. *International Journal of Pediatric Otorhinolaryngology, 59,* 187–194.

El-Kashian, H. K., Ashbaugh, C., Zwolan, T., & Telian, S. A. (2003). Cochlear implantation in prelingually deaf children with ossified cochleae. *Otology and Neurotology, 24,* 596–600.

Ell, K. (2006). Depression care for the elderly: Reducing barriers to evidence based practice. *Home Health Care Services Quarterly, 25,* 115–148.

Elliot, L. B., Stinson, M. S., McKee, B. G., Everhart, V. S., & Francis, P. J. (2001). College students' perceptions of the C-Print-Speech-to-Text Transcription System. *Journal of Deaf Studies and Deaf Education, 6,* 285–298.

English, K., Kooper, R., & Bratt, G. (2004). Informing parents of their child's hearing loss: "Breaking bad news": Guidelines for audiologists. *Audiology Today, 16*(2), 10–12.

English, K. M. (2002). *Counseling children with hearing impairment and their families.* Boston: Allyn & Bacon.

Erber, N. P. (1988). *Therapy for adults with sensory loss* (2nd ed.). Victoria, Australia: Clavis.

Erber, N. P. (1996). *QUEST?AR: Communication practice.* Clifton Hill, Victoria, Australia.

Erber, N. P. (2002). Hearing, vision, communication, and older people. *Seminars in Hearing, 23,* 35–42.

Erber, N. P. (2003a). Use of hearing aids by older people: Influence of non-auditory factors (vision and manual dexterity). *International Journal of Audiology, 42,* 2S 21–25.

Erber, N. P. (2003b). *Communication and adult hearing loss.* Melbourne, Australia: Clavis Publishing.

Erber, N. P. (2006). *Hearing, vision, communication and older people.* Melbourne, Australia: Clavis Publishing.

Erber, N. P., Holland, J., & Osborn, R. R. (1998). Communicating with elders: Effects of speaker-listener distance. *British Journal of Audiology, 32,* 135–138.

Erikson, E. (1968). *Identity: Youth and crisis.* New York: Norton.

Erlandsson, S. (2000). Psychological profiles of tinnitus in patients. In R. S. Tyler (Ed.), *Tinnitus handbook* (pp. 25–58). San Diego, CA: Singular/Delmar Cengage Learning.

Erler, S. F., & Garstecki, D. C. (2002). Hearing loss- and hearing aid-related stigma: Perceptions of women with age-normal hearing. *American Journal of Audiology, 11,* 83–91.

Estabrooks, W. (1994). *Auditory-verbal therapy for parents and professionals.* Washington, DC: Alexander Graham Bell Association for the Deaf.

Eye Diseases Prevalence Research Group. (2004a). The prevalence of refractive errors among adults in the United States, Western Europe, and Australia. *Archives of Ophthalmology, 122,* 195–205.

Eye Diseases Prevalence Research Group. (2004b). Causes and prevalence of visual impairment among adults in the United States. *Archives of Ophthalmology, 122,* 477–485.

Eye Diseases Prevalence Research Group. (2004c). Prevalence of age-related macular degeneration in the United States. *Archives of Ophthalmology, 122,* 564–572

Fahy, C. P., Carney, A. S., Nikolopoulos, T. P., Ludman, C. N., & Gibbin, K. P. (2001). Cochlear implantation in children with large vestibular aqueduct syndrome and a review of the syndrome. *International Journal of Pediatric Otorhinolaryngology, 59,* 207–215.

Fallowfield, L., & Jenkins, V. (2004). Communicating sad, bad, and difficult news in medicine. *Lancet, 363,* 312–319.

Federal Communication Commission (FCC) (2006). *FCC consumer advisory: FCC acts to promote accessibility of digital wireless phones to individuals with hearing disabilities.* Retrieved from http://www.fcc.gov/cgb/consumerfacts/accessiblewireless.html

Ferguson, N. M., & Nerbonne, M. A. (2003). Status of hearing aids in nursing homes and retirement centers in 2002. *Journal of the Academy of Rehabilitative Audiology, 36,* 37–44.

Field, M. J., & Lohr, K. N. (1990). *Clinical practice guidelines: Directions for a new program, Institute of Medicine.* Washington, DC: National Academy Press.

Filipo, P., Mancini, P., Ballantyne, D., Bosco, E., & D'Elia, C. (2004). Short-term study of the effect of coding strategy on the auditory performance of pre- and post-lingually deafened adults implanted with the Clarion CII. *Acta Otolaryngologica, 124,* 368–370.

Filipo, R., Bosco, E., Mancini, P., & Ballantyne, D. (2004). Cochlear implants in special cases: Deafness in the presence of disabilities and/or associated problems. *Acta Otolaryngologica Supplement, 552,* 74–80.

Finitzo, T., & Crumley, W. (1999). The role of the pediatrician in hearing loss: From detection to connection. *Pediatric Clinics in North America, 46,* 15–34.

Fishman, G. A., Bozbeyoglu, S., Massof, R. W., & Kimberling, W. (2007). Natural course of visual field loss in patients with Type II Usher syndrome. *Retina, 27,* 601–608.

Fligor, B. J., & Cox, L. C. (2004). Output levels of commercially available portable compact disc players and the potential risk to hearing. *Ear and Hearing, 25,* 513–527.

Fligor, B. J., & Ives, T. (2006). *Does earphone type affect risk of recreational noise-induced hearing loss?* Paper presented at the Noise-Induced Hearing Loss: Children at Work and Play Meeting, Covington, KY.

Flores, P., Martin, F. N., & Champlin, C. A. (1996). Providing audiological services to Spanish speakers. *American Journal of Audiology, 5,* 69–73.

Flynn, M. C. (2003). *Sailing out of the windless sea of monosyllables: The use of speech perception tests in aural rehabilitation.* Retrieved from http://www.hearingreview.com/issues/articles/2003-04_02.asp

Folstein M. F., Folstein S. E., & McHugh P. R. (1975). "Mini-mental state": A practical method for grading cognitive state of patients for the clinician. *Journal of Psychiatric Research, 12,* 189–198.

Forner, L. L., & Hixon, T. J. (1977). Respiratory kinematics in profoundly hearing-impaired speakers. *Journal of Speech and Hearing Research, 20,* 373–408.

Foster, S., & Brown, P. (1989). Factors influencing the academic and social integration of hearing impaired college students. *Journal of Postsecondary Education and Disability, 7,* 78–96.

Frattali, C. M. (1998). Outcomes measurement: Definitions, dimensions, and perspectives. In C. M. Frattali (Ed.), *Measuring outcomes in speech-language pathology* (pp. 1–27). New York: Thieme.

Freeman, B. A. (2006). Ethics and professionalism. In T. A. Hamill (Ed.), *Ethics in audiology* (pp.7–9). Reston, VA: American Academy of Audiology.

Fretz, R. J., & Fravel, R. P. (1985). Design and function: A physical and electrical description of the 3M House cochlear implant system. *Ear and Hearing, 6*(Suppl.), 14S–19S.

Friedmann, N., & Szterman, R. (2006). Syntactic movement in orally trained children with hearing impairment. *Journal of Deaf Studies and Deaf Education, 11,* 56–75.

Friend, M. (2005). *Special education: Contemporary perspectives for school professionals.* Boston: Allyn & Bacon.

Frye, G. (2005). *FONIX: ANSI '03 Workbook.* Tigard, OR: Frye Electronics.

Fudala, J. B. (2000). *Arizona articulation proficiency scale, third edition (Arizona-3).* Los Angeles, CA: Western Psychological Services.

Gallaudet Research Institute. (November 2008). *Regional and national summary report of data from the 2007-2008 Annual Survey of Deaf and Hard of Hearing Children and Youth.* Washington DC: Gallaudet University.

Gantz, B. J., Hansen, M. R., Turner, C.W., Oleson, J. J., Reiss, L. A., & Parkinson, A. J. (2009). Hybrid 10 clinical trial: Preliminary results. *Audiology and Neurotology, 14*(Suppl. 1), S32–S38.

Gantz, B. J., Tye-Murray, N., & Tyler, R. S. (1989). Word recognition performance with single-channel and multichannel cochlear implants. *American Journal of Otology, 10,* 91–94.

Gantz, B. J., Tyler, R. S., Knutson, J. F., Woodworth, G., Abbas, P., McCabe, B. F., . . . Brown, C. (1988). Evaluation of five different cochlear implant designs: Audiologic assessment and predictors of performance. *Laryngoscope, 98,* 1100–1106.

Garahan, M. B., Waller, J. A., Houghton, M., Tisdale, W. A., & Runge, C. F. (1992). Hearing loss prevalence and management in nursing home residents. *Journal of the American Geriatrics Society, 40,* 130–134.

Garstecki, D. C, & Erler, S. F. (1999). Older adult performance on the Communication Profile for the Hearing Impaired: Gender difference. *Journal of Speech, Language, and Hearing Research, 42,* 785–796.

Gatehouse, S. (1999). The Glasgow Hearing Aid Benefit Profile: Derivation and validation of a client-centered outcome measure for hearing aid services. *Journal of the American Academy of Audiology, 10,* 80–103.

Gatehouse, S., Naylor, G., & Elberling, C. (2003). Benefits from hearing aids in relation to the interaction between the user and the environment. *International Journal of Audiology, 42(Suppl.),* S77–S85.

Geers, A. E., & Moog, J. S. (1978). Syntactic maturity of spontaneous speech and elicited imitation of hearing-impaired children. *Journal of Speech and Hearing Disorders, 43,* 380–391.

Geers, A. E., Nicholas, J. G., & Sedey, A. L. (2003). Language skills of children with early cochlear implantation. *Ear and Hearing, 24*(Suppl. 1), 46S–58S.

Gelfand, S. A., & Silman, S. (1993). Apparent auditory deprivation in children: Implications of monaural versus binaural amplification. *Journal of the American Academy of Audiology, 4,* 313–318.

Gelfand, S. A., Silman, S., & Ross, L. (1987). Long-term effects of monaural, binaural, and no amplification in subjects with bilateral hearing loss. *Scandinavian Audiology, 16,* 201–207.

Giangiacomo, J., & Morey, S. S. (2005). Improving preschool vision screening programs. *Missouri Medicine, 102,* 55–58.

Giles, L. C., Glonek, G. F., Luszcz, M. A., & Andrews, G. R. (2005). Effects of social networks on 10 year survival in very old Australians: The Australian longitudinal study of aging. *Journal of Epidemiology and Community Health, 59,* 574–579.

Gillespie, L. D., Robertson, M. C., Gillespie, W. J., Lamb, S. E., Gates, S., Cumming, R. G., & Rowe, B. H. (2009). Interventions for preventing falls in older people living in the community. *Cocrane Database of Systematic Reviews,* CD007146.

Giolas, T. J., Owens, E., Lamb, S. H., & Schubert, E. D. (1979). Hearing Performance Inventory. *Journal of Speech and Hearing Disorders, 44,* 169–195.

Glass, T. A., De Leon, C. F., Bassuk, S. S., & Berkman, L. F. (2006). Social engagement and depressive symptoms in late life: Longitudinal findings. *Journal of Aging and Health, 18,* 604–628.

Gold, T. (1980). Speech production of hearing-impaired children. *Journal of Communication Disorders, 13,* 397–418.

Goldberg, D. M., & Flexer, C. (2001). Auditory-verbal graduates: Outcome survey of clinical efficacy. *Journal of the American Academy of Audiology, 12,* 406–414.

Golding, M., Taylor, A, Cupples, L., & Mitchell, P. (2006). Odds of demonstrating auditory processing abnormality in the average older adult: The Blue Mountains Study. *Ear and Hearing, 27,* 129–138.

Goldman, R., & Fristoe, M. (2000). *Goldman-Fristoe test of articulation competence (G-FTA-2),* (2nd ed.). San Antonio, TX: AGS/ Pearson Assessment.

Goldstein, D. P., & Stephens, S. D. (1981). Audiological rehabilitation: Management Model I. *Audiology, 20,* 432–452.

Good-Lite. (2006). *Pediatric vision screening from Good-Lite.* Elgin, IL: Author.

Govaerts, P. J., De Beukelaer, C., Daemers, K., De Ceulaer, G., Yperman, M., Somers, T., . . . Offeciers, F. E. (2002). Outcome of cochlear implantation of children at different ages from 0 to 6 years. *Otology and Neurotology, 23,* 885–890.

Grantham, R. B. (1997). ASHA and the schools. In P. F. O'Connell (Ed.), *Speech, language, and hearing programs in the schools: A guide for students and practitioners* (pp. 24–65). Gaithersburg, MD: American Speech-Language-Hearing Association.

Gravel, J. S., & O'Gara, J. (2003). Communication options for children with hearing loss. *Mental Retardation Developmental Disabilities Research Review, 9,* 243–251.

Greer Clark, J., & English, K. M. (2004). *Counseling in audiologic practice: Helping patients and families adjust to hearing loss.* Boston: Allyn & Bacon.

Håkanssön, B., Carlsson, P. U., Tjellström, A., & Lidén, A. (1994). The bone-anchored hearing aid: Principal design and audiometric results. *Ear, Nose, and Throat Journal, 73,* 670–675.

Hallahan, D. P., & Kauffman, J. M. (2006). *Exceptional learners: An introduction to special education* (10th ed.). Boston: Allyn & Bacon.

Hallam, R., Ashton, P., Sherbourne, K., & Gailey, L. (2006). Acquired profound hearing loss: Mental health and other characteristics of a large sample. *International Journal of Audiology, 45,* 715–723.

Halpern, A. S. (1993). Quality of life as a conceptual framework for evaluating transition outcomes. *Exceptional Children, 59,* 486–489.

Hammerman-Rozenberg, R., Maaravi, Y., Cohen, A., & Stressman, J. (2005). Working late: The impact of work after 70 on longevity, health and function. *Aging Clinical and Experimental Research, 17,* 508–513.

Hamzavi, J., Baumgartner, W., Egelierler, B., Franz, P., Schenk, B., & Gstoettner, W. (2000). Follow up of cochlear-implanted handicapped children. *International Journal of Pediatric Otorhinolaryngology, 56,* 169–176.

Hamzavi, J., Baumgartner, W. D., Pok, S. M., Franz, P., & Gstoettner, W. (2003). Variables affecting speech perception in postlingually deaf adults following cochlear implantation. *Acta Otolaryngologica, 123,* 493–498.

Hanavan, P. C., Greer Clark, J., & Abrahamson, J. (2006). *AR specialty certification: An idea whose time has come?* Paper presented at the 2006 Academy of Rehabilitative Audiology Institute, Louisville, KY.

Hanson, M. J. (1997a). Ethic, cultural, and language diversity in intervention settings. E. W. Lynch & M. J. Hanson (Eds.), *Developing cross-cultural competence: A guide for working with children and their families* (2nd ed., pp. 3–22). Baltimore, MD: Brookes.

Hanson, M. J. (1997b). Families with Anglo-European roots. In E. W. Lynch & M. J. Hanson (Eds.), *Developing cross-cultural competence: A guide for working with children and their families* (2nd ed., pp. 93–126). Baltimore, MD: Brookes.

Harris, A. H., & Thoresen, C. E. (2005). Volunteering is associated with delayed mortality in older people: Analysis of the longitudinal study of aging. *Journal of Health Psychology, 10,* 739–752.

Harvey, M. (2004). *Psychosocial aspects of hearing loss.* Elkins Park, PA: Pennsylvania College of Optometry.

Harvey, M. A. (1998). *Odyssey of hearing loss: Tales of triumph.* San Diego, CA: Dawn Sign Press.

Haskins, H. A. (1949). *A phonetically balanced test of speech discrimination for children.* Unpublished master's thesis, Northwestern University, Evanston, IL.

Hawkins, D., Larkin, M. & Tedeschi, T. J. (2006). Relationships with hearing aid manufacturers. In T. A. Hamill (Ed.), *Ethics in audiology* (pp.25–36). Reston, VA: American Academy of Audiology.

Hawkins, D. B. (2005). Effectiveness of counseling-based adult group aural rehabilitation programs: A systematic review. *Journal of the American Academy of Audiology, 16,* 485–493.

Hawkins, D. B., & Mueller, H. G. (1992). Test protocols for probe-microphone measurements. In H. G. Mueller, D. B. Hawkins, & Northern, J. L. (Eds.), *Probe microphone measurements* (pp. 269–278). San Diego, CA: Singular/Delmar Cengage Learning.

Hawkins, D. B., & Schum, D. J. (1991). LDL measures: An efficient use of clinic time? *American Journal of Audiology, 8*–10.

Haynes, W. O., & Johnson, C. E. (2009). *Understanding research and evidence-based practice in communication disorders. A primer for students and practitioners.* Boston: Allyn & Bacon.

Hazell, J. (2007). *Tinnitus Retraining Therapy: Guidelines and exercises for patients.* Retrieved from http://www.tinnitus.org/home/frame/THC1.htm

Hazell, J. W., & Jastreboff, P. J. (1990). Tinnitus I: Auditory mechanisms: A model for tinnitus and hearing impairment. *Journal of Otolaryngology, 19,* 1–5.

Hearing Instrument Manufacturers' Software Association. (2007). *About HIMSA.* Retrieved from http://www.himsa.com/AboutHIMSA/tabid/79/language/en-US/Default.aspx

Hearing Loss Association of America. (2010). Retrieved from http://www.hearingloss.org/

Heavner, K. (2007). Changing trends in the educational placement for children with cochlear implants. *Advanced Bionics: Loud and Clear,* Issue 2, November. Retrieved from http://www.advancedbionics.com/UserFiles/File/2-091702%20Loud-Clear-FINAL%20Issue%202%202007.pdf.

Hehar, S. S., Nikolopoulos, T. P., Gibbin, K. P., & O'Donoghue, G. M. (2002). Surgery and functional outcomes in deaf children receiving cochlear implants before age 2 years. *Archives of Otolaryngology—Head and Neck Surgery, 128,* 11–14.

Heine, C., & Browning, C. J. (2002). Communication and psychosocial consequences of sensory loss in older adults: Overview and rehabilitation directions. *Disabilities and Rehabilitation, 24,* 763–773.

Helm, H. M., Hayes, J. C., Flint, E. P., Koenig, H. G., & Blazer, D. G. (2000). Does private religious activity prolong survival? A six-year follow-up study of 3,851 older adults.*The Journals of Gerontology Series A: Biological Sciences and Medical Sciences, 55,* M400–405.

Helpguide.org. (2006). *Depression.* Retrieved from http://www.helpguide.org/topics/depression.htm

Helpguide.org (2010). *Understanding senior housing care.* Retrieved from http://www.helpguide.org/elder/senior_housing_residential_care_types.htm

Henderson Sabes, J. H., & Sweetow, R. W. (2007). Variables predicting outcomes on listening and communication enhancement (LACE) training. *International Journal of Audiology, 46,* 374–383.

Henry, J. A., Loovis, C., Montero, M., Kaelin, C., Anselmi, K. A., Coombs, R., . . . James, K. E. (2007). Randomized clinical trial: Group counseling based on Tinnitus Retraining Therapy. *Journal of Rehabilitation Research and Development, 44,* 21–32.

Henry, J. A., Schechter, M. A., Zaugg, T. L., Griest, S., Jastreboff, P. J., Vernon, J. A., . . . Stewart, B. J. (2006). Outcomes of a clinical trial: Tinnitus masking versus tinnitus retraining therapy. *Journal of the American Academy of Audiology, 17,* 104–132.

Henry, J. A., Trune, D. R., Robb, M. J. A., & Jastreboff, P. J. (2007a). Tinnitus retraining therapy: Clinical guidelines. San Diego, CA: Plural Publishing.

Henry, J. A., Trune, D. R., Robb, M. J. A., & Jastreboff, P. J. (2007b). Tinnitus retraining therapy: Patient counseling guide. San Diego, CA: Plural Publishing.

Henry, J. L., & Wilson, P. H. (2001). *The psychological management of chronic tinnitus: A cognitive-behavioral approach.* Boston: Allyn & Bacon.

Herdman, A. T., & Stapells, D. R. (2001). Thresholds determined using the monotic and dichotic multiple auditory steady-state response technique in normal-hearing subjects. *Scandinavian Audiology, 30,* 41–49.

Hérraiz, C., Hernandez, F. J., Toledano, A., & Aparicio, J. M. (2007). Tinnitus retraining therapy: Prognosis factors. *American Journal of Otolaryngology, 28,* 225–229.

Hill, R. D., Allen, C., & Gregory, K. (1990). Self-generated mnemonics for enhancing free recall performance in older learners. *Experimental Aging Research, 16,* 141–145.

Hill, T. D., Burdette, A. M., Angel, J. L., & Angel, R. J. (2006). Religious attendance and cognitive functioning among older Mexican Americans. *The Journals of Gerontology Series B: Psychological Sciences and Social Sciences, 61,* P3–9.

Hilton, M., & Pinder, D. (2004). The Epley canalith repositioning manoeuvre for benign paroxysmal positional vertigo. *Cochrane Database of Systematic Reviews, 2.* CD003162.

Hilton, M., & Stuart, E. (2004). Ginkgo biloba for tinnitus. *Cochrane Database of Systematic Reviews, 2.* CD003852.

Hipskind, N. (2007). Visual stimuli in communication. In R. L. Schow and M. A. Nerbonne (Eds.), *Audiologic rehabilitation* (5th ed., pp. 139–182). Boston: Allyn & Bacon.

Hladek, G. A. (2002). Cochlear implants, the deaf culture, and ethics: A study of disability, informed surrogate consent, and ethnocide. *Monash Bioethics Review, 21,* 29–44.

Hnath-Chisolm, T., & Abrams, H. (2008). Outcome measures and evidence-based practice. In H. Hosford-Dunn, R. Roeser, & M. Valente (Eds.), *Audiology practice management* (2nd ed., pp. 171–194). New York, NY: Thieme.

Hochmair, E. S., & Hochmair-Desoyer, I. J. (1983). Precepts elicited by different speech-coding strategies. In C. W. Parkins & S. W. Anderson (Eds.), *Cochlear prostheses: An international symposium* (pp. 268–279). New York: Raven Press.

Hodges, A. V., Dolan, A. M., Balkany, T. J., Schloffman, J. J., & Butts, S. L. (1999). Speech perception results in children with cochlear implants: Contributing factors. *Otolaryngology, Head, and Neck Surgery, 121,* 21–34.

Hoffman, R. A., Downey, L. L., Waltzman, S. B., & Cohen, N. L. (1997). Cochlear implantation in children with cochlear malformations. *American Journal of Otology, 18,* 184–187.

Hogan, C. A., & Turner, C. W. (1998). High-frequency audibility: Benefits for hearing-impaired listeners. *Journal of the Acoustical Society of America, 104,* 432–441.

Hol, M. K., Spath, M. A., Krabbe, P. F., van der Pouw, C. T., Snik, A. F., Cremers, C.W., & Mylanus, E. A. (2005). The bone-anchored hearing aid: Quality-of-life assessment. *Archives of Otolaryngology, Head, and Neck Surgery, 130,* 394–399.

Hollins, P. (2005). How to get the most out of college. *Hearing Loss Magazine, 26*(4), 10–15.

Hollis, S., & Campbell, F. (1999). What is meant by intention to treat analysis? Survey of published randomized controlled trials. *British Medical Journal, 319,* 670–674.

Hood, R. B., & Dixon, R. F. (1969). Physical characteristics of speech rhythm of deaf and normal-hearing speakers. *Journal of Communication Disorders, 2,* 20–28.

Hosford-Dunn, H., Roeser, R. J., & Valente, M. (2008). *Audiology practice management.* New York, NY: Thieme.

Hospice Foundation of America. (2006). *What is hospice?* Retrieved from http://www.hospicefoundation.org/pages/page.asp?page_id=47055

House Ear Institute. (2006). *Auditory brainstem implant—HEI fact sheet.* Retrieved from http://www.hei.org/news/facts/abifact.htm

Huch, J. L., & Hosford-Dunn, H. (2000). Inventories of self-assessment measurements of hearing aid outcome. In R. Sandlin (Ed.), *Textbook of hearing aid amplification,* (2nd ed., pp. 489–521). Clifton Park, NY: Delmar Thomson Learning.

Iezzoni, L. I., O'Day, B. L., Killeen, M., & Harker, H. (2004). Communicating about health care: Observations from persons who are deaf or hard of hearing. *Annals of Internal Medicine, 140,* 356–362.

Individuals with Disabilities Education Improvement Act. (2004). Public Law No. 108–446, 118 Stat. 2647.

Isaacson, G. (2000). Universal newborn hearing screening in an inner city, managed care environment. *Laryngoscope, 110,* 881–894.

Jacobson, G. P., & Newman, C. W. (1990). The development of the Dizziness Handicap Inventory. *Archives of Otolaryngology, Head, and Neck Surgery, 11,* 424–427.

Jacobson, G. P., Newman, C. W., Hunter, L., & Balzer, G. K. (1991). Balance function test correlates of the Dizziness Handicap Inventory. *Journal of the American Academy of Audiology, 2,* 253–260.

Jakobsson, P., Kvarnström, G., Abrahamsson, M., Bjernbrink-Hörnblad, E., & Sunnqvist, B. (2002). The frequency of amblyopia among visually impaired persons. *Acta Ophthalmologica Scandinavica, 80,* 44–46.

Jastreboff, P. J. (2000). Tinnitus habituation therapy (THT) and tinnitus retraining therapy (TRT). In R. S. Tyler (Ed.), *Tinnitus handbook* (pp. 357–376). San Diego, CA: Singular/Delmar Cengage Learning.

Jastreboff, P. J., & Hazell, J. W. (1993). A neurophysiological approach to tinnitus: Clinical implications. *British Journal of Audiology, 27,* 7–17.

Jeng, F. C., Brownt, C. J., Johnson, T. A., & Vander Werff, K. R. (2004). Estimating air-bone gaps using auditory-state responses. *Journal of the American Academy of Audiology, 15,* 67–78.

Jerger, J. (2007). Editorial: Do hearing aids really improve quality of life? *Journal of the American Academy of Audiology, 18,* 96.

Jerger, J. F., Chmiel, R., Florin, E., Pirozzolo, F., & Wilson, N. (1996). Comparison of conventional amplification and an assistive listening device in elderly persons. *Ear and Hearing, 17,* 490–504.

Jerger, J. F., & Hayes, D. (1976). The cross-check principle in pediatric audiometry. *Archives of Otolaryngology, 102,* 614–620.

Joe, J. R., & Malach, R. S. (1997). Families with Native American roots. In E. W. Lynch & M. J. Hanson (Eds.), *Developing cross-cultural competence: A guide for working with children and their families* (2nd ed., pp. 127–164). Baltimore, MD: Brookes.

John, J. E., & Howarth, J. N. (1965). The effect of time distortion on the intelligibility of deaf children's speech. *Language and Speech, 8,* 127–134.

Johnson, C. (2000). *How the Individuals with Disabilities Education Act (IDEA) applies to deaf and hard of hearing students.* Washington, DC: Laurent LeClerc National Deaf Education Center, Gallaudet University.

Johnson, C. D., Benson, P. V., & Seaton, J. B. (1997). *Educational audiology handbook.* San Diego, CA: Singular/Delmar Cengage Learning.

Johnson, C. E. (1999). Dimensions of multiskilling: Considerations for educational audiology. *Language, Speech, and Hearing Services in Schools, 30,* 4–10.

Johnson, C. E., & Danhauer, J. L. (1982). Attitudes towards severely hearing-impaired geriatrics with and without hearing aids. *Australian Journal of Audiology, 4,* 41–45.

Johnson, C. E., & Danhauer, J. L. (1997a). CIC instruments: Cosmetic issues. In M. Chasin (Ed.), *CIC handbook* (pp. 151–167). San Diego, CA: Singular/Delmar Cengage Learning.

Johnson, C. E., & Danhauer, J. L. (1997b). The "Hearing Aid Effect" revisited: Can we meet the needs of cosmetically sensitive patients? *High Performance Hearing Solutions, 1,* 37–44.

Johnson, C. E., & Danhauer, J. L. (1999). *Guidebook for support programs in aural rehabilitation.* San Diego, CA: Singular/Delmar Cengage Learning.

Johnson, C. E., & Danhauer, J. L. (2002a). *Handbook of outcomes measurement in audiology.* Clifton Park, NY: Thomson Delmar Learning.

Johnson, C. E., & Danhauer, J. L. (2002b). A transdisciplinary holistic approach to hearing health care. *Geriatric Times, 3*(5). 10–11.

Johnson, C. E., Danhauer, J. L., & Edwards, R. G. (1982). The "Hearing Aid effect" on geriatrics—Fact or fiction? *Hearing Instruments, 33*(10), 21, 24, 36.

Johnson, C. E., Gavin, R. B., & Reith, A. C. (2004). Hearing aid compatibility: Are cell phone retailers ready? Poster presented at the Annual Convention and Exposition of the American Academy of Audiology, Salt Lake City, UT.

Johnson, C. E., Stein, R. L., Gorman, S., & Tracy, L. (1997). Noise and hearing conservation: Students' habits, knowledge, and attitudes. *HEARSAY: The Journal of the Ohio Speech and Hearing Association, 11*(2), 29–34.

Joint Committee on Infant Hearing: American Academy of Audiology; American Academy of Pediatrics; American Speech-Language-Hearing Association; Directors of Speech and Hearing Programs in State Health and Welfare Agencies. (2000). Year 2000 position statement: Principles and guidelines for early hearing detection and intervention programs. *Pediatrics, 106,* 798–817.

Joint Committee on Infant Hearing. (2007). Year 2007 position statement: Principles and guidelines for early hearing detection and intervention programs. *Pediatrics, 120,* 898–921.

Jönsson, R., Sixt, E., Landahl, S., & Rosenhall, U. (2004). Prevalence of dizziness and vertigo in an urban elderly population. *Journal of Vestibular Research, 14,* 47–52.

Jordan, B. (2001a). *Adult services referral checklist for transition-age young adults who are deaf blind.* Paper presented at the Kansas University Summer Transition Institute.

Jordan, B. (2001b). *Considerations when teaching students who are deaf-blind.* Retrieved from http://projects.pepnet.org/downloads/TPSHT_Deaf_Blind.pdf

Jupiter, T. (2009). Screening for hearing loss in the elderly using distortion product otoacoustic emissions, puretones, and a self-assessment tool. *American Journal of Audiology, 18,* 99–107.

Kalcioglu, M. T., Miman, M. C., Toplu, Y., Yakinci, C., & Ozturan, O. (2003). Anthropometric growth study of normal human auricle. *International Journal of Pediatric Otorhinolaryngology, 67,* 1169–1177.

Kanowitz, S. J., Shapiro, W. H., Golfinos, J. G., Cohen, N. L., & Roland, J. T. Jr. (2004). Auditory brainstem implantation in patients with neurofibromatosis type 2. *Laryngoscope, 114,* 2135–2146.

Kaplan, D. M., Shipp, D. B., Chen, J. M., Ng, A. H. C., & Nedzelski, J. M. (2003). Early-deafened adult cochlear implant users: Assessment of outcomes. *The Journal of Otolaryngology, 32,* 245–249.

Kaplan, H. (1996). Speechreading. In M. J. Moseley & S. Bally (Eds.), *Communication therapy: An integrated approach to aural rehabilitation* (pp. 229–250). Washington, DC: Gallaudet University Press.

Kates, J. M. (2008). *Digital hearing aids.* San Diego, CA: Plural.

Kaye, H. S., Yaeger, P., & Reed, M. C. (2008). Disparities in usage of assistive technology among people with disabilities. *Assistive Technology, 20,* 194–203.

Keller, B. K., Martin, J. L., Thomas, V. S., & Potter, J. F. (1999). The effect of visual and hearing impairments on functional status. *Journal of the American Geriatric Society, 47,* 1319–1325.

Kemperman, M. H., Hoeflsoot, L. H., & Cremers, C.W. (2002). Hearing loss and connexin 26. *Journal of the Royal Society of Medicine, 95,* 171–177.

Kennedy, C., McCann, D., Campbell, M. J., Kimm, I., & Thornton, R. (2005). Universal newborn hearing screening for permanent childhood hearing impairment: An 8-year follow-up of a controlled trial. *Lancet, 366,* 660–662.

Kennedy, C. R., McCann, D. C., Campbell, M. J., Law, C. M., Mullee, M., Petrou, S., . . . Stevenson, J. (2006). Language ability after early detection of permanent childhood hearing impairment. *New England Journal of Medicine, 354,* 2131–2141.

Kenneth Burger Hearing Aid Museum. (2009). Retrieved from http://www.kent.edu/ehhs/spa/museum/index.cfm

Kent, R. D., Osberger, M. J., Netsell, R., & Goldschmidt-Hustedde, C. (1987). Phonetic development in identical twins. *Journal of Speech and Hearing Disorders, 52,* 64–75.

Kentish, R. C., Crocker, S. R., & McKenna, L. (2000). Children's experience of tinnitus: A preliminary survey of children presenting to a psychology department. *British Journal of Audiology, 34,* 335–340.

Kerr, M. J., Savik, K., Monsen, K. A., & Lusk, S. L. (2007). Effectiveness of computer-based tailoring versus targeting to promote use of hearing protection. *Canadian Journal of Nursing Research, 39,* 80–97.

Kessels, R. P. C. (2003). Patients' memory for medical information. *Journal of the Royal Society of Medicine, 96,* 219–222.

Killion, M. (2004). Unlocking knowledge; debunking myths: Translating audiological research into clinical applications. *The Hearing Review, 11*(9), 14, 16, 18–20, 66.

Kirk, K. I. (2001). Challenges in the clinical investigation of cochlear implants. In J. K. Niparko, N. K. Mellon, A. M. Robbins, D. L. Tucci, & B. S. Wilson (Eds.), *Cochlear implants: Principles and practices* (pp. 225–258). Baltimore, MD: Lippincott Williams & Wilkins.

Kirk, K. I., Diefendorf, A. O., & Robbins, A. M. (1997). Assessing speech perception in children. In L. L. Mendel & J. L. Danhauer (Eds.), *Audiological evaluation and management and speech perception assessment* (pp.101–148). San Diego, CA: Singular/ Delmar Cengage Learning.

Kirk, K. I., Firszt, J. B., Hood, L. J., & Holt, R. F. (2006, November 28). New directions in pediatric cochlear implantation: Effects on candidacy. *The ASHA Leader.*

Kirk, K. I., Pisoni, D. B., & Osberger, M. J. (1995). Lexical effects on spoken word recognition by pediatric cochlear implant users. *Ear and Hearing, 16,* 470–481.

Kirkwood, D. H. (2009). Resilient hearing aid industry despite a troubled economy. *The Hearing Journal, 62*(12), 11–14, 16.

Klop, W. M., Briaire, J. J., Stiggelbout, A. M., & Frijns, J. H. (2007). Cochlear implant outcomes and quality of life in adults with prelingual deafness. *Laryngoscope, 117,* 1982–1987.

Knecht, H. A., Nelson, P. B., Whitelaw, G. M., & Feth, L. L. (2002). Background noise levels and reverberation times in unoccupied classrooms: Predictions and measurements. *American Journal of Audiology, 11,* 65–71.

Koch, D. B., Osberger, M. J., Segel, P., & Kessler, D. (2004). HiResolution and conventional sound processing in the HiResolution bionic ear: Using appropriate outcome measures to assess speech recognition ability. *Audiology and Neurotology, 9,* 214–223.

Kochkin, S. (1990). Introducing MarketTrak: A consumer tracking survey of the hearing instrument market. *The Hearing Journal, 43*(5), 17–27.

Kochkin, S. (1991). Part I: Why don't people buy hearing instruments? Hearing professionals' views on market expansion. *Hearing Instruments 42*(12), 6–8.

Kochkin, S. (1994). MarkeTrak IV: Impact of purchase intent of cosmetics, stigma, and style of hearing instrument. *The Hearing Journal, 47*(9), 29–36.

Kochkin, S. (1997). MarketTrak norms: Subjective measures of satisfaction and benefit. *Seminars in Hearing, 18,* 37–48.

Kochkin, S. (2000). Binaural hearing aids: The fitting of choice for bilateral loss subjects. Itasca, IL: Knowles Electronics.

Kochkin, S. (2006). *Hearing solutions—Expectations—A key to success.* Retrieved from http://www.betterhearing .org/hearing_solutions/expectations.cfm

Kochkin, S., & Rogin, C. (2000). Quantifying the obvious: The impact of hearing instruments on quality of life. *The Hearing Review, 7*(1), 6–35.

Knowles, M., Holton, E. E. III, & Swanson, R. A. (2005). *The adult learner, sixth edition.* Burlington, MA: Elsevier.

Koch, M. (1999). *Bringing sound to life.* Baltimore, MD: York.

Kompis, M., Vibert, D., Senn, P., Vischer, M. W., & Haüsler, R. (2003). Scuba diving with cochlear implants. *Annals of Otology, Rhinology, & Laryngology, 112,* 425–427.

Kopun, J. G., & Stelmachowicz, P. G. (1998). Perceived communication difficulties of children with hearing loss. *American Journal of Audiology, 7,* 30–38.

Kosma-Spytek, L. (2003). *Digital cell phones and hearing aid FAQ.* Retrieved from http://tap.gallaudet.edu/ voice/DigitalCellFAQ.asp

Kozak, E. A. (1993). Preparing for surgery: This practical workup pinpoints preoperative dangers. *Geriatrics, 48,* 39–40, 45.

Kramer, S. E., Kapetyn, T. S., Kuik, D. J., & Deeg, D. J. (2002). The association of hearing impairment and chronic diseases with psychosocial health status in older age. *Journal of Aging and Health, 14,* 122–137.

Krefting, L. H., & Krefting, D. V. (1991). Cultural influences on performance. In C. Christiansen, & C. Baum (Eds.), *Occupational therapy.* Thoroughfare, NJ: Slack.

Kricos, P. B. (2006a). *Minimizing the effects of non-audiological variables on hearing aid outcome.* Retrieved from http://www.audiologyonline.com/articles/ article_detail.asp?article_id=1527

Kricos, P. B. (2006b). *Audiologic rehabilitation with the geriatric population.* Retrieved from http:// www.audiology online.com/articles/article_detail.asp? article_id=1673

Kricos, P. B., & Lesner, S. A. (1997). Evaluating the success of hearing aid orientation groups. Instructional course presented at the Ninth Annual Convention of the American Academy of Audiology, Fort Lauderdale, FL.

Kricos, P. B., & Lesner, S. A. (2000). Evaluating the success of adult audiologic rehabilitation support programs. *Seminars in Hearing, 21,* 267–279.

Kübler-Ross, E. (1969). *On death and dying.* New York: Macmillan.

Kühn-Inacker, H., Shehata-Dieler, W., Müller, J., & Helms, J. (2004). Bilateral cochlear implants: A way to optimize auditory perception abilities in deaf children? *International Journal of Pediatric Otorhinolaryngology, 68,* 1257–1266.

Kukula, J. M. (2006). Ethics 101. In T. A. Hamill (Ed.), *Ethics in audiology* (pp. 133–135). Reston, VA: American Academy of Audiology.

Kumar, M., Hickey, S., & Shaw, S. (2000). Manual dexterity and successful hearing aid use. *Journal of Laryngology and Otology, 114,* 593–597.

Kuntzman G. (2007) *Stop 'iPod oblivion.'* Retrieved from http://www.brooklynpaper.com/stories/30/6/30_06ipods.html

Kuo, S. C., & Gibson, W. P. (2005). The role of the promontory stimulation test in cochlear implantation. *Cochlear Implants International, 3,* 19–28.

Labadie, R. F., Carrasco, V. N., Gilmer, C. H., & Pillsbury, H. C. III. (2000). Cochlear implant performance in senior citizens. *Otolaryngology, Head, and Neck Surgery, 123,* 419–424.

Lam, B. L., Lee, D. J., Gómez-Marin, O., Zheng, D. D., & Caban, A. J. (2006). Concurrent visual and hearing impairment and risk of mortality: The National Health Interview Survey. *Archives of Ophthalmology, 124,* 95–101.

Lamb, S. H., Owens, E., & Schubert, E. D. (1983). The revised form of the Hearing Performance Inventory. *Ear and Hearing, 4,* 152–157.

Landis, B., & Landis, E. (1992). Is biofeedback effective for chronic tinnitus? An intensive study with seven subjects. *American Journal of Otolaryngology, 13,* 349–356.

Lane, H., & Bahan, B. (1998). Ethics of cochlear implants in young children: A review and reply from a Deaf World perspective. *Otolaryngology, Head, and Neck Surgery, 119,* 297–313.

Lane, H., Hoffmeister, R., & Bahan, B. (1996). *A Journey into the Deaf-world.* San Diego, CA: Dawn Sign Press.

Lane, H. L. (1999). The mask of benevolence: Disabling the Deaf community. San Diego, CA: Dawn Sign Press.

Lankford, J. E., & Hopkins, C. M. (2000). Ambient noise levels in nursing homes: Implications for audiometric assessment. *American Journal of Audiology, 9,* 30–35.

Larson, V. S., Williams, D. W., Henderson, W. G., Luethke, L. E., Beck, L. B., Noffsinger, D., . . . Rappaport, B. Z. (2000). Efficacy of 3 commonly used hearing aid circuits: A crossover trial. *Journal of the American Medical Association, 284,* 1806–1813.

Laufer, S. (2000a). Taking the initiative in meeting and dealing with challenges of acquiring a college education: Part I. *Hearing Loss Magazine, 21*(1) 8–12.

Laufer, S. (2000b). Taking the initiative in meeting and dealing with challenges of acquiring a college education: Part II. *Hearing Loss Magazine, 21*(2).

Layton, T. & Holmes, D. W. (1985). *Carolina picture vocabulary test. For deaf and hearing-impaired children.* Austin, TX: Pro-Ed.

Lederman, N., & Hendricks, P. (2003). *Induction loop assistive listening system: A venerable technology meets the new millennium.* Retrieved from http://www.ovalwindowaudio.com/articles/selectloop.htm

Lee, D. J., Gómez-Marin, O., Lam, B. L., Zheng, D. D., Arheart, K.L., Christ, S. L., & Caban, A. J. (2007). Severity of concurrent visual and hearing impairment and mortality: The 1986–1994 National Health Interview Survey. *Journal of Aging and Health, 19,* 382–396.

Lee, D. J., Gómez-Marin, O., & Lee, H. M. (1996). Sociodemographic correlates of hearing loss and hearing aid use in Hispanic adults. *Epidemiology, 7,* 443–446.

Lee, J. (1997). *Speech reading in context: A guide for practice in everyday settings.* Washington, DC: Laurent Clerc National Deaf Education Center, Gallaudet University.

Lee, J. C., Yoo, M. H., Ahn, J. H., & Leek, K. S. (2007). Value of the promontory stimulation test in predicting speech perception after cochlear implantation. *Laryngoscope, 117,* 1988–1992.

Lenarz, T., Battmer, R. D., Frohne, C., Büchner, A., & Parker, J. (2000). The Nucleus Double Array cochlear implant for obliterated cochleae. *Advances in Otorhinolaryngology, 57,* 354–359.

Lesner, S. A., & Kricos, P. B. (1995). Audiologic rehabilitation assessment: A holistic approach. In P. B. Kricos & S. A. Lesner (Eds.), *Hearing care for the older adult: Audiologic rehabilitation* (pp. 21–58). Boston: Butterworth-Heinemann.

Leveque, M., Labrousse, M., Seidermann, L., & Chays, A. (2007). Surgical therapy in intractable benign paroxysmal positional vertigo. *Otolaryngology, Head, and Neck Surgery, 136,* 693–698.

Levitt, H. (2006). *Computer assisted tracking.* Paper presented at the State-of-the-Science (SOS) Conference on Hearing Enhancement, Gallaudet University held September 18–20, 2006.

Levitt, H., Stromberg, H., Smith, C., & Gold, T. (1980). The structure of segmental errors in the speech of deaf children. *Journal of Communication Disorders, 13,* 419–441.

Lew, H. L., Jerger, J. F., Guillory, S. B., & Henry, J. A. (2007). Auditory dysfunction in traumatic brain injury.

Journal of Rehabilitation Research and Development, *44,* 921–928.

Lewis, J., Stephens, D., & Huws, D. (1992). Suicide in tinnitus sufferers. *Journal of Audiological Medicine, 1,* 30–37.

Li, J. C., & Epley, J. (2010). *Benign paroxysmal positional vertigo.* Retrieved from http://emedicine.medscape.com/article/884261-overview

Li, W., Keegan, T. H., Sternfeld, B., Sidney, S., Quesenberry, C. P. Jr, & Kelsey, J. L. (2006). Outdoor falls among middle-aged and older adults. A neglected public health problem. *American Journal of Public Health, 96,* 1192–1200.

Li, Y., Bain, L., & Steinberg, A. G. (2004). Parental decision-making in considering cochlear implant technology for a deaf child. *International Journal of Pediatric otorhinolaryngology, 68,* 1027–1038.

Light, L. L., & Singh, A. (1987). Implicit and explicit memory in younger and older adults. *Journal of Experimental Psychology: Learning, Memory, & Cognition, 13,* 531–541.

Litovsky, R. Y., Johnstone, P. M., & Godar, S. P. (2006). Benefits of bilateral cochlear implants and/or hearing aids in children. *International Journal of Audiology, 45,* 578–591.

Litovsky, R. Y., Johnstone, P. M., Godar, S. P., Agrawal, S., Parkinson, A., Peters, R., & Lake, J. (2006). Bilateral cochlear implants in children: Localization acuity measured with minimum audible angle. *Ear and Hearing, 27,* 43–59.

Litovsky, R. Y., Parkinson, A., Arcaroli, J., Peters, R., Lake, J., Johnstone, P., & Yu, G. (2004). Bilateral cochlear implants in adults and children. *Archives of Otolaryngology, Head, and Neck Surgery, 130,* 648–655.

Loh, K. (2000). Professionalism, where are you? *Ear, Nose, and Throat Journal, 79,* 242–246.

Lukomski, J. (2007). Deaf college students' perceptions of their social-emotional adjustment. *Journal of Deaf Studies and Deaf Education, 12,* 486–494.

Lundeen, C. (1996) Count-the-Dot audiogram in perspective. *American Journal of Audiology, 5*(3), 57–58.

Lusk, S. L., Ronis, D. L., Kazanis, A. S., Eakin, B. L., Hong, O., & Raymond, D. M. (2003). Effectiveness of a tailored intervention to increase factory workers' use of hearing protection. *Nursing Research, 52,* 289–295.

Lynch, E. W. (1997a). Conceptual framework: From culture shock to cultural learning. In E. W. Lynch & M. J. Hanson (Eds.), *Developing cross-cultural competence: A guide for working with children and their families* (2nd ed., pp. 23–46). Baltimore, MD: Brookes.

Lynch, E. W. (1997b). Developing cross-cultural competence. In E. W. Lynch & M. J. Hanson (Eds.), *Developing cross-cultural competence: A guide for working with children and their families* (2nd ed., pp. 47–89). Baltimore, MD: Brookes.

Lynch, E. W., & Hanson, M. J. (1997). *Developing cross-cultural competence: A guide for working with children and their families* (2nd ed.). Baltimore, MD: Brookes.

MacKenzie, D. J., Mueller, H. G., Ricketts, T. A., & Konkle, D. F. (2004). The hearing aid occlusion effect: Measurement devices compared. *The Hearing Journal, 57*(9), 30, 34–36, 38–39.

MacLeod-Gallinger, J.E. (1992). The career status of deaf women. A comparative look. *American Annals of the Deaf, 137,* 315–325.

Madell, J. (1978). Amplification for hearing-impaired children: Basic considerations. *Journal of Communication Disorders, 11,* 125–135.

Magnuson, M., & Hergils, L. (1999). The parents' view on hearing screening in newborns. Feelings, thoughts, and opinions on otoacoustic emissions screening. *Scandinavian Audiology, 28,* 47–56.

Mahoney, D. F. (1993). Cerumen impaction. Prevalence and detection in nursing homes. *Journal of Gerontological Nursing, 19,* 23–30.

Majdani, O., Bartling, S. H., Leinung, M., Stöver, T., Lenarz, M., Dullin, C., & Lenarz, T. (2008). A true minimally invasive approach for cochlear implantation: High accuracy in cranial base navigation through flat-panel-based volume computed tomography. *Otology and Neurotology, 29,* 120–123.

Margolis, R. (2004). Audiology informational counseling. *Audiology Today, 16*(2), 14–15.

Margolis, R. H. (2004, August 3). Boosting memory with informational counseling: Helping patients understand the nature of disorders and how to manage them. *The ASHA Leader.*

Marill, K. A. (2009). *Vestibular neuronitis.* Retrieved from http://www.emedicine.com/EMERG/topic637.htm

Markides, A., & Ayree, D.T.-K. (1978). The effect of hearing aid use on the user's hearing: A follow-up study. *Scandinavian Audiology, 7,* 19–23.

Markides, A., & Ayree, D. T.-K. (1980). The effect of hearing aid use on the user's hearing II: A follow-up study. *Scandinavian Audiology, 9,* 55–58.

Marschark, M. M., Leigh, G., Sapere, P., Burnham, D., Convertino, C., Stinson, M., Knoors, H., . . . Noble, W. (2006). Benefits of sign language interpreting and text alternatives for deaf students' classroom learning. *Journal of Deaf Studies and Deaf Education, 11,* 421–437.

Martin, F. N., & Clark, J. G. (2008). *Introduction to audiology* (10th ed.). Boston: Allyn & Bacon.

Martin, R. L. (1999). A troubleshooting guide for your patients and families. *The Hearing Journal, 53*(2), 66.

Massachusetts Eye and Ear Infirmary (2005). *Taking care of the hearing aid, advice from the hearing aid, and cochlear implant center.* Retrieved from http://www.meei .harvard.edu/shared/oto/audiology/ha_careofaid.php

Mathews, M. R., Johnson, C. E., & Danhauer, J. L. (2009). Pediatricians' knowledge of, experience with, and comfort levels for cochlear implants in children. *American Journal of Audiology, 18,* 129–143.

Mathiowetz, V., & Weber, K. (1985). Adult norms for the 9-hole peg test of finger dexterity. *Occupational Therapy Journal of Research, 5,* 24–38.

May, A. E., Upfold, L. J., & Battaglia, J. A. (1980). The advantages and disadvantages of ITC, ITE, and BTE hearing aids: Diary and interview reports from elderly users. *British Journal of Audiology, 24,* 301–309.

Mayne, A. M., Yoshinaga-Itano, C., Sedey, A. L., & Carey, A. (2000). Expressive vocabulary development of infants and toddlers who are deaf or hard of hearing. *Volta Review, 100,* 1–28.

McArdle, R., Chisolm, T. H., Abrams, H. R., Wilson, R. H., & Doyle, P. J. (2005). The WHO-DAS II: Measuring outcomes of hearing aid intervention in adults. *Trends in Amplification, 9,* 127–143.

McClearn, G. E., Johansson, B., Berg, S., Pedersen, N. L., Ahern, F., Petrill, S. A., & Plomin, R. (1997). Substantial genetic influence on cognitive abilities in twins 80 or more years old. *Science, 276,* 1560–1563.

McConkey-Robbins, A. (1998). Two paths of auditory development for children with cochlear implants. *Loud and Clear: A Cochlear Implant Rehabilitation Newsletter, 1,1.* Retrieved from http://www.advancedbionics .com/printables/archive/April_98.pdf

McConkey-Robbins, A., Koch, D. B., Osberger, M. J., Zimmerman-Phillips, S., & Kishon-Rabin, L. (2004). Effect of cochlear implantation on auditory skill development in infants and toddlers. *Archives of Otolaryngology, Head, and Neck Surgery, 130,* 570–574.

McGowan, R. S., Nittrouer, S., & Chenausky, K. (2008). Speech production in 12-month-old children with and without hearing loss. *Journal of Speech, Language, Hearing Research, 51,* 879–888.

McKibbon, A., Easy, A., & Marks, S. (1999). *PDQ: Evidence-based principles and practice.* St. Louis, MO: Decker.

McPherson, B., Hickson, L., & Baumfield, A. (1992). Clinical reliability of insertion gain measurements with assistive listening devices. *Scandinavian Audiology, 21,* 51–54.

McReynolds, L. V., & Thompson, C. K. (1986). Flexibility of single-subject experimental designs. Part I: Review of the basics of single-subject designs. *Journal of Speech and Hearing Disorders, 51,* 194–203.

McSpaden, J. B. (1990). One approach to a unilateral "dead" ear. *Audecibel, 38,* 10–14.

Meador, J. A. (1995). Cerumen impaction in the elderly. *Journal of Gerontological Nursing, 21,* 43–45.

Med-El (2005). *Communication options and educational placements.* Retrieved from http://www.medel.at/US/ Information-for-Candidates/Solutions-for-Children/ Communication-Options.php

Medicine.Net. (2006). *Definition of primary care.* Retrieved from http://www.medterms.com/script/main/ art.asp?articlekey=5042

Medicine.Net (2010). *Definition of respiration.* Retrieved from http://www.medterms.com/script/main/art.asp? articlekey=5328

Medwetsky, L. (2002). Central auditory processing testing: A test battery approach. In J. Katz (ed.) *Handbook of clinical audiology* (5th ed., pp. 510–524). Baltimore, MD: Lippincott, Williams & Wilkins.

Megerian, C. A., & Murray, G. S. (2010). *Cochlear implants, surgical techniques: Multimedia.* Retrieved from http:// emedicine.medscape.com/article/857242-overview

Meier, G. (2006). *Hearing aid warranties.* Retrieved from http://www.audiologyawareness.com/ha_warranty.asp

Meister, H., Lausberg, I., Kiessling, J., von Wedel, H., & Walger, M. (2002). Identifying the needs of elderly hearing-impaired persons: The importance and utility of hearing aid attributes. *European Archives of Otolaryngology, 259,* 531–534.

Mejstad, L., Heiling, K., & Svedin, C. (2009). Mental health and self-image among deaf and hard of hearing children. *American Annals of the Deaf, 153,* 504–515.

Mendel, L. L., & Danhauer, J. L. (1997). Characteristics of sensitive speech perception tests. In L. L. Mendel & J. L. Danhauer (Eds.), *Audiological evaluation and management and speech perception assessment* (pp. 59–100). San Diego, CA: Singular/Delmar Cengage Learning.

Merriam-Webster's Medical Dictionary Online. (2008). *Magnetic resonance imaging.* Retrieved from http:// medical.merriamwebster.com/medical/medical?book= Medical&va=magnetic+resonance+imaging

Middlebrooks, J. C. (2008). Cochlear-implant high pulse rate and narrow electrode configuration impair transmission of temporal information to the auditory cortex. *Journal of Neurophysiology, 100,* 92–107.

Miller, J. F. (2010). *Systematic analysis of language transcripts (SALT).* Retrieved from http://www.saltsoftware .com/company/

Miller, W. R., & Rollnick, S. (2002). *Motivational interviewing: Preparing people for change* (2nd ed.). New York, NY: Guilford Press.

Mississippi Project START. (2002). *About Project START: Assistive Technology Act.* Retrieved from http://www.msprojectstart.org/techact.html

Mitchell, R. E. (2006). How many deaf people are there in the United States? Estimates from the Survey of Income and Program Participation. *Journal of Deaf Studies and Deaf Education, 11,* 112–119.

Miyamoto, R. T., Bichey, B. G., Wynne, M. K., & Kirk, K. I. (2002). Cochlear implantation with large vestibular aqueduct syndrome. *Laryngoscope, 112,* 1178–1182.

Moeller, M. P. (2010). Baby babble: Optimizing early word learning in infants and toddlers. *Audiology Today, 22*(3), 19–27.

Moeller, M. P., Hoover, B., Peterson, B., & Stelmachowicz, P. G. (2009). Consistency of hearing aid use in infants with early-identified hearing loss. *American Journal of Audiology, 18,* 14–23.

Moeller, M. P., Hoover, B., Putman, C., Arbataitis, K., Bohnenkamp, G., Peterson, B., . . . Stelmachowicz, P. (2007). Vocalizations of infants with hearing loss compared with infants with normal hearing: Part I: Phonetic development. *Ear and Hearing, 28,* 605–627.

Moeller, M. P., Hoover, B., Putman, C., Arbataitis, K., Bohnenkamp, G., Peterson, B., . . . Stelmachowicz, P. (2007). Vocalizations of infants with hearing loss compared with infants with normal hearing: Part II—Transition to words. *Ear and Hearing, 28,* 628–642.

Moeller, M. P., White, K. R., & Shisler, L. (2006). Primary care physicians' knowledge, attitudes, and practices related to newborn hearing screening. *Pediatrics, 118,* 1357–1370.

Mohr, P. E., Feldman, J. J., Dunbar, J. L., McConkey-Robbins, A., Niparko, J. K., Rittenhouse, R. K., & Skinner, M. W. (2000). The societal costs of severe to profound hearing loss in the United States. *International Journal of Technology Assessment in Health Care, 16,* 1120–1135.

Mojtabai, R., & Olfson, M. (2004). Major depression in community-dwelling middle-aged and older adults: Prevalence and 2-year and 4-year follow-up symptoms. *Psychological Medicine, 34,* 623–634.

Moller, A. R. (2006). History of cochlear implants and auditory brainstem implants. *Advances in Otorhinolaryngology, 64,* 1–10.

Möller, K. (2003). Deaf blindness: A challenge for assessment—Is the ICF a useful tool? *International Journal of Audiology, 42*(Suppl. 1), S140–S142.

Monsen, R. B. (1979). Acoustic qualities of phonation in young hearing-impaired children. *Journal of Speech and Hearing Research, 22,* 270–288.

Monsen, R. B., Engebretson, A. M., & Vermula, N. R. (1979). Some effects of deafness on the generation of voice. *Journal of the Acoustical Society of America, 66,* 1680–1690.

Moog, J. S., & Kozak, V. J. (1983). *Teacher assessment of grammatical structures (TAGS).* St. Louis, MO: Central Institute for the Deaf.

Moog, J. S., Kozak, V. J., & Geers, A. E. (1983). *Grammatical analysis of elicited language—presentence level (GAEL-P).* St. Louis, MO: Central Institute for the Deaf.

Moore, A. M., Voytas, J., Kowalski, D., & Maddens, M. (2002). Cerumen, hearing, cognition, and the elderly. *Journal of the Medical Directors Association, 3,* 136–139.

Morata, T. C. (2007). Young people: Their noise and music exposures and the risk of hearing loss. *International Journal of Audiology, 46,* 111–112.

Mormer, E., & Palmer, C.P. (1997). *The developmental index of Audition and Listening.* Westminister, CO: Educational Audiology Association.

Moxley, A., Mahendra, N., & Vega-Barchowitz, C. (2004, April 13). Cultural competence in health care. *The ASHA Leader.*

Mueller, H. G. (2006). Open is in. *The Hearing Journal, 59*(11), 11,12–14.

Mueller, H. G., & Bentler, R. A. (2005). Fitting hearing aids using clinical measures of loudness discomfort levels: An evidence-based review of effectiveness. *Journal of the American Academy of Audiology, 16,* 461–472.

Mueller, H. G., Hawkins, D. B., & Northern, J. L. (1992). *Probe microphone measurements: Hearing aid selection and measurement.* San Diego, CA: Singular/Delmar Cengage Learning.

Mueller, H. G., Johnson, E. H., & Strouse-Carter, A. (2002). Hearing aids and assistive devices. In R. L. Schow & M. A. Nerbonne (Eds.), *Audiologic rehabilitation* (5th ed., pp. 31–76). Boston: Allyn & Bacon.

Mueller, H. G., & Killion, M. C. (1990). An easy method for calculating the articulation index. *The Hearing Journal, 43*(9), 14–17.

Mueller, H. G., & Ricketts, T. A. (2005). Digital noise reduction: Much ado about something. *The Hearing Journal, 2*(1), 10–18.

Mulac, A., Danhauer, J. L., & Johnson, C. E. (1983). Young adults' and peers' attitudes towards elderly hearing aid wearers. *Australian Journal of Audiology, 5,* 57–62.

Muñoz, K., Shisler, L., Moeller, M. P., & White, K. R. (2009). Improving the quality of early hearing detection and intervention programs through physician outreach. *Seminars in Hearing, 30,* 184–192.

Murphy, J. S., & Newlon, B. J. (1987). Loneliness and the mainstreamed hearing impaired college student. *American Annals of the Deaf, 132,* 21–25.

Musick, M. A., Herzog, A. R., & House, J. S. (1999). Volunteering and mortality among older adults: Findings from a national sample. *The Journals of Gerontology Series B: Psychological Sciences and Social Sciences, 54,* S173–S180.

Musiek, F. E., & Chermak, G. D. (2007). *Handbook of (central) auditory processing disorders: Auditory neuroscience and diagnostics – volume 1.* San Diego, CA: Plural.

Mylanus, E. A., Snik, A. F., & Cremers, C. W. (1995). Patients' opinions of bone-anchored conventional hearing aids. *Archives of Otolaryngology, Head, and Neck Surgery, 121,* 421–425.

Mylanus, E. A. M., Rotteveel, L. J. C., & Leeuw, R. L. (2004). Congenital malformation of the inner ear and pediatric cochlear implantation. *Otology and Neurotology, 25,* 308–317.

National Academy on an Aging Society (NAOAS). (1999). Hearing loss: A growing problem that affects quality of life. *Challenges for the 21st Century: Chronic and Disabling Conditions: 1*(2), 1–6.

National Acoustics Laboratories. (2009). *Client oriented scale of improvement for children.* Retrieved from http://www.nal.gov.au/pdf/COSI-C-Questionnaire.pdf

National Association of the Deaf. (2010a). *Position statement on cochlear implants.* Retrieved from http://www.nad.org/issues/technology/assistive-listening/cochlear-implants

National Association of the Deaf. (2010b). *Closed captioning requirements.* Retrieved from http://www.nad.org/issues/television-and-closed-captioning/closed-captioning-requirements

National Cancer Institute. (2010). *Pancreatic cancer.* Retrieved from http://www.cancer.gov/cancertopics/types/pancreatic.

National Captioning Institute. (2005). *Various pamphlets.* Vienna, VA: National Captioning Institute.

National Captioning Institute. (2006). *NCI real-time captioning.* Retrieved from http://www.ncicap.org/livecap.asp

National Center for Injury Prevention and Control, Centers for Disease Control and Prevention. (2010). *Traumatic brain injury.* Retrieved from http://www.cdc.gov/traumaticbraininjury/

National Center on Birth Defects and Disabilities, Office of Minority Health, U.S. Department of Health and Human Services. (2009). *Bringing early hearing detection and intervention programs to minority populations.* Retrieved from http://www.cdc.gov/ncbddd/ehdi/documents/Minority_Tips.pdf

National Center on Elder Abuse. (2007). Retrieved from http://www.elderabusecenter.org/

National Council on the Aging. (1999). *The consequence of untreated hearing loss in older persons.* A study conducted by the Seniors Research Group, an alliance between the National Council on the Aging and Market Strategies, Inc., Washington, DC.

National Heart, Lung, and Blood Institute. (2010). *High blood pressure.* Retrieved from http://www.nhlbi.nih.gov/health/dci/Diseases/Hbp/HBP_WhatIs.html

National Institutes of Health. (1993). *Quality of life assessment: practice, problems, and promise—Proceedings of a workshop.* Washington, DC: U.S. Department of Health and Human Services.

National Institutes of Health. (2001). *NIH policy on reporting race and ethnicity data: Subjects in clinical research- NOT-OD-01-053.* Retrieved from http://grants.nih.gov/grants/guide/notice-files/not-od-01-053.html

National Institute on Aging. (2010). *Alzheimer's disease fact sheet.* Retrieved from http://www.nia.nih.gov/alzheimers/publications/adfact.html

National Institute on Deafness and other Communication Disorders. (2003). *Sudden deafness.* Retrieved from http://www.nidcd.nih.gov/health/hearing/sudden.htm

National Institute on Deafness and other Communication Disorders. (2009). *Usher syndrome.* Retrieved from http://www.nidcd.nih.gov/health/hearing/usher.html

National Institute on Deafness and other Communication Disorders. (2010). *Quick statistics.* Retrieved from http://www.nidcd.nih.gov/health/statistics/quick.htm

National Institute on Neurological Disorders and Stroke (NINDS). (2009). *Neurofibromatosis information page.* Retrieved from http://www.ninds.nih.gov/disorders/neurofibromatosis/neurofibromatosis.htm

National Library of Medicine. (2010a). *Fact Sheet: MEDLINE.* Retrieved from http://www.nlm.nih.gov/pubs/factsheets/medline.html

National Library of Medicine. (2010b). *Fact Sheet: Medical subject hearings (MeSH).* Retrieved from http://www.nlm.nih.gov/pubs/factsheets/maisonettes

National Library of Medicine. (2010c). *Fact Sheet: What is the difference between MEDLINE and PubMed?* Retrieved from http://www.nlm.nih.gov/pubs/factsheets/dif_med_pub.html

National Public Website on Assistive Technology (2006). *AT report – Assistive listening technology.* Retrieved from http://www.assistivetech.net/at_reports/assistive_listening_devices.php#q3

Nelson, H. D., Bougatsos, C., Nygren, P., & the 2001 U.S. Preventive Services Task Force. (2008). Universal newborn hearing screening: Systematic review to update the 2001 US Preventive Services Task Force Recommendation. *Pediatrics, 122,* 266–276.

Newman, C. W., Weinstein, B., Jacobson, G. P., & Hug, G. A. (1990). The Hearing Handicap Inventory for Adults: Psychometric adequacy and audiometric correlates. *Ear and Hearing, 11,* 430–433.

Newman, C. W., Weinstein, B., Jacobson, G. P., & Hug, G. A. (1991). Test-retest reliability of the Hearing Handicap Inventory for Adults. *Ear and Hearing, 12,* 355–357.

Newman, T. B., Browner, W. S., Cummings, S. R., & Hulley, S. B. (2007). Designing cross-sectional and case-control studies. In S. B. Hulley, S. R. Cummings, W. S. Browner, D. G. Grady, & T. B. Newman (Eds.), *Designing clinical research, An epidemiologic approach* (3rd ed.; pp. 109–126). Baltimore, MD: Lippincott Williams & Wilkins.

Nilsson, M., Soli, S. D., & Sullivan, J. A. (1994). Development of the Hearing in Noise Test for the measurement of speech reception thresholds in quiet and in noise. *Journal of the Acoustical Society of America, 95,* 1085–1099.

Nilsson, M. J., Soli, S. D., & Gelnett, D. J. (1996). *Development of the hearing in noise test for children (HINT-C).* Los Angeles, CA: House Ear Institute.

Nilsson, M. J., Soli, S. D., & Sumida, A. (1996). *Development of norms and percent of intelligibility functions for the HINT.* Los Angeles, CA: House Ear Institute.

Niparko, J. K., & Wilson, B. S. (2001). History of cochlear implants. In J. K. Niparko, N. K. Mellon, A. M. Robbins, D. L. Tucci, & B. S. Wilson (Eds.), *Cochlear implants: Principles and practices* (pp. 103–108). Baltimore, MD: Lippincott Williams & Wilkins.

Niskar, A. S., Kieszak, S. M., Holmes, A. E., Esteban, E., Rubin, C., & Brody, D. J. (2001). Estimated prevalence of noise-induced hearing threshold shifts among children 6 to 19 years of age: The Third National Health and Examination Survey, 1988–1994, United States. *Pediatrics, 108,* 40–43.

Nittrouer, S., & Burton, L. T. (2001). The role of early language experience in the development of speech perception and language processing abilities in children with hearing loss. *The Volta Review, 103,* 5–37.

Nondahl, D. M., Cruickshanks, K. J., Wiley, T.L., Klein, R., Klein, B. E., & Tweed, T. S. (2000). Recreational firearm use and hearing loss. *Archives of Family Medicine, 9,* 352–357.

Norcross, J. C., & Prochaska, J. O. (2002). Using the stages of change. *Harvard Mental Health Newsletter, 18*(11), 5–7.

Northern, J. L., & Downs, M. P. (2002). *Hearing in children* (5th ed.). Baltimore, MD: Lippincott Williams & Wilkins.

Northrup, B. (1985). Audiologic assessment and multicultural populations. In *Communication disorders in multicultural populations* (pp. 1–22). Rockville, MD: American Speech-Language-Hearing Association.

Northrup, B. (2009a). *English-to Spanish translations of common words used in audiology.* Dallas, TX: Author.

Northrup, B. (2009b). *Spanish-to-English translations of common words used in audiology.* Dallas, TX: Author.

Nosrati-Zarenoe, R., Hansson, M., & Hultcrantz, E. (2010). Assessment of diagnostic approaches to idiopathic sudden sensorineural hearing loss and their influence on treatment and outcome. *Acta Otolaryngologica, 130,* 384–391.

Nott, P., Cowan, R., Brown, P. M., & Wigglesworth, G. (2009). Early language development in children with profound hearing loss fitted with a device at a young age: Part I—The time period to acquire first words and word combinations. *Ear and Hearing, 30,* 526–540.

Nussbaum, D. (1999). *Factors influencing performance: the benefits and limitations of cochlear implants.* Retrieved from http://clerccenter.gallaudet.edu/x18061.xml

Occupational Safety and Health Administration (OSHA). (1983, March 3). Occupational noise exposure: Hearing conservation amendment: Final rule. *Federal Register, 46,* 9738–9785.

Occupational Safety and Health Administration (OSHA). (2007). *About OSHA.* Retrieved from http://www.osha.gov/about.html

Office of Minority Health, U.S. Department of Health and Human Services (2009). *National standards on culturally and linguistically appropriate services (CLAS).* Retrieved from http://minorityhealth.hhs.gov/templates/browse.aspx?lvl=2&lvlID=15

Ogden, P. W. (1996). *The silent garden: Raising your deaf child.* Washington, DC: Gallaudet University Press.

O'Hara, R., Brooks, J. O. III, Friedman, L., Schröder, C. M., Morgan, K. S., & Kraemer, H. C. (2007). Long-term effects of mnemonic training in community-dwelling older adults. *Journal of Psychiatric Research, 41,* 585–590.

Olson, A. D., & Shinn, J. B. (2008). A systematic review to determine the effectiveness of using amplification in conjunction with cochlear implantation. *Journal of the American Academy of Audiology, 19,* 657–671.

Omnibus Reconciliation Act (OBRA). (1987: Suppl. 1989). Public Law 100–203, 101 Stat. 1330 (Codified at 42 U.S.C.A. Sec. 1396).

O'Neill, C., O'Donoghue, G. M., Archbold, S. M., Nikolopoulos, T. P., & Sach, T. (2002). Variations in gains in auditory performance from cochlear implantation. *Otology and Neurotology, 23,* 44–48.

Osberger, M. J., & Levitt, H. (1979). The effect of timing errors on the intelligibility of deaf children's speech. *Journal of the Acoustical Society of America, 66,* 1316–1324.

Osberger, M. J., Robbins, A. M., Lybolt, J., Kent, R. D., & Peters, J. (1986). Speech evaluation. In M. J. Osberger (ed.), *Language and learning skills of hearing-impaired students* (pp. 24–31). *ASHA Monograph #23.* Rockville, MD: American Speech Language-Hearing Association.

Osberger, M. J., Zimmerman-Phillips, S., Barker, M., & Geier, L. (1999). Clinical trial of the CLARION cochlear implant in children. *Annals of Otology, Rhinology, and Laryngology Supplement, 177,* 88–92.

Paden, E., & Brown, C. (1992). *Identifying early phonological needs in children with hearing impairment.* Washington, DC: Alexander Graham Bell Association.

Palazzoli, M. S., Boscolo, L., Cecchin, G. F., & Prata, G. (1977). Family rituals a powerful tool in family therapy. *Family Processes, 16,* 445–453.

Palmer, C. V., Adams, S. W., Bourgeois, M., Durrant, J., & Rossi, M. (1999). Reduction in caregiver-identified problem behavior in patients with Alzheimer disease post hearing aid fitting. *Journal of Speech, Language, and Hearing Research, 42,* 312–328.

Pappas, D. G., Flexer, C., & Shackelford, L. (1994). Otological and habilitative management of children with Down Syndrome. *Laryngoscope, 104,* 1065–1070.

Parkhurst, B. G, & Levitt, H. (1978). The effect of certain prosodic errors on the intelligibility of deaf speech. *Journal of Communication Disorders, 11,* 249–256.

Parving, A., & Philip, B. (1991). Use and benefit of hearing aids in the tenth decade—and beyond. *Audiology, 30,* 61–69.

Patterson, M. B., & Ballough, B. J. (2006). Review of pharmacological therapy for tinnitus. *International Tinnitus Journal, 12,* 149–159.

Paul, P. (1996). Reading vocabulary knowledge and deafness. *Journal of Deaf Studies and Deaf Education, 1,* 3–15.

Peck, J. E. (1980). The use and misuse of hearing aids. *Annals of Otology, Rhinology, and Laryngology, 89,* 70–73.

Peck, J. E. (2001). Noise-induced hearing loss in shooters of shoulder firearms. *American Family Physician, 63,* 1053.

Pediatric Working Group of the Conference on Amplification for Children with Auditory Deficits. (1996) Amplification for infants and children with hearing loss. *American Journal of Audiology, 5,* 53–68.

Pekkarinen, J., Iki, M., Starck, J., & Pyykkö, I. (1993). Hearing loss risk from exposure to shooting impulses in workers exposed to occupational noise. *British Journal of Audiology, 27,* 175–182.

Penn, J. P. (1955). Voice and speech patterns of the heard of hearing. *Acta Otolaryngologica,* (Suppl. 124), 1–69.

Perigoe, C. (2009). The Auditory-Verbal approach. Presentations to the faculty and students of the Department of Communication Disorders, Auburn University, November 2009.

Pichora-Fuller, M. K., & Benguerel, A. P. (1991). The design of CAST (Computer-Aided Speechreading Training). *Journal of Speech, Language, and Hearing Research, 34,* 202–212.

Plant, G. (1994). *ANALYTIKA: Analytical testing and training lists.* Somerville, MA: Hearing Rehabilitation Foundation.

Plant, G. (2000a). *Hear at home: A home training program for adults: Receiver's manual.* Somerville, MA: Hearing Rehabilitation Foundation.

Plant, G. (2000b). *Hear at home: A home training program for adults: Speaker's manual.* Somerville, MA: Hearing Rehabilitation Foundation.

Pleis, J. R., & Coles, R. (2003). Summary health statistics for U.S. adults: National Health Interview Survey. *Vital Health Statistics.* Washington DC: National Center for Health Statistics.

Plomin, R., Pedersen, N. L., Lichtenstein, P., & McClearn, G. E. (1994). Variability and stability in cognitive abilities are largely genetic later in life. *Behavioral Genetics, 24,* 207–215.

Podashin, L., Ben-David, Y., Fradis, M., Gerstel, R., & Felner, H. (1991). Idiopathic subjective tinnitus related by biofeedback, acupuncture, and drug therapy. *Ear, Nose, and Throat Journal, 70,* 284–289.

Poissant, S. F., Beaudoin, F., Huang, J., Brodsky, J., & Lee, D. J. (2008). Impact of cochlear implantation on speech understanding, depression, and loneliness in the elderly. *Journal of Otolarngology, Head, and Neck Surgery, 37,* 488–494.

Pollack, D. (1983). Teaching the child with hearing impairment by the Acoupedic approach. In W. Perkins (Ed.), *Current therapy of communication disorders: Hearing disorders* (pp. 47–60). New York: Thieme-Stratton.

Pollack, D. (1993). Reflections of a pioneer. *The Volta Review, 95,* 197–204.

Population Resource Center. (2006) *Executive summary: A population perspective of the United States.* Retrieved from http://www.prcdc.org/summaries/uspopperspec/uspopperspec.html

Portnuff, C. D. F. (2010). *Teenage MP3 player use: A hazard to hearing?* An Audiology Online continuing education course.

Portnuff, C. D. F., & Fligor, B. J. (2006). *Output levels of portable digital music players.* Children at Work and Play Meeting, Covington, KY.

Power, D. J., & Quigley, S. P. (1973). Deaf children acquisition of the passive voice. *Journal of Speech and Hearing Research, 16,* 5–11.

Powerhouse Museum (2006). *Cochlear implants: The future.* Retrieved from http://www.powerhousemuseum.com/hsc/cochlear/cochlear_future.htm

Pratt, S. K. & Tye-Murray, N. T. (2009). Speech impairment secondary to hearing loss. In M. R. McNeil (Ed.), *Clinical management of sensorimotor speech disorders* (2nd ed., pp. 204–234). New York: Thieme.

Pressnell, L. M. (1973). Hearing-impaired children's comprehension and production of syntax in oral language. *Journal of Speech and Hearing Research, 16,* 12–21.

Prochaska, J. O., DiClemente, C. C., & Norcross, J. C. (1992). In search of how people change. Applications to addictive behaviors. *American Psychologist, 47* 1102–1114.

Prosser, S., Tartari, M. C., & Arslan, E. (1988). Hearing loss in sports hunters exposed to occupational noise. *British Journal of Audiology, 22,* 85–91.

Pruitt, J. (1990). Assistive listening device versus conventional hearing aid in an elderly patient: Case report. *Journal of the American Academy of Audiology, 1,* 41–43.

Pugh, K. C., & Crandell, C. C. (2002). Hearing loss, hearing handicap, and functional health status between African-American and Caucasian-American seniors. *Journal of the American Academy of Audiology, 13,* 493–502.

Puisieux, F., Pardessus, V., & Bombois, S. (2005). Dementia and falls. *Psychology and Neuropsychiatry Visions, 3,* 271–279.

Punch, J. F. (1988, February). CROS revisited. *Asha, 30,* 35–37.

Punch, R., Creed, P. A., & Hyde, M. B. (2006). Career barriers perceived by hard-of-hearing adolescents: Implications for practice from a mixed-methods study. *Journal of Deaf Studies and Deaf Education, 11,* 224–237.

Purdy, S. C., Farrington, D. R., Moran, C. A., Chard, L. L., & Hodgson, S. A. (2002). A parental questionnaire to evaluate children's auditory behavior in everyday life (ABEL). *American Journal of Audiology, 11,* 72–82.

Quigley, S., Jenne, W., & Phillips, S. B. (1968). *Deaf students in colleges and universities.* Washington, DC: Alexander Graham Bell Association for the Deaf.

Quigley, S. P., Steinkamp, M., Power, D., & Jones, B. (1978). *Test of syntactic abilities.* Beaverton, OR: Dormac.

Rabinowitz, P. M. (2000). Noise-induced hearing loss. *American Family Physician, 61,* 2749–2756, 2759–2760.

Rabinowitz, P. M., & Duran, R. (2001). Is acculturation related to use of hearing protection? *American Industrial Hygiene Association Journal, 62,* 611–614.

Rall, E. (2007, September 25). Psychosocial development of children with hearing loss. *The ASHA Leader.*

Ramkissoon, I., & Kahn, F. (2003, February 18). Serving multicultural clients with hearing loss: How linguistic diversity affects audiologic management. *The ASHA Leader.*

Ramsden, J. D., Papaioannou, V., Gordon, K. A., James, A. L., & Papsin, B. C. (2009). Parental and program's decision making in pediatric simultaneous bilateral cochlear implantation: Who says no and why? *International Journal of Pediatric Otolaryngology, 73,* 1325–1328.

Ramsden, J. D., Papsin, B. C., Leung, R., James, A., & Gordon, K. A. (2009). Bilateral simultaneous cochlear implantation in children: Our first 50 cases. *Laryngoscope, 129,* 2444–2448.

Rance, G., & Barker, E. J. (2009). Speech and language outcomes in children with auditory neuropathy/dys-synchrony managed with either cochlear implants or hearing aids. *International Journal of Audiology, 48,* 313–320.

Randell-David, E. (1989). *Strategies for working with culturally diverse communities and clients.* Washington, DC: Association for the Care of Children's Health.

Rao, S. S (2005). Prevention of falls in older patients. *American Family Physician, 72,* 81–88.

Rayovac. (2006). *Batteries: Frequently asked questions.* Retrieved from http://www.rayovac.com/batteries/faq.htm

Read, S., Pedersen, N. L., Gatz, M., Berg, S., Vuoksimaa, E., Malmberg, B., . . . McClearn, G. E. (2006). Sex differences after all those years? Heritability of cognitive abilities in old age. *The Journals of Gerontology Series B: Psychological Sciences and Social Sciences, 61,* P137–P143.

Reichman, J., & Healey, W. C. (1989). Amplification monitoring and maintenance in the schools. *Asha, 31,* 43–45.

Revicki, D. A. (1989). Health-related quality of life in the evaluation of medical therapy for chronic illness. *Journal of Family Practice, 29,* 377–380.

Reynell, J. K., & Gruber, C. P. (1999). *Reynell developmental language scales.* Los Angeles, CA: Western Psychological Services.

Ricketts, T. A. (2005). Directional hearing aids: Then and now. *Journal of Rehabilitation Research and Development, 42,* 133–144.

Ricketts, T. A., Bentler, R. A., & Mueller, G. (2010). *Modern hearing aids.* San Diego, CA; Plural.

Ricketts, T., & Henry, P. (2002). Evaluation of an adaptive, directional-microphone hearing aid. *International Journal of Audiology, 41,* 100–112.

Ries, P. W. (1994). *Prevalence and characteristics of persons with hearing trouble: United States, 1990–1991, Series 10, No. 188.* Washington, DC: National Center for Health Statistics.

Ringdahl, A., & Grimby, A. (2000). Severe-profound hearing impairment and health-related quality of life among post-lingual deafened Swedish adults. *Scandinavian Audiology, 29,* 266–275.

Robbins, A. M. (2002). Empowering parents to help their newly diagnosed child gain communication skills. *The Hearing Journal, 55*(11), 55–56, 59.

Robbins, A.M. (2005; Issue 1). Clinical red flags for slow progress in children with cochlear implants. *Advanced Bionics: Loud and Clear.* Retrieved from http://www.advancedbionics.com/userfiles/File/Issue1-2005.pdf

Roberson, J. R. Jr., O'Rourke, C., & Stidham, K. (2003). Auditory steady-state responsetesting in children: Evaluation of a new technology. *Otolaryngology-Head and Neck Surgery, 129,* 107–113.

Robey, R. R., & Dalebout, S. D. (1998). A tutorial on conducting meta-analysis of clinical outcome research. *Journal of Speech, Language, and Hearing Research, 41,* 1227–1241.

Robin, N. (2008). *Medical genetics: Its application to speech, hearing, and craniofacial disorders.* San Diego, CA: Plural.

Robson, G. (2008). *Real-time captioning.* Retrieved from http://www.dcmp.org/caai/nadh28.pdf

Rocchiccioli, J. T., Sanford, J., & Caplinger, B. (2007). Polymedicine and aging. Enhancing older adult care through advanced practitioners. GNPs and elder care pharmacists can help provide optimal pharmaceutical care. *Journal of Gerontological Nursing, 33,* 19–24.

Rochester Institute of Technology Libraries. (2003). *FAQs and general TTY etiquette tips for new TTY users.* Retrieved from http://www.library.rit.edu/depts/ref/research/deaf/ttyuse.html

Roland, J. T. (2008). *Interview with Dr. J. Thomas Roland, Jr., Director of Otology and Neurotology, Co-director of the New York University Cochlear Implant Center.* Retrieved from http://www.audiologyonline.com/interview/interview_detail.asp?wc=1&interview_id=457

Roland, J. T., Jr., Cossetti, M., Wang, K. H., Immerman, S., & Waltzman, S. B. (2009). Cochlear implantation in the very young child: Long-term safety and efficacy. *Laryngoscope, 119,* 2205–2210.

Roland, P. S., Kutz, J. W., & Marcincuk, M. C. (2010). *Inner ear presbycusis.* Retrieved from http://www.emedicine.medscape.com/article/855989-overview

Ross, M. (2004). Today's debate: Over-the-counter hearing aids. *Hearing Loss, 25*(3), 18–23.

Ross, M. (2005). Home-based auditory and speechreading training. *Hearing Loss, 26*(3), 30–34.

Ross, M. (2006). *Troubleshooting your hearing aid.* Retrieved from http://www.healthyhearing.com/articles/7835-troubleshooting-your-hearing-aid

Ross, M. (2009). *Mark Ross on veterans and aural rehabilitation.* Retrieved from http://www.hearinglossweb.com/Issues/Services/ar/ross2.htm

Ross, M., Brackett, D., & Maxon, A., (1991). *Assessment and management of mainstreamed hearing-impaired children.* Austin, TX: Pro-Ed.

Rothstein, R., & Everson, J. M. (1994). Assistive technology for individuals with sensory impairments. In F. F. Flippo, K. J. Inge, & J. M. Barcus (Eds.), *Assistive technology: A resource for school, work, and community* (pp. 105–132). Baltimore, MD: Brookes.

Roush, J., & Harrison, M. (2002). What parents want to know at diagnosis and during the first year. *The Hearing Journal, 55*(11), 52–54.

Rubenstein, L. Z. (1997). Preventing falls in the nursing home. *Journal of the American Medical Association, 278,* 595–596.

Rubenstein, L. Z., & Josephson. K. R. (2002). The epidemiology of falls and syncope. *Clinics in Geriatric Medicine, 18,* 141–58.

Rubenstein, L. Z., Robbins, A. S., Schulman, B. L., Rosado, J., Osterweil, D., & Josephson, K. R. (1988). Falls and instability in the elderly. *Journal of the American Geriatrics Society, 36,* 266–278.

Runge, J. W. (1993). The cost of injury. *Emergency Medicine Clinics of North America, 11,* 241–253.

Rvachew, S., Slawinski, E. B., Williams, M., & Green, C. L. (1996). Formant frequencies of vowels produced by infants with and without otitis media. *Canadian Acoustics, 24,* 19–28.

Sackett, D. L., Rosenberg, W. M. C., Gray, J. A. M., Haynes, R. B., & Richardson, W. S. (1996). Evidence-based medicine: What it is and what it isn't. *British Medical Journal, 312,* 71–72.

Sackett, D. L., Straus, S. E., Richardson, W. S., Rosenberg, W., & Haynes, R. B. (2005). *Evidence-based medicine: How to practice and teach EBM* (3rd ed.). New York: Churchill Livingstone.

Saeed, S. R., Ramsden, R. T., & Axon, P. R. (1998). Cochlear implantation in the deaf-blind. *American Journal of Otology, 19,* 774–777.

Sahyoun, N. R., Lentzer, H., Hoyert, D., & Robinson, K. N. (2001). *Trends in aging and health: Trends in cause of death among the elderly.* Atlanta, GA: Centers for Disease Control and Prevention: National Center for Health Statistics.

Salvinelli, F., Trivelli, M., Casale, M., Firrisi, L., DiPeco, V., D'Ascanio, L., . . . Bernabei R. (2004). Treatment of benign positional vertigo in the elderly: A randomized trial. *Laryngoscope, 114,* 827–831.

Sandridge, S. A. (1995). Beyond hearing aids: Use of auxiliary aids. In P. B. Kricos, & S. A. Lesner (Eds.), *Hearing care for the older adult: Audiologic rehabilitation* (pp. 127–166). Boston: Butterworth-Heinemann.

Sandridge, S., Newman, C., Bea, S., Charian, N., Kahn, K., & Cherian, K. (2010). *Multidisciplinary clinical model for managing patients with tinnitus.* A webinar on e-Audiology from the American Academy of Audiology.

Saunders, G. H., & Echt, K. V. (2007). An overview of dual sensory impairment in older adults: Perspectives for rehabilitation. *Trends in Amplification, 11,* 243–258.

Schafer, E. C., & Thibodeau, L. M. (2003). Speech recognition performance of children using cochlear implants and FM systems. *Journal of Educational Audiology, 11,* 13–26.

Schafer, E. C., & Thibodeau, L. M. (2004). Speech recognition abilities of adults using cochlear implants interfaced with FM systems. *Journal of the American Academy of Audiology, 15,* 678–691.

Scheetz, N. A. (2004). *Psychosocial aspects of deafness.* Boston: Allyn & Bacon.

Schein, J. (1989). *A home among strangers.* Washington, DC: Gallaudet University Press.

Schiavetti, N., & Metz, D. E. (2002). *Evaluating research in communicative disorders* (4th ed.). Boston: Allyn & Bacon.

Schmuziger, N., Patscheke, J., & Probst, R. (2006). Hearing in nonprofessional pop/rock musicians. *Ear and Hearing, 27,* 321–330.

Schmuziger, N., Schimmann, F., á Wengen, D., Patscheke, J., & Probst, R. (2006). Long-term assessment after implantation of the Vibrant Soundbridge device. *Otology and Neurotology, 27,* 183–188.

Schönberger, J., Wang, L., Shin, J. T., Kim, S. D., Depreux, F. F., Zhu, H., . . . Seidman, C.E. (2005). Mutation in the transcriptional coactivator EYA4 causes dilated cardiomyopathy and sensorineural hearing loss. *Nature Genetics, 37,* 418–422.

Schopmeyer, B. (2001). Professional roles in multidisciplinary assessment of candidacy. In J. K. Niparko, N. K. Mellon, A. M. Robbins, D. L. Tucci, & B. S. Wilson (Eds.), *Cochlear implants: Principles and practices* (pp. 178–180). Baltimore, MD: Lippincott Williams & Wilkins.

Schow, R. L. (1982). Success of hearing aid fitting in nursing homes. *Ear and Hearing, 3,* 173–177.

Schow, R. L., & Nerbonne, M. A. (1982). Communication screening profile: Use with elderly clients. *Ear and Hearing, 3,* 135–147.

Schow, R. L., & Nerbonne, M. A. (2002). *Introduction to audiologic rehabilitation* (4th ed.). Boston: Allyn & Bacon.

Schreiber, B. E., Agrup, C., Haskard, D. O., & Luxon, L. M. (2010). Sudden sensorineural hearing loss. *Lancet, 375,* 1203–1211.

Schroedel, J., & Geyer, P. (2000). Long-term career attainments of deaf and hard of hearing college graduates: Results from a 15-year follow-up survey. *American Annals of the Deaf, 145,* 303–314.

Schuknecht, H. F. (1964). Further observations on the pathology of presbycusis. *Archives of Otolaryngology, Head, and Neck Surgery, 80,* 369–382.

Schuknecht, H. F., & Gacek, M.R. (1993). Cochlear pathology in presbycusis. *Annals of Otology, Rhinology, and Laryngology, 102,* 1–16.

Schultz, D., & Mowry, R. B. (1995). Older adults in long-term care facilities. In P. B. Kricos & S. A. Lesner (Eds.), *Hearing care for the older adult: Audiologic rehabilitation* (pp. 167–184). Boston: Butterworth-Heinemann.

Schulz, K. E., Altman, D. G., Moher, D. & CONSORT group. (2010). CONSORT 2010 Statement: Updated guidelines for reporting parallel group randomized trial. *Journal of Clinical Epidemiology, 63,* 834–840.

Schum, D. J. (1992). Responses of elderly hearing aid users on the Hearing Aid Performance Inventory. *Journal of the American Academy of Audiology, 3,* 308–314.

Scientific Learning. (2010). *Fast ForWord® program.* Retrieved from http://www.scilearn.com/products/

Scollie, S., Ching, T. Y., Seewald, R., Dillon, H., Britton, L., Steinberg, J., & Corcoran, J. (2010). Evaluation of the NAL-NL1 and DSL v4.1 prescriptions for children: Preference for real world use. *International Journal of Audiology, 49* (Suppl. 1), S49–S63.

Scollie, S., Seewald, R., Cornelisse, L., Moodie, S., Bagatto, M., Laurnagaray, D., . . . Pumford, J. (2005). The Desired Sensation Level Multistage Input/ Output Algorithm. *Trends in Amplification, 9,* 159–197.

Scottish Intercollegiate Guidelines Network. (2008). SIGN-50: *A guideline developer's handbook.* Edinburgh, Scotland: Author.

Scudder, S. G., Culbertson, D. S., Waldron, C. M., & Stewart, J. (2003). Predictive validity and reliability of adult hearing screening techniques. *Journal of the American Academy of Audiology, 14,* 9–19.

Semel, E., Wiig, E. H., & Secord, W. A. (2003). *Clinical evaluation of language fundamentals—preschool* (2nd ed.) San Antonio, TX: Harcourt Assessment.

Senge, J. C., & Dote-Kwan, J. (1998). Responsibilities of colleges and universities to provide print access for students with visual impairments. *Journal of Visual Impairments and Blindness, 92,* 269–275.

Seyfried, D. N., Hutchinson, J. M., & Smith, L. L. (1989). Language and speech of the hearing impaired. In R. L. Schow and M. A. Nerbonne (Eds.), *Introduction to aural rehabilitation* (2nd ed., 181–239). Austin, TX: Pro-Ed.

Shallop, J. K., Peterson, A., Facer, G. W., Fabry, L. B., & Driscoll, C. L. (2001). Cochlear implants in five cases of auditory neuropathy: Postoperative findings and progress. *Laryngoscope, 111,* 555–562.

Shapiro, D. E., Boggs, S. R., Melamed, B.G., & Graham-Pole, J. (1992). The effect of varied physician affect on recall, anxiety, and perceptions in women at risk for breast cancer: An analogue study. *Health Psychology, 11,* 61–66.

Shargorodsky, J., Curhan, S. G., Curhan, G. C. & Favey, R. (2010). Change in prevalence of hearing loss in US adolescents. *Journal of the American Medical Association, 304,* 772–778.

Sharifzadeh, V. S. (1997). Families with Middle Eastern roots. In E. W. Lynch & M. J. Hanson (Eds.), *Developing cross-cultural competence: A guide for working with children and their families* (2nd ed., pp. 441–482). Baltimore, MD: Brookes.

Sheyte, A., & Kennedy, V. (2010). Tinnitus in children: An uncommon symptom? *Archives of Disease in Children, 95,* 645–648.

Shiffman, R. N., Shekelle, P., Overhage, J. M., Slutsky, J., Grimshaw, J., & Deshpande, A. M. (2003). Standardized reporting of clinical practice guidelines: A proposal from the Conference on Guidelines Standardization. *Annals of Internal Medicine, 139,* 493–498.

Shohet, J. A. (2010). *Implantable hearing devices.* Retrieved from http://emedicine.medscape.com/article/860444-overview

Silman, S., Gelfand, S. A., & Silverman, C. A. (1984). Late-onset auditory deprivation: Effects of monaural versus binaural hearing aids. *Journal of the Acoustical Society of America, 76,* 1357–1362.

Silverman, S. R., & Hirsh, I. J. (1955). Problems related to the use of speech in clinical audiometry. *Annals of Otology, Rhinology, & Laryngology, 64,* 1234–1244.

Simon, J. W., & Kaw, P. (2001). Commonly missed diagnoses in the childhood eye examination. *American Family Physician, 64,* 623–628.

Sininger, Y., Marsh, R., Walden, B., & Wilber, L. A. (2003). Guidelines for ethical practice in research for audiologists. *Audiology Today, 15*(6), 14–17.

SKI-HI Institute (2010). *SKI-HI Institute.* Retrieved from http://www.skihi.org

SKYPE. (2010). *SKYPE.* Retrieved from http://www.skype.com

Sloane, P. D., Dallara, J., Roach, C., Bailey, K. E., Mitchell, M., & McNutt, R. (1994). Management of dizziness in primary care. *Journal of the American Board of Family Practitioners, 7,* 1–8.

Smith, C. R., (1975). Residual hearing and speech production in deaf children. *Journal of Speech, Language, and Hearing Research, 18,* 795–811.

Smith, P. K., & Monks, C. P. (2008). Concepts of bullying: Developmental and cultural aspects. *International Journal of Adolescent Medicine and Health, 20,* 101–112.

Smith, S. L., Bennett, L. W., & Wilson, R. N. (2008). Prevalence and characteristics of dual sensory impairment (hearing and vision) in a veteran population. *Journal of Rehabilitation, Research and Development, 45,* 597–609.

Smith, S. L., & Kricos, P. (2003). Acknowledgement of hearing loss by older adults. *Journal of the Academy of Rehabilitative Audiology, 36,* 23–35.

Smith, S. L., & West, R. L. (2006). The application of self-efficacy principles to audiologic rehabilitation: A tutorial. *American Journal of Audiology, 15,* 46–56.

Solodar, H., & Chappell, J. (2005) "Welcome to Medicare" preventative exam includes hearing and balance screening. *Audiology Today, 17*(1), 49.

Sommers, M. S., Tye-Murray, N., & Spehar, B. (2005). Auditory-visual speech perception and auditory-visual enhancement in normal-hearing younger and older adults. *Ear and Hearing, 26,* 263–275.

Sorenson Communications. (2010). *Sorenson communications.* Retrieved from http://www.sorenson.com

Sorkin, D. L., & Zwolan, T. A. (2004). Trends in educational services for children with cochlear implants. In R. T. Miyamoto (Ed.), *Cochlear implants: Proceedings of the VIII International Cochlear Implant Conference* (pp. 417–421). Amsterdam, Netherlands: Elsevier B.V.

Sparkle. (2010). *Project SPARKLE.* Retrieved from http://www.sparkle.usu.edu/

Spencer, L. J., Barker, B. A., & Tomblin, J. B. (2003). Exploring the language and literacy outcomes of pediatric cochlear implant users. *Ear and Hearing, 24,* 236–247.

Spencer, L. J., Gantz, B., & Knutson, J. (2004). Outcomes and achievement of students who grew up with access to cochlear implants. *Laryngoscope, 114,* 1576–1581.

Spencer, L. J., Tye-Murray, N., Kelsay, D. M. R., & Teagle, H. (1998). Learning to use the cochlear implant: A child who beat the odds. *American Journal of Audiology, 7,* 24–29.

Spiers, E., & Hammett, R. (1995). *Students who are deafblind on campus.* Washington, DC: HEATH Resource Center, American Council on Education.

Spilker, B. (1996). Introduction. In B. Spilker (Ed.), *Quality of life and pharmaeconomics in clinical trials, second edition* (pp. 1–10). Philadelphia, PA: Lippincott-Raven.

Spitzer, J. B., Leder, S. B., & Giolas, T. G. (1993). *Rehabilitation of late-deafened adults: Modular program manual.* St. Louis, MO: Mosby.

Staab, W. J. (1991). *Hearing aids: A user's guide.* Phoenix, AZ: Author.

Staab, W. J., Dennis, M., Schweitzer, C., & Weber, J. E. (2004). *Measuring the occlusion effect in a deep-fitting hearing device.* Retrieved from http://www.hearingreview.com/issues/articles/2004-12_05.asp

Stach, B. A. (2008). *Clinical audiology: An introduction* (2nd ed.). Clifton Park, NY: Cengage Learning.

Stelmachowicz, P., Pittman, A., Hoover, B., Lewis, D., & Moeller, M. (2004). The importance of high-frequency audibility in the speech and language development of children with hearing loss. *Archives of Otolaryngology, Head and Neck Surgery*, *130,* 556–562.

Stelmachowicz, P. G., Pittman, A. L., Hoover, B. M., & Lewis, D. E. (2001). Effect of stimulus bandwidth on the perception of /s/ in normal- and hearing-impaired children and adults. *Journal of the Acoustical Society of America*, *110*, 2183–2190.

Stephens, D. (2002). The International Outcome Inventory for Hearing Aids (IOI-HA) and its relationship to the Client-Oriented Scale of Improvement (COSI). *International Journal of Audiology, 41,* 42–47.

Sterkers, O., Boucarra, D., Labassi, S., Bebear, J. P., Dubreuil, C., Frachet, B., . . . Vaneecloo, C. M.. (2003). A middle ear implant, the Symphonix Vibrant Soundbridge: Retrospective study of the first 125 patients implanted in France. *Otology and Neurotology, 24,* 427–436.

Sterkers, O., Mosnier, I., Ambert-Dahan, E., Herelle-Dupuy, E., Bozorg-Grayeli, A., & Bouccara, D. (2004).

Cochlear implants in the elderly: Preliminary results. *Acta Otolaryngologica Supplementum, 552,* 64–67.

Stewart, A. P. (1994). The comprehensive hearing conservation program. In D. Lipscomb (Ed.), *Hearing conservation in industry, schools, and the military* (pp. 203–230). San Diego, CA: Singular/Delmar Cengage Learning.

Stewart, D. A., & Kluwin, T. N. (2001). *Teaching deaf and hard of hearing students: Content, strategies, and curriculum.* Boston: Allyn & Bacon.

Stewart, M., Pankiw, R., Lehman, M. E., & Simpson, T. H. (2002). Hearing loss and hearing handicap in users of recreational firearms. *Journal of the American Academy of Audiology, 13,* 160–168.

Stinson, M., Chase, K., & Kluwin, T. (1990). *Self-perceptions of social relationships in hearing-impaired adolescents.* Paper presented at the American Educational Research Association, Boston.

Stockman, I. J., Boult, J., & Robinson, G. (2004, July 20). Multicultural issues in academic and clinical education: A cultural mosaic. *The ASHA Leader.*

Stoel-Gammon, C. (1998). Role of babbling and phonology in early linguistic development. In A. Wetherby, S. F. Warren, & J. Reichle (Eds.) *Transitions in prelinguistic communication* (pp. 87–110). Baltimore, MD: Paul H. Brookes Publishing.

Stoel-Gammon, C., & Otomo, K. (1986). Babbling development of hearing-impaired and normally hearing subjects. *Journal of Speech and Hearing Disorders, 51,* 33–41.

Stone, R. I. (2000). *Long-term care for the elderly with disabilities: Current policy, emerging trends, and implications for the twenty-first century.* New York: Millbrank Memorial Fund.

Stredler-Brown, A. (2004). *Developing a treatment program for children with auditory neuropathy.* Retrieved from http://www.arlenestredlerbrown.com/docs/Auditory_Neuropathy.pdf

Stredler-Brown, A., & Johnson, C. (2004). *Functional auditory performance Indicators: An integrated approach of auditory development*, Colorado Department of Education, Special Education Services Unit. Retrieved from http://www.cde.state.co.us/cdesped/download/pdf/FAPI_3-1-04g.pdf

Stuart, A., Moretz, M., & Yang, E.Y. (2000). An investigation of maternal stress after neonatal hearing screening. *American Journal of Audiology, 9,* 135–141.

Stueve, M. P., & O'Rourke, C. (2003). Estimation of hearing loss in children: Comparison of auditory steady-state response, auditory brainstem response, and behavioral test methods. *American Journal of Audiology, 12*, 125–136.

Susac, J. O. (1994). Susac's syndrome: The triad of microangiopathy of the brain and retina with hearing loss in young women. *Neurology, 44,* 591–593.

Suter, A. H., & Berger, E. H. (2002). *Hearing conservation manual.* Milwaukee, WI: Council for Accreditation in Hearing Conservation.

Svirsky, M. A., Robbins, A. M., Kirk, K. I., Pisoni, D. B., & Miyamoto, R. T. (2000). Language development in profoundly deaf children with cochlear implants. *Psychological Science, 11,*153–158.

Swartz, R., & Longwell, P. (2005). Treatment of vertigo. *American Family Physician, 71,* 1115–1122.

Sweetow, R. W. (1999). *Counseling for hearing aid fittings.* San Diego, CA: Singular/Delmar Cengage Learning.

Sweetow, R. W., & Sabes. J. H. (2006). The need for and the development of an adaptive Listening and Communication Enhancement (LACE™) program. *Journal of the American Academy of Audiology, 17,* 538–558.

Sweetow, R. W., & Sabes, J. H. (2007). Technological advances in aural rehabilitation: Applications and innovative methods of service delivery. *Trend in Amplification, 11,* 101–111.

Tait, M., Nikolopoulos, T. P., Archbold, S., & O'Donoghue, G. M., (2001). Use of the telephone in prelingually deaf children with a multichannel cochlear implant. *Otology and Neurotology, 22,* 47–52.

Taylor, A., Booth, S., & Tindell, M. (2006). *Deaf-blind communication devices.* Retrieved from http://www.nfb.org/Images/nfb/Publications/bm/bm06/bm0609/bm060913 .htm.

Teagle, H. F. B., Roush, P. A., Woodard, J. F., Hatch, D. R., Zdanski, C. J., Buss, E., & Buchman, C. A. (2010). Cochlear implantation in children with auditory neuropathy spectrum disorder. *Ear and Hearing, 31,* 325–335.

Teoh, S. W., Pisoni, D. B., & Miyamoto, R. T. (2004). Cochlear implantation in adults with prelingual deafness: Part I: Clinical results. *Laryngoscope, 114,* 1536–1540.

Tharpe, A. M. (1998). Treatment fads versus evidence-based practice. In F. H. Bess (Ed.), *Children with hearing impairment: Contemporary trends* (pp. 179–188). Nashville, TN: Vanderbilt Bill Wilkerson Center Press.

Thibodeau, L., & Schafer, E. (2005, November). *Optimal arrangements for cochlear implant users.* Paper presented at the Annual Convention of the American Speech-Language-Hearing Association, San Diego, CA.

Thibodeau, L. M. (1993). Counseling for pediatric amplification. In J. G. Clark & F. N. Martin (Eds.), *Effective counseling in audiology: Perspective and practice* (pp. 147–183): Englewood Cliffs, NJ: Prentice Hall.

Thibodeau, L. M., & Schmitt, L. (1988). A report on condition of hearing aids in nursing homes and retirement centers. *Journal of the Academy of Rehabilitative Audiology, 21,* 113–119.

Thompson, D. C., McPhillips, H., Davis, R. L., Lieu, T. L., Homer, C. J. & Helfand, M. (2001). Universal newborn hearing screening: Summary of evidence. *Journal of the American Medical Association, 286,* 2000–2010.

Tiffin, J., & Asher, E. (1948). The Purdue Pegboard: Norms and studies of reliability and validity. *Journal of Applied Psychology, 32,* 234–247.

Tjellström, A., & Håkanssön, B. (1995). The bone-anchored hearing aid. Design principles, indications, and long-term clinical results. *Otolaryngology Clinics of North America, 28,* 53–72.

Tobey, E. A., Rekart, D., Buckley, K., & Geers, A. E. (2004). Mode of communication and classroom placement impact on speech intelligibility. *Archives of Otolaryngology, Head, and Neck Surgery, 130,* 639–643.

Torre, P. III. (2008). Young adults' use and output level settings of personal music systems. *Ear and Hearing, 29,* 791–799.

Torre, P. III, Cruickshanks, K. J., Klein, B. E., Klein, R., & Nondahl, D. M. (2005). The association between cardiovascular disease and cochlear function in older adults. *Journal of Speech, Language, and Hearing Research, 48,* 473–481.

Tremblay, K., Kraus, N., McGee, T., Ponton, C., & Otis, B. (2001). Central auditory plasticity: Changes in the N1-P2 complex after speech-sound learning. *Ear and Hearing, 22,* 79–90.

Tremblay, K. L., & Kraus, N. (2002). Auditory training induces asymmetrical changes in cortical neural activity. *Journal of Speech, Language, and Hearing Research, 45,* 564–572.

Trychin, S., & Eckhardt, J. (2004). *Vocational rehabilitation and workers with hearing loss.* Retrieved from http://www.audiologyonline.com/articles/article_detail.asp?article_id=727

Tufts, J. B., Vasil, K. A., & Briggs, S. (2009). Auditory fitness for duty: A review. *Journal of the American Academy of Audiology, 20,* 539–557.

Turner, C. W., & Hurtig, R. R. (1999). Proportional frequency compression of speech for listeners with sensorineural hearing loss. *Journal of the Acoustical Society of America, 106,* 877–886.

Turunen-Rise, I., Flottorp, G., & Tvete, O. (1991). A study of the possibility of acquiring noise-induced hearing loss by the use of personal cassette players (Walkman). *Scandinavian Audiology, 34,* 133–144.

Tye-Murray, N. (1997). *Communication training for older teenagers and adults: Listening, speechreading, and using conversational strategies.* Austin, TX: Pro-Ed.

Tye-Murray, N. (2002). *Conversation made easy: Speechreading and conversation strategies training for adults and teenagers with hearing loss (CD-ROM).* St. Louis, MO: Central Institute for the Deaf.

Tye-Murray, N. T. (2008). *Foundations of aural rehabilitation: Children, adults, and their family members, 3rd edition.* Clifton Park, NY: Delmar Cengage Learning.

Tye-Murray, N., Spencer, L., & Woodworth, G. G. (1995). Acquisition of speech by children who have prolonged cochlear implant experience. *Journal of Speech, Language, and Hearing Research, 38,* 327–337.

Tye-Murray, N., Tyler, R. S., Bong, B., & Nares, T. (1988). Computerized laser videodisc programs for training speechreading and assertive communication behaviors. *Journal of the Academy of Rehabilitative Audiology, 21,* 143–152.

Tyler, R. S. (1993). Cochlear implants and Deaf culture. *American Journal of Audiology, 2,* 26–32.

Tyler, R. S., Gantz, B. J., McCabe, B. F., Lowder, M. W., Otto, S. R., & Preece, J. P. (1985). Audiological results with two single channel cochlear implants. *Annals of Otology, Rhinology, and Laryngology, 94,* 133–139.

Tyler, R. S., Tye-Murray, N., Moore, B. C., & McCabe, B. F. (1989). Synthetic two-formant vowel perception by some of the better cochlear implant recipients. *Audiology, 28,* 301–315.

Uhlmann, R. F., Larson, E. B., Rees, T. S., Koepsell, T. D., & Duckert, L. G. (1989). Relationship of hearing impairment to dementia and cognitive dysfunction in older adults. *Journal of the American Medical Association, 261,* 1916–1919.

Understanding and Coping with Macular Degeneration. (2006a). *Encyclopedia category: Disease.* Retrieved from http://www.macula.org/encyclopedia-disease

Understanding and Coping with Macular Degeneration. (2006b). *Low vision aids and rehabilitation.* Retrieved from http://www.macula.org/low_vision/index.html

U.S. Census Bureau. (2010). *2010 census data.* Retrieved from http://2010.census.gov/2010census/data.

U.S. Department of Health Education and Welfare. (1998). *The challenge and the charge. A report on the National Conference on the Education of the Deaf.* Washington, DC: United States Government Printing Office.

U.S. Food and Drug Administration. (2000). *Nucleus 24 auditory brainstem implant system.* Retrieved from http://www.fda.gov/MedicalDevices/ProductsandMedical Procedures/DeviceApprovalsand Clearances/Recently-ApprovedDevices/ucm089750.htm.

U.S. Preventive Services Task Force. (2008). *Clinical summary of the U.S. Preventive Services Task Force recommendation on newborn hearing screening.* Retrieved from http://www.uspreventiveservicestask force.org/uspstf08/newbornhear/newbhear sum.htm

University of Michigan Kellogg Eye Center [UMKEC]. (2006a). *Amblyopia.* Retrieved from http://www.kellogg.umich.edu/patientcare/conditions/amblyopia.html

University of Michigan Kellogg Eye Center [UMKEC]. (2006b). *Strabismus.* Retrieved from http://www.kellogg.umich.edu/patientcare/conditions/strabismus.html

University of Michigan Kellogg Eye Center [UMKEC]. (2006c). *Astigmatism.* Retrieved from http://www.kellogg.umich.edu/patientcare/conditions/astigmatism.html

University of Michigan Kellogg Eye Center [UMKEC]. (2006d). *Hyperopia.* Retrieved from http://www.kellogg.umich.edu/patientcare/conditions/hyperopia.html

University of Michigan Kellogg Eye Center [UMKEC]. (2006e). *Myopia.* Retrieved from http://www.kellogg.umich.edu/patientcare/conditions/myopia.html

University of Michigan Kellogg Eye Center [UMKEC]. (2007). *Eye conditions.* Retrieved from http://www.kellogg.umich.edu/patientcare/conditions/index.html

University of Washington Center for Technology and Disability Studies. (2003). *Paying for the assistive technology you need: A consumer guide for funding sources in Washington State.* Retrieved from http://uwctds.washington.edu/resources/legal/funding%20manual/index.htm

Upfold, L. J., May, A. E., & Battaglia, J. A. (1990). Hearing aid manipulation skills in the elderly population: A comparison between ITE, BTE, and ITC aids. *British Journal of Audiology, 24,* 311–318.

Utley, J. (1946). A test of lipreading ability. *Journal of Speech Disorders, 11,* 109–116.

Valente, M., Abrams, H., Chisolm, T., Citron, D., Hampton, D., Loavenbruck, A., . . . Sweetow, R. (2006). *Guidelines for the audiologic management of adult hearing impairment.* Retrieved from http://www.audiology.org/resources/documentlibrary/Documents/haguidelines.pdf

Valente, M., Potts, L. G., Valente, M., & Goebel, J. (1995). Wireless CROS versus transcranial CROS for unilateral hearing loss. *American Journal of Audiology, 4,* 52–59.

Valente, M., Valente, M., & Mispagel, K. (2006). *Fitting options for patients with single sided deafness.*

Retrieved from http://www.audiologyonline.com/articles/article_detail.asp?article_id=1629

Vander Werff, K. R., Brown, C. J., Gienapp, B. A., & Schmidt Clay, K. M. (2002). Comparison of auditory steady-state response and auditory brainstem response thresholds in children. *Journal of the American Academy of Audiology, 13,* 227–235.

Van Hecke, M. L. (1993). Emotional responses to hearing loss. In J. G. Clark & F. N. Martin (Eds.), *Effective counseling in audiology: Perspective and practice* (pp. 92–115): Englewood Cliffs, NJ: Prentice Hall.

Vaughan, N., James, J., McDermott, D. Griest, S., & Fausti, S. (2005). A 5-year prospective study of diabetes and hearing loss in a veteran population. *Otology and Neurotology, 27,* 37–43.

Ventry, I. M, & Weinstein, B. E. (1982). The hearing handicap inventory for the elderly: A new tool. *Ear and Hearing, 3,* 128–134.

Ventry, I. M., & Weinstein, B. E. (1983). Identification of elderly people with hearing problems, *ASHA, 25,* 37–42.

Vermeire, K., Brokx, J. P., Van de Heyning, P. H., Cochet, E., & Carpentier, M. (2003). Bilateral cochlear implantation in children. *International Journal of Pediatric Otorhinolaryngology, 67,* 67–70.

Wagner, A. L. (2008). *Neurofibromatosis type 2.* Retrieved from http://emedicine.medscape.com/article/342667-overview

Wall, T. C., Peralta-Carcelen, M., Fargason, C. A. Jr., Evans, H. H., Snyder, E. D., & Woolley, A. L. (2001). Support of universal newborn hearing screening among mothers and health care providers. *Ambulatory Child Health, 7,* 283–295.

Wall, T. C., Senicz, E., Evans, H. H., Woolley, A., & Hardin, J. M. (2006). Hearing screening practices among a national sample of primary care pediatricians. *Clinical Pediatrics, 45,* 559–566.

Waltzman, S. B., & Cohen, N. L. (1999). Implantation of patients with prelingual long-term deafness. *Annals of Otology, Rhinology, and Laryngology Supplement, 177,* 84–87.

Waltzman, S. B., Robbins, A. M., Green, J. E., & Cohen, N. L. (2003). Second oral language capabilities in children with cochlear implants. *Otology and Neurotology, 24,* 757–763.

Waltzman, S. B., Scalchunes, V., & Cohen, N. L. (2000). Performance of multiply handicapped children using cochlear implants. *American Journal of Otology, 21,* 329–335.

Ware, J. E. Jr., & Sherbourne, C. D. (1992). The MOS 36-item short-form health survey (SF-36). I. Conceptual framework and item selection. *Medical Care, 30,* 473–483.

Washington University School of Medicine, Bernard Backer Medical Library (WSSM-BBML) (2006). *WUSM-BBML: Concealed hearing devices of the 19th and 20th centuries.* Retrieved from http://beckerexhibits.wustl.edu/did/

Watkins, S. (2004). *The SKI-HI language development scale.* Logan, UT: SKI-HI Institute.

Wayner, D. S. (2005). Aural rehabilitation adds value, lifts satisfaction, cuts returns. *Hearing Journal, 58*(12), 30, 32, 34–35, 38.

Wayner, D. S., & Abrahamson, J. E. (2001). *Learning to hear again: An audiologic rehabilitation curriculum, 2nd edition.* Latham, NY: Hear Again, Inc.

Wayner, D. S., Abrahamson, J. E., & Casterton, J. (1998). *Learning to hearing again with a cochlear implant.* Latham, NY: Hear Again, Inc.

Weichbold, V., & Welzl-Mueller, K. (2001). Maternal concern about positive test results in universal newborn hearing screening. *Pediatrics, 108,* 1111–1116.

Weichbold, V., Welzl-Mueller, K., & Mussbacher, E. (2001). The impact of information on maternal attitudes towards universal neonatal hearing screening. *British Journal of Audiology, 35,* 59–66.

Weiner, M. T., & Miller, M. (2006). Deaf children and bullying: Directions for future research. *American Annals of the Deaf, 151,* 61–70.

Weinstein, B. E. (1995). Auditory testing and rehabilitation of the hearing-impaired. In R. Lubinski (ed.) *Communication and dementia* (pp. 223–237). San Diego, CA: Singular/Delmar Cengage Learning.

Weinstein, B. E. (2000). *Geriatric audiology.* New York: Thieme.

Weinstein, S. (1993). Fifty years of somatosensory research: From the Semmes-Weinstein Monofilaments to the Weinstein Enhanced Sensory Test. *Journal of Hand Therapy, 6,* 11–22.

Weisel, A., & Cinamon, R. G. (2005). Hearing, deaf, and hard-of-hearing Isaeli adolescents' evaluations of deaf men and deaf women's occupational competence. *Journal of Deaf Studies and Deaf Education, 10,* 376–389.

Wessex Universal Neonatal Screening Trial Group (1998). Controlled trial of universal neonatal screening for early detection of childhood deafness. *Cochrane Database of Systematic Reviews,* CD003731.

White, S., Dancer, J., & Burl, N. (1996). Speechreading and speechreading tests: A survey of rehabilitative audiologists. *American Annals of the Deaf, 141,* 236–239.

Whitehead, R. L., & Whitehead, B. H. (1985). Acoustic characteristics of vocal tension/harshness in the speech of the hearing impaired. *Journal of Communication Disorders, 18,* 351–361.

Wilkerson, D. L. (1998). Program evaluation. In C. M. Frattali (Ed.), *Measuring outcomes in speech-language pathology* (pp. 151–171). New York: Thieme.

Wilson, A., & Childs, S. (2006). The effect of interventions to alter the consultation length of family physicians: A systematic review. *British Journal of General Practice, 58,* 876–882.

Wilson, B. C., Finley, C. C., Lawson, D. T., Wolford, R. D., Eddington, D. K., & Rabinowitz, W. M. (1991). Better speech recognition with cochlear implants. *Nature, 352,* 236–238.

Wilson, B. S. (1997). The future of cochlear implants. *British Journal of Audiology, 31,* 205–225.

Wilson, C., & Stephens, D. (2003). Reasons for referral and attitudes toward hearing aids: Do they affect outcome? *Clinical Otolaryngology Allied Sciences, 28,* 81–84.

Witte, T. N., & Kuzel, A. J. (2000). Elderly deaf patients' health care experiences. *Journal of the American Board of Family Practice, 13,* 17–22.

Wolf, K. (2004, April 13). Cultural competence in audiology. *The ASHA Leader.*

Wolff, J. L., Starfield, B., & Anderson, G. (2002). Prevalence, expenditures, and complications of multiple chronic conditions in the elderly. *Archives of Internal Medicine, 162,* 2269–2276.

Wong, T. W., Van Hasselt, C. A., Tang, L. S., & Yiu, P. C. (1990). The use of personal cassette players among youths and its effects on hearing. *Public Health, 104,* 327–330.

World Health Organization. (1999). *World Health Organization Disabilities Assessment Schedule II.* Geneva, Switzerland: World Health Organization.

World Health Organization. (2001). International classification of functioning, disabilities, and health. Geneva, Switzerland: World Health Organization.

World Health Organization. (2002). *Towards a common language for functioning, disability, and health.* Geneva, Switzerland: World Health Organization.

Wrightslaw. (2010). *Procedural safeguards and parent notice.* Retrieved from http://www.wrightslaw.com/info/safgd.index.htm

Wu, C. S., Lin, H. C., & Chao, P. Z. (2006). Sudden sensorineural hearing loss: Evidence from Taiwan. *Audiology and Neurootology, 11,* 151–156.

Yakel, D. A., Rosenblum, L. D., & Fortier, M. A. (2000). Effects of talker variability on speechreading. *Perception and Psychophysics, 62,* 1405–1412.

Yeager, P., Kaye, S., & Reed, M. (2007). Tools for living: Assistive technology experiences of Californians with disabilities. Retrieved from http://www.atnet.org/downloads/Tools%20for%20Living%20Assistive%20Technology%20Experiences%20of%20Californians%20with%20Disabilities.htm

Yellin, M. W., & Johnson, T. W. (2000). A case of Susac syndrome. *Journal of the American Academy of Audiology, 11,* 484–488.

Yoshinaga-Itano, C. (2000). Assessment and intervention with preschool children who are deaf and hard of hearing. In J. G. Alpiner & P. A. McCarthy (Eds.), *Rehabilitative audiology: Children and adults* (pp. 140–177). Philadelphia: Lippincott Williams & Wilkins.

Young, K. T., Davis, K., Schoen, C., & Parker, S. (1998). Listening to parents: A national survey of parents with young children. *Archives of Pediatric and Adolescent Medicine, 152,* 255–262.

Youse, K., Lei, K., Cannizzaro, M., & Coelho, C. (2002; June 25). Traumatic brain injury. *The ASHA Leader.*

Yueh, B., Souza, P., McDowell, J. A., Collins, M. P., Loovis, C. F., Hedrick, S. C., . . . & Deyo, R. A. (2001). Randomized trial of amplification strategies. *Archives of Otolaryngology Head, and Neck Surgery, 127,* 1197–1204.

Zahn, S. B., & Kelly, L. J. (1995). Changing attitudes about the employability of the deaf and hard of hearing. *American Annals of the Deaf, 140,* 381–385.

Zazove, P., Niemann, L. C., Gorenflo, D. W., Carmack, C., Mehr, D., Coyne, J. C., & Antonucci, T. (1993). The health status and health care utilization of deaf and hard-of-hearing persons. *Archives of Family Medicine, July 2(7),* 745–752.

Zeng, F. G., & Liu, S. (2006). Speech perception in individuals with auditory neuropathy. *Journal of Speech, Language, and Hearing Research, 49,* 367–380.

Zimmerman, I. L., Steiner, V. G., & Pond, R. E. (2002). Preschool language scale (4th ed.), (PLS-4). San Antonio, TX: Psychological Corporation.

Zimmerman-Phillips, S., Robbins, A. M., & Osberger, M. J. (2000). Assessing cochlear implant benefit in very young children. *Annals of Otology, Rhinology, & Laryngology Supplement, 185,* 42–43.

Zogby International. (2005). *Survey of teens and adults about the use of personal electronic devices and headphones.* Retrieved from http://www.asha.org/uploadedFiles/about/news/atitbtot/zogby_survey2006.pdf

Zuniga, M. E. (1997). Families with Latino roots. In E. W. Lynch & M. J. Hanson (Eds.), *Developing cross-cultural competence: A guide for working with children and their families* (2nd ed., pp. 209–250). Baltimore, MD: Brookes.

Zwerling, C., Whitten, P. S., Davis, C. S., & Sprince, N. L. (1998). Occupational injuries among older workers with visual, auditory, and other impairments: A validation study. *Journal of Occupational and Environmental Medicine, 40,* 720–723.

Zwolan, T. A., Ashbaugh, C. M., Alarfaj, A., Arts, H. A., Kileny, P. R., El-Kashlan, H. K. & Telian, S. A. (2004). Pediatric cochlear implant patient performance as a function of age at implantation. *Otology and Neurotology, 25,* 112–120.

Zwolan, T. A., Kileny, P. R., & Telian, S. A. (1996). Self-report of cochlear implant use and satisfaction by prelingually deafened adults. *Ear and Hearing, 17,* 198–210.

Zwolan, T. A., & Sorkin, D. L. (2006; November 28). Cochlear implant collaborations aid school success: Parents, schools, and implant centers build winning partnerships. *The ASHA Leader.*

Index